Speech pathology

An applied behavioral science

Speech pathology

An applied behavioral science

William H. Perkins, Ph.D.

Professor, Speech Communication, Graduate Program
in Communicative Disorders, Otolaryngology,
University of Southern California,
Los Angeles, California

SECOND EDITION

with 132 illustrations

The C. V. Mosby Company

Saint Louis   1977

Second edition

Copyright © 1977 by The C. V. Mosby Company

Previous edition copyrighted 1971

Printed in the United States of America

Distributed in Great Britain by Henry Kimpton, London

Library of Congress Cataloging in Publication Data

Perkins, William Hughes, 1923-
    Speech pathology: an applied behavioral science.

    Bibliography: p.
    Includes index.
    1. Speech, Disorders of. I. Title. [DNLM:
1. Speech disorders. WM475 P451s]
RC423.P43   1977   616.8′55   76-25839
ISBN 0-8016-3785-6

GW/CB/B 9 8 7 6 5 4 3 2 1

In remembrance of
ALIZON

Preface

The original conception of *Speech Pathology: an Applied Behavioral Science* as an overview of speech pathology has been retained. Some experience with early development of the National Examinations in Speech Pathology and Audiology was the impetus for this conception. These examinations grew out of the efforts of clinicians whose backgrounds and interests ranged across the spectrum of speech pathology and audiology. In a real sense, the philosophy they formulated spoke for the profession. Before they could begin, they had to agree on answers to such questions as, "Why give an examination in the first place?" and "What information should be examined?" Their answers were these*:

If certification of clinical competence is to protect the public, then certification procedures must involve some mechanism for insuring that individual clinicians know the best information and techniques available. . . .
Clinical practice, it seems, is often a matter of conjecture and opinion. Points of view about best methods of assessment and therapy of disorders of speech and hearing are many and varied. The NESPA subcommittees concluded, early in the development of these examinations, that opinion questions should not be a part of the examinations since the effect of including them might be to set permanently as "facts" those points of view tested, and no one was willing to assert that current clinical practices are the best that we can ever hope to achieve. Nor have many practices held as best by one "school of thought" proved better than those held by another.
With opinions excluded, a written test of clinical competence, at least insofar as it deals directly with current clinical procedures, became all but

*From Perkins, W., Shelton, R., Studebaker, G., and Goldstein, R., The National Examinations in Speech Pathology and Audiology: philosophy and operation. *Asha*, **12**, 176-177 (1970).

impossible. The basic purpose for such an examination was thereby brought into sharp focus as being distinctly separate from a test of practical skills.

What became increasingly apparent was that to prepare for these examinations, students would have to turn to our journals rather than to our books. Clinical applications, especially in speech pathology texts, have been written with few exceptions from the author's personal experience. Although often rich in human interest and clinical wisdom, personal statements are what the profession, through its National Examinations, has attempted to supplant with statements of greater generality and certainty. In effect, the same standards of evidence were to be applied to the information expected of our future clinicians as are applied to information considered acceptable for our journals.

The first edition of this book was not written as a study guide for the National Examination. If some have used it for that purpose, I hope it has been helpful. The need seen originally, which has also directed this revision, is for a text that speaks to the same philosophy as that reflected in the profession's publications and examinations.

My attempt has been to provide an even-handed account of the best information available. The biggest challenge has been to make a comprehensive statement about the full scope of speech pathology that is also comprehensible. The course for which I envisioned this text being used would be populated by interested students who can read English and would have sufficient depth to stay off the "Mickey Mouse" list.

This profession is rooted in phonetics and linguistics, in the psychology of learning and emotion, in education, in neurology and sensory physiology, in acoustics, and in psychophysics. This is far from a definitive catalog. The ideal speech pathologist would be a Renaissance man with profound knowledge of all the ways that speech permeates our nature. Then he might have a glimmering of the human condition of the person he is seeking to help, as well as of ways in which he could be of greatest service.

I have tried to meet this challenge by steering a course between definitive analyses on one side and a mere outline of topics on the other. What I have sought are the most responsible statements I can make that will permit the student to have at least a rudimentary grasp of each topic. Rather than bury students in an avalanche of encyclopedic details, I have provided references to which they can turn for definitive elaboration. My hope is that from this text, students will have sufficient understanding of each topic so that they can read about it in our literature with comprehension.

My decision to undertake this task as a single author was dictated by my desire to present the structure of this profession as clearly as possible. I thought that the student would have a better chance of following a single writer's conception of how all the parts of this field fit together than he would have if he tried to piece several authors' views together. To this end I have retained the chapter outlines and summaries as providing the clearest view of the framework of speech pathology.

Information in all chapters has been updated. Those containing areas in which considerable work has been done, such as stuttering and language, are the ones I have rewritten most extensively. Much work has been done on language involvement in autism, childhood aphasia, and mental retardation that I decided must be included. The chapter on therapy has also been heavily revised. It reflects that growing concern clinicians are showing for knowledge of how well techniques work and how thoroughly they have been tested. Throughout, I have attempted to avoid personal opinion and have relied, instead, on verifiable evidence. Finally, thanks to the efforts of Jody Bell, a glossary has been appended to aid the student in mastering the complex array of behavioral terms indigenous to speech pathology. Space did not permit extending the list to the vast array of anatomic, physiologic, and disease conditions related to our concerns.

My gratitude goes to all who have helped in ways they may not suspect. Linda Johnson, for example, has carried the bulk of responsibility for our intensive stuttering therapy research during this trial of authorship. I am especially indebted to Rheta Hirsch for her invaluable assistance in preparing the revisions of the effects of childhood autism and aphasia on language development. Similarly, Barbara Dabul and Glenda Bachman were most helpful in providing materials and advice on adult aphasia. And I thank Janice Stocks for her willing assistance in the research for this revision. Above all, though, I am grateful to Mary Gerlitz, without whom my professional life would have fallen apart years ago.

William H. Perkins

Contents

Foundations of speech pathology

Chapter 1

Prologue

WHAT IS SPEECH PATHOLOGY?

Early in this century rivulets of interest in communicative disorders began to flow from several wellsprings. Psychology was a fountainhead, as in many ways were education and medicine. Over subsequent years, other disciplines and professions joined in contributing to what is now the mainstream of speech pathology, an interdisciplinary profession rapidly developing an identity of its own.

A profession by any other name

Like all youth, speech pathology has suffered from, and periodically is still agonized by, growing pains. What is probably a major source of strength for this young field, its multiple roots, has at the same time been a major source of its chief conflict: identity. Who is a speech pathologist? From the answers to this question, two types of bias are often visible.

From one, we can generally sort academicians from clinicians. Those who prefer academic identity may label their area of concern *communication sciences*. This recently developed hybrid has had sufficient vitality to survive and sufficient breadth to include areas that would otherwise be called *experi-*

mental phonetics, speech science, and *voice science*. Those interested in these areas are closest to being the "pure" scientists of speech pathology. In fact, some are so pure that they do not want to be speech pathologists at all. Their interests tend to focus on normal processes of communication.

On the other side of this bias are the academicians' applied brethren, the clinicians who dispense service to the speech handicapped. They, too, have preferred identities that often reveal bias toward the related profession with which they are most closely aligned. In public schools are *speech correctionists, speech improvement teachers*, and, more recently (with some relief to the profession), well-qualified *speech specialists*. *Speech therapists* are a vanishing breed. This label is onerous to the profession only because it implies that as therapists they work under medical prescription. These clinicians seek medical consultation regarding somatic conditions and, in turn, provide consultation for physicians regarding the adequacy of a patient's speech performance. Theirs is therefore a consultative, not a prescriptive, relationship. Finally, reflecting preference for medical affiliation is the *speech clinician* and his more exalted colleague, the *speech pathologist*. It is this name with its obvious, and somewhat erroneous, medical connotation that has been taken as generic for the profession.

This proliferated jumble of titles has been the subject of much discussion—at times approaching contest proportions. Speech

---

Wendell Johnson (1968), one of speech pathology's most distinguished scholars, attempted to bring order out of this search for a name. What did he propose?

---

pathology's counterpart in hearing, *audiology*, being blessed with an adequate moniker for its scientific and clinical aspects, generously offered its name as an umbrella under which to include speech and its disorders. The offer was declined. Speech pathology seems to be as much with us as ever as a surname for the family of scientists and clinicians interested in normal and disordered processes of speech. Still, out of this great introspective effort are emerging a few general terms that encompass audiology as well as speech pathology: *speech and hearing,* historically accepted as connoting interest in normal as well as disordered processes of communication; *communicative disorders,* a newcomer that is spreading rapidly; and *communicology,* a name with the proper spirit but little enthusiastic support to nourish it.

So much for what this fledgling among health professions chooses to call itself. The question still remains: what is it? It is an *applied interdisciplinary behavioral science.* This term denotes that, on one side, the profession is an interdisciplinary field of study of disordered oral communication, and, equally important on the other, it is an interprofessional area of clinical practice in which knowledge of problems of speech is applied in their remediation. Let us glimpse first what speech pathologists study.

Disorders of oral communication

What speech pathologists seek, first and last, is an understanding of the disorders of oral communication. These disorders afflict a larger portion of our population than are deaf, blind, and crippled. In fact, at 11:00 A.M. on November 20, 1967, when the Census Bureau's population clock recorded 200 million citizens of the United States, we had in this nation, by conservative estimate, over 12 million speech-handicapped persons (National Advisory Neurological Diseases and Stroke Council, 1969). Prevalence estimates, none too reliable (especially for adults), generally range from 4% to 10% but often extend upward to 20% (Milisen, 1971). Disorders of speech are not respectful of age, sex, or position. The young, though, during growing years are especially susceptible. Their numbers exceed the population of the entire state

of Kansas or Mississippi, even when we include only those who, as Johnson and his colleagues (1967) said, "are certain to go through life at a serious disadvantage vocationally, socially, and in intimate personal ways if not given appropriate corrective attention."

What is defective speech? The term *speech* has been used in the layman's sense to mean any aspect of oral communication. For terminologic economy, let us retain this meaning and agree on what disorders of speech are and are not. Just as speaking is a behavioral endeavor, so too are disorders of speech defective forms of behavior. They are not anatomic disorders, although structural flaws in the speech apparatus may contribute to defectiveness. They are not physiologic disorders, although we must assume, to avoid becoming enmeshed in mysticism, that all behavior can be reduced to physiologic correlates. They are not acoustical disorders, although sound waves are physical phenomena that carry information to our ears about defective speech. Instead, they are disorders of oral language behavior. Defined, *speech is defective when it is ungrammatical, unintelligible, culturally or personally unsatisfactory, or abusive of the speech mechanism.*

From here on, we must delineate the terms used to distinguish various aspects of speech. First is *language,* the symbolic formulation of ideas according to semantic and grammatical rules. Since these rules are in the mind, we must observe them indirectly through their effects on speaking and writing. Defective use of linguistic rules is seen mainly in delayed speech development and aphasia. These neurologically based problems are included in the language disorders estimate of 2.1 million shown in Fig. 1-1. By contrast, Myklebust (1964) and Wood (1969) estimate that 5% of school-age children have language problems severe enough to interfere with education. That estimate would involve 10 million children, almost 8 million more than are estimated in Fig. 1-1. That difference probably results largely from a difference in definition: articulatory disorders

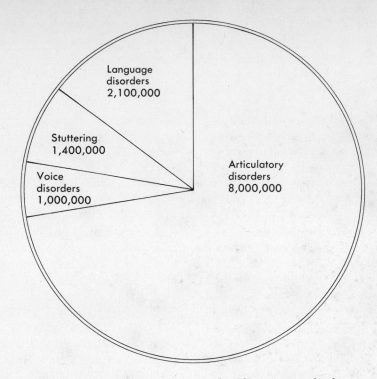

Fig. 1-1. Estimated prevalence of communicative disorders. (National Advisory Neurological Diseases and Stroke Council, 1969.)

are often counted among language disorders, and vice versa.*

We will use the term *speaking* to identify observable processes of oral language. *Speech* is often used in this technically restricted

---

Cutting and Kavanagh (1975) make a case for speech and language as being separate entities in a symbiotic relationship.

---

sense as well as in a broad sense to include covert thinking processes of language and

---

*Results of studies on frequency of occurrence vary widely, probably because of varying definitions of speech disorders and the adequacy of sampling procedures. Accordingly. Fig. 1-1 has been constructed as a compromise estimate from such sources as the report of the ASHA Committee on the White House Mid-century Conference (1952), Milisen's (1957) review of incidence data, and the recent report of the National Advisory Neurological Diseases and Stroke Council (1969). This compromise, based on a population assumption of 200 million is gross at best and should be taken none too seriously.

overt phonetic processes of speaking. To use the same term both ways is confusing. Therefore we will use *speaking* to denote the motor act of uttering speech sounds.

Historically, speaking processes have been the major focus of speech pathology. Only in recent years has the profession begun to delve seriously into language to obtain a better understanding of disorders of speech. Past tendency has been to view defective speech as a neuromuscular or perceptual problem, or even a problem of learning, but not as one of language formulation. The trend has shifted, and that shift will be reflected in this text.

Speaking is composed of three processes: phonation, articulation-resonance, and speech-flow. Phonatory processes are basic to production of voice. Fig. 1-1 shows the estimated prevalence of persons having voice problems to be between 5% and 15% of the speech handicapped, or about 1% of the general population.

Articulatory-resonatory processes are basic

to production of the different sounds of speech. They are far and away the most prevalent type of defective speaking behavior. They generally comprise about 75% of speech handicaps and are found in from 20% of schoolchildren in lower grades to 2% in upper grades. But they overlap the delayed speech category to such an extent that both categories are inflated considerably.

Speech-flow processes are basic to prosody (stress, inflection, rhythm), to pronunciation (arranging sounds in proper sequence), to rate, and to the fluency with which sounds are initiated and joined together. The major defect of speech-flow with which speech pathologists have been concerned is *stuttering*, the incidence of which usually hovers around 1% of the total population (Milisen, 1971). With the possibility that 80% of stutterers recover, prevalence of stuttering in

---

Young (1975) argues that either an 80% recovery rate is too high, or a 1% prevalence of stuttering in adults is too high, or both. What is the basis of his argument?

---

adults is obviously much lower than in children (Sheehan and Martyn, 1966). Another speech-flow disorder, *cluttering*, has been discussed more often by European phoniatrists but is of growing interest to American speech pathologists. Although cluttering is presumably rare, data on frequency of occurrence are virtually nonexistent.

Where sciences converge

Nothing so marks man at the pinnacle of the phylogenetic hierarchy as speech. At the simplest instant of existence as a single fertilized egg, the past experience of our species is transmitted by molecular DNA codes that are estimated to contain as much information as a thousand printed volumes, each the size of a volume of the Encyclopaedia Britannica —and all packed into an egg one millionth the size of a pinhead! If this problem is basic to understanding the simplest beginnings of human life, may we not speculate that man's most complex achievement, speech, offers an even greater challenge to those who would

unravel it? For any one science to lay claim to study of such an intricate enterprise would be sheer folly.

Fortunately for speech pathology, with its aggregation of multiple identities, it is anything but a closed science. Quite the contrary, much of its strength is in open-armed welcome of other fields of study as they converge on normal and disordered speech. Its academic relatives are scattered across the spectrum of knowledge. They range from behavioral to biologic and physical sciences to the humanities. Psychologists, with interest in development, learning, sensation, perception, and thinking; psycholinguists and linguists; geneticists and biochemists; physiologists and anatomists; acousticians; electrical engineers; anthropologists—these representatives of various areas of knowledge do not exhaust by any means the range of scholarly interests brought to bear on communication and its problems. Even a partial list extends beyond four dozen professions (National Advisory Neurological Diseases and Stroke Council, 1969).

Thus a speech pathologist is responsible primarily for understanding behavioral aspects of speech. Understanding is approached scientifically, and there is heavy reliance on related disciplines to bolster the study of communicative processes. In addition, knowledge is applied to the intricately involved problems of the speech handicapped. Clearly, as a field of study, speech pathology is an applied interdisciplinary behavioral science.

That a field can be identified as a science imputes certain merits to it, not the least of which is virtuous social status. Among more solid credits attributable to a scientific approach is the ability to estimate how certain we are of what we think we know. With reasonably exact knowledge, one can predict and control the course of events, which in the final analysis is an ultimate test of how well we understand a phenomenon.

A price is exacted, though, for scientific certainty. Science requires an analytic operation that dissects a phenomenon into component parts. Granted, these parts can be put back together. But if we are to know how much of each to reassemble into the whole, we must first pull the apparatus asunder, measure it piece by piece, and specify how each piece functions in relation with every other piece. Then, Providence willing, we may understand it well enough to reconstruct it and make it work.

As advantageous as an analytic approach is, the fact remains that the whole is obscured by analysis of the parts. For some fields this price may be small, but for speech pathology, with its ultimate interest in applied problems of the speech handicapped, it is large. We need a scheme for classifying the parts that fall out from an analysis of speech, but we risk losing sight of the person whose parts are being catalogued into their appropriate pigeonholes. Because analysis must precede synthesis, this text will be organized around an analytic exploration of what is known about disorders of communication. Remember, though, that these separate aspects of the speech handicapped have no practical meaning until reassembled to make a whole person with special problems in which we are interested.

Where professions converge

Just as speech pathology is a field of interdisciplinary study, so too is it an area of interprofessional clinical practice. A multitude of problems can impair the ability to communicate orally. A person may be cerebral palsied or aphasic, or have Parkinson's disease or multiple sclerosis—typical neurologic disabilities; he may have a cleft palate, a cleft lip, or any number of dental abnormalities—orofacial problems; he may have vocal nodules, polyps, contact ulcers, laryngeal paralysis, or worse yet, a laryngectomy—common disabilities of the vocal mechanism; he may be an "exceptional" child (often an inverted euphemism for "mentally retarded"); or he may be so emotionally disturbed as to be neurotic, sociopathic, or even psychotic.

Obviously, no one professional specialty claims knowledge about such an abundance of disabilities. Moreover, speech disorders are treated in college and university clinics,

dental clinics, private agencies, and especially public schools, as well as in hospital clinics. The clinical speech pathologist practices his profession as a consultant to, and in consultation with, almost all health, education, and welfare professions; the list can reach staggering proportions.

Clinical artistry. As the scientific approach is marked by use of logical analysis, so the clinical approach is marked by intuitive artistry of the clinician. This is not to say that

---

What does Beveridge (1957) say about science as art?

---

clinical artistry is an unknowable, mystical amalgam or that science is entirely analytic and not creative. That the scientist's analytic and the clinician's intuitive approaches in some ways are polar opposites, however, can be demonstrated. The difference lies in how time is used, a difference elaborated by Langer (1951) as "discursive" and "presentational" forms of symbolism. By "discursive" she means the type of symbolism used in language, and by "presentational," the type used in a painting. Her distinction, based on philosophic studies of Wittgenstein and Carnap, is that in discursive symbolism ideas are developed through time, whereas in presentational symbolism meaning is embodied in perception of an integrated whole. A picture is a form of presentational symbolism in which relations among all of the parts are immediately apparent. Discursive description of these relations in language might take hours of explication—an instance of the adage, "A picture is worth a thousand words."

Thus laws of discursive thought are laws of language reasoning: to obey them requires that one follow syntactic rules that govern sequential arrangement of symbols. In application, discursive language of words is constructed in sentences, of mathematics in formulas; to read a sentence or a formula one must begin at the beginning and follow the logical sequence. Language does not make sense if arrangement of its parts in temporal order (its syntax) is violated. Obviously, this is the form of symbolism characteristic of scientific analysis that proceeds through a sequence of logically reasoned steps.

Contrast how time is used discursively for analysis with its presentational use in clinical practice. The difference between listening to a person with impaired speech and studying his impairment analytically is in many ways like the difference between listening to music performed and studying it as written. A musical score is in discursive form; the more it is analyzed and its parts studied, the more its rich texture can be discerned.

But artistic impact is not in the parts; it is in their relation to the whole. If one listens only for notes, he will miss the melody. So, too, will the clinician risk missing the essence of the patient's problem if he attempts to analyze each moment of therapy as it occurs. Detailed analysis of the defective performance is appropriate for scientific study, but if the clinical relationship is approached as an analytic rather than an artistic endeavor, the risk is in not keeping pace with the patient, who, to paraphrase Thoreau, will march to a different drummer.

Questions define scope of field

A prevailing assumption will be that a field of study is defined by the questions asked. The identity of a discipline does not reside in objects studied but in questions asked about the objects. Behavioral sciences ask questions about the behavior of an organism, biologic sciences about the organism's biology, physical sciences about the physical aspects of its existence. The primary thrust of this text is toward behavioral questions. A counterpart is Mysak's (1976) recent text, which is addressed to questions about the biologic systems that underlie speech and its disorders.

We can divide the scope of speech pathology, and this text, into five major categories, each of which is distinguished by characteristic questions. In Part I, questions are about how we know what we know and about processes and development of speech. In Part II, questions are about various disabilities that limit acquisition or use of oral language skills. Part III is defined by questions about behavioral characteristics of impaired speech. Part IV deals with clinical questions about assessment and therapy of disorders of speech.

REFERENCES

ASHA Committee on the Midcentury White House Conference, Speech disorders and speech correction. *J. Speech Hearing Dis.*, **17**, 129-137 (1952).

Beveridge, W., *The Art of Scientific Investigation.* New York: W. W. Norton & Co., Inc. (1957).

Cutting, J., and Kavanagh, J., On the relationship of speech to language. *Asha*, **17**, 500-506 (1975).

Johnson, W., Communicology? *Asha*, **10**, 43-56 (1968).

Johnson, W., and others, *Speech Handicapped School Children.* New York: Harper & Row, Publishers (1967).

Langer, S., *Philosophy in a New Key.* New York: Mentor Books (1951).

Milisen, R., The incidence of speech disorders. In Travis, L. E. (Ed.), *Handbook of Speech Pathology and Audiology.* New York: Appleton-Century-Crofts (1971).

Myklebust, H., Learning disorders: psychoneurological disturbances in childhood. *Rehabil. Lit.*, pp. 354-360, Dec. (1964).

Mysak, E., *Pathologies of Speech Systems.* Baltimore: The Williams & Wilkins Co. (1976).

National Advisory Neurological Diseases and Stroke Council, *Human Communication and its Disorders —an Overview.* Bethesda, Md.: National Institute of Neurological Diseases and Stroke (1969).

Sheehan, J., and Martyn, M., Spontaneous recovery from stuttering. *J. Speech Hearing Res.*, **9**, 121-135 (1966).

Wood, N., *Verbal Learning.* Dimensions in early learning series. San Rafael, Calif.: Dimensions Publishing Co. (1969).

Young, M., Onset, prevalence, and recovery from stuttering. *J. Speech Hearing Dis.*, **40**, 49-58 (1975).

Speech science

Part I deals with the scientific roots from which applications of speech pathology are drawn. The major objective is to identify explicitly the behavioral processes of speech which, when defective, must be corrected. Such correction requires knowledge of methods of study to gain understanding of the processes, of the nature of the processes, and of the manner in which they develop.

Chapter 2

Speech pathology: a behavioral science

Questions

1. What are the bases of knowledge of communicative disorders?
2. What are the data of speech pathology?
3. How can speech be observed and measured?
4. What methods are applicable for the study of speech?

BASES OF KNOWLEDGE

Speech pathology is an applied behavioral science responsible for habilitation and rehabilitation of speech-handicapped persons. Knowledge of defective speech must be in a form that will permit modification of these disorders—hence the necessity of following precepts of science in gaining understanding. To predictably improve disorders of speech, problems must be analyzed to determine important variables, precise relations among them must be revealed, crucial questions must be asked, and definitive answers must be produced. These issues for speech pathology are but a special instance of issues for all of science.

Questions guide knowledge

The product of formal education would seem to be answers. If science points to one abiding conclusion, however, it is that answers are fickle: those we "know" today will stand in jeopardy tomorrow. By contrast, good questions abide—witness the philosophic questions of the ancient Greeks that still guide much of modern scientific inquiry. The course of advancing knowledge is marked by the questions asked. That course may be paved with answers (the quality of the paving will be no better than the validity and reliability of the blocks of facts fit together), but the route of the course will be determined by the questions. Silly questions breed silly answers; trivial questions, trivial answers. Only crucial questions that open vistas of essential relationships can lead to crucial answers. As Frye (1966) said: "The simplest questions are those that only great genius can answer, because it takes great genius to become aware of them as questions."

The structure of knowledge: strategies of inquiry

Hans Selye's (1950) monumental treatise, *Stress*, begins with an enumeration of ways of studying life: facts of the world can be tabulated, intricate relationships among events described, or building blocks of knowledge erected into a unified scientific structure.

Cataloging. Tabulation, or cataloging, is safe, uninspired, and dull, but for those who see knowledge as an encyclopedic collection of facts, such bookkeeping of nature may be sufficient. Although accumulated "facts" are essential for other strategies of inquiry, they must be arranged in a structure of knowledge to have meaning (Fig. 2-1).

Description. The second way of studying life, to describe it in its rich complexity, has considerably more merit than mere cataloging of data. In this approach the structure of knowledge is recognized; understanding involves more than an accumulation of formless facts. As Hanson (1965) said of Galileo, he would have been disturbed deeply by the notion that observations can occur in a perceptual vacuum. Nothing is seen in isolation; everything that can be observed has form of some sort. If the conception changes, so do observations of facts about it, as seen in Fig. 2-2, which, when viewed one way, is a vase; viewed another way it is a nose-to-nose confrontation.

The value of description of complex events is limited only by the genius of the observer. Giants of the stature of a Galileo, a Newton, or an Einstein could see the universe in a grain of sand. The less gifted can piece together as sweeping and as accurate a description of the shape of reality as powers of observation and reasoning will permit. With a descriptive approach, the observer does not have the benefit of the experimental method (the bulwark of science) to guide his observations. He is free not to think, a disciplined endeavor of considerable difficulty; he can pontificate; he can produce pronouncements untrammeled by ugly facts. If he is to avoid seeing the world through his own biases, he must rely on his own resources for being rigorously objective.

Scientific method. The third way of studying life fortifies an investigator with the method of science. It provides a procedural blueprint that permits systematic construction of an explanation of whatever segment of reality interests him. First, he confronts his phenomenon, becomes curious about it, observes it, records observations of it, asks how

GRIN AND BEAR IT BY LICHTY
FIGBY RESEARCH IN MEDICINE
NEW GRANTS
FIGBY RESEARCH INSTITUTE
PRES.
12-19
© Field Enterprises, Inc., 1969
"Big deal, awarding the Nobel Prize to Dr. Sneedby for his research in viruses... He merely counted the exact number of them going around!"

Fig. 2-1. The low road of knowledge: cataloging. (Courtesy Publishers-Hall Syndicate.)

it works, and poses a problem that can be solved with empirical evidence. Second, he formulates hypotheses about how one fact is related to another (here creative genius pays off). Third, he deduces from each hypothesis a prediction of what he would expect to observe if his understanding were accurate (here hardheaded logic is required). Finally, he conducts a crucial experiment to attempt to disprove his idea. If it survives the test, he can have reasonable confidence that he knows what he knows with some certainty.

It has been this third way of studying life that has dominated scientific effort and that has accounted for most technologic advances of this century. Impressive as progress has been on all fronts, some fields (such as high-energy physics with its revelations of a subatomic world and molecular biology with its discovery of the genetic code of life) have advanced at phenomenal rates. They have used

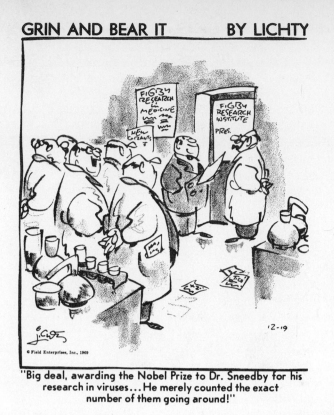

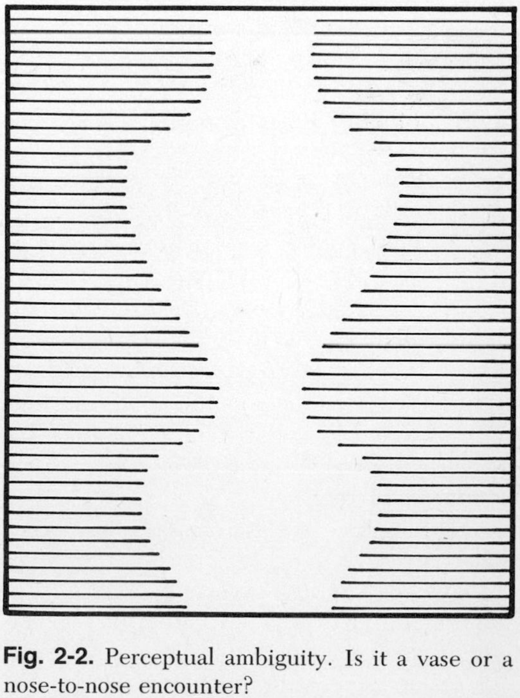

Fig. 2-2. Perceptual ambiguity. Is it a vase or a nose-to-nose encounter?

problem-oriented approaches. Others have chugged along steadily and undramatically with method-oriented approaches. Neophytes such as the social and behavioral sciences have toddled awkwardly in the footsteps of their seniors, uncertain at times as to whether they even belong in the family of sciences.

Why, if all fields use the same scientific method, do they progress at different rates? Many arguments could be advanced: Some sciences are better than others (an argument that would be vehemently denied by those at the bottom of the pecking order, but if all sciences are equal, the fact remains that some are more equal than others). Some have more measurable phenomena than others. Some can control their variables better than others. Or, perish the thought, some have brighter scientists than others.

Strong inference. Platt (1964), a biophysicist, eschews these arguments for one that can produce more light and less heat. He points to use of an accumulative method of inductive inference (he calls it *strong inference*) by those fields that have moved forward fastest. He argues that regular systematic application of strong inference makes the difference. Not new, it goes back to the early seventeenth century, when Francis Bacon replaced Aristotle's deductive approach to knowledge with a method of inductive inference.

Strong inference involves a three-step cycle that can be repeated endlessly:

Step 1. Devise alternate explanations, which lessens a theorist's natural inclination to develop paternalistic affection for his brainchild.

Step 2. Devise crucial experiments with alternative possible outcomes, each of which is intended to exclude the possibility that one or more of the hypothesized explanations is correct.

Step 3. Conduct the experiment to obtain a clean result.

At this point the procedure is recycled, but one is farther down the road of knowledge, albeit by exclusion; he knows one or more leads that are not worth following. This is a system that branches like a tree, and in fact it is sometimes called an "inductive tree." It works like the game of twenty questions, each question corresponding to an alternate hypothesis designed to exclude, ideally, half of the possible answers that could be guessed. An experimental result that does not exclude a possible answer is insecure; it must be rechecked. Any delay in recycling to the next set of hypotheses is wasteful. It is a powerful method, a fast method for exploring the unknown—hence the name "*strong* inference."

The crux of this approach deserves emphasis. Speech pathology, and behavioral sciences generally, could profit from its use. Its effectiveness can be seen from Newton's work to Fermi's. Pasteur's successes as he moved from one biologic problem to another every 2 or 3 years were testimonials to his inductive method. In each problem many experts were infinitely superior in their encyclopedic knowledge; yet each time Pasteur solved problems in a few months that others had not been able to solve in years. His secret was to formulate questions that could be tested and hypotheses that could be excluded (Platt, 1964).

As Rushton said: "A theory which cannot be mortally endangered cannot be alive." The crux is to emphasize the problem, not its method of solution. The method-oriented man succumbs to the busy work of methodologic housekeeping. He may be praised for a lifetime of study of more and more about less and less. He may measure, define, compute, analyze—but he does not exclude. His studies may continue indefinitely, but the problems he studies could often be solved in a few short months, or even weeks, of incisive inductive inferential thinking that sharply excludes profitless directions of inquiry.

Great scientists from Galileo to Einstein have decried method-oriented research. Hyman (1963) called it "knob-twirling research." The investigator holds no clear expectation of what he seeks or what he will find. He often proceeds on a "what if" basis: what would happen if one variable, chosen at random, were compared with another? Important knowledge *can* fall out from random research by virtue of serendipity, but the combination of variables that could be compared by twirling knobs is infinite, and the cost of research is high. Without a question to pursue, joy goes from the hunt; a random search for any stray quarry soon bores an intelligent observer.

Incisive thinking: the strategy of giants. "My way of discovering sciences goes far to level men's wit and leaves but little to individual excellence, because it performs everything by the surest rules and demonstrations." These words of Bacon were prophetic. His way of discovering the structure of knowledge by inductive analysis, by systematically constructing the relationship of one empirical event with another, has guided the bulk of scientific effort for more than four centuries. But in rare instances stupendous leaps in the conception of the world have been accomplished without apparent reference to the diligent constructive work in progress at the time. Few have been capable of these leaps—the genius of a Galileo, Newton, or Einstein stands outside the range of most mortals. What strategy did these giants use to make their contributions?

Their genius is marked by incisive thinking that cut deeply to the essence of a problem. These men could and did perform great experiments, but this was not how they turned the course of science. Galileo, for example, viewed experiments only as demonstrations of what reason, reflection, and argument had already revealed. He saw observations as intelligible only to the extent that they were informed by laws. For the most part, all that these men saw had long been seen by earlier natural philosophers: that water rises only to 32 feet in a suction pump, or, for Newton, that an apple falls from the tree—unremarkable observations. Yet from these commonplace events their philosophic visions synthesized the order of the physical world.

Similarly, Einstein had remarkable facility for designing crucial conceptual experiments aimed at capturing some paradoxic or contradictory feature of quantum theory or thermodynamics. Like Galileo and Newton, he could make inductive inferential leaps from such commonplace observations as the nonexistence of perpetual motion to principles that resolved inconsistencies in the foundation of physics. He started with such a question as: "What must the laws of nature be like not to permit construction of a perpetual motion machine?" He then moved to the question: "What must the laws of nature be like so that there are no specially privileged observers?" By sheer rigor of logical thought, he was able to deduce as part of the answer the whole structure of his theory of special relativity (Klein, 1967).

Which strategy is best? Strategies of inquiry are roads of knowledge; some permit faster travel than others. The low road, cataloging, is one that must be traveled without a map. With only an atlas of facts available, there are no directions as to location of one fact in relation to another. The middle road, description, offers a map of sorts. It would correspond to the route you would sketch after having traveled from one place to another. Crude and inaccurate, it would probably be better than no map at all for anyone unfamiliar with the terrain. The high road of the scientific method, strong inference, and incisive thinking would correspond to the road for which maps have been systematically assembled. Offering the most elaborate design of the structure of knowledge, it permits traveling farthest fastest.

To erect a structure of knowledge is to integrate existing data into a unified conception and to provide a basis for predicting as yet unobserved relationships. Difference in size of the structure is a difference in level of abstraction. A higher-order theory integrates a wider range of facts than does a lower-order theory, or than does a low-order hypothesis that frequently specifies only the relation between two facts (Fig. 2-3). As Fairbanks (1966) once said, a hypothesis "is simply a guess. . . . A theory then becomes a state-

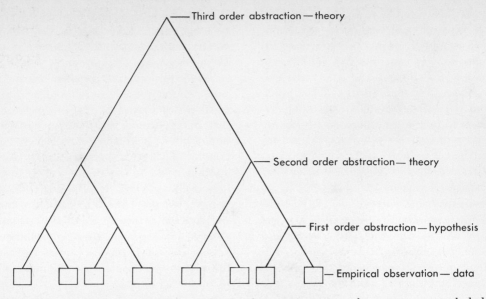

Fig. 2-3. Three levels of explanation of eight observations. More observations are included in a theory of high-level abstraction than in a low-level hypothesis.

ment of policy, an integrated set of good guesses, if you like."

Because accurate hypotheses are more within the range of most scientists, they are the safest and most useful maps for day-in, day-out investigation of the unknown. To build a solid theory requires an invariant relationship (some solid facts) and a genius capable of erecting hypotheses on this foundation within rigorous inductive logic. He devises a principle that unifies in one simplified conception what before had appeared to be a vast array of unrelated complexities. Such is the law of gravity. Such is the principle of evolution. Such is the principle of reinforcement, which comes as close to the elite theories of the natural sciences as any produced in the behavioral sciences.

STRATEGIES OF INQUIRY IN SPEECH PATHOLOGY
Physical model borrowed

Strategies of inquiry in speech pathology are those used by all behavioral sciences. Borrowed from our scientific forefathers, especially physicists, their appropriateness for

biologic sciences, let alone behavioral or social sciences, has been questioned.

Limitations of a physical model. In physics, when more than one variable is loose, and if that one is not observed with minute precision, the effort is not even considered by some as science. As the distinguished biologist, Szent-Györgyi (1964), observed when he joined the Institute for Advanced Studies in Princeton:

I did this in the hope that by rubbing elbows with those great atomic physicists and mathematicians, I would learn something about living matter. But as soon as I revealed that in any living system there are more than two electrons, the physicists would not speak to me. With all of their computers they could not say what the third electron might do.*

Science developed as our principal means of changing common sense (waggishly defined as the sense that tells us the earth is flat) into closer correspondence with objec-

---

*Szent-Györgyi, A., Teaching and the expanding knowledge. *Science*, **146**, 1278-1279 (1964).

tive reality. Its rise depended on the belief that the universe can be explained without recourse to miracles or mysticism. Out of this belief developed a conception of the material universe as a deterministic, self-contained, self-regulating physical system. Only much later did scientists come to the idea that living systems, too, can be studied within the conception of self-regulation and do not require recourse to ineffable spiritual explanations. The model of the physical world has been borrowed as a means of looking at the biologic world.

The life sciences, by adopting a physical model of reality, unintentionally acquired a tacit set of assumptions, some of which do not fit. Living systems—and especially the culmination of their development, speech and language—are incomparably more complex than physical systems. The material world can be reduced to two properties, mass and energy. When these physical dimensions have been specified, a physicist can proceed with confidence that he is in control of all the factors that can affect his observations. Not so in the life sciences. Especially is it not so for psychologists and speech pathologists, who concern themselves with motivation, emotion, intellect, cognition, perception, or any of the other unobservable processes of the mind. In fact, the deterministic cornerstone of behavioral science—that mind is a mentalistic figment reducible to neurophysiologic matter—is now being shaken. Sperry (1969) has concluded from his pioneering work with "split-brain" subjects that consciousness does indeed affect patterns of neurophysiologic performance, which reopens the issue of free will as a determinant of behavior.

Imperfect use of an imperfect model. Imperfect as a physical model is for understanding man and his speech, it is nonetheless what we have inherited. Speech pathology is a young science that has not yet developed a better way of knowing about communicative processes. It is just emerging from its "descriptive" period of development, through which all sciences pass. As von Békésy (1960) observed: "When a field is in its early stage of development, the selection of good problems is a more hazardous matter than later on, when some general principles have begun to be developed."

This period for speech pathology was dominated by shrewd observers who attempted to describe as accurately as they could the nature of disordered speech as they saw it. To make sense of why speech is defective, they constructed theories. Interestingly, theories did not proliferate around problems associated with organic disabilities. It was as though the physical impairment explained the "cause" of the disorder adequately. Around so-called "functional" problems that do not have an "obvious cause," however, one authority's explanation was about as good as another's. Lacking evidence from which to reason, schools of thought developed in which each authority had his followers, who, as much by debate as by scientific inquiry, attempted to prove that his school possessed the "truth."

With notable exceptions, clinical questions asked and answers propounded have tended to be inherently incapable of being tested. Paternalistic theorists have too often been unwilling to subject their progeny to rigorous attempts to disprove their right to exist as valid conceptions. That speech pathologists still argue over theories spawned more than 30 years ago proclaims failure to exclude less profitable from more profitable research leads; it proclaims imperfect use of scientific tools at hand for shaping credible ideas that can be held with confidence. Fairbanks' (1966) observation is apropos: "We are often guilty of clothing our problems in the trappings of science, and deceiving ourselves with the belief that this is science since it sounds like science."

Mind-bending versus back-bending. Compared with sciences that have progressed most, behavioral sciences, speech pathology included, have been concerned with backbending more than mind-bending, with exact answers more than probing questions (Bakan, 1967). Surveys have been done, experiments conducted, equipment designed, and systematic measurements made. All are proper and honorable when fit into a chain of precise reasoning that leads to understanding, but too often, elaborate statistical manipulation has been substituted for strong inductive thinking. Paraphrasing Woodford, even a lively idea has been choked to death with stately abstractions and statistical permutations, drained of lifeblood with passive constructions, the remains embalmed in polysyllables, the corpse wrapped in a veil of jargon, and the stiff old mummy buried with academic pomp in the most distinguished journal that will take it—all with a claim of contributing to knowledge.

An approach such as strong inference, with its multiple hypotheses and sharp inductive reasoning, has not been much used. Such an approach has been more prevalent when investigating acoustical or physiologic correlates of speech. As far as understanding clinical aspects of speech behavior is concerned, development of hard facts is in its infancy. Granted, the approach requires systematic exclusion of unprofitable alternative explanations, and we are not sufficiently certain of enough about speech to afford the luxury of categoric exclusion. Still, even if sharp exclusions are not possible, it is an approach that permits sorting of better from poorer leads.

If communicative behavior is lawful, then nothing about it is unalterably unknowable. The challenge is to continue to discover its laws. That challenge will be met as improved questions are asked. As they are, speech pathology will then progress toward maturity.

ANSWERS IN SPEECH PATHOLOGY: THE DATA

Whereas questions guide the search for knowledge, data produced and answers inferred from the search constitute our fund of knowledge. As wrong questions lead research astray, so do uncertain answers lead it into endless unproductive circles. A question not answered definitively is not answered. A possible explanation is not excluded.

Basic to obtaining clear answers is a clear idea of exactly what is to be measured. Phenomena observed and measured are the data

of science. Obviously, a fundamental necessity is that we know the nature of what is being observed.

Psychologic data are primary

Levels of organization. The primary observations of speech pathology are of psychologic processes. This statement identifies the level in the hierarchy of organization of phenomena for which we hold major interest and responsibility. The phrase "the level in the hierarchy of organization of phenomena" has an awesome ring, but it is not a mystifying idea. If it were applied to automobiles, we could talk at the highest level of organization about different makes of cars. At this level, each car functions as an integrated system, as a whole. We have Fords, Chevrolets, and Plymouths, as well as sedans, coupes, and convertibles, but all have their identities as cars. This level corresponds roughly in the life sciences to the psychologic, the level at which each organism has its unique identity as a whole, functioning system.

From this level down, we can engage in what is called *reductionism.* Unfortunately, some are inclined to believe that the greater the reduction and the smaller the unit of measure, the more profound the truth and the better the science. As Waterman (1961) observed of molecular biologists, they sometimes "give the impression that their truths are somehow deeper and more meaningful than those of other biologists." Reducing a car to its component parts (chassis, body, en-

---

What do Perkins and Curlee (1969) say about reductionistic thinking? Do they maintain that a "basic" cause can be found?

---

gine block, lights, pistons, carburetor) corresponds to reducing man to his anatomy. Parts of the car function in the electrical system, carburetion system, and transmission system; similarly, anatomic parts of man function physiologically in his nervous system, muscular system, respiratory system, circulatory system, digestive system, and endocrine system. But notice that we are no longer talking about a car or a man. We are talking about parts and how they function (Sperry, 1969).

These levels of organization of phenomena offer possibilities for descriptive economy. The simplest psychologic event, say waggling the tongue, involves the whole organism and all its systems at any given instant (Fig. 2-4, Level I). All systems must be described for that instant to account physiologically (Level II) for the event that can be described economically at a psychologic level (for example, the tongue moved a given distance and direction at a given rate). Matters get worse the farther reductionism is carried. The physiologic level can be reduced to levels of biochemistry and molecular biology (Level III). Merits of reductionism for the speech pathologist pale, however, when we consider that the number of molecules in a teaspoon of water, if they were grains of sand, would fill a trough 1 foot wide and 1 foot deep stretching from New York to San Francisco. The prospect of describing molecular, let alone atomic or subatomic, correlates of each instant of speech behavior stupifies the imagination.

Two classes of psychologic data. A psychologic analysis of movement of your tongue as you start to speak could describe either the *behavior* of moving the tongue or the *cognition* (thinking) involved in deciding what to say and how to say it. These make up the two classes of psychologic data: behavior is open to inspection—it can be observed directly and publicly; cognition is a private process within the estate of the mind—the public is not admitted and can only guess at what goes on inside by observing what comes out. These distinctions can be confusing, especially when psychology is defined as the science of behavior. When "behavior" is used in this generic sense, cognitive processes are considered as *implicit covert behavior,* and observable acts as *explicit overt behavior.* Regardless of the terms, the distinctions are the same.

Cognitive data. Many questions in speech pathology require cognitive answers. "How does a cerebral-palsied child feel?" "Is a stutterer anxious?" "Is a child with defective speech motivated?" "Does a hard-of-hearing child perceive speech normally?" "How is the thinking of an aphasic adult impaired?" "How do the mentally retarded learn?" These are questions about private operations; observers can infer what the person thinks only by what he does.

Since feeling, anxiety, motivation, perception, thinking, and learning cannot be observed directly, we refer to these cognitive phenomena by such names as *hypothetical constructs, intervening variables,* and *mediating responses.* Cognitive observations are necessarily indirect and inferential. They are subject to distortion by the person observed. Who has not on occasion disguised his motives by deceptive acts? They are also subject to distortion by the observer. An apocryphal indictment of projective tests of personality is that they reveal more about tester than

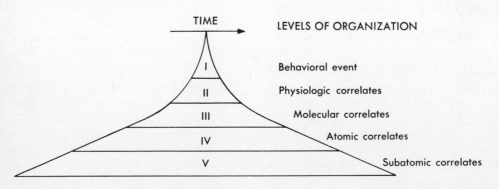

Fig. 2-4. Schematic representation of a behavioral event. The lower the level of organization, the greater the number of relationships among more phenomena to be described at any instant.

testee. Admittedly, cognition is difficult to measure, but the alternative to not measuring it is to discard it as an area for study.

Behavioral data. Many speech pathologists, especially clinicians, argue that the subjective world of feeling and thought is a vital area of concern. Others hold that cognition is a scientific dead end. Both have a point. To discard cognition discards man's psyche. To retain it limits what can be observed and known about it. Those who take the latter position content themselves with speech and language behavior that can be measured. They do not deny that cognition exists, but because it cannot be dealt with directly and precisely, they simply build psychologic conceptions of man that account for how he behaves.

B. F. Skinner, a major force behind this approach, has taken the position that because all that we know about cognition must be inferred from observable behavior, if we explain behavior, we explain all that can be known psychologically. On the face of it, this seems a cold-blooded approach that divests humans of their humanity. (A case can be made against this criticism, but this is not the place for it.) Still, behavioral analysis does yield hard data on which have been built psychologic conceptions that permit remarkable prediction and control of human as well as animal behavior.

Biologic and physical data are supportive. To say that the primary data of speech pathology are psychologic is not to say that other classes of data are irrelevant. Anatomic structures and their physiologic functioning in the production of speech represent biologic levels of vital importance to speech pathologists. Likewise, acoustical characteristics of sound waves generated in speech provide essential physical data. Crucial as these classes of biologic and physical phenomena are, they are typically involved as correlates of speaking behavior that the speech pathologist attempts to predict and control. Were they his prime interest and responsibility, he would study speech as a physiologist, an anatomist, or an acoustician. In fact, speech pathology draws vitality from many such members. For the majority, however, biologic and physical data are supportive.

ANSWERS IN SPEECH PATHOLOGY: CONDITIONS FOR OBSERVATION
Quantification of observation

How much impairment of language has an aphasic person suffered? How much better is a stutterer after a year of therapy? How much must the aperture of a cleft palate be reduced to relieve nasality? How much is respiratory difficulty disruptive of speech of a cerebral-palsied child? Meaningful answers to such questions require quantification. Intuitive answers are not enough. Cloaked behind general impressions is imprecise observation. If a thing exists, it exists in some amount. The problem of science in general and of speech pathology in particular is to find ways of measuring that amount.

To determine the quantity of a thing requires placing the thing you do *not* know about in relation to something you *do* know about. A wheezy old admonition in astronomy is that you must clean the eyepiece of your telescope carefully lest you mistake a flyspeck on the lens for a stellar object. The point of this absurdity is well taken: without a frame of reference for measuring a thing, you have no way of knowing that it exists, much less of knowing in what amount.

All measurement implicitly or explicitly involves comparison and discrimination. So far, so good—but tread gingerly. As a distinguished member (Campbell, 1938) of that most distinguished science, physics, said: "The most distinguished physicists, when they attempt logical analysis, are apt to gibber; and probably more nonsense is talked about measurement than about any other part of physics." Measurement, common as it is, involves profound assumptions that need concern us to the extent that we not violate them.

Scales of measurement. To have more than a vague impression of a comparison requires assignment of numerals to things to be compared in order to quantify them and discriminate among them. Numerals always fit into some scale of measurement. Scales deter-

THE WIZARD OF ID   by Brant parker and Johnny hart

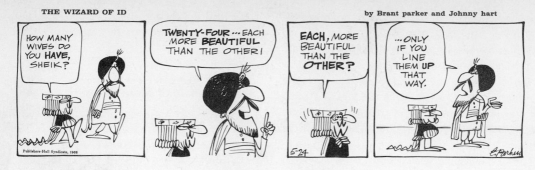

Fig. 2-5. Order of merit method of measurement. Rank ordering of observations is the basis for use of ordinal scale measurement. (Courtesy Johnny Hart and Field Enterprises, Inc.)

mine the nature of comparison and the significance of numbers in quantifying comparisons. Different scales permit use of different statistics and are also necessary to answer different types of questions.*

Nominal scale. If we asked, "How many different classes of speech disorders can be categorized?" a numeral could be assigned to each category to make a nominal scale. This is the basis for codes. We could, for instance, assign code number "1" to articulation disorders, "2" to language disorders, "3" to voice disorders, and "4" to stuttering. A nominal scale is considered the most primitive, and because it only distinguishes separate categories—category numbers cannot be added or subtracted—one can object to its being considered a scale of measurement. Yet classifying categories is a first step if a phenomenon is to be analyzed.

Ordinal scale. To answer the question, "What types of speech disorders are most fre-

quently encountered?" another type of scale would be needed that would permit us to rank speech handicaps in order from most to least prevalent: disorders of articulation would rank first, stuttering second, and so on. The ordinal scale accomplishes this purpose. With it numerals are assigned according to which categories are largest in comparison with each other (Fig. 2-5).

Interval scale. Suppose we wanted to measure changes that occur in attitude toward speech as a consequence of therapeutic modification of an impairment. We would need to quantify how much change occurs, which would require that each unit on the attitude scale be equal to every other unit. A person whose attitude had improved 2 points, say from 1 to 3, could be compared with another who, say, had also changed 2 units, from 4 to 6. An interval scale would be needed in which distances between intervals (units of measurement) are equal. Without equal intervals, effects of one condition could not be compared with another.

Ratio scale. Clearly, interval scales are considerably more useful than ordinal and certainly of more value than nominal scales. What they do not reveal, though, is the absolute value of a unit, essential information for a ratio scale. Knowing exactly how heavy a unit of weight is (a pound, a ton, a gram), how long a unit of length is, or for that matter, knowing the exact quantity of most physical properties, permits use of a ratio scale. This scale is not appropriate, though, for measuring such things as attitude, personal-

---

*Having seen the terms *statistics, measurement, numbers, scale,* and *quantification,* you may be bracing for an onslaught of mathematical symbols and algebraic equations. Be of good cheer. We will look only at the logic of these problems, so that you can better evaluate available information about disorders of oral communication. Although mathematics is logic in its purest form, and although mathematical symbols provide the most efficient means of carrying out logical maneuvers, still, many of us capable of understanding logic do not know the symbols well enough to think easily in the language of mathematics. English is not an ideal language for logic, but at least it is a language that all of us understand reasonably well.

ity, or intelligence, for which no absolute values exist. The reason is that we cannot find zero. Absolute zero is known for most physical scales, but the idea of having no attitude, no personality, or no intelligence seems almost too silly to contemplate. About the best we can do with cognitive phenomena is to establish relative values of their units of measure on an equal interval scale.

Ratio scales are used frequently, however, in the realm of *psychophysics*. This is a formidable term that refers to the relationship between *psycho*logic response, let us say hearing, and the *physic*al stimulus, in this case acoustical sound waves. Any sound has energy on which perception of loudness depends. Such energy can range, theoretically, from none at all, zero, to infinitely large amounts—the Saturn rocket makes a nearby airplane sound like a whisper, but the sound of that airplane has more than a trillion times the energy of a rustling leaf. Similarly, pitch of tones depends on frequency of vibration that can range from zero to the upper limit of pitch perception (about 20,000 Hz—short for *hertz*, meaning cycles per second—for healthy human ears). Acoustically, a ratio scale can be established that permits us to say, for instance, that a frequency of 200 Hz is twice that of 100 Hz.

Can we also measure the psychologic attributes, pitch and loudness, so that they can be compared proportionately? From such a question has come a *ratio scale* of pitch in which the unit of measure, the *mel*, has an absolute ratio value. That is, a sound of two mels is heard twice as high as a sound of one mel, three mels three times as high, four mels four times as high, and so on. Similarly, a ratio scale of loudness has been devised in which the unit of measure is the *sone*. Notice that in both interval and ratio scales, units can be added and subtracted, whereas only in ratio scales can they be multiplied and divided. The most sophisticated scale, the ratio scale, allows the widest range of statistical applications.

A helpful way of thinking about scales of measurement is to remember that they merely offer a convenient system for recording and analyzing observations. The appropriate scale is the one that permits meaning-

---

S. S. Stevens (1951, 1968) discusses problems of measuring psychologic phenomena. Does he say that the scale of measurement determines the statistic that can be used, or vice versa?

---

ful mathematical operations on the observations. Were we to look for differences between apples and oranges, we would not measure them with an interval scale; observations about these categories could be placed on a nominal scale. Alternatively, apples and oranges could be ranked in order of size, for which an ordinal scale should be used, or they could be compared for exact measurements of their weights (we might find an orange twice as heavy as an apple), a comparison that requires multiplication— hence a ratio scale.

Methods of measurement. A big problem in quantifying observations is obtaining stable measures, technically a problem of *reliability*. Repeated observations that yield different measures cast doubt on their accuracy. Let us look at a sampling of methods by which reliability of measures for the different scales can be improved.

Rating scale. A frequently used measure for such things as parental attitude and speaker personality is the rating scale. With it, a number is assigned to quantify the amount of the thing observed. A rating scale is easy to construct. It is also easy to use, especially when many judgments must be made, as on a multiple-item personality inventory. It is also the most subjective and consequently least reliable of methods. Still, it can be, and is, used to judge rank order on ordinal scales, establish equal intervals on interval scales, and determine proportions on ratio scales.

Minimal change. The method of minimal change involves varying a stimulus, such as a speech sound, in relation to some criterion. Suppose we wanted to know how much acoustical variation is possible in the /s/ sound before we begin to hear a lisp. We could find out by making minimal changes in spectrograms of normal productions of /s/. Since reliable distinctions among categories can be made with this method, it is used with the nominal scale.

Order of merit. Were you to listen to a group of defective speech sounds presented simultaneously and then attempt to rank them in order of impairment, you would be using the method of order of merit. It would have the difficulty of forcing you to remember all the sounds while you sort and compare them in your mind before ranking them on an ordinal scale (Fig. 2-5).

Paired comparison. A more cumbersome but considerably more reliable means of establishing an ordinal scale is the use of the method of paired comparison. Suppose you were to rank order a group of tones in terms of vocal quality. You would pair each tone with every other tone and judge which one in each pair you liked best. After all pairs had been compared, you would be able to rank each in relation to all the others.

Adjustment. The method of adjustment is a popular and useful technique for assigning numbers on any scale but the ordinal. With it a stimulus is adjusted (perhaps a pitch level that is too high) until it is matched subjectively in some desired relation to a criterion (possibly a lower pitch level). If the method of adjustment were used to develop ability to distinguish optimal pitches from those too high or too low, you would be using it to establish categories of a nominal scale. If used to measure how far habitual pitch is from a desired pitch, it would be for establishing an interval scale. If it were said that one pitch is twice that of another, a ratio scale would be established.

Fractionation. Fortunately, humans have the ability to judge accurately how much of a thing, say a pitch, is half of another thing, in this case another pitch (judgments of other fractions can be made, but not as accurately). This judgment of a ratio of two to one is a wonderfully simple psychologic operation; it is the basis of the method of fractionation. Although used to determine equal intervals, its chief value is for construction of ratio scales, such as those for pitch (the mel) and

for loudness (the sone). The ratio scale for pitch, as an example, was worked out by adjusting tones until they were half as high in pitch as standard tones. After a series of pitches had been found that stood in known ratio to each other, all were numbered according to their ratios to a reference pitch.

Magnitude estimation. Another procedure for determining proportions of a ratio scale is magnitude estimation. As the term suggests, an observer estimates stimulus magnitude proportional to other stimuli. A vocal tone of given loudness, for instance, could be assigned a number, say 10, as a reference. An observer would then assign numbers to tones of other loudness levels proportional to their apparent magnitude. The procedure can also be used by allowing the observer to work out his own reference system for proportional magnitudes.

This discussion is far from an exhaustive account of methods by which observations can be quantified in the various scales of measurement. These methods are familiar tools for the psychophysicist. Neither exotic nor

---

Stevens (1958) provides a thorough analysis of these psychophysical methods and their use with various scales of measurement.

---

difficult to master, they can be of immense value to the clinician in converting vague impressions into relatively exact observations.

Behavioral observation

Direct measurement. The speech pathologist is concerned primarily with behavioral (overt behavior) and cognitive (covert behavior) data. Since behavioral data are public, they can be observed and measured directly. They would include movements of lips, tongue, jaw, and other speech organs in the production of speech sounds. Although physiologic processes underlying speaking behavior and acoustical characteristics of speech sounds produced can also be measured directly, they should not be confused with the speaking behavior with which they are correlated.

Fallible observers. Because much of the direct observing of behavior, especially in a clinical setting, is done by one person noting what another is doing, the bugaboo of human fallibility looms large. The vexation of observer bias is ever present. Try as we may to

---

What problems do psychologists (Rosenthal, 1968; Bugelski, 1951) encounter when they attempt "objective" measurement?

---

be scrupulously objective, we cannot help leaning one way or another in our observations. When we suspect ourselves of succumbing to a halo effect, we may bend over backward to compensate, and the halo becomes a noose. Worse yet is the observer who filters all direct observations through the mesh of motivational interpretations. This observer fails to sort out what is done from the *reasons* ascribed for the doing. A statement such as, "He was angry because his clinician made him sit up straight," is not an observation; it is a pronouncement of the observer's interpretation of motive—an interpretation that could easily be a misperception of acute indigestion. Research points consistently to an alarming lack of reliability among clinical judgments for just such reasons (Goldberg, 1968).

Cognitive observation

Introspection. One of the oldest forms of observation of inner experience is introspection. As practiced by Wundt, it was anything but casual subjectivity. It involved a rigorous attempt to describe subjective experiences of thinking and feeling as objectively as possible in terms of basic perceptual attributes. A pencil would not be a pencil but a round, hard, yellow object, 6 inches long, with a red rubber tip at one end and a black lead point at the other. Objective as an introspectionist may attempt to be, the fact remains that no one can verify his observations. Too, it is not a very helpful technique with children, and many nonintrospective adults may be less than enthralled with it. Still, it does offer the most direct access to the much-valued private life of the mind.

Operational definitions. Lacking direct evidence of mental processes such as are involved in language, observable operations are defined as evidence of these processes—hence the term *operational definition*. Too, operational definitions are used to make categories explicit. Failure to define disfluent speech characteristics subjectively judged as stuttering, for example, has led to confusing research results (Bloodstein, 1975). Since there is no universally accepted operational definition, it is difficult to decide without ambiguity when an act of stuttering occurs. We could say that palmar sweat, for which various measuring techniques have been used, is evidence of anxiety, an aversive feeling presumed to prevail with many disorders of speech. One investigator built a "twitch meter" to record the twitch rate of an entire audience as an operational definition of anxiety. True, the behavior chosen to operationally define a cognitive condition may be disputed, but at least the definition involves a known, verifiable phenomenon (Underwood, 1957).

Logical constructs. The terms *hypothetical constructs*, *intervening variables*, and *mediating responses* are all closely related to logical constructs, and are so named to represent an attempt to construct a logical explanation for what goes on in the mind when we listen, think, speak, feel, learn, and so on. Such logical lifting of oneself by the bootstraps is not scientific larceny; it must be practiced by all sciences. Physicists would know nothing of electromagnetic force, gravitational force, or nuclear force if they had restricted themselves to direct observation. Who has ever seen any field of force? Only its effects (as operationally defined) are visible. Speech pathologists are in good company when they resort to logical constructs to explain such phenomena as how we learn the rules of a language, or how we learn any aspect of speech, for that matter.

ANSWERS IN SPEECH PATHOLOGY: METHODS OF STUDY

Methods of studying normal and defective speaking processes are modified versions of the various strategies of inquiry already considered. Certainty of what we know depends in large part on the methods by which we study a problem. All methods do not produce equally good answers.

Descriptive methods

Descriptive methods are just what the term implies: methods for describing what is observed. They differ mainly in the rigor of conditions for observation, and also in the nature of conditions that they are designed to explore. If utilized for the exclusive purpose of describing facts, they would be a low road of knowledge, the road of cataloging. If utilized to describe how one thing seems to function in relation to another, they would be a middle road, the road of describing the apparent structure of reality. This road is the highest one that can be traveled with descriptive methods. Because conditions of observation are all that can be controlled with these methods—they do not permit control of causal factors—one cannot make statements with them about cause and effect. The chief value of descriptive methods lies in searching out what look like cause-and-effect relationships that can then be investigated with more powerful, and frequently more costly, research methods.

Field-study method. A major descriptive tool of any science is the field-study method, often called the method of *naturalistic observation* and less frequently the *empirical method*. It is especially useful in early stages of development of knowledge in a field. As one might expect, it has been widely used in speech pathology. It has involved direct, systematic observations of defective speech in a natural clinical setting, with no attempt to alter or control behavior observed.

Because the field-study method cannot give a strong answer to why what has been observed functions as it does, it is not a substitute for experimental methods. But often experimentation is impossible. In fact, astronomy is a science that (with the exception of moon studies) cannot use it at all, for obvious reasons. Because astronomers cannot control their stars, they must do the next best

thing: control conditions of observation as carefully as possible. Similarly, speech pathologists may often ask important clinical questions that cannot be answered by experimentation in the artificial setting required for laboratory control. Naturalistic observation is sometimes the only ethical method. Removal of the larynx to determine its effects on stuttering, for example, would be a dubious operation. A caution, though: because it may be the only sensible method, certainty of answers produced is not better than it would be if experimentation were possible.

Life-history methods
Longitudinal study. Often we want to know the history of behavior observed: how normal speech develops, and how defective speech develops in specific individuals with specific impairments. An investigator who had enough time, energy, and money could trace development of normal speech by direct observation of children over a period of years. This study would be longitudinal, a type widely used to acquire much of the information we have about developmental norms.

Case history. The clinical investigator as well as the clinician is hampered in the use of longitudinal studies. We are only beginning to predict with accuracy which 5% of all toddlers will develop impaired speech—and no investigator has yet dedicated his life to studying a large enough segment of the population over a long enough period to obtain accurate information about the course of acquisition of defective speech. The next best solution has been to obtain case history information from the person himself and often from parents, relatives, and teachers. Since direct observation is impossible, life history must be reconstructed from selective recall, wishful thinking, recollections, and records subject to bias. This solution is hazardous for those who value accuracy of knowledge.

Test and questionnaire methods. Gathering of large quantities of data from large groups of people is usually not feasible by any direct means of observation. Much cognitive information is collected by tests or questionnaires on everything from sex life to speech habits. Tests, to be useful, must be standardized, whereas questionnaires are for eliciting specific information about individual characteristics. To remove ambiguity from test items or questions is exceedingly difficult. Even more difficult is test standardization (and test items interpreted out of standardized context are useless).

In fact, the apparent ease with which these instruments can be constructed is deceptive. They are fraught with possibilities for abuse. They often abuse assumptions about scales of measurement when data from them are tabulated and interpreted. They often abuse the privacy of individuals asked to fill them out; this abuse has irritated the federal government enough to restrict their use. They often abuse a person's time by inclusion of questions that are irrelevant to the inquiry but that would be "nice to know about."

Nonetheless, if done with consummate skill, a test or questionnaire type of inquiry may produce reasonably valid and reliable information. Many such instruments exist, and many of the important tests have been standardized and are utilized extensively in clinical assessment and research. Probably the most useful but not necessarily the most exact questionnaire information produced for speech pathology has been about incidence of communicative disorders.

Interview method. One school of thought maintains that a carefully planned interview technique will net more valid and reliable information than can be scooped up with questionnaires. This point of view is doubtlessly true, especially if questions are being asked about sensitive areas in one's life. Interviews require considerably more time from a research team, and their results are still far from being as exact as those produced by direct observation.

Clinical method. The clinical method, a loose term, has been saved until last because it can involve all descriptive methods and an experimental method, the analysis of behavior. Normally, a clinician will observe speech behavior—the field-study method; obtain a case history—a life-history method; conduct a structured interview to determine

attitudes; and probably administer tests. Finally, the clinician may obtain a base rate for, say, frequency of response of correct production of a sound produced incorrectly most of the time. The base rate would be used for later comparison to determine change in speech during and after therapy—experimental analysis of behavior. The keynote of the clinical method is flexibility: use the best that is available to solve the immediate problem at hand.

Experimental methods

We come now to the high road of knowledge: experimentation. Not a road to be followed casually or with little preparation, it is tortuous and demanding. The competition on it is fierce. Blunders are torn to shreds before the eyes of scientific colleagues in the arena of scholarly publications. But with the mind, stomach, and stamina for the game, the rewards can be mighty. The researcher can follow twistings and turnings of nature's riddles farther into the unknown than with any other method.

Granted, no riddle can be tracked to its ultimate end; science does not *prove*—it proceeds by disproof, so final answers are never reached. Granted, some riddles important clinically would be distorted if put into the laboratory for experimental solution. Granted, too, some riddles that theoretically could be answered with experimentation are automatically excluded for lack of volunteers.

Do Goldstein and his colleagues (1966) maintain that imaginative research of therapeutic processes could surmount typical problems of lack of rigor?

(Who would be willing to have portions of his brain removed to determine effects on his speech? A vital issue, but one that society precludes answering experimentally, thank goodness!) Still, a challenge of this road is to devise strategies for obtaining definitive answers to meaningful questions.

Experimental method. One method of experimentation is called the *experimental method.* The equivalent in speech pathology of the classical scientific method, it is applicable to any class of data: behavioral, cognitive, physiologic, acoustical. Not only conditions of observation but also conditions affecting behavior to be observed are controlled. Therefore, it is a method that permits replication. The ability to repeat an experiment under equivalent conditions is essential. Only as early observations are later confirmed can they be accepted with confidence, can they become "facts." Finally, it is a method that, like a high-power telescope, allows for detailed analysis of a limited field. Since definitive answers to only very limited questions can be produced, it is not a method with which one searches at random for a stellar problem to investigate.

Hypothesis testing. For the experimental method to be used economically, and to capitalize on its explanatory power, an investigator needs a clear conception of the question on which this method would be focused. He must therefore have a clear conception of what he *thinks* is the structure of knowledge in the area he is investigating. Furthermore, he either must have a theory that interrelates functions of many variables, or he must have at minimum a *hypothesis* about the relationship between two variables.

Regardless of the scope of his conception, he must be in a position to predict what he would find were he to look to reality to verify what his concept says he would find. And this means that the number of variables he can control with precision will be limited. Thus his inquiry is typically concerned with only two or three at a time—the level of hypothesis testing. Finally, this means that to conduct an effective experiment, he should test (by attempting to disprove) a prediction about a crucial functional relationship in the conception.

A theory is useless unless it can be put to the test of disproof. The better the theory, the more tightly it is integrated, and hence the more of it that can be put into jeopardy by a crucial experiment. Unprovable theories never die; they just fade away into ritualistic pronouncements. For those that are tested and fail in part, their fate is often a patch job. Rarely abandoned or reformulated in terms

of all evidence available—the job that is really required—they evolve with ad hoc qualification tacked onto ad hoc qualification until parsimony vanishes, internal consistency is contorted, and explanatory power diminishes. Fairbanks* (1966) said it best:

> There is an extraordinary amount of sheer aesthetics or beauty in science. We often speak about a beautiful theory, where we mean beauty in the purely aesthetic sense. We refer to a thought as being elegant, and when we do, we mean that it has a kind of parsimonious inevitability about it, not to be tinkered with any more than we would tinker with a painting.

Speech pathology and the behavioral sciences have few well-integrated disprovable theories; they are more the property of mature sciences. Nonetheless, this is the type of theory toward which speech pathology is striving.

Variables in experimentation. A dimension that can be measured directly or indirectly is a *variable.* Whether these dimensions are behavioral, cognitive, acoustical, physiologic, or anatomic, for experimentation the speech pathologist deals with them as *independent, dependent,* and other *relevant variables.* The researcher works from the premise that by controlling all but one relevant variable that could affect behavior being observed, he will exclude the important extraneous factors that might influence the experiment. With everything under experimental control, he watches effects on the *dependent* variable when he manipulates the only important one not being held constant, the *independent* variable. It is independent because it is free of effects other than those which the experimenter knows he is controlling. Conversely, the variable being influenced is dependent in that any changes in it can be attributed to manipulations of the independent variable made by the experimenter. The more consistently accurate are predictions about the dependent variable, the more support there is for the hypothesis.

Loose ends in experimentation are a pe-

---

*Fairbanks, G., *Experimental Phonetics: Selected Articles.* Urbana: University of Illinois Press (1966).

rennial problem. One would think, with all important variables controlled, observed, or manipulated, that we could be reasonably certain of results. But interaction arises to plague us (McGuigan, 1960). Variables have a way of influencing each other. Were we to investigate the relationship between subglottal air pressure (the dependent variable) and vocal pitch (the independent variable), loudness would need to be controlled as one of several relevant variables—it interacts with pitch. The relationship between subglottal pressure and pitch at one loudness level would probably be different than at another. Nature offers endless challenge to those who would unravel her complexities and permutations. As Nobel Laureate Feynman* (1965) said to his students in physics:

> One does not, by knowing all of the fundamental laws as we understand them today, immediately obtain an understanding of anything much. It takes a while, and even then it is only partial. Nature, as a matter of fact, seems to be so designed that the most important things in the real world appear to be a kind of complicated accidental result of a lot of laws.

Experimental and control groups. Much work done in speech pathology has been to determine ways in which the speech handicapped differ from those whose speech is normal. Lacking an independent variable under direct control, the experimenter approximates it by dividing subjects according to whether or not they exhibit the speech problem in question. If they do, they join the *experimental* group; if not, they go into the *control* group. The operation of the dependent variable is presumed to be different in the experimental group from that in the control group.

Use of experimental and control groups is deemed good scientific practice when the experimental method is employed. The difference between the two groups is always limited to whether or not the independent variable is present. In all other respects, the groups are intended to be equivalent either by selection or statistical manipulation. For example, assume that we were interested in the effects on speech of damage in the dominant temporal lobe of the brain. We would select persons with injury in this location for the experimental group. For the control group, we would choose persons without such injury who matched the experimental group in all other respects as closely as possible. The purpose of a control group is to assure probability that effects of experimentation are indeed attributable only to manipulation of the independent variable and not to some irrelevant, unobserved factor. In fact, use of a control group is essential with the experimental method if one is to hazard statements of cause and effect with much certainty.

Experimental design. A distinguishing feature of the experimental method is advance planning. Not a little something whipped up in spare time, it may take months of planning of the most minute detail. The blueprint for the research is called the experimental design. Just as correction of a faulty blueprint is too late once building construction begins, so correction of a faulty design is too late once experimentation is under way. The design includes specification of the problem to be investigated; exact predictions of hypotheses that would be excluded with each possible result; important variables to be observed, manipulated, and controlled; conditions, procedures, and instruments to be used for observation, manipulation, or control; subject requirements for experimental and control groups; and statistical procedures to be used for describing and interpreting results.

Experimental analysis of behavior. The other experimental method, the experimental analysis of behavior, is particularly relevant for applied purposes of speech pathology. It is a paradoxic method. On one hand, it is the quintessence of experimentation; it more closely approximates the model of physics for scientific investigation than any other in the behavioral sciences. Since it is designed for analysis of invariant relationships with the individual, inferential statistics

*Feynman, R.: *The Character of Physical Law.* Cambridge, Mass.: The M.I.T. Press (1965).

is of limited value. Its data are exclusively behavioral. They can be defined explicitly and measured objectively. It provides for more than just experimental control of relevant variables. It extends control directly to behavior. Its trademark is establishment of a stable *base line* for the most measurable aspect of behavior: rate of responding—hence the other term, *base rate*.

Rate of behavioral response, then, is the dependent variable. Effects produced by systematic manipulation of experimental conditions, one independent variable at a time, can then be observed directly on deviations of observed behavior from the base rate. Effects are immediately apparent, if they occur at all. Let us say, for example, that we obtained a base rate of stuttering during reading. Then if we discovered that syllable disfluency decreased in frequency each time syllables were prolonged and increased when speech was rapid, we would have a strong basis for suspecting a cause-and-effect relationship. In fact, it would be so apparent that statistics would be unnecessary to describe it. If response rate does not deviate from base line, loss of behavioral (to say nothing of experimental) control is presumed. Experimentation does not continue until control is reestablished. No purpose would be served by continuing otherwise. If experimental manipulations do not produce readily observable consequences, the presumed relation between independent and dependent variables is quickly revealed as more presumption than reality. Experimental analysis of behavior offers prompt feedback about accuracy of an investigator's conception of behavioral relationships (Sidman, 1960).

So far, so good. This system for a functional analysis of behavior is elegantly simple. The criticism arises from the fact that it seems to be a sort of "Johnny-one-note" system; it repeatedly demonstrates its basic premise: the future of any behavior is a function of its consequences. Still, this premise has already proved to be a germinal concept for what started as a drizzle of operant conditioning studies with the early work of B. F. Skinner. It soon reached deluge proportions, and the monsoon season has now spread to speech pathology. The concept may even prove to

---

Does Brookshire (1967) apply experimental analysis of behavior to only selected types or to all types of communicative disorders?

---

be one of the very few solid rocks on which speech pathology and all other behavioral sciences can be built.

Immensely impressive as this functional concept of behavior is for anyone seeking lawful invariant relationships, it is far from satisfying for those who would construct theories of such cognitive phenomena as learning, emotion, perception, and language. Skinner lays no claim to having sired a theory. He claims only to have developed a powerful method of analysis. Yet science utilizes methods for erection of integrated structures of knowledge—and these structures are its theories. Here, we confront the paradox: a functional analysis of behavior utilizes the finest method of experimentation developed in behavioral science, but its advocates have not yet shown much inclination, with a few notable exceptions, to use it for construction of a sturdy theoretical edifice of behavioral knowledge. The probability seems good that whatever the structure proves to be, one of its cornerstones will include the concept that in large measure the functional consequences of behavior determine its future.

Value for speech pathology. The payoff to society from speech pathology is service to the speech handicapped. When grouped, they are plentiful enough to constitute an army, but when helped, each person's uniqueness must be confronted. Little wonder that a functional analysis of behavior has such charismatic appeal for clinicians. It is an approach designed to study individuals, not groups. It reveals directly, simply, and quickly the functions of an individual's behavior. The system works as well for those who respond differently to the same circumstances as it does for those who respond identically.

The experimental analysis of behavior is concerned with *operant* responses. The term was coined by Skinner to designate responses that operate on the environment to produce consequences. If consequences are *reinforcing,* likelihood that the response will recur increases, and it is learned. If consequences are aversive, the response is unlikely to occur as frequently. It will be replaced by other, more successful operants and may disappear from the behavioral repertoire—which, incidentally, is not the same as saying that it is unlearned. All speaking behavior can be thought of as operant responses. To control an operant, consequences following it must be manipulated. Therefore the operant must occur before it can be controlled. Since operants cannot be made to happen reflexively, we say that they are *emitted.*

Skinner also coined the term *respondents* to describe another class of behavior characterized by responses that occur reflexively each time certain stimuli are presented. The form of the response seems predetermined; it apparently does not depend on consequences produced. Respondent behavior is more typical of the vegetative than of the skeletal muscular system. After all, certain stable gastrointestinal responses are essential to healthy digestion, regardless of what one is doing or saying. To control a respondent, one must manipulate the stimuli preceding it; thus we say that respondents are *elicited.* Note that this temporal arrangement of independent and dependent variables is classic for studies using the experimental method.

Contingencies of reinforcement. Analysis of operant speech is an analysis of effects of contingencies of reinforcement on a stable base rate of speech responses. A fundamental premise of this conception is that emitted speech behavior is acquired by reinforcement. Four basic procedures involving two types of *reinforcement* and two types of *punishment* are utilized as shown in the accompanying diagram to accomplish *operant conditioning,* a name often used interchangeably with analysis of behavior. Probably nothing is less absolute than reward and punishment. Pleasure for one is revulsion for another. Yet, pleasure reinforces and punishment repels. Scientific analysis of behavior is doomed if these types of consequences cannot be distinguished. The dilemma is resolved in operant conditioning by defining consequences in terms of their behavioral effects, as follows:

positive reinforcement Presentation of an event (presumably pleasurable) contingent on a response, followed by an increase in frequency of that response.
negative reinforcement Removal of an aversive condition (presumably unpleasant) contingent on a response, followed by an increase in frequency of that response.
punishment I Removal of a positive reinforcer contingent on a response, followed by a decrease in frequency of that response.
punishment II Presentation of an aversive condition contingent on a response, followed by a decrease in frequency of that response.

Positive and negative reinforcement both increase response rate, but positive rein-

---

Contingencies of reinforcement and punishment

Response frequency	Contingent stimulus	
	Presented	Removed
Increases	Positive reinforcement	Negative reinforcement
Decreases	Punishment II	Punishment I

forcement increases approach responses, whereas negative reinforcement increases avoidance responses. Curiously, even in operant conditioning two negatives can make a positive. By making aversive stimuli contingent on avoidance behavior, a condition is established in which avoiding avoidance is negatively reinforced. The result equals emission of approach responses. To illustrate, suppose that you are a stutterer and, like many people with this problem, you detest using the telephone. Suppose further that you have finally been offered the job that you have been seeking for years, only to discover that it would require extensive use of the telephone. The aversive price of continued avoidance of the telephone will be the coveted position. If you want the job badly enough, you will have to avoid a pet avoidance. You will have to substitute an approach response—and use the telephone.

Schedules of reinforcement. We have seen procedures by which consequences contingent on a response can be managed. Now let us look at schedules by which these consequences can be applied. Called *schedules of reinforcement*, they produce characteristic patterns of rate of response. They are plentiful, ranging from schedules of *continuous reinforcement* (crf) to *differential reinforcement of rate* (dr), from *fixed interval* (FI) and *fixed ratio* (FR) to *variable interval* (VI) and *variable ratio* (VR), and included is an *extinction* (ext) schedule.

Effects of these schedules are much as one would expect. If a child were given a bite of candy each time after a correct articulatory response (crf), rate of responding would be increased if he wanted candy. If suddenly the candy were withdrawn (ext), he would quickly suspect that the arrangement had ended; thus responding might stop. If, instead, he discovered that tidbits were dispensed after 2 minutes of correct articulation (FI), or after, say, twenty correct responses (FR), response rate would probably increase as the payoff approached and decrease with receipt of a bonbon. But were goodies dispensed at random, either at unpredictable times (VI) of after an unpredictable number of responses (VR), he would be uncertain as to when reinforcement might occur. He would probably plug along steadily at a fairly constant rate of response, an essential condition if carryover of corrected speech to everyday life is to be achieved. Management of schedules of reinforcement and of contingent consequences is the essence of analysis of behavior. These schedules determine contingencies of reinforcement by which behavioral as well as experimental control can be demonstrated and functions of behavior discovered.

Statistical methods

Often with the experimental method, so many variables are involved that to control even a portion would be impossible or to match a control with an experimental group for all variables would leave no subjects. Clearly, these circumstances call for a solution other than experimental control. Here, statistical methods, such as *analysis of variance*, can be substituted. Instead of studying effects of the independent variable against constant values of controlled variables, it is studied against randomized values of the freely operating variables held "constant" by mathematical manipulation.

Not only is statistical control substituted for experimental control of relevant variables, but it is used as a partial substitute for experimentation. For instance, in research on defective speech associated with neurologic disabilities, we cannot manipulate the independent variable, the brain; thus we must settle for statistical correlations of different amounts and locations of accidental damage to the brain and concomitant disorders of speech. This approach, the method of *concomitant variation*, is not preferable to the experimental method, with its greater precision of control, but where experimentation is not possible, the general logic of experimentation can be approximated through use of correlation.

Often, too, we want to know factors involved in performance of speech or language tasks. For instance, lively disputes have blossomed over whether or not a common language ability runs through all forms of symbolic impairment in brain-injured adults. The argument hinges in large measure on *factor analysis*, a statistical tool for analyzing intercorrelations among test items, the assumption being that high positive correlations between items indicate that they are measuring much the same thing. Thus statistics can be used for analysis as well as for control.

Complicated as statistical methods seem at first glance, they are actually a means of reducing volumes of data to a form simple enough for the mind to grasp. Although statistics has been defined facetiously as the art of stating precisely what one does not know, and a statistician as one who draws mathematically precise lines from unwarranted assumptions to foregone conclusions, statistical methods are in reality designed to help make the best guess possible in the face of uncertain facts. Therefore statistics "is the study and informed application of methods for reaching conclusions about the world from fallible observations" (Kruskal, 1967). For raw data the speech pathologist records his observations in numbers on some scale of measurement. Until cooked with descriptive or inferential statistical procedures, however, they are generally indigestible for human consumption.

Statistics used for description. A descriptive statistic is a single number that summarizes a characteristic of a collection of measurements on a group. Three characteristics can be described: *central value* of the measures, their *variability*, and *correlations* among them. Need for these statistical descriptions is dictated by the questions to be answered, but the scale of measurement used to gather the data may rule out the preferred statistic. This is an admonition to design research with the necessary statistics in mind from the start. We will look at various descriptive statistics to see for which scales they are appropriate.

Statistics descriptive of central value. The descriptive characteristic always of concern is the central value of a set of measures. Implied in an "average performance" is the central tendency of repeated measures of individual or group responses. *Average* is not a precise term, although it generally is used as a synonym for the *mean*. The most useful measure of central value available, means are computed by addition of all scores and division by their total number. These arithmetic operations are not meaningful, however, with nominal or (speaking strictly) ordinal scales. Adding or subtracting numbers is the same as adding or subtracting units, and only interval and ratio scales involve units. Only with them are means appropriate.

Suppose, however, you ask the question: "What is a typical speech disorder?" Computation of a mean to answer it would be silly—the answer might come out something like 3/17. Obviously, the answer must be a category, not some fraction of an interval. A sensible answer would be selection of the category with highest incidence of defective speech on a nominal scale: for instance, disorders of articulation. This measure of central tendency is called the *mode*.

Suppose, now, that you want to determine the most typical type of disfluency of a particular stutterer. One approach would be to rank disfluencies of his stuttered speech in order of frequency. The type of disfluency in the middle of the ranking would be "typical." The answer in this instance still involves selection of a category: a type of disfluency (for example, repetition of sounds) cannot be chopped into fractions, added, subtracted, or anything else. The middle position in the rank-order on an ordinal scale can be specified, and that is all. This measure of central value is a *median*.

Statistics descriptive of variability. Another characteristic of a set of measures that we often wish to describe is their variability. If different results were obtained with repeated measures of nasal air escape during cleft palate speech, one would have to decide how much credence to give the different measures. Usually several measures are obtained to permit a defensible general statement, such as: "Nasal air escape varies proportionately with size of palatal cleft."

Certainty of this conclusion, however, will depend on how much the different measures vary. Making general statements, then, requires description of how measures differ. A convenient descriptive device is a statistic that summarizes variability.

As we have different measures of central value appropriate for different scales of measurement, so we have different measures of variability. The simplest is *range*. If the lowest value observed is 7 and the highest is 97, the range would be 90. This figure was obtained by subtracting 7 from 97, an arithmetic operation that requires manipulation of equal intervals. Nominal and ordinal scales therefore do not allow for description of variability. Perhaps you have already leaped ahead to the conclusion that follows: generalizations cannot be inferred legitimately when observations are measured on nominal or ordinal scales—that is, if variability cannot be described, inferences cannot be drawn. Again, we see the need to know before beginning observations whether scales of measurement to be used will permit the type of research information needed.

Suppose, in the illustrative range of 90 just mentioned, that a total of thirty measures were made, of which all but two were between 70 and 97. One was, perhaps, 23, and the other was the lowest, 7, that we subtracted from 97 to obtain the range of 90. Obviously, the *range* does not represent the variability of these measures very well; the majority of scores are wagged badly by the tail of the single minority score, 7. Needed is a description of variability that will reflect all scores. Such a statistic is the *standard deviation*. Based on the amount that each score varies from the mean (standard deviations cannot be computed with modes or medians), it is a description of how much the mean fails to be representative of all measures. It is a *standard* for the set of scores of how much the average measure *deviates* from their means.

Were the standard deviation computed by subtracting each score from the mean, half would be above and half below it—they would cancel each other out. The standard deviation would always be zero, regardless of how much the scores varied. The solution is easy. Since negatives multiplied by negatives give positive numbers, all deviation scores are squared. Now, all variation, irrespective of whether above or below the mean, can be summed. The average of that sum is *variance*. When the square root of variance is taken to get the variability index back to original scale, the result is the *standard deviation*.

Often, we want to assess adequacy of individual performances on a battery of tests. Raw scores would be useless because they must be related to normal performance to have meaning. The most representative measure of normal performance is the mean, and the best description of an average variation from a mean is a standard deviation. It is such a good measure that it is used as a score, the *standard score*, to describe adequacy of an individual performance in comparison with an average performance. We can say, then, that a person scores so many standard deviations above or below the mean—this figure is his standard score.

Statistics descriptive of correlations. Most of science is concerned with how one variable relates to another. If only naturalistic observations are available, the statistic with which co-relations among variables are described is *correlation*. Again, the scale of measurement imposes limitations on how correlations can be calculated, but considerable flexibility is available. A set of scores on any scale can be correlated with another set on any other scale.

For correlations of nominal scales, we might be interested in relations between types of disabilities associated with speech disorders and age groups—both involve categories, hence, nominal scales. For lack of formal research results, we will pretend that a study of incidence of selected disabilities in children of different ages attending a speech

Table 2-1. Hypothetical study of correlations between speech disorders and age groups

Type of disability	Age					
	0-5	5-12	12-18	18-50	50-80	Total
Cerebral palsy	27	23	19	12	2	83
Cleft palate	24	21	11	11	5	72
Mental retardation	38	45	49	33	14	179
Asphasia	0	2	3	17	29	51
Laryngectomy	0	0	0	6	21	27
Total	89	91	82	79	71	412

clinic has been done, and we will fabricate a set of figures that would seem sensible. They might look like those shown in Table 2-1.

Even casual inspection of this hypothetical table reveals what speech pathologists know: that a fairly high correlation exists between age and type of disability—cerebral palsy, cleft palate, and, to a lesser extent, mental retardation are predominantly children's disabilities that affect speech, whereas aphasia and laryngectomy are characteristic of the waning years. A statistic that describes this correlation between scores on nominal scales is the *coefficient of contingency*. It is the degree to which scores in each cell (a cell is formed by the intersection of two categories: the score where aphasia and the 18- to 50-year age group intersect is 17) depart from what might be expected by chance.

Similarly, a statistic called *rank-difference correlation* can be used to describe the relation between scores on ordinal scales. Suppose we are trying to determine how functions of the vocal mechanism differ when a pleasant tone is produced from when a rough and harsh sound is made. A good suspicion would be that rough sound correlates with irregular vocal cord vibration ("jitter"). Because vocal jitter cannot be controlled directly by the experimenter, naturalistic observation of vocal cord vibration is left as an independent variable that could be quantified on ordinal, interval, or ratio scales. An ordinal scale could be used by ranking vibratory patterns in order of amount of jitter. Similarly, judgments of roughness would possibly be ranked by the method of paired comparison. With two scores for each sound, jitter and roughness rankings, the problem is set for solution by rank-difference correlation. Had the method of fractionation been used to develop equal interval scales for jitter and perceived roughness, the arithmetic operations of addition and subtraction would be permissible. A more useful measure of the relationship would be possible with the *product-moment correlation coefficient*. Only the ability to make a meaningful correlational statement would be improved—not the ability to make a causal statement.

A good text in statistics, such as Guilford's (1956), will help you to explore these problems in greater depth.

Statistics used for inference. That speech pathology is an applied behavioral science carries several statistical implications. Being "applied" means that the value of "pure" knowledge lies in its usefulness, usually in the solution of clinical problems. Being a "behavioral" more than a "social" science means that the applied problems to be solved are those of the individual, not of the group. That we can predict with confidence that some difference will be found when groups are compared is of little value if that difference is not present for the specific individual for whom we have clinical responsibility. The fact, for example, that many stutterers seem to anticipate words to be stuttered is of little consequence if you are working with one in the minority group who does not anticipate his occurrences of stuttering.

The uniqueness of each speech-handicapped person poses an idiographic challenge to a clinician's artistry. The scientist, however, must seek commonality in this uniqueness. Scientific laws are applicable irrespective of the individual. All science seeks that which is crucial for speech pathology, with its responsibility for individuals with handicapped speech: invariant relationships and general knowledge that can be applied appropriately without exception.

This preamble to *statistical inference* has been written to prepare you for its limits and merits. It will reveal whether or not a factor is operating in enough people in a group to justify predicting its presence in a similar group. It will not reveal a factor's presence in a specific individual in the group. It will permit testing of factors hypothesized to be operating in groups. It will not discriminate whether they are big or little factors.

Humans are so unlimited in their ways of being complex that few if any laws hold for them without exception. In speech pathology the search for invariant relationships on which to erect a solid structure of knowledge must contend with the most complex of all human activities—speech. Were laws available that would be consistently applicable to individuals, inferential statistics would be unnecessary. Lawful effects would be readily apparent without statistics. Lacking knowledge of such laws, we must look for signs of them wherever they can be teased out, frequently in groups—hence, statistical inference.

Parametric statistics. If, on the basis of a limited number of observations of a limited number of speech-handicapped persons, general statements were made about a large *population* of speech-handicapped individuals, the assumption would be that the *sample* of individuals observed was typical of the population. Just as you assume that the bite of food you sample in the kitchen gives an accurate estimate of what you will eat at the table, so the statistical sample, when properly selected, can be assumed to give an accurate estimate of how people perform in the population sampled. When this assumption can be made, parametric statistics can be used to draw inferences.

A *parameter* is a number that describes a characteristic of a population. A *statistic*, the counterpart of a parameter, is a number derived from a sample that is an estimate of a characteristic of a population. For statistical inference this characteristic is *distribution* of scores. With the sophisticated formulas for

sampling distributions available to statisticians, loss of precision in estimating a population of scores is slight even with small samples. As with any estimate, though, it will always be off a bit. To determine how far off and to correct for sampling error, an ideal abstract model, the *normal distribution*, is used as a standard for comparison. This is the distribution described by the *bell-shaped curve*, a curve whose fame (or infamy, depending on your success as a student) pervades grading throughout education. It is simply a description of the distribution of scores that would be expected theoretically if an infinitely large, normally distributed population were measured.

Characteristics of the normal distribution are described precisely by two parameters: mean and standard deviation. Given numbers for these two parameters, the ideal bell-shaped curve can be plotted. Therefore, the closer a sample approximates the normal distribution, the more confidence that it was drawn from a normally distributed population described accurately by the mean and standard deviation. If the sample does not approximate a normal distribution, the error that would be made in estimating the mean and standard deviation can be corrected by a variety of techniques.

With examination grades used as an example, the farther out on the "curve," the higher or lower is the score. Grades on the bell-shaped curve of a normal distribution typically look like the display in Fig. 2-6. Were the numerical score the exact average for the class, it would be the mean. Variability above and below the mean would be measured by the standard deviation (symbolized by s in a sample). Frequently, if a student's score varies above the mean by one standard deviation $(+1s)$, he is in line for at least a B. If above by two or more standard deviations $(+2s, +3s,$ and so on), he is entering the rarefied atmosphere of the upper 2½% of the class. Similarly, for those who may have partied instead of studying, the dubious honor of being in the lower 2½% of the class will earn an F. Lying between this 5%, half of whom are average-raisers and the other half

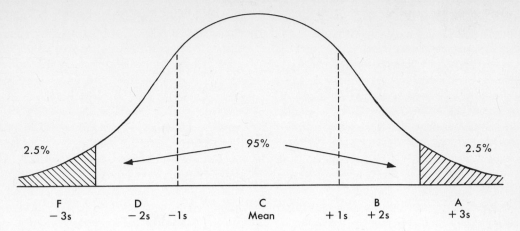

Fig. 2-6. Bell-shaped curve of a normal distribution. The number of standard deviations (s) above or below the mean is typically the basis for assigning test grades.

flunkees, will be roughly 95% who earned B, C, or D.

Generalizing from grade curves, the problem is to determine whether or not a difference between one set of scores and another is of sufficient significance to say that something is operating differently in one group than in the other. The criterion used to determine significance is the probability that the difference is not a result of chance. To help guard against confirming expectations, you set up a *null hypothesis* with which you predict that any difference *is* a result of chance. The null hypothesis is the alternate guess that something is nothing. To test the research hypothesis, you must be able to reject the probability that the null hypothesis is correct. If lenient, you may reject it when it could be correct in five instances out of one hundred. If strict, you may insist on the odds being only one in 100 that chance could account for the difference.

Suppose that two forms of an intelligence test were available, with one suspected of being more difficult than the other. To minimize bias in testing this suspicion, the null hypothesis would be predicted that any difference found would result from some chance factor: weather, time of day, ski conditions, location of pretty girls in class—students can be distracted by so many things. When the two forms, A and B, were administered to the same class, let us say that the mean score

for Form B is twelve points higher than for Form A. The question is whether this difference is accidental or a result of the test. The question could be answered by repeated testing. If the difference occurred time after time, suspicion of the tests would grow stronger. Undoubtedly, though, the difference would vary from administration to administration, so that after many repetitions, a *sampling distribution* of difference scores would become available. Like all distributions, it could be described with a mean as the most representative score and with a standard deviation that, for a sampling distribution, is called the *standard error*, or in this case the *standard error of the mean.* In practice, variability of sampling distributions is so well known that the standard error can be estimated by statistical formulas.

The question would still remain whether the difference is accidental or a function of the test. Translated for statistical answer, the question is: what is the probability that this difference would not be accidental and therefore that the null hypothesis should be rejected? The bell-shaped curves of Fig. 2-7 provide the answer. We know that to go toward both tails of a normal curve about two standard deviations (two standard errors in this case) would leave roughly 95% of the scores in the middle (Fig. 2-6). These scores could be predicted by chance. Thus, odds are only five out of 100 that a difference be-

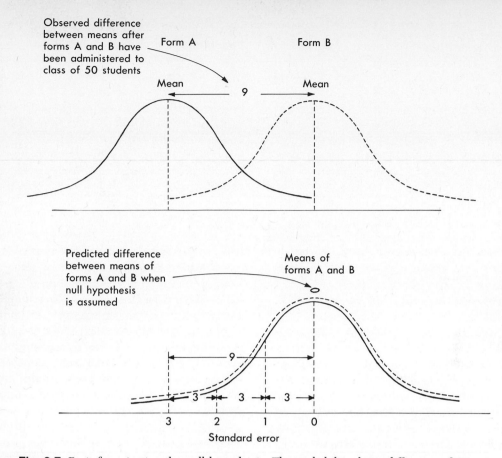

Fig. 2-7. Basis for rejecting the null hypothesis. The probability that a difference of 9 in test forms A and B could be an accident is slight. Fewer than 5% of the scores are 3 standard errors (standard deviations) from the mean.

tween tests that is more than two standard errors in either direction from the mean would be accidental—odds that even cautious gamblers would like. If this remaining 5% were not to be attributed to chance, presumably it would be evidence of some factor that works differently in one group than the other.

To determine whether the two tests are different, the twelve-point difference between them must be translated into standard errors. If three were used as the size of the standard error (a likely size if the examinations were given to a class of fifty), we could compute the number of standard errors from the mean that the difference of twelve would be by setting up a ratio: 12/3. This ratio is critical for determining the significance of a

difference between two sets of scores— hence it is a *critical ratio*. It tells us that a difference of twelve equals four standard errors from the mean, and the bell-shaped curve tells us that odds are much less than five to 100 that this difference of three standard errors would result from chance. We would then reject the null hypothesis and conclude that the tests, in fact, are different.

Because much of the research in speech pathology involves relatively small samples, a more realistic and refined test of statistical significance is the *t ratio*. Essentially the same as the critical ratio, the t ratio takes into account the size of a small sample. For the critical ratio, the standard error is estimated on the assumption of a large, normally distributed sample. With such a sample, estimate of the standard error is reasonably accurate, thereby permitting a correspondingly accurate test of significance.

With small samples, however, this estimate is less reliable. To offset the greater likelihood of discrepancies in estimating the standard error for small samples, a t ratio is used that must be slightly greater than the critical ratio that would be required to reject the null hypothesis at any specified level of significance. For example, a critical ratio of 1.96 would be required for an infinitely large sample to establish a difference significant at the 5% level of confidence. To establish the same difference with the same significance from a small sample of thirty would require a bit larger t ratio of 2.04.

A brief review may help to clarify basic steps in the statistical machinations used to infer that a difference between groups is a real difference.

Step 1. Define the population of measures that you plan to sample, to describe, and to draw statistical inferences about. Clarity of definition will probably be a function of clarity of the research question. If you do not know what you are asking, you probably will not know what you are measuring.

Step 2. Draw a sample from the population. Whatever procedure is used, random or otherwise, it must offer assurance of giving a sample that is representative of the population.

Step 3. Conduct research on the sample. Observe variables to be compared. Record observations on an appropriate scale of measurement.

Step 4. Compute the necessary descriptive statistics: for example, mean, standard deviation, standard error.

Step 5. From these statistics descriptive of the sample and from known characteristics of the ideal normal distribution, logically infer characteristics of the population. These inferences will be your generalizations.

Nonparametric statistics. The discussion of statistics used for inference has proceeded on four assumptions: (1) that samples drawn are representative of the population as a whole; (2) that the population is normally distributed in the fashion of the bell-shaped curve; (3) that large critical ratios for differences between samples indicate that the samples are drawn from different populations; and (4) that the scales of measurement used for gathering data permit computation of means and standard deviations: equal-interval or ratio scales. These assumptions are necessary to describe various parameters of the distribution of scores in a population. That is, they are essential to the use of parametric statistics.

If violations of these assumptions cannot be corrected adequately, the alternative is to use statistics that make few, if any, assumptions about the form of distribution of scores in the population sampled. These are called *distribution-free* or *nonparametric* statistics. Various nonparametric techniques are available both for statistical description and inference. In fact, we have already considered two nonparametric techniques descriptive of correlations that can be used with nominal and ordinal scales: the coefficient of contingency and the rank-difference correlation. Since this discourse is intended only to provide a glimmering of the overall logic behind various statistical tactics, we will not delve further into individual tests.

A few general comments are in order, however, about relative merits of parametric and nonparametric statistics used for inference. The utility of nonparametric statistics as time-savers will be accorded minimal importance, but it is a fringe benefit to be enjoyed. More substantial is the answer to which is the lesser of two evils: parametric tests weakened by invalidated assumptions, or nonparametric tests that sacrifice available information. Differences in scales of measurement hold a key. Equal-interval and ratio scales provide more information that permits more exact description of central value and variability than do ordinal or nominal scales. Whereas all that is known for a median on an ordinal scale is ranking of scores, size of interval between ranks must also be known for a mean on an equal-interval or ratio scale. This information about intervals is wasted in nonparametric statistics that utilize at best the level of information found in ordinal scales.

Practically, the relative merits of para-

Siegel (1956) elaborates on the nature, the values, and the limits of nonparametric statistics.

---

metric and nonparametric statistics add up to the following: When samples are small, the various assumptions underlying parametric statistics cannot be tested adequately. Since their inferential power is dependent on validity of these assumptions, their use with small samples is risky. Fortunately, nonparametric statistics, being relatively free of assumptions that could be violated, are nearly as powerful with small samples, for which they are often a useful statistic of choice. They lose out to parametric statistics, however, as sample size increases. Inferential power increases more rapidly with parametric than with nonparametric tests. Similarly, distribution-free methods are no alternative to parametric methods for analysis of interactions among several variables.

The answers–résumé

1. What are the bases of knowledge of communicative disorders?

Speech pathology is an applied behavioral science responsible for habilitation and rehabilitation of the speech handicapped as well as for understanding disorders of communication. Knowledge of these disorders, therefore, must be in a useful form; it must permit accurate prediction of what causes what, and effective control of conditions that will yield helpful changes for persons with speech problems. This objective requires that knowledge be obtained by the approaches of science; intuition alone is not sufficient. Problems must be analyzed to determine important variables. Precise relationships among the variables must be described. Crucial questions must be asked that pierce to the essence of problems. And definitive answers must be produced that provide solid facts on which a sturdy structure of knowledge can be erected.

2. What are the data of speech pathology?

The answer is less ambiguous for the clinician than for the scientist. The clinician is limited by law, by training, and by professional responsibility to psychologic data. His primary concern is with utilization of learning to effect improvement in communicative behavior. The scientist, on the other hand, may be interested in various correlates of cognitive and behavioral processes: he may also study acoustical and physiologic aspects of speaking.

3. How can speech be observed and measured?

Speech output and observable behavior of speaking can be measured directly. Rules by which ideas are formulated into language, however, involve cognitive processes that cannot be observed directly; these operations are therefore defined by observable consequences. Recording observations in a form that permits accurate comparison requires measurement; the more precise the measurement, the more precise the comparison that is possible. A variety of methods can be used to increase the reliability and validity of observations. Moreover, four scales of measurement are available that differ in the types of quantification they permit: nominal scales permit the assignment of observations to categories, ordinal scales permit ranking, interval scales permit addition and subtraction, and ratio scales permit all these operations plus multiplication and division.

4. What methods are applicable for the study of speech?

All experimental, descriptive, and statistical methods, in one way or another, are applicable. Aside from the limitations of time and money, two other practical considerations weigh heavily in selection of a method: conditions for observation and ethical feasibility. The clinician, with greatest opportunity for extended observation of disordered speech, is generally ethically pledged to use methods that will provide service in a manner that will be in the best interests of his client. Since he is obligated to use techniques of demonstrated effectiveness, naturalistic observation of the speech handicapped in a clinical setting is usually his chief method for discovering new relationships. Although the scientist is not limited to clinical conditions of observation, he, too, is restricted by ethical considerations. He cannot experimentally manipulate pathologic conditions of the speech apparatus (such as clefts in the palate, neurologic defects, laryngeal pathologies) to determine speech effects. He can, however, use any method that will not be harmful to study persons with normal or abnormal speech. Ideally, the method that would yield the most accurate estimate of what causes what would be used.

As with all of science, causal relationships can only be disproved. The possibility always remains that an unknown condition intervenes between suspected cause and observable effect. The sun could be said to rise because the cock crows if high correlations were sufficient. To demonstrate that one thing changes only as the result of another requires experimentation. That a change in one variable is a result of a change in another is more of a certainty if the independent variable can be controlled directly. Assigning sunrise to a cock's crow would be likely only with naturalistic observation. With experimental manipulation of the independent variable (decapitating the cock) we would soon discover that the sun still rises, rooster or no rooster. But experimental control of variables can still fall short. Use of the experimental method does not require (or preclude) that changes in the dependent variable occur in temporal proximity to manipulations of the independent variable. The longer the delay between manipulation and observed effect, the greater the possibility for intrusion of some intervening variable that could account for the changes noted. Requirements for a causal statement—high correlation, direct control of the independent variable, control of relevant variables, and temporal proximity of experimental manipulation and observed effect—are met more consistently by experimental analysis of behavior than by any other method. Yet, the best that can be demonstrated legitimately is not that we can cause behavior but that we can control it. Production of "hard facts" is a grueling endeavor. Speech pathology has done its share of grueling, but it is far from being able to demonstrate conclusively the *causes* of many disorders of speech.

REFERENCES

Bakan, D., *On Method*. San Francisco: Jossey-Bass, Inc., Publishers (1967).

Bloodstein, O., *A Handbook on Stuttering*. Chicago: National Society for Crippled Children and Adults (1975).

Brookshire, R., Speech pathology and the experimental analysis of behavior. *J. Speech Hearing Dis.*, 32, 215-227 (1967).

Bugelski, B., *First Course in Experimental Psychology*. New York: Holt, Rinehart & Winston (1951).

Campbell, N., *Symposium: Measurement and Its Importance for Philosophy*. Aristotelian Society Supplement (Vol. 17). London: Harrison (1938).

Fairbanks, G., *Experimental Phonetics: Selected Articles*. Urbana: University of Illinois Press (1966).

Feynman, R., *The Character of Physical Law*. Cambridge, Mass.: The M.I.T. Press (1965).

Frye, N., Introduction. In Frye, N. (Ed.), *Blake: a Collection of Critical Essays*. Englewood Cliffs, N.J., Prentice-Hall, Inc. (1966).

Goldberg, L., Simple models or simple processes? *Am. Psychol.*, 23, 483-496 (1968).

Goldstein, A., Heller, K., and Sechrest, L., *Psychotherapy and the Psychology of Behavior Change*. New York: John Wiley & Sons, Inc. (1966).

Guilford, J., *Fundamental Statistics in Psychology and Education*. New York: McGraw-Hill Book Co. (1956).

Hanson, N., Galileo's discoveries in dynamics. *Science*, 147, 471-478 (1965).

Hyman, C., . . . Therefore, let us be tolerant of each other's research. *Am. Scient.*, 51, 367A-380A (1963).

Klein, M., Thermodynamics in Einstein's thought. *Science*, 157, 509-516 (1967).

Kruskal, W., Statistics, Molière, and Henry Adams. *Am. Scient.*, 55, 416-428 (1967).

McGuigan, F., *Experimental Psychology: a Methodological Approach*. Englewood Cliffs, N.J., Prentice-Hall, Inc. (1960).

Perkins, W., and Curlee, R., Causality in speech pathology. *J. Speech Hearing Dis.*, 34, 231-238 (1969).

Platt, J., Strong inference. *Science*, 146, 347-353 (1964).

Rosenthal, R., Self-fulfilling prophecy. *Psychology Today*, 2, 46-51 (1968).

Selye, H., *Stress*. Montreal: Acta, Inc. (1950).

Sidman, M., *Tactics of Scientific Research*. New York: Basic Books, Inc. (1960).

Siegel, S., *Nonparametric Statistics for the Behavioral Sciences*. New York: McGraw-Hill Book Co. (1956).

Sperry, R., A modified concept of consciousness. *Psychol. Rev.*, 76, 532-536 (1969).

Stevens, S., Mathematics, measurement, and psychophysics. In Stevens, S. (Ed.), *Handbook of Experimental Psychology*. New York: John Wiley & Sons, Inc. (1951).

Stevens, S., Problems and methods of psychophysics. *Psychol. Bull.*, 55, 177-196 (1958).

Stevens, S., Measurement, statistics, and the schemapiric view. *Science*, 161, 849-856 (1968).

Szent-Györgyi, A., Teaching and the expanding knowledge. *Science*, 146, 1278-1279 (1964).

Underwood, B., *Psychological Research*. New York: Appleton-Century-Crofts (1957).

Von Békésy, G., *Experiments in Hearing*. New York: McGraw-Hill Book Co. (1960).

Waterman, A., Science in the sixties. *Am. Scient.*, 49, 1-8 (1961).

Chapter 3

Processes of speech

Questions

1. What are the linguistic and psychologic dimensions of language processes?
2. What are the behavioral dimensions of speaking processes?

PROCESSES OF SPEECH AS A BODY OF KNOWLEDGE

Several years ago, Gordon Peterson and Grant Fairbanks (1963), two of the field's most distinguished scientists, argued that a clinical profession not anchored in a scientific discipline is unlikely to achieve attractive status. Imagine a physician trained only in techniques of managing a scalpel and dispensing pills who, without knowledge of biology and chemistry, treats children. Such would be the parallel to a speech pathologist armed with inspiration to aid those with communication handicaps and trained in a variety of remedial techniques who, without solid knowledge of speech processes and a reasonable understanding of psychology, human biology, and acoustics, would try to help those who stutter or are cerebral palsied or are aphasic or have a cleft palate.

A profession needs a discipline

All professions borrow from more than a single discipline, yet each is identified with a core discipline. Medicine is built on biology, yet it is supported by chemistry as a strong buttress. Clinical psychology is built on academic psychology, yet physiology is of considerable importance. On what foundation has speech pathology been erected? Some members have veered toward psychology, others toward medicine; some toward engineering, others toward education; some toward linguistics, others toward dentistry. But pulling all these diverging interests toward the same center has been a primary concern for speech. The foundation for speech pathology, as Peterson and Fairbanks maintained, is *speech science,* or as it is now more popularly called, *communication sciences* (a term covering all aspects of communication, including speech).

This conclusion prevails whether one approaches the issue scientifically or clinically. Persons interested in studying processes of speech are of necessity primarily concerned with language formulation and speaking behavior, the subject matter of speech science. Clinically, deviant behavior for which the speech pathologist assumes therapeutic responsibility also involves speaking and linguistic processes. We need not hold that the clinician is concerned exclusively with speech any more than we would hold that a physician should deal exclusively with physical complaints and leave our feelings about it alone. Still, the minimal competence expected of a physician is ability to alleviate somatic distress. Similarly, skill in understanding, identifying, and modifying speech processes is the minimal competence expected of a speech pathologist.

Simplicity belies complexity. Without expert knowledge of linguistic and speaking behavior, the speech pathologist has little to offer not available in larger measure from members of other professions. To gain such knowledge is no small challenge. A complication is the deceptive simplicity of speech. It is so universal, so natural, and so easy for most that we are lulled into looking at it with the dullest tools for knowing reality: casual observation and common sense. Generally, the result is that we look for obvious connections between cause and effect. Yet speech is immensely complex—it is probably the most complicated activity in which humans engage. Those cause-and-effect relationships that seem obvious on the surface most often prove treacherously misleading when pursued in depth.

Without deep understanding of speech processes, the clinician is ill prepared to distinguish between those problems which will yield to relatively simple therapeutic procedures and those which will resist modification for the most complex reasons. Moreover, without solid knowledge the clinician will be hard pressed to evaluate therapeutic effectiveness. How much was he responsible for whatever improvement occurred? Would some who improved have outgrown their problem without help? Why do some who receive therapy not improve? Why do some become worse? These are among the most troublesome questions in speech pathology. The answers must be drawn from widely scattered sources of knowledge. All the answers, though, pivot on speech processes. What does the person with defective speech *do* that must be modified if he is to speak normally?

Explicit speech behavior can be modified. This chapter is about what one does when he speaks. At the simplest practical level, a tenable working assumption for the clinician is that any emitted behavior must be identified specifically if it is to be systematically modified. The crux of the speech clinician's responsibility is his ability to make explicit the defective aspects of speech, and to be equally explicit about the desired communicative behavior to be achieved. In a word, the clinician must be able to specify what a person does to produce defective speech, and what he should do to produce correct speech.

Phonetic and linguistic behavior

The processes of speech have been the focus of mounting interest and inquiry. These processes are being studied by psychologists and linguists, by biologists and physicists, by communications engineers and mathematicians, and, of course, by speech scientists and speech pathologists. What has been learned stems from two quite different research strategies. The output aspect of speech, the speaking process, permits direct observation for *phonetic* studies. The language formulation aspect of speech is covert. Since it cannot be observed directly, *linguistic* studies are necessarily inferential. Language processes in the mind must be deduced from observations of speaking and writing.

A clinical implication. Phonetic behavior has been the traditional focus of corrective techniques. Defective speaking behavior is so obvious that it all but demands therapeutic attention. Not surprisingly, the most successful therapeutic procedures have been designed for the most explicit aspect of speaking behavior: articulation. We have a much clearer image of how *phonemes* (the smallest units of speech) should sound than of any other feature of speaking behavior. This clear phonetic conception provides a target against which articulatory errors can be compared and toward which corrections can be aimed.

In fact, so many articulatory disorders can be readily modified that the clinicians sometimes speak of "simple" articulation problems. Such statements reflect simplistic understanding more than simplicity of the problem. The point here is that any behavior that could be identified as specifically as can articulation of speech sounds would probably be as easy to modify, regardless of how complicated it is in reality. Chances are good that if the defective behavior in voice problems and stuttering (both notoriously difficult to correct) were made as explicit as that of articulation, clinicians might also speak of "simple" voice and stuttering problems.

The possibility of achieving clinically adequate specification of major aspects of speaking behavior is within reach. Specification of language behavior is another matter. Two current views of language are very much in conflict. If the descriptions of structural linguists, learning theorists, and behavioral psychologists are correct, then linguistic behavior can be specified in terms of language units (phonemes, morphemes, and sentences) or of psychologic operations (sentences as conditioning devices). From attempts to teach speech to the mentally retarded, evidence shows that modifications in overt utterances can be made: articulation of phonemes can be improved, and words, phrases, and sentences appropriate to various situations can be acquired. These gains can be substantial and of clinical importance, but they are limited to speech behavior that can be made explicit.

Opposition to this view is led by cognitive psychologists and the modern generative grammarians. With Chomsky as a forceful spokesman, they have mustered powerful arguments against the adequacy of structural or behavioral explanations of language. Basically, their argument is that the essence of any language is the ability to make original statements. Man has the capacity to think and speak ideas never thought or spoken before. They hold that the underlying uniquely human ability to generate innovative statements cannot be explained in behavioral terms. They do not deny that a physical explanation may eventually be possible, but they maintain that whatever it proves to be will be profoundly different from those now used. Let us examine these arguments about language processes more closely.

LANGUAGE PROCESSES
A descriptive view of language

Anything that one would understand with reasonable accuracy must first be observed. Linguists have applied this dictum to language to build the science of *descriptive linguistics*. The unit of speech that they have described as their building block is the *phoneme* (for example, /s/). Although meaningless alone, phonemes are used to construct *morphemes* that are meaningful combinations of sounds from which words are built (for instance, /ræts/ has two morphemes, /ræt/ and /s/; the first means one rodent, the second, plural). Individual words are described *semantically* in terms of their referents. When properly selected and arranged in *syntactic* order to form a sentence, words relate one idea to another.

Implicit in this description of language is the conception of structural relations among these linguistic parts; hence, another name for this view is *structural linguistics*. The structural linguist has taken as his premise that language is a system and that the only observable evidence of how the system functions is seen in what happens to phones. Accordingly, he takes the sounds of a language (*phonology*) as the observable events from which he infers rules of word formation (*morphology*) and word combination (*syntax*). That is, the morphologic and syntactic structure of grammar is erected on the foundation of phonology.

The structural linguist goes about describing a language system in much the same way that a naive spectator would figure out rules of a sporting event. Suppose an Eskimo on his first trip away from the Arctic had ventured for some unknown reason into the Los Angeles Coliseum on a Thursday night in late September, 1957. He would have seen about 50,000 people leaping in and out

of their seats in various states of madness: some gesticulating joyously, some in agony, some screaming "murder the bums." On the field would have been anywhere from ten to thirteen men, all dressed much alike, who for the most part just stood around watching one man throw a ball at another man with a club. Let us say that, puzzled but intrigued, our Eskimo decides to return the next night to try to decipher this strange ritual.

He returns Friday night at the same time to find 50,000 people still performing their same rites of autumnal madness. The only difference is that on the field this night are twenty-two men dressed quite differently from those of the preceding night. More baffling, they line up facing each other about once every minute and then run wildly around the field knocking each other down. Occasionally, one of the men can be seen with an odd-shaped ball.

How can one make sense of this chaos? Were our Eskimo sufficiently observant and persistent, he would eventually have noted that two different games were being played: baseball on Thursday night, football on Friday. Furthermore, the apparently chaotic behavior of players on the field would become orderly as the complicated patterns became apparent. But the structure of these patterns would never be seen directly. The rules of the game could only be inferred by observing behavior of the players.

Phonology: phonetics and phonemics. Just as the difference in the rules of baseball and football can be detected from behavior of the players, so can rules of various languages be detected in the way sounds are used to change meaning. Furthermore, although only players can be observed directly, the positions they play determine their patterns of behavior. Because different players carry out assignments of these different positions differently, an observer would have to record the performance of many players at each position in order to separate each performer's idiosyncrasies from the general assignments. Similarly, only sounds actually spoken (*phones*) can be observed directly and measured physiologically and acoustically. These sounds, like individual players, are unique; they never occur exactly the same way twice. Only those differences that native speakers hear that make a difference in word meaning are of linguistic importance.

Phonetic description. Because a linguist who sets out to describe a language has no prior knowledge of rules of that particular language nor of differences among sounds that make differences in meaning, he must be prepared to record what he hears as accurately as possible. His first requirement is a *phonetic* transcription that takes account of all differences that can be significant in any language. He will put his symbols in brackets to indicate that he is making a *close* or *narrow* transcription of phonetic differences ([s] as in "sit"). As anyone who has attempted to learn to speak a foreign language without an accent knows, differences in sound systems can be subtle. Thus the phonetic transcription should be sufficiently refined to be free of cultural bias.

Originally, the International Phonetic Alphabet (I.P.A.) was intended to be an inventory of all elementary speech sounds used in all languages of the world. Each I.P.A. symbol was to provide a distinct sign for every distinct speech sound and a gross physiologic recipe by which the sound could be produced. As originally created, the I.P.A. has proved to be an insufficient tool for the phonetic transcription task of descriptive linguists. Still, the basic idea of a phonetic system for describing significant sounds and the physiology of their production for any particular language remains valid. The most complete notational system to date provides eighty-six phonetic symbols to represent sounds that can be produced with over one-hundred physiologic adjustments (Peterson and Shoup, 1966b).

Phonemic description. Were most native Americans asked whether the first sound in "hot" is the same as the first in "huge," they would probably agree that it is. Listen to that sound in the two words carefully and observe how the lips are adjusted, however, and you will detect that /h/ looks, feels, and sounds

differently in the two words. Despite these differences, /h/ functions linguistically as a single sound and is heard by native American speakers as the same sound. Of the infinite number of sounds that can be produced and of the multitude of categories that can be transcribed phonetically, most languages use only a few dozen differences among these sounds (American speakers use over forty, as shown in Table 3-1) to make differences in the meaning of words. Groups of sounds that make these differences are called *phonemes,* from the Greek "phon" for sound and "eme" for meaningful unit. Notice that phonemic symbols are shown by slant lines, called *virgules,* to show that broad differences are being transcribed.

Although a phoneme is sometimes said to be a sound family, this metaphor needs a bit of correction, especially if it is to help clarify the differences among phones, phonemes, and phonemic subdivisions called *allophones.* Let us make the phoneme /i/ (as in "se*a*t") analogous to, say, the McTavish clan of Scots. Just as McTavish families belong to the same clan, so do families of /i/ allophones belong to the same phoneme. Clans and families, however, are abstract categories. They actually exist only as they have live members. If one were to study behavioral or biologic characteristics of the McTavish clan, some living McTavishes would have to be available. Similarly, phonemes and their subcategories, allophones, are abstract classifications. They exist and can be studied physically only as they occur as phones.

The correction needed in the "sound family" metaphor is in the basis for membership in a phoneme. Whereas a McTavish belongs to his family and clan by virtue of birth, a phone can be put into its phoneme only by the ear of the listener, not by the mouth of the speaker. A McTavish need not look like a McTavish to be a McTavish, but an /i/ phone must have a distinctive sound of /i/ to the native speaker to be in the /i/ phoneme. The /i/ is not distinctively different from /I/ (as in "sit") for the Japanese, for example, which explains their confusion with words like "meal" and "mill." Thus a phonetic difference, to be a phonemic difference, must make a distinctive difference. Speakers utter only phones; listeners hear only phonemes.

The unit of language. Now we are brought to a fundamental question that will recur to plague us time and again. What is the basic unit of language? Is it a phone? No one has argued explicitly that it is; yet most attempts to improve language proceed on the implicit assumption that a modification of phonetic behavior provides access to language performance. For the moment, let us recognize that the phone is a unit comparable to the player in a baseball or football game, or to a living member of a family; a phone exists (albeit briefly). It is the only aspect of spoken

Table 3-1. Comparative chart of phonetic alphabets*

IPA	Webster's New Collegiate	Webster's New World	American College	NBC Handbook
i	ē	ē	ē	ee
ɪ	ĭ	i	ĭ	i
e	ā	ā	ā	ay
ɛ	ĕ	e	ĕ	ai e
æ	ă	a	ă	a
ɑ	ŏ	ä o	ä	ah
ɔ	ô	ô	ô	aw
o	ō	ō	ō	oh
ʊ	o͞o	oo	o͞o	oo
u	o͞o	o͞o	o͞o	oo:
ʌ	ŭ	u	ŭ	uh
ɝ	ûr	ūr	ûr	er
ə	(italics)	ə	ə	uh
ɚ	ēr	ēr	ər	er
aɪ	ī	ī	ī	igh
ɔɪ	oi	oi	oi	oi
ju	ū	ū	ū	yoo:
aʊ	ou	ou	ou	ow
p	p	p	p	p
t	t	t	t	t
b	b	b	b	b
d	d	d	d	d
k	k	k	k	k
g	g	g	g	g
tʃ	ch tū͝	ch	ch	ch
dʒ	j dū͝	j	j	j
f	f	f	f	f
v	v	v	v	v
θ	th	th	th	th
ð	th	th	th	th:
s	s	s	s	s
z	z	z	z	z
ʃ	sh	sh	sh	sh
ʒ	zh	zh	zh	zh
h	h	h	h	h
m	m	m	m	m
n	n	n	n	n
ŋ	ng	ŋ	ng	ng
l	l	l	l	l
w	w	w	w	w
hw	hw	hw	hw	hw
j	y	y	y	y
r	r	r	r	r

*From Carrell, J., and Tiffany, W., *Phonetics: Theory and Application to Speech Improvement*, New York: McGraw-Hill Book Co. (1960). Used with permission of McGraw-Hill Book Co.

language that can be directly observed. Hence, it is the aspect most available for alteration and improvement through learning.

The descriptive linguist, however, has built his linguistic structure with phonemic, not phonetic, units. These units are comparable to families and clans, not to people; to game positions, not to individual players. Phonemic units reveal functional relationships in the language system. They are governed by rules of language. Knowing this the linguist, proceeding inductively, reasons that if he observes phonemic patterns, he will be able to infer morphemic, syntactic, and semantic rules of the language he is describing.

Language communicates discriminative relations. The purpose of language, of course, is to communicate information about how one thing is related to another. Add to this the precept of science that if a thing exists, it exists in some amount. Taken together, language can be seen as a system by which we can compare how much of one thing is related to how much of another. The essence of this comparison is a discrimination, and, as Guilford (1967) maintains, discriminations comprise the information that is processed in intellectual functions (Chapter 9).

Most languages are designed to show certain *indispensable relations.* Sentences must be able to show who or what is acting on whom or what; this is the subject-object relation. Too, every language must be able to show how a thing has attributes, which is done in English by the noun-adjective relation. In addition, there are a variety of *dispensable relations* that can be shown, but need not be. Time, for example, is a relation built into the tense of verbs used in English and in most other western languages. In Chinese, however, it is dispensable; time of an action cannot be *signaled* by a feature of the verb system. A Chinese speaker who wishes to make a statement about time must select an appropriate word equivalent to "today," "noon," or "8:37 P.M." Another relation signaled by most western languages that is dispensable in Chinese is number. This is the idea of plural or singular, which we specify with the form of most nouns and pronouns. English, however, has its dispensable relationships that can be signaled by other languages. A Cree Indian, for instance, can use his language to signal that the listener is either included or excluded in the Cree version of the word "our."

Signaling devices for relations. Indispensable relationships are signaled in practically all languages by word order. Take this sentence as an illustration: "Wolves pursued a black sheep." Who is doing what to whom (the basic subject-object relation) is specified by word order that places "wolves" ahead of "sheep." Turn that order around and the resulting sentence would be as newsworthy as "Man bites dog." The other indispensable noun-adjective relation is signaled by the position of "black" before "sheep." Placed before "wolves" it would assign the attribute of blackness to these animals.

Dispensable relations found only in some languages can be signaled in any of three ways: by *word order,* by *inflectional endings,* and by *structure words.* The preceding wolves-pursued-sheep sentence contains examples of the latter two. "Wolves," an inflected form of "wolf," denotes more than one. By contrast, "sheep" does not have an inflected form to distinguish number, so the structure word "a" in "a black sheep" signals that several wolves were ganging up on only one black sheep. Finally, the inflected "ed" ending of "pursued" tells us that this deed is past history.

Grammar and its functions. Often, when one with little knowledge of language sets out to learn a new one—for example, French—his initial search is for vocabulary equivalents of familiar English words. He will soon discover that a sizable supply of French words have been transplanted intact into English. Though key words in the following sentence, "The beige cigarettes are in the garage," are lifted directly from French, still the statement bears no resemblance to French. Why? Because English and French language systems are different. This is equivalent to saying that the grammars are different. Grammar can be defined as the system in a language by which meanings are changed and relationships are signaled. These functions

---

Does Gleason (1961) agree with Allen and his associates (1966) that phonology should be included as a part of grammar?

---

are accomplished at three levels of grammatical structure: phonemic, morphemic, and syntactic.

Segmental phonemes. Though many languages use almost the same sounds, these languages differ widely in ways in which these sounds are organized to make words. Even regional dialects of the same language can vary considerably in sound systems used to represent the same words. It is difficult to know, for instance, whether a native of East Texas has said, "I'm concerned about Texas" or "I'm concerned about taxes."

The major method used by all languages to change meaning is with segmental phonemes, which is merely a technical way of specifying speech sounds. Remember that phonemes are categories into which phones of speech are sorted as sounds flow from the speaker. Phonemic categories, then, are segments in the continuum of speech. The manner in which phonemic segments are combined is the primary means of building words. Systematically changing segments one at a time in a word such as "let" (/lɛt/) yields results such as "net" (/nɛt/), "lit" (/lɪt/), and "led" (/lɛd/). American speakers typically use about forty-five phonemic segments in lawful combinations to produce the half million words of English.

Suprasegmental phonemes. A moment's reflection on how you shift meaning in everyday speech will reveal use of more than phonemic segments. Sometimes you do it with stress: "*pre*sent" (/'prɛzənt/) is what you receive, whereas "pre*sent*" (/prɪ'zɛnt/) is what you do. Or stress may change meaning in less obvious but equally important ways. If someone said, "She's a German teacher," stress on "German" or on "teacher" would help you determine whether she is German by birth and teaches or whether the subject

she teaches is German. Frequently, you signal by pitch whether you mean to ask a question, make a statement, or express uncertainty, as in "yes" spoken with a rising reflection, a falling inflection, or a rising and falling inflection. Too, when pitch is used in *terminal juncture,* a technique of pauses and inflections used by speakers to end phrases, intent is made clear whether more is to be said (by use of level pitch at the phrase end), or, if the idea is complete, whether it is a statement or a question. Finally, you use *internal juncture* to put "joints" between words in ways that control meaning. The following example is resurrected from childhood memory. One morning at breakfast, my aunt, aghast at how my uncle was shoveling eggs into his mouth, admonished him: "You'll have eggs past your eyes." Without missing a stroke, and with a slight alteration in internal juncture, my uncle echoed her with: "Pasteurized eggs. Hmmm."

As you can see, because stress, pitch, and juncture are all effective techniques for changing meaning, some linguists consider them just as phonemic as sound segments. Unlike segmental phonemes, however, stress, pitch, and juncture extend over segments. Hence, when they make distinctive differences they are called *suprasegmental phonemes.*

Units of meaning: morphemes. We have seen that a primary function of grammar is to signal relationships. We also saw that dispensable relationships that occur in English, such as time and number, are often signaled by inflection (meaning to vary or bend a word). The grammatical level at which inflections are accomplished is that of the *morpheme.* Composed of any combination

---

Gleason (1961) devotes five chapters to morphemes. Why are they so complex?

---

of phonemes, a morpheme is the smallest unit of language that *has* meaning, whereas the phoneme, which may be meaningless alone, is the basic unit in linguistics for *changing* meaning.

You may have discerned that we have

suprasegmental phonemes
stress, pitch, juncture

been alluding to two types of meaning, lexical and grammatical. _Lexical meaning_ is found in the dictionary: the root meaning of vocabulary words. The words themselves are constructed of morphemes. In _free form,_ morphemes are identical to words: "pin," "come," "go." In _bound form,_ morphemes cannot stand alone: "ren" in "children," "un" in "unsung." Unlike lexical meaning, which is concerned with the relation between symbol and referent, _grammatical meaning_ (also called _structural meaning_) has to do with relations among ideas, the types of relations already discussed. Thus every statement has both lexical and grammatical meaning. Each word within the utterance "German a teacher she's" has lexical meaning, but the utterance violates structural rules for showing relations meaningfully. Put the words in grammatical order, but pronounce each one backward, "Seh's a Namreg rehcaet," and the result would have structural meaning were the words not lexical nonsense.

Units of complete ideas: sentences. The issue of structural meaning brings us to the highest level of grammar: syntax. This is the level at which word order is used to signal all indispensable and some dispensable relations. The basic unit for signaling those relations necessary to express a complete idea is the _sentence._

Though infinitely varied, basic patterns of subject-predicate sentences are few. Only the predicate determines the pattern. The subject can remain the same, as you can see in Table 3-2. The simplest possible sentence, Pattern I, can be two words, but the predicate must be a verb that can stand alone and imply the object of action, if any. In other patterns, the verb must be complemented with at least one additional word to complete the idea of what is predicated for the subject. The complement to the verb in Pattern II specifies, rather than implies, the object of what is predicated (this is the indispensable relation shown by both Patterns I and II). In the remaining patterns, an attribute of the subject (the other indispensable relation) is predicated by a complementary noun (Pattern III), adjective (Pattern IV), or adverb (Pattern V).

Although the simplicity of these patterns is generally obscured in the convolutions of everyday speech, we still intuitively use these patterns to test the completeness of most sentences. Any can be transformed into incredibly complicated statements, but if, after elaborate transformations have been peeled away, the skeleton of one of the five fundamental patterns is not laid bare, we would know that the sentence is incomplete. As an example: "Warriors of old, tillers of the soil, conquerors of frontiers, defenders of the faith, men, who with brawn and brain have bent nature to human purpose, are in such short supply as to be desperately needed." Shorn of transformations, those thirty-six words translate into our three-word Pattern V sentence: "Men are needed." What transformations add to the basic pattern is information about relationships (dispensable and indispensable) over and above the primary relation between subject and predicate (Allen and others, 1966).

**Words and meaning.** Language is but one tool for communicating that elusive, intangible something that we devote our lives to pursuing and that conveys our intent: _meaning._ Philosophers study the meaning of meaning. Psychologists study the processes that make meanings meaningful. Linguists study the formal system for transmitting meaning. Speech pathologists repair the system when it does not work properly. Yet meaning is not the exclusive property of language. Nonverbal modes of communication can weigh so heavily that we even have the folk-expression, "Actions speak louder than words."

A language system is embedded in the

Table 3-2. Basic subject-predicate sentence patterns

Pattern	Subject	Predicate	
I	Men	eat.	
II	Men	like	women.
III	Men	are	leaders.
IV	Men	are	tough.
V	Men	are	needed.

context of its culture. To communicate effectively one must estimate from his listener's background, the nature of the speaking situation, and myriad other contextual conditions how much meaning is needed and how much can be absorbed when transmitted formally in language. We have looked at the grammar system used for communicating structural meaning of relations among ideas and have seen that it operates lawfully. Now we will look at the semantic basis for communicating lexical meaning of the relation between the word and its referent.

Symbols and signs. To say that something has meaning is to say that it has significance beyond itself. To say that a man's life has meaning implies that he has produced some effect on the world independent of his existence, an effect that will survive after he is gone. Extend this logic to any communication system and you can see why its essential commodity is meaning. Things used to refer to something else are trivial in themselves; their worth is in what they mean. Sounds, gestures, markings, and other such events as used for communication are of little consequence taken alone. When they stand for something else, however, they can assume significance of towering proportions, as in Einstein's formula: $e = mc^2$. The relation between term and referent gets at the nature of meaning.

Not all systems of communication are systems of language. Animals have elaborate schemes for transmitting information, but does this mean that all animals use language (Von Frisch, 1950; Wenner, Wells, and Johnson, 1969; Smith, 1969)? Not in the human sense, and one basic difference lies in

---

Dolphins, chimpanzees, and even honeybees are suspected of having linguistic ability. Does the work of Lilly (1962), Premack (1970), and Gould (1975) support this suspicion?

---

the distinction that Langer (1951) makes between *symbol* and *sign*.

The meaning of signs, according to Langer, is simple, direct, and universal. A sign and its object stand in a one-to-one relation; they form a pair. A sign signifies something —past, present, or future. Natural signs are symptomatic of a state of affairs: puddles signify that it has rained, patters on the roof that it is raining, and lightning that it is going to rain. Sounds and gestures are signs that animals usually employ for signification: dogs have "let-me-out" barks, "chase-the-cat" barks, "time-for-a-walk" tail waggings, and "save-me-from-thunder-and-lightning" slinking postures. The communication system of young children, prior to language acquisition, relies exclusively on signs: children cry, yell, scream, and point to obtain what they want. Even adults in emergencies revert to sign systems: pointing, waving, yelling to get the message across quickly. Thus, communication by signification must have present the subject who uses the sign, the signal itself, and the object signified.

Symbols function entirely differently. If someone shouts "Duck!" the word operates as a sign at which one immediately pulls in his head and then peers around for the source of danger. The object of a sign is always close at hand. Were that same word, "duck," to be mentioned casually in conversation, no one would be likely to ask, "Where?" The word "duck," used as a symbol, does not signal the presence of the object but serves as a vehicle for the conception of a class of objects that waddle and quack. As signs announce their objects, symbols announce conceptions that can exist independent of their referents.

Denotation and connotation. What do words used as symbols mean? The portion of their meaning commonly accepted in the culture is found in a dictionary definition. Again following Langer, where three terms are needed for signification (subject, sign, and object), four are needed for symbolization: subject, symbol, conception, and object. What a symbol *denotes* is the relation to its object as defined in a dictionary: "spinach" is an "annual potherb with edible leaves used as greens." What it *connotes* is the conception it holds for the subject who hears it, thinks it, or speaks it: what "spinach" connotes for children is "yuk!" Thus the words we speak can serve several functions. They can be used as signs to signal meaning. For this purpose, signaling devices of grammar are irrelevant. More typically, words are used symbolically in language to denote the objective meaning of the referent and to connote the subjective meaning of the concept. The meaning of "meaning" can be signification, denotation, or connotation. All are legitimate meanings, but they are not interchangeable.

A psychologic view of language

Near the midpoint of this century, after a Social Science Research Council seminar on language, psychology discovered descriptive linguistics. They courted, soon joined in a new research venture dubbed "psycholinguistics," and together have been expanding vigorously ever since (Saporta, 1961). For their part, psychologists found a "new" science that had long been working diligently to erect a body of empirical knowledge about the very subject on which psychology was weakest: language behavior. With the various models of learning and perception available, the possibility of teaching animals to talk seemed within reach. Why they could not be taught to talk and how children acquire speech perplexed psychologists. Linguistic research offered new light on such puzzles.

To the extent that the partners in this psycholinguistic endeavor are still discernibly different, descriptive linguists have attended to erection of a formal structure of language. They have observed and described language, but they have not explained in any psychologic or biologic sense why it occurs as it does. Psychologists, on the other hand, have attended to *functions* of a formal language system in human communication. They have attempted to explain the determining behavioral and biologic conditions of language. Where linguists have been concerned with "what," psychologists have been concerned with "why." Those interested in learning theory have, for the most part, focused on how word meaning is acquired, with some attention given to the psychologic function of sentences. Those interested in experimental analysis of behavior have attempted to demonstrate how the functional properties of a language system are controlled. Dominating the scene recently are those interested in cognitive processes. They have no precise answers as to how grammatical meaning is learned but some very disturbing doubts about the adequacy of anyone else's answer.

The psychologist's view of language is of special value to the speech pathologist because it is a view of how information is processed and of how behavior is acquired and modified—all being the substance of the speech pathologist's applied concerns. When language functioning is defective, linguistic theory provides the structure by which we can find the parts needing correction. Is the problem one of limited vocabulary that restricts the person handicapped in lexical meaning, or is it one of grammatical inability to handle structural meaning? This linguistic information is essential, but without psychologic explanations of how the language processes operate and how they can be altered by learning, the speech pathologist's rehabilitation efforts falter.

A psychologic view of word meaning: semantic processes. Though concepts connoted by words are unique to each speaker and listener, still, words denote features that exist demonstrably in the real world. This arrangement permits one to hold private views in his concepts, and yet use denotational meaning to transmit information to others about the reality in which they live. If words had no referents by which they could be defined, we could not use symbols to share and preserve knowledge. Lexical meaning is obviously essential to interpersonal communication.

What is not so obvious is the value of symbols for *intra*personal communication, for remembering and thinking. In the most thoroughgoing form of *linguistic relativity* proposed by Whorf (1956), a speaker's language determines in large measure his view of the world. In Whorf's hypothesis, not the empirical conditions themselves but the language used to symbolize reality shapes how one thinks. Though this view is probably extreme, evidence does indicate that one can remember best those details of the world for which he has words.

Brown and Lenneberg (1954) demonstrated this in an elegantly simple experiment. They collected a set of twenty-four color samples that a group of people had named. Some colors were easily identified with the same name by everyone. Others were ambiguous. When these twenty-four colors were presented to experimental subjects who were asked to select immediately a matching sample, the selections were as accurate for easily named colors as for ambiguous ones. When the subjects were delayed for some time in selecting a matching color, however, their accuracy was much better for those colors easily named than for those which were ambiguous.

What do such results suggest? They suggest that we can remember physical details of our environment only briefly, and that we preserve our memory of color, at least, more easily with words. This conception implies that ability to discriminate is facilitated by having an abundance of words that denote shades of difference in their referents. Thus we should find many words for important objects and conditions, and few for those which are trivial. It is perhaps for this reason that Eskimos have at least eleven words for snow, whereas we have only a few (Krauss, 1968).

Acquisition of meaning. Words may not be the only means, but they are certainly the major means by which, holding the world symbolically in our heads, we can solve problems abstractly without having to confront the real world concretely. How do words acquire meaning? Because words function in a language system primarily as symbols, and seldom as signs (following Langer's distinction), we can focus on how they acquire denotative and connotative meaning. For denotation, focus is on acquisition of connections between symbol and referent; for connotation, on connections between symbol and concept. Furthermore, in the psychologic analysis that follows, we must distinguish between learning the meaning of words

as listeners and learning the use of words as speakers.

Psychologists have been vigorously concerned with verbal learning for nearly two decades. Attempts by learning theorists and especially by behaviorists to explain language have, however, been criticized severely by the linguists and cognitive psychologists identified as psycholinguists. Staats (1968) has shown, though, that this criticism should not tar all learning approaches to language with the same brush. He maintains that previous attempts to explain how complex language behavior is learned have been open to criticism because they are incomplete and have oversimplified the problem. He argues, for example, that too few learning principles have been used. Skinner (1957) relied on an operant analysis of verbal behavior. Osgood (1953, 1957) used instrumental conditioning, mainly of connotative word meaning as measured by his *semantic differential* scale. Mowrer (1954) relied on higher-order classical conditioning to explain transfer of meaning from word to word within the sentence. It is not that these theorists were wrong, but that they tried to explain too much with too few principles.

Staats maintains that a pluralistic conception of word meaning is needed. To explain meaning in listening and speaking and in denotation and connotation, for instance, requires more than just *classical conditioning* or just *instrumental conditioning*. (In classical conditioning, the connection between a response and its stimulus is reinforced by virtue of stimulus and response [S-R] occurring together; in instrumental conditioning, the connection between a response and the stimulus conditions preceding it is strengthened by virtue of the reinforcing consequences that follow the response.) The difference between these two learning principles is vital to an understanding of the learning of speech.

Thus instrumental conditioning (also called *operant conditioning*) can explain acquisition of verbal behavior that produces consequences. Words such as "the," "of," and "an" have only grammatical meaning; they function as structural signaling devices. They occur only in conjunction with words having lexical meanings, such as nouns and adjectives. We pay little attention to structure words and inflectional endings except as grammatical signaling devices. Since structure words produce consequences in altering the meaning of a sentence, their acquisition can be explained reasonably by instrumental conditioning. They are learned when the child's language development reaches the stage of complexity at which he must resort to using structure words and inflectional endings to make clear discriminations in ideas he is trying to express.

Instrumental conditioning may also be pivotal to sharpening socially useful denotational referents of lexical meaning. Because all objects have many names by which they can be described, Krauss (1968) became interested in how children learn to select names that will communicate their meanings successfully. He and his colleagues devised a block-stacking task in which blocks of unusual shape would be difficult to describe verbally. The task was for two people with identical blocks, who could hear but not see each other, to build their stacks in the same order—a neat little communicative microcosm. The task was trivial for adults, even dull-normal adults with meager education. For children it was difficult, especially for preschool children, regardless of how alert and clever they were. The difference in difficulty proved not to be difference in vocabulary or grammatical ability, but difference in what Sullivan (1953) called *consensual validation,* that is, consensus with others about the meaning of a word. For example, my son at a tender age called scrambled eggs "shragments." When we finally deciphered his private code, it was quite sensible. The egg scrapings looked like a combination of shreds and fragments. Although "shragments" is now consensually validated within our family, outsiders find it of little communicative value. Ability to select meanings that can be received on listeners' wavelengths is clearly a product of social learning by instrumental conditioning.

But how can we explain connotative meaning in which the connection learned is between symbol and concept? Or how can we explain the child's earliest understanding of speech months before he utters his first meaningful word? Or how can we explain the sensory imagery and emotional loads that many lexical words carry? These examples do not appear to be the result of instrumental conditioning; no response is clearly evident that produces a reinforcing consequence. Instead, they seem to be the result of learning by classical conditioning: "ball" is learned in the presence of a ball, "mother" in relation to mother. Sensory and emotional events that accompany the word are learned in connection with the word. Initially, then, classical conditioning is probably responsible for the child's earliest denotative and connotative meanings.

The sentence as a conditioning device. Some years ago, Mowrer (1954) planted a germinal idea that is still awaiting full bloom. He suggested that what the sentence does is to transfer meaning from the predicate to the subject by the principle of classical conditioning. He points out that this type of transfer can be accomplished at four levels. The two lowest levels, *thing-thing* "sentences" and *thing-sign* "sentences," are the ones at which most animals communicate. At the thing-thing level, a dog (subject) scratches the door (predicate) to get out; a mother slaps her son's hand after it has been in the cookie jar. At the thing-sign level, similar conditioning can be accomplished if the dog barks at the door instead of scratching it, or if the mother, catching her son in the act, scolds instead of slapping him. Note that at both levels the subject of the sentence is physically present as a *thing.* Thus, following Langer's distinction, the predicate *sign* operates as a signal rather than as a symbol. Most animals do not progress beyond this level because they apparently do not master the "noun-idea" essential to abstract speech.

At the next highest level, the *sign-thing* "sentence," the mother, discovering the cookie scandal after the fact, calls her son in, tells him what she knows he did (sign), and then spanks him (thing). At the highest level of the true sentence, the *sign-sign* level, the mother might say, "Herkimer, don't let me catch you in the cookie jar again." The signs for both subject and predicate both serve as symbols.

All four levels function as conditioning arrangements, but at the highest levels, where signs serve as symbols, Mowrer posits a *mediating response* (roughly analogous to Langer's "concept") that stands between symbol and referent. Transfer of meaning is from one mediating response to another; a change in mediating response changes the meaning not only of the symbol but also of the referent. Elaborating on Mowrer's sample sentence, "Tom is a thief," if Tom were mayor of the community and the statement were made by the chief of police, the name "Tom" would lose some luster, and the person, Tom, would probably lose more than that. The predicate idea of "thief" would "rub off" on the mediating response for "Tom."

Mowrer's proposal that sentences transfer meaning from one lexical symbol to another has lain dormant, possibly because soon after it was presented, psycholinguists launched a wholesale attack on behavioral explanations of language. Staats (1968) is among those who have recently sought to salvage learning theory from the shambles left by the assault of linguists and cognitive psychologists. By using classical as well as instrumental conditioning principles, he demonstrates that many of the salvos fired at learning theory explanations could have been avoided. Furthermore, by recognizing that words have reinforcing value, he has shown that by talking to oneself, an individual's own verbal behavior can shape his conception of a situation as forcefully as would external events. Such self-determination of action would give the appearance of spontaneity and freedom of choice, but in point of fact it would reflect transfer of meaning in the mind by conditioning of one mediating response under the influence of other mediating responses.

Information and redundancy. Were the

police chief to have spoken Mowrer's sentence, "Tom is a thief," with a twinkle in his eye, and if he had said it at the Policemen's Ball, to which Tom had been invited as master of ceremonies, the conditioning effects would probably have been negated. Information in the sentence would have been cancelled by information from the social context and from the nonverbal communication of a twinkling eye. Meaning must somehow hinge on information.

What is information? *Communication theory*, in vogue now for over two decades, has provided a mathematical definition that makes measurement possible. Information is defined mathematically as a measure of freedom of choice in selection of a message. Although this concept may ultimately prove to be of immense value to the measure of information in the everyday sense of "meaning," it was not designed to meet this need at all. It was developed by scientists at Bell Telephone Laboratories and elsewhere to

---

Why do Shannon and Weaver (1964) caution against confusing "information" as defined in communication theory with "meaning"?

---

give communication engineers a method by which they could measure the amount of information in signals to be transmitted and the capacity of telephone and telegraph circuits to carry these signals (Cherry, 1957).

Shannon and Weaver (1964) were responsible for seeing the fundamental parallel between information and the concept of *entropy*—the second law of thermodynamics —that has been said to hold "the supreme position among the laws of Nature." Entropy is the tendency of all matter to become less and less organized, to become randomly arranged, to become "shuffled." To overcome this entropic tendency, energy must be expended to organize matter into structured forms. It is this tendency that defeats perpetual motion, that gives time its arrow that flies only forward, that makes return to dust with death the inevitable end of life when energy to rebuild is depleted. And it is the measure of entropic randomness that equals the measure of information as used in communication theory (Shannon and Weaver, 1964).

Measurable information has to do with structure versus randomness, with the predictable versus the unpredictable, with redundancy versus novelty. If you were to start reciting the alphabet or a nursery rhyme to an adult, you would hardly get to "A, B, C" or past "Mary had a little . . ." before anything else said would be so predictable as to be completely redundant. The structure of the alphabet and the syntax of nursery rhymes makes them high in redundancy and low in entropy. The *unit of information* that strikes a balance between these polar opposites can be loosely defined in nonmathematical terms as the amount of freedom of choice between two equally probable events.

This unit, called a *bit* (short for *bi*nary di*git*), gives engineers a precise measure by which they can calculate communication channel capacity, and from which some intriguing comparisons become apparent. For example, man, the supreme communicator, has puny communication channel capacity, at least as far as output is concerned. Even when speaking rapidly he produces only about fifty bits per second, at which rate, if he spent a 60-year lifetime talking, he would yield about 60 billion bits. A television channel, operating at 4 billion bits per second, could transmit this lifetime of information in about 15 seconds. Worse yet, if a man performed at his usual rate of about 15 bits per second, his life's output could be transmitted via television in 5 seconds.

How can man be such an effective communicator, and yet be so limited in channel capacity? The answer lies in our fantastic ability to load the symbols we transmit with abstract meaning (Miller, 1956). Words identify categories, not individual instances: "man" refers to all men, not an individual man. Ironically, far more words are needed to describe a specific object than to describe a class of objects. By being able to say, for instance, "Man uses speech," we transmit relatively few speech signals through our output channels; yet from that message our

listener can infer linguistic ability for all men. The same inference could be reached by obtaining a census of all persons in the world and reading from it the names of those who use speech. After filling the oral output channels of several generations of readers with endless redundancy, as much would be known about man's linguistic ability as is contained in the three-word sentence, "Man uses speech."

Actually, we encode messages so efficiently (to make maximum use of what little channel capacity we have) that we use only a small fraction of our total capacity for transmitting the entropic, unpredictable, novel portions of speech. A much larger proportion of channel capacity is devoted to transmitting redundancy. Why waste space on redundancy? Because without it, the probability of receiving the message is low. Redundancy provides a safety factor for message reception. If you have ever tried to decipher a telephone conversation carried on with a bad connection, you know the difficulty of understanding the words being spoken. If you did not know the structure, rules, and probabilities of language, you probably could never sort out the speech signals from the noise.

What is learned with speech are techniques for increasing redundancy, for ensuring that messages will be received as spoken. Since you know the sounds of speech, coughing and sneezing sounds, as an example, can be ignored as irrelevant to linguistic meaning. Since you know the statistical probability of speech sound combinations intuitively, you are able to catch any part of syllables such as "ing" or "tion," and the whole syllable is grasped, but "tzfbrw" never occurs and has no linguistic importance.

Similarly, you know that some morphemes occur frequently, whereas others that could occur never do so at all. Too, morphemes occur only in certain sequences, to say nothing of the syntactic restrictions that dictate which word sequences are sentences and which are not. "Was from pad a blast-off Apollo's launch Cape Kennedy" is unpredictable grammatical gibberish. When rearranged according to linguistic rules, it becomes "Apollo's blast-off was from a Cape Kennedy launch pad," a prosaic, normally redundant sentence for anyone of our generation. Had this sentence been spoken a century ago, it would have still been grammatically predictable, but being semantic nonsense in that era, it would have been far less redundant than it would be today. Not only linguistic, social, and cultural contexts contribute to one's expectation of what is likely to be said; so also do nonlinguistic signals. If one were trying to overhear what a leering lad was saying to an indignant lass, one would not expect to hear: "The square of the hypotenuse is equal to the sum of the squares on the other two sides."

What does information as used in communication theory have to do with word meaning and its acquisition? Nothing explicitly, yet much implicitly. Remember that what has been worked out mathematically for communication engineers is a measure of freedom of choice in selection of signals for a message; it matters not at all whether the message is meaningful, utter nonsense, or a mere string of sounds. What has not been worked out for psycholinguists is a similar system for quantifying information in the sense of meaning. Still, intuitively one sees a basic relation between meaning and the unpredictable, the novel, the entropic portion of the content of a message (Gleason, 1961; Shannon and Weaver, 1964).

Ideas that seem meaningful strike a balance between redundancy and novelty. Clichés are trite and dull because they are so predictable. They are hackneyed perceptions of life that have become so obvious that as Lionel Trilling said: "They seem to close for us the possibility of thought and imagination." Conversely, abstruse statements are so freighted with incomprehensible information that the idea is largely unpredictable, and hence meaningless. Not only do concepts of redundancy and novelty appear applicable to linguistic meaning, but they seem relevant to information used in the sense of discriminations for intellectual functioning and learning. For discriminations to be learned, they must have some novelty, but not so much as

to make them unpredictable and therefore indiscriminable.

A cognitive view of structural meaning: grammatical processes. The general nature of the battle lines of psycholinguists' attacks on behavioristic explanations of language are drawn along some profound philosophic issues that go to the heart of scientific understanding of reality. Chomsky (1968) sees in the structure of language endless complexities stretching to infinity, possibly touching ultimate reality, which science admittedly is unequipped to handle. Language makes infinite use of finite means. It is creative and innovative; with a few dozen sounds, it permits endless statements never heard or thought before. The question is whether science with its current concepts, indeed, whether science itself, is adequate to explain as profound a phenomenon as language.

Chomsky traces modern postulates of science, from which behavioral explanations are drawn, back to the fundamental separation of newtonian empiricism from cartesian philosophy. Descartes (whose deductive method of science more nearly approximates the procedures of the advanced physical sciences today than does the inductive system of Francis Bacon, who is considered the father of the experimental method) argued that mind, particularly thought and language, cannot be explained in physical terms. Accordingly, Descartes concluded on logical grounds that the substance of mind, the essence of which is thought, must exist alongside body, the essence of which is behavior. Reflecting his position in his famous dictum, "Cogito ergo sum"—I think, therefore I am—Descartes forecast twentieth-century computer technology. He argued that the only convincing evidence that a body (other than one's own) possesses a human mind and is not merely a cleverly contrived automaton is its ability to use language normally.

Ironically, newtonian physics, from which the assumptions of behavioral psychology descend, was spawned in an assumption about gravity that troubled Newton almost as much as it did the cartesian philosophers. Newton could not accept Descartes' mechanical explanation of gravity as adequate, but the alternative was a mystical postulate that gravity is a force acting at a distance. Newton's notion that all matter was endowed with such an occult force was as jarring to common sense as was Descartes' postulate that mind is separate from body. With the prestige of mathematical physics and the predictive success of the gravitational hypothesis, objections to the occult nature of gravity waned. The mystical force of gravity became an integral part of scientific "common sense." Mind, on the other hand, has remained mystical and unacceptable to the "hardnosed" empiricism of behavioral scientists.

Just as Newton was forced to reject a mechanical explanation of gravity, so are humanistic psychologists (Robb, 1969) and psycholinguists questioning the adequacy of behavioral explanations of the nature of man, especially as revealed by his ability to think and use language. Royce (1964) holds that it would take egotistic gall to believe that man can ultimately describe reality with his newly developed tools of science. The universe is estimated at 6 billion years of age, our sun at 5 billion, the earth at 4 billion, life at 2 billion to 3 billion, man at little more than 1 million, and recorded history at 5,000 to 6,000 years of age. From the earliest records around 4,000 B.C. to about 500 A.D., man's conception of the universe was formulated as mythology. Then through the influence of such prophets and thinkers as Confucius in China, Buddha in India, Zarathustra in Persia, Moses in Palestine, and Homer and Plato in Greece, the spiritual outlook of the ptolemaic view (that the world is the center of creation) held sway until the Renaissance. With the advent of the copernican view in the fifteenth century of the earth as a satellite of the sun, man's conception of himself has shrunk and science has prevailed. Seen in historical perspective, one can find little evidence that science will not eventually be supplanted by better ways of knowing about reality.

The fact that Chomsky and psycholinguists of his outlook have demonstrated the apparent inadequacy of behavioral explanations of language in no way demonstrates that a better answer has been offered. So far, they have done a more effective job of posing the problem than of providing the solution (Staats, 1968). Whether that solution will fit within the framework of science remains to be seen. Unless a mystical concept such as "mind" can be demonstrated to have predictive power similar to Newton's concept of "gravitational force," it probably will not survive inside or outside the framework of science.

The speech pathologist cannot dodge these philosophic issues. They set the perimeter for the amount of help that can be offered to persons whose language is impaired. To proceed blindly on the assumption that one has the therapeutic tools to habilitate or rehabilitate language, when, in point of fact, we do not even know the dimensions of the problem, would be of service to no one. Of all the disorders of speech, those of language must be confronted with the greatest uncertainty—and hence the greatest humility.

Chomsky's (1968) advice is to describe language and thought as accurately as possible, develop the best theoretic account possible of the mental apparatus for linguistic organization and function, and not attempt at present to relate hypothetic mental structures to physiologic processes. He does not deny that physical bases for cognitive processes of language may be found, but he cautions that if they are discovered, they may bear little resemblance to physical processes with which we are currently familiar. This advice is reminiscent of Robb's (1969) caution that we not confuse correlation with identity. The fact that bodily functions may be cor-

---

Would Perkins and Curlee (1969) maintain that the cause of language and its disorders can never be properly attributed to physiologic processes? Why?

---

related with mental functions can never be taken as proof that they are identical, that mind is "nothing but" an aggregation of bio-logic processes. Imperfect as psycholinguistic explanations may be, they nonetheless comprise challenging concepts that we will now examine.

Universal grammar. How can a polyglot (one having facility in many languages) express essentially the same idea in any of them? How can a translator, say at the United Nations, listen to a speech in one language and, with little distortion of meaning, speak it in another? At the root of a psycholinguistic conception of language is recognition of the fundamental similarity of all languages. No human language exists that does not provide a formal grammatical structure for systematically relating a subject idea to a predicate idea. Languages vary widely, of course, in how they organize this relation. As an example, Japanese and English go about it in an almost exactly opposite manner: "Miyazaki of airport at stepped down when exceedingly of sunshine at be (was) amazed" is a literal translation of a Japanese comment. When the same subject-predicate idea is arranged in normal English, it would be expressed: "I was amazed at the intensity of the sunshine when I stepped down at Miyazaka Airport" (Kolers, 1969). Generative grammarians maintain that as much as particular grammars may vary, they are only cultural instances of an underlying universal grammar with which all humans are endowed.

Although the notion of universal grammar is not universally accepted, the observations on which it is based demand explanation. All normal children in a normal environment will manage to learn the rules of a "perfect" grammar in about 2 years. Since they will rarely hear "perfect" grammar spoken, conceivably the possible grammars that they could learn are endless. Yet they learn only the natural language that they hear spoken.

These observations are not disputed. Disputes arise over explanations of the observations. Cognitive theorists maintain that if humans were not born with a "knowledge" of universal grammar, with an innate biologic

capacity to learn the structure of a particular language, they would never be able to focus on necessary linguistic discriminations that behavioral theorists explain with learning principles. The cognitive view is that particular grammars develop from a universal human capacity for language, a capacity that has to do with general properties of human intelligence, a capacity that presumably sets man apart from lower animals.

Deep structure versus surface structure. Although universal grammar is fraught with profound philosophic issues, abilities required for a particular grammar are of practical concern to the speech pathologist. Once a particular language is learned, how is it that we can transform thoughts into a stream of meaningful sounds and conversely, acquire meaning when we listen to speech? Knowledge of a language, *linguistic competence*, involves knowledge of rules that relate sound and meaning in a particular way. Observe yourself briefly to see how you go about formulating a spoken statement. You probably did not rehearse what you were going to say before you said it. More likely, at some deep level you put a subject and a predicate idea together in an abstract form too amorphous to describe. Yet, that form fit the structure of the language you spoke. Had you used a different language, you would probably have arranged the ideas in your mind differently, reflecting the oft-heard observation that people think differently in different languages (Kolers, 1968). Ability to arrange an infinite combination of ideas that can be spoken reflects knowledge of the *deep structure* of one's language.

By contrast, phonetic organization of sounds spoken and sounds heard reflects the *surface structure* of language. This is the level of the physical signal actually produced, the level of the phone, the level that the structural linguist describes, the level that the behavioral psychologist manipulates in learning experiments, and the level at which the speech pathologist works in his remedial efforts. Surface structure characterizes *linguistic performance.*

Linguistic competence, then, requires the ability to make *grammatical transformations* from deep structure to surface structure, to

---

Williams and Cairns (1973) offer a readable account of the organization of language. How do they explain the operation of transformational rules?

---

generate an infinite set of subject-predicate combinations in abstract deep structure form that can be transformed by syntactic, morphemic, and phonemic rules into phonetic arrangements of surface structure that express the intended meaning (Fig. 3-1). This ability is central to the normal creative use of any particular language. It goes beyond any known cognitive or behavioral system. Furthermore, since innate capacity for universal grammar goes far beyond any known mental organization, no aspect of linguistic ability, as Chomsky sees it, can be explained adequately with existing knowledge.

A behavioral view of grammatical functions. The shot heard round the psycholinguistic world was fired when Chomsky (1959) reviewed Skinner's (1957) book, *Verbal Behavior*. In a critique that has not been answered, Skinner's operant analysis of verbal

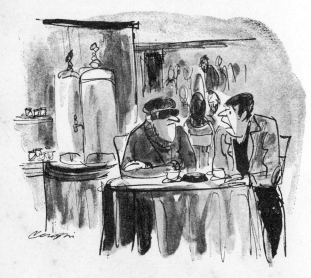

"I have deep perceptive thoughts, but I can't get them into sentences."

Fig. 3-1. An instance of limited linguistic competence. (Courtesy Robert Censoni. Copyright 1969 Saturday Review, Inc.)

behavior was challenged as a sufficient explanation of language.

Operant view. Skinner (1957) attempted to save language from itself by freeing it from the mentalistic mysticism of "meaning." Eschewing a linguistic analysis with its traditional terms, such as "speech" and "language," he proposed a psychologic analysis of the function of *verbal behavior*. He demonstrated forcefully that "meaning," when stripped of mentalistic circumlocutions (such as defining words with other words that mean the same thing), has no existence of its own, nor is it a property of behavior. Instead, it describes the relation between verbal behavior and the conditions under which that behavior occurs.

A person who understands what a statement means is able to infer stimulus conditions to which the statement is a response. To say, "The room is green," is to respond verbally to a condition of the room. If the shade of green evokes a subjective feeling of nausea, the response might be altered to: "The room is bilious green." Thus, verbal behavior is dependent on internal and external stimulus conditions. If the stimulus is altered independently, say you moved on to a red room, then a statement about room color would have to change to reflect the new color denoted and one's feeling about it that is connoted.

As you can see, Skinner analyzes the relation between stimulus and verbal response as identical to the relation between independent and dependent variables. In a functional analysis of language, meaning is embedded in the stimulus condition rather than in the verbal response, where it is traditionally assigned in linguistic analyses. To the extent that one can specify all independent stimulus variables on which the verbal response is dependent, one can specify meaning. Much of Skinner's effort was to make verbal behavior explicit and measurable.

Because his analysis was functional, not linguistic, Skinner ignored syntactic, morphemic, and phonemic structures. Instead, he examined the psychologic function of verbal utterances irrespective of linguistic function. He observed that different types of verbal responses were under different types of stimulus control. In all types described, though, verbal behavior operated on the environment to produce consequences; thus he viewed all utterances as *verbal operants*.

Skinner noted that some responses are demands, and he called that type of verbal operant a *mand*. Mands could be words ("There!"), phrases ("Right there!"), or sentences ("Put it right there!"). Functionally they are equivalent, each being reinforced or punished by the effect produced on the listener. Other types of verbal operants include *echoic* behavior, which echoes a stimulus; *textual* behavior, which is under control of the material being read; and *intraverbal* behavior, which involves completion of a stereotyped response, such as completing "Hickory, dickory, _____."

Of the basic verbal operants, responses controlled by contact with the environment (hence called *tacts*) form the largest group. Tacts describe some property of the stimulus condition. Verbal operants can be of any linguistic size and can serve any functional purpose. Using Skinner's example, "fire" can be a tact for a roaring conflagration, a mand to a firing squad, an intraverbal response to "Ready, aim, _____," an echoic response of incredulity when told that your house is on fire, and a textual response when reading a news account of your disaster.

Skinner's functional conception of language has been of inestimable value in making verbal behavior explicit, measurable, and controllable. All these conditions are essential for scientific analysis and for clinical modification of behavior. Not surprisingly, speech pathologists have found much merit in this approach. Vulnerability of the analysis

---

What success was achieved in teaching language to mentally retarded children when a skinnerian model of verbal behavior was used (Schiefelbusch, 1963)?

---

lies not in the fact that it is wrong, but in the constricted limits within which it is right. Persons who look only for verbal behavior as types of operant responses can be per-

suaded greatly by his work. This is precisely what he offered, no more.

Persons who seek a complete analysis of language in all of its grammatical complexity, however, will be frustrated. Skinner speaks only of those verbal responses that must be emitted and reinforced to be acquired. He thereby excludes for practical purposes the abundance of innovative statements that comprise the bulk of most speakers' comments. Not only does he not explain how these original statements that occur only once, never to recur, can be reinforced sufficiently to be preserved, but he also does not explain how they occurred in the first place. He speaks of how syntactic functions are reinforced in terms of *autoclitics*, but on the subject of the structure of language and how it is acquired, he is silent.

Learning theory view. Learning principles have foundered, not in explanations of how words acquire meaning, but when used to explain how the grammatical structure of language is acquired. Staats (1968) has taken a long step toward resolving this inadequacy. He borrowed a key concept of *privileges of occurrence* from Brown and Berko (1960). These authors demonstrated that different classes of words occur only in certain relations to other classes of words. The nature of the structure of language affords the privilege of occurrence to any word in the appropriate grammatical class whether it makes semantic sense or not. Any noun can occur where subject or object is required, any verb can be placed in the predicate slot, and so on. For instance, "The moon jumped over the cow" is nonsense, but it is grammatical because all parts of speech are privileged to occur where they do. On the other hand, "The jumped the over cow moon" is ungrammatical nonsense because it violates grammatical sequences that are privileged to occur in English. Granted that children rarely hear "perfect" grammar. Conversely, they probably rarely hear violations of privileges of occurrence.

Working from this premise, Staats proposed that the prelinguistic child learns through classical conditioning to distinguish privileges of occurrence of major parts of speech that he hears, starting with the basic distinction between subject and predicate. When he begins to use speech, instrumental conditioning, too, helps to shape his intuitive sense of grammar. He learns conditions under which certain word sequences are permitted. From these sequences, he can deduce privileges of occurrence. By listening, speaking, and reading, the child learns how grammatical rules of his language operate, even though he cannot state the rules formally.

This conception of how grammar is learned appears to meet one of the major challenges that any explanation must meet: the normal human ability to generate novel statements. Once privileges of occurrence of parts of speech are learned, the child knows the rules of grammar. He would then be able to apply these rules to generate endless combinations of original grammatical statements. Concurrently, he learns meanings of words and is therefore able to fill the privileged grammatical slots with semantically appropriate words. Thus he is able to speak and to understand sensible statements. Too, he is able to talk to himself, to use sentences as conditioning devices to shape his own thinking, thereby contributing to the apparent originality of what he has to say.

The cloud on the horizon of Staats' analysis may or may not dampen the value of his conception. Whether this integrated use of learning principles is sufficient to explain how a child learns rules of his native language in a relatively brief span of about 2 years remains to be seen. Considering the complexity of linguistic rules, considering the infinite number of wrong rules that could be learned, and considering a child's unerring ability to select the proper rules, one question is paramount: "What is the guidance system that children use normally to navigate their way through language learning?" It could be by observing and learning privileges of occurrence, provided the child rarely hears exceptions to these principles.

Psychologic reality of linguistic rules. How much the acquisition of linguistic rules can

be explained by learning principles and how much by innate capacity to learn only a natural language remains an open issue. No matter; the important consideration for speech pathologists is to identify those linguistic rules that, however acquired, come closest to having psychologic reality. If rules by which language is used can be made explicit, we would have a foundation for understanding and improving it. The four levels of rules of generative grammar come as close as any yet developed to having psychologic relevance.

The lowest level involves rules governing use of a pool of vocabulary words, morphemes, and phonemes. This is the semantic and morphophonemic level at which words have meaning and physical reality by virtue of being pronounced. Therefore, it is a level at which performance can be observed directly and measured physiologically and acoustically as well as behaviorally. For this reason, if for no other, it is the easiest level at which the speech pathologist works: pronunciation and articulation can be observed and corrected, and new words can be given meaning by associating them with appropriate objects, pictures, or other words, all of which can be made explicit. Of course, teaching the meaning of function words (such as prepositions and connectives) that have no observable referent is a more challenging task.

The next level involves rules for determining the grammatical class of a word. The traditional parts of speech (nouns, verbs, adjectives, and so on) are replaced by a much larger set of grammatical classes in a generative grammar. Normally, we comprehend and organize speech in phrases, not in individual words that can be classified by traditional grammar. Thus, for words that function in phrases, the large list of classes of a generative grammar seems to have more psychologic relevance than the shorter list of traditional grammar (Miller, 1962).

The level of phrase structure involves rules for generation of syntactic sentences. Here, arguments among linguists mount higher. Which theory has the most elegant simplicity? The most economy? Miller (1962) holds that an understanding of how speech is used can be found in the psychologic processes involved, not in the formal structure of linguistic theory. For speech pathologists as for psychologists, the important issue is: which theory best explains how we understand and utter grammatical sentences?

Psychologically, normal speech is perceived in larger units than words (much less morphemes or phonemes). Are particular types of phrase structure also preferred psychologically? Yes. This preference excludes sentences that are linguistically grammatical but psychologically incomprehensible. As an example, consider the following sentence: "The race that the car that the people whom the obviously not very well-dressed man called sold won was held last summer." Difficult to understand and remember, it is just as grammatical as when phrase structure is rearranged this way: "The obviously not very well-dressed man called the people who sold the car that won the race that was held last summer."

Why is the latter structure so much easier to grasp than the former? Because, as Miller points out, the first sentence places much greater demand on the very limited temporary storage capacity of our memories. The latter sentence is a *right-recursive* phrase-structure that could be described as a *Markov chain* (a sequence of events in which the probability of each event is determined by those that have preceded it). If all phrase-structures employed associational probabilities of a Markov chain, the strain on our temporary memory storage ability would be lessened and grammar would be simpler. But natural languages cannot be explained so easily. They permit *left-recursive* structures (such as "The obviously not very-well dressed man is here") with their possibility of unlimited *self-embedding*, a type of phrase structure that makes this example so horrendous.

Beyond rules of grammatical categories and rules of phrase-structure are transformational rules. Here, arguments among linguists reach their peak. How to explain what seem to be

variations of the same idea, such as in these sentences: "John pushed Mary." "Mary was pushed by John." "Did John push Mary?" "Mary was not pushed by John." Linguists of one opinion hold that we learn separate *sentence frames* for each type of sentence. With this view, we should expect to find our memories filled with unrelated rules for constructing such active, passive, declarative, interrogative, affirmative, negative sentence types as those just given.

The alternative to a long list of short transformational rules is a short list of long transformational rules of the sort that generative grammarians propose. Their rules are quite complicated. Still, from a psychologic standpoint they seem to hold considerable explanatory power (Braine, 1963). The essence of a transformational theory of grammar is a set of rules by which the basic sentence patterns,

Chomsky (1957) describes the rules of generative grammar in his oft-cited text. How do these rules for transformation, phrase-structure, and grammatical class differ from those of traditional grammar?

kernel sentences, can be transformed into various sentence types. According to this theory, transformational rules are applied in a certain order. For instance, to get from an active negative sentence ("Mary did not slap John") to its passive negative form ("John was not slapped by Mary"), the sentence must first be "untransformed" to its kernel ("Mary slapped John"), then changed to passive form ("John was slapped by Mary") before the final negative transformation can be applied.

Let us again turn to Miller's (1962) work for a test of these alternative explanations of transformational ability. Miller reasoned that the more complicated a transformation, the longer it would take to perform. If each type of sentence has its own separate sentence frame, we should be able to make one transformation as quickly as another. But if the transformational theory of generative grammarians is correct, transformations are accomplished sequentially, so that some should take longer than others. This is exactly what Miller found: more than twice as much time is required to go from a kernel sentence to its passive negative than to its active nega-

---

What counterarguments do Williams and Cairns (1973) offer to the sequential application of transformational rules? How do they explain sentence comprehension?

---

tive form, and even more time is required to transform an active negative sentence into passive affirmative form. Miller suspects that people decipher speech they hear by extracting the kernel sentence and adding a footnote in their memories about the transformational form in which it occurred.

Behavioral units of language. What we have reviewed are aspects of language that seem closest to describing how it is produced and perceived. Unfortunately, psychology has far less understanding of how internal rules operate in governing behavior than it has of how external conditions affect overt behavioral responses. If rules of language could be converted into functional behavioral units, disorders of language could be managed with confidence in results that could be achieved.

Johnson (1965) is one of the few psychologists who has attempted to convert rules of generative grammar into functional units of language behavior. In his preliminary effort, he suggests a method of attack that could prove profitable. Johnson starts by establishing functional properties that characterize any behavioral unit: on one hand, the response unit either exists or it does not, so it can be scored as having occurred or not occurred; on the other, the response is integral—it changes as a whole unit, not in parts. Normally, psychologists want to stipulate the behavioral unit that they observe, but with language the response unit is an internal rule defined by the subject, not the observer. Still, if subjectively defined response units can be identified empirically, the prospect is within reach of determining functional units of language behavior.

By determining units of language, speech pathologists as well as psychologists could deal with the four levels of generative gram-

mar as two basic behavioral issues. First to be identified would be language units; second would be operations used to manipulate the units. How can this be done? Johnson (1965) proposes that the first three levels of grammar have to do with size of linguistic units and how they are formed. Formation of a vocabulary pool of morpheme and word units into various syntactic categories differs from formation of phrase-structure units mainly in terms of size of the unit. At the fourth level, Johnson views transformational rules as a set of operations by which these various language units are manipulated into meaningful, hence syntactic, statements.

The feasibility of this solution for making language disorders operationally manageable rests on the feasibility of making rules explicit. Whereas responses that actually exist can be observed directly, rules can be observed only by the effect they produce on responses, and that effect is to determine the class of response required. For example, certain phonemic sequences occur frequently in English (such as /pl/, /sp/, /gr/), whereas others never occur at all (/pz/, /sd/, /gt/). Similarly, certain morphemic and syntactic sequences occur with regularity but others are prohibited by rules of a language—the privileges of occurrence. Such sequences appear to constitute classes of responses that are functional units. Operations that govern occurrence of these classes apparently comprise rules learned when one acquires a language. If this is the case, as Johnson (1965) suspects, then associations utilized for producing speech are not between functional units of language, the response class of various sizes, but between operations by which these units are manipulated to transform kernel sentences into various types of syntactic statements.

Strategies for mastering language. Various strategies can be utilized in attempts to cope with grammatical rules, some of which are far more likely to lead to language mastery than others. In a recent experiment subjects were given samples of an artificial grammar and were to try to construct new sentences according to that grammar. Some tried by rote.

They memorized samples and had little success dealing with new sentences. Some tried by determining positions of words in sample sentences. Their system broke down for new sentences when word order was reversed. Those who succeeded best abstracted word classes and rules for their combination from the samples. Not only did subjects differ in how they went about solving the problem, but they also differed in ability to generalize when they tried to abstract response classes (Saporta and others, 1965).

These issues suggest crucial questions about factors that determine selection of strategies for language learning and ability to generalize once a productive strategy is selected. Do these factors depend primarily on innate capacity? If so, prospects for the language impaired are limited. Are these factors subject to modification? Humane concerns alone demand that we pursue this possibility. It is the source of hope for the linguistically handicapped.

Nor is it an idle hope. What determines discovery that language involves lawful relations that cannot be mastered by imitating stereotyped responses? Discovery of details of those relations could depend on how extensively and directly a child must be confronted with the inadequacy of his misconception of rules before he will attempt to work out a more accurate generalization. It could depend on the availability of a speech

---

Winitz (1966) describes examples of how children normally progress in learning morphologic rules and syntactic privileges of occurrence of class words and function words. What implications does he see for children with delayed language?

---

model who speaks often enough and in long-enough utterances to permit contemplation, speculation, and generalization about what patterns do recur. It could depend on who is chosen as a model for shaping one's identity and on strength of identification: the "strong, silent" type would not be a very helpful speech model. It could depend on how long and how successfully one has lived with an inaccurate conception of grammatical rules.

SPEAKING PROCESSES

All that can be seen of linguistic principles at work is in surface expressions of phonetic performance. We now turn to the three major processes for producing this overt speaking behavior: *articulatory-resonatory*, *phonatory*, and *speech-flow*. Some unraveling of intricate intertwining of phonation, resonance, and articulation must be undertaken first.

Sound generation and transmission

Generation. Much as a potter molds a blob of clay on his wheel into a finished pot, so does a speaker modulate the breath stream into an intelligible flow of speech. Three types of sound can be generated: *waves*, *turbulence*, and *pulses*.

Waves are generated by *phonation*. When vocal folds vibrate they release a series of pulses of air pressure, a *voiced* sound. Pulses of energy are released by laryngeal vibrations in a fashion similar to that of an inflated balloon when the neck is stretched to emit a "Bronx cheer." The rate of this *glottal* vibration (opening and closing of the glottal space between the vocal cords), called the *fundamental frequency*, is the main determinant of what is heard as *pitch*. If the larynx were disconnected from the vocal tract so that it spewed glottal pulses into open air, the energy in these pulses would be expended rapidly as all of the surrounding molecules were set to vibrating at many rates. This process of generating repetitive glottal pulses without benefit of resonators, when displayed graphically as in Fig. 3-2, would reveal a sharp increase in energy as glottal pressure is released and a rapid decrease as energy is quickly expended or, technically, *damped*.

When the larynx opens as in breathing, the folds do not vibrate, so a *voiceless* breath stream is released with which turbulence or pulses can be produced. Turbulence is generated at points of constriction in the *vocal tract*, such as for friction sounds (fricatives) such as /s/. Pulses are generated by abrupt release of closures in the vocal tract, such as for explosion sounds (plosives), such as /t/, that begin with a clicklike pulse.

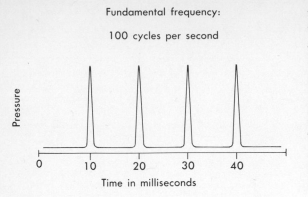

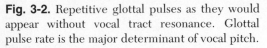

Fig. 3-2. Repetitive glottal pulses as they would appear without vocal tract resonance. Glottal pulse rate is the major determinant of vocal pitch.

Transmission. Whether the breath stream is voiced or voiceless, airflow normally must be transmitted through cavities of the vocal tract and out the mouth or the nose. Air molecules in these throat, mouth, and nose cavities will vibrate *(resonate)* when energy is available to give them a push. Much as a child sitting in a swing needs a push, so do air molecules in resonators need a source of energy to set them to vibrating. That source for voiced sounds is phonation. Repetitive pressure pulses of phonation push resonator molecules vigorously, with each pulse giving the resonator a sharp beat of pressure. With a voiceless stream of air, energy may be generated by turbulence or isolated pulses. Voiced sounds are louder than voiceless ones because resonator molecules are pushed with more energy by waves of pressure than by turbulence or isolated pulses.

The rate at which resonator molecules will vibrate depends largely on size, shape, and surface texture of the cavity. To appreciate effects of these cavity features on molecular vibration, stretch your imagination a bit and visualize a room full of electric cars, such as are driven at amusement parks, that bang into one another and bounce off railings. Let each car be an air molecule and the room be the resonating cavity. Now imagine (and this will stretch things a bit) that you want to see how fast you can get the cars in and out of the room through one exit that we will make analogous to the shape of the opening of a resona-

tor. The larger the exit (the larger the resonator aperture), the faster the cars can move in and out (the higher the frequency at which a resonator will vibrate). The larger the room (the resonator), and the more cars (air molecules) that move in and out through the exit, the slower the process will be (the lower the frequency at which a resonator will vibrate). The springier the railings (the more tense the tissue of the vocal tract), the faster will cars bounce off the walls (the more conducive to high-frequency vibration). Finally, the greater variety of rates at which cars mill around trying to go in and out of the room (the wider the range of frequencies at which molecules vibrate in a resonator), the more they use energy banging into each other (the faster will energy in a resonator be expended).

This analogy would hold if vocal tract resonators functioned separately. Oral, nasal, and pharyngeal resonators would contribute independently to the speech sound produced. In reality, these cavity resonators are *coupled* from trachea to lips. That is, they interact in their effects on air molecule movement, much as would happen if our electric cars had to move through several rooms and exits of different sizes. The result is that resonance frequencies of speech cannot be assigned to specific cavities in the vocal tract.

Fortunately, the larynx is normally connected with the vocal tract, an arrangement that does not significantly alter sharpness with which the phonatory process puts energy into each glottal pulse but that does alter how that energy is spent. Instead of being used up very quickly by pushing molecules into vibration at many possible frequencies, energy is used more slowly to force molecules to vibrate at frequencies determined by the coupled resonators, as shown in Fig. 3-3. Note that the fundamental frequency of glottal pulse rate at 100 Hz (*Hz* is the symbol for "cycles per second") is the same as in Fig. 3-2. The difference lies in how quickly each pulse is damped. In Fig. 3-3, only one resonator is shown using energy at 1,000 Hz (Ladefoged, 1962).

We now have three points established. First, the *phonatory process* controls release

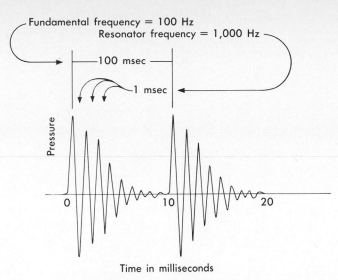

Fig. 3-3. Repetitive glottal pulses with vocal tract resonance. Frequency of resonator response can be seen as energy in each glottal pulse is utilized.

of a voiced or voiceless breath stream with which energy will be generated as waves, turbulence, or pulses. Second, this breath stream is transmitted through cavities of the vocal tract, where energy is expended by pushing molecules into vibration. Third, characteristics of the coupled resonators will determine frequency of resonance of the vocal tract. From these points, you can see that the more that molecules are set to vibrating, the faster will their energy be expended. You can see, too, that resonators have no way of adding energy to a sound. They can only use energy at frequencies at which air in them will vibrate. They *modulate* energy transmitted through them, filtering it out at all frequencies at which they do not vibrate. Those resonance frequencies at which peaks of energy are expended in greatest vibrations are called *formants* (F).

Modulation: articulation-resonance. We must now clarify potential terminologic confusion between resonance and articulation. *Articulation* identifies vocal tract movements for speech sound production. For the many *consonants* characterized by generation of turbulence or pulses, these movements constrict or stop either a voiced or voiceless breath stream. For *vowels* (such as /i/ in "he"), *diphthongs* (two vowels blended tightly such

as /aɪ/ in "h*igh*"), and *semivowels* (vowel-like consonants such as /m/ in "hi*m*"), these movements adjust resonance characteristics of the vocal tract. By these adjustments, generated waves of the voiced breath stream (unless speech is whispered) are *modulated* into speech sounds. Resonator adjustments are an unavoidable consequence of articulatory movements. Thus articulatory and resonatory processes are inseparable. Hence, we will follow Darley's (1964) lead by using the hyphenated hybrid *articulation-resonance* as synonymous with *articulation*.

Sound perception and production

For analysis of each of the three aspects of the speaking process, a distinction will be necessary between the perception of sounds as a listener and their production as a speaker. Superficially, the difference is reflected in the phenomena with which they are correlated. As a listener, one's ear responds to acoustical events, to physical changes in air pressure in a sound wave. As a speaker, sound is produced by physiologic processes. But the difference is more complicated, however. Dimensions by which a sound can be conveniently described perceptually can seriously mislead efforts to describe how that same sound was produced. Furthermore, the difficulty of correlating the acoustics of speech with the perception of speech dims hope for the immediate future of correlating the physiology of speech production with the acoustics of speech perception (Peterson and Shoup, 1966b).

Perhaps most impenetrable is the difference in requirements for establishing control over sound perception processes in contrast to sound production processes. The stimuli to which sense organs respond can be controlled physically. Change the acoustical properties of a sound and the ear will respond differently. This is not to say that the way a sound is perceived will be completely controlled acoustically, but physical properties of a stimulus are certainly a major source of perceptual control. In fact, those who hear sounds without benefit of acoustical stimulation are likely to be candidates for a mental hospital. For listening, the physical properties of a sound can be viewed as an independent variable on which perception of that sound is dependent (Chapter 2).

With sound production, the problem of stimulus is far more nebulous. The dependent variable is all that can be observed: it is the sound produced. The independent variables that directly control sound production are in the mind, inaccessible to observation or measurement. What little you know of them must be inferred from sensory feedback of the sound and from the feel of what is produced in the first place. To guide production requires that you already have a reasonably clear idea of the sound to be produced. Notice that this "clear idea" is an auditory image of how you should hear the sound after it is produced, and a somesthetic image (much of which you are unaware) of how the speech mechanism would "feel" while producing it.

Now change the problem from how one guides production of sounds with which he is already familiar to how unfamiliar sounds are acquired. The speech clinician must deal with this very practical problem. How does one teach a speech-handicapped person to change his defective performance? Here we face a key question.

Suppose you are a native Midwesterner, have never learned any language other than your native tongue, and now for whatever reason are intent on learning to speak French without an accent—a problem akin to that of correcting a speech disorder. How do you proceed? One necessity would be to listen to French as spoken by native Frenchmen. This activity would provide a vague notion of how you should sound to others, but it would reveal little about how you would sound to yourself—a self-evident point if you have ever heard a recording of your own speech. Sound that travels by air from mouth to ear is heard quite differently from sound that travels to the ear by both bone and air. Listeners are privileged to hear the former type of sound, whereas only speakers are privy to the latter. Therefore, to obtain an auditory image of how you should sound when speaking French properly requires that you hear yourself speak French properly, which would require that your performance be checked and corrected by a knowledgeable listener.

Too, speech apparatus movements are guided by "feel": of tongue against teeth, of lips compressed, of tongue grooved along the midline, and so on. Generally, the deeper in the vocal tract that movements occur, the less accessible they are to awareness. In phonation, for example, laryngeal adjustments are not felt directly at all but are guided indirectly by vague sensations of tonal "placement." Human sound is speech apparatus movements made audible, so the essence of learning a new performance comes down to learning the feel and sound of a new set of movements that must occur before their feedback can be established.

The speech mechanism as a servosystem. One of the most viable theories in speech and hearing science describes interaction between speech perception and production. It is Fairbanks' (1954) conception that the speech mechanism functions as a servosystem. Where Wiener (1948) extended the principles of automatic control of machines to biologic systems under the banner of *cybernetics,* Fairbanks applied the idea of cybernetics to the speaking process. He viewed

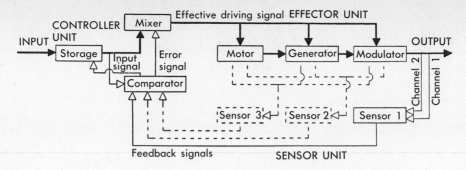

Fig. 3-4. Model of a closed cycle control system for speaking. Input consists of instructions to the effector unit for production of a sound. The sensor unit feeds back output information that is compared with original instructions to determine corrections, if any, that are needed. (From Fairbanks, G., Systematic research in experimental phonetics. I. A theory of the speech mechanism as a servosystem. *J. Speech Hearing Dis.*, **19**, 136, 1954.)

speech as an example of automatic control in which the acoustical output and the somesthetic "feel" of speech feed back for comparison with the intended output. If performance does not match intent, then future output is corrected on the basis of *negative feedback* until desired performance is achieved.

That Fairbanks presented his concept in the form of the model seen in Fig. 3-4 rather than as a replica of the speaking system attests to his recognition that it would need refinement as knowledge advanced. Because the model demonstrates operational principles rather than anatomic structures, it contains such terms as "controller unit," "motor," "generator," and "sensor," rather than brain, lungs, larynx, and ear. Among principles demonstrated was that of *closed-cycle control*. Any self-regulating system that controls its own performance to achieve a goal is a closed-cycle system. By contrast, in an *open-cycle system* the goals, or *set points*, are imposed from outside the system rather than from within it, as is the case in socializing the young. Another principle is that of negative feedback, which is basic to correcting the performance of any homeostatic system. Whereas *positive feedback* is illustrated by the population explosion (the greater the output of babies, the greater will be the supply of adults to produce more babies), negative feedback is illustrated by a thermostat that controls furnace output in a *steady state* by

reducing heat output to counteract high temperature and by increasing output to correct a low temperature.

Several important inferences can be drawn from this model. First, to disrupt auditory, tactile, or kinesthetic feedback would be to disrupt speech output. Second, *set points* (articulatory targets) to guide sound production are established initially by open-cycle control when the child acquires the speech patterns of his culture. Third, once set points that match cultural norms are *stabilized*, the child can guide future speech performance automatically by closed-cycle control. Conversely, if he stabilizes set points that do not match cultural standards, he must be either unable or unwilling to discriminate and correct the difference between his defective performance and acceptable sound production.

Articulatory-resonatory processes: segmental analysis

Approximately forty-five phonemes are used in American English—some regional dialects use more, some less. Remember that a phoneme is a psychologic, not a physical, reality. A word such as "sit" can be spoken many ways and still be understood. The speaker may be a child, a wrestler, a breathy-voiced seductress, a Casper Milquetoast, or a hoarse victim of laryngeal pathology. No matter how different these people may sound, they are still able to produce phones that a

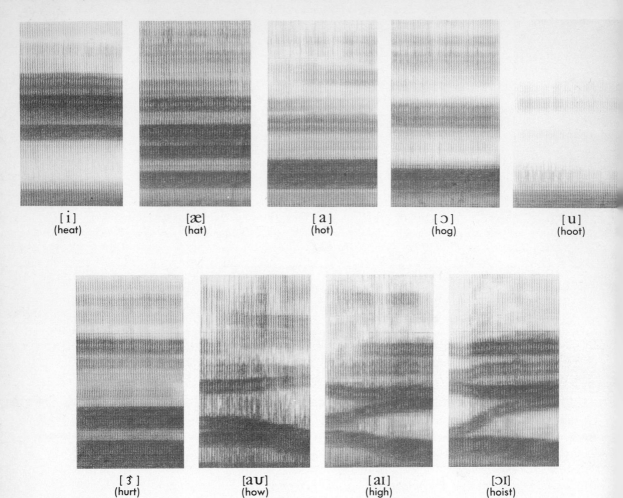

Fig. 3-5. Spectrograms of vowels and diphthongs spoken by the same speaker at the same pitch.

listener can interpret phonemically as "sit." The test of articulatory adequacy is how well a speaker produces phonemic segments intelligible to his listeners.

Processes of speech perception. After World War II, with the advent of computer technology, communication theory, and "visible speech" recordings of the sound spectrograph, the prospect seemed imminent of being able to convert speech into writing and writing into speech automatically. Even the possibility of machine translation from one spoken language to another was just around the corner. Equipment and mathematical tools were available to extract acoustical characteristics of phonemic segments. Since speech is perceived as a string of phonemes,

the ability to record, store, and transmit acoustical properties of each phonemic segment made extension of automation to the speaking process seem feasible.

Acoustical phonetics. Over two decades later, despite diligent effort, that prospect remains largely unrealized. Although the acoustics of speech have been studied intensively with remarkable precision, what acoustical phonetics has revealed as much as anything is the incredible complexity of speech perception. Not that these studies have been unproductive—far from it. Acoustical properties of segments of sustained vowels, for instance, are now known with reasonable certainty. As you can see from the *spectrograms* of Fig. 3-5, different vowels and diphthongs

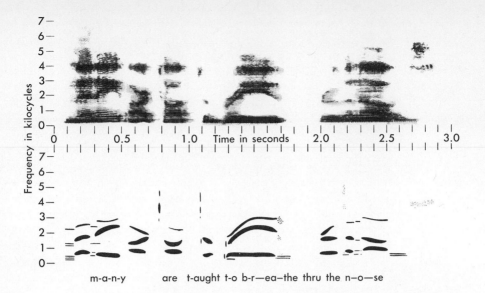

Fig. 3-6. Pattern-playback synthesized speech. The upper portion is a spectrogram of the sentence below as spoken naturally. The lower portion is a painted pattern of the first three formants, which can be played on a pattern-playback to synthesize the same sentence. (From Denes, P., and Pinson, E., *The Speech Chain*. Murray Hill, N. J.: Bell Telephone Laboratories (1963). Courtesy Bell Telephone Laboratories, Inc.)

have different formant frequencies for their resonator adjustments.

So much is known about acoustical phonetics that speech synthesizers have been built that can simulate speech that is all but indistinguishable from human performance. A much bigger challenge has been to build equipment that can recognize speech. Rudimentary computer recognition systems have been devised, but speech flows at forty times the rate at which they operate. Perhaps the only assurance that such a system can be built is the fact that one has been—man himself (Denes and Pinson, 1963; Reddy, 1967).

Limits of segmental analysis. The difficulty of simulating human ability to recognize speech attests to how extraordinary is this ability that all of us use with casual ease. Much of the complexity lies in the fact that speech is not produced one isolated sound at a time. It is a continuously flowing stream of phones that the listener sorts into phonemic categories. A segment of a "pure" *steady-state* phone is hard to find in normal speech. In fact, if speech were a string of "pure" phones arranged in proper linguistic order, it

would be almost unintelligible. It would sound like a jerky series of isolated sounds that would bear little resemblance to comprehensible words. Much of speech perception hinges on acoustical *transitions* heard as one sound flows into the next. This is especially true of consonants that depend on frequency patterns of friction noises, and even more heavily on frequency changes and timing of transitions (O'Connor, 1961).

With plosive consonants such as /p/, /t/, and /k/, for instance, when frequency of noise of the explosive burst is the same, a listener will hear /k/ when the transition is to one vowel, /t/ when it is to another, and so on. Fricative consonants depend mainly on frequency of friction noise (the difference between "see" and "she" depending on whether the frequency is above 4,000 Hz or between 2,000 to 3,000 Hz). Still, they also depend on time. Reduce the fricative segment of "see" from 0.1 to 0.01 second and you would tend to hear "tee." As you can see in Fig. 3-6, formants are in almost constant transition from one frequency to another. The marvel of speech perception is our capacity to detect various cues in this acoustical flux that permit understanding of what has been spoken (Denes and Pinson, 1963).

Motor theory of speech perception. That speech is not perceived one sound at a time has become abundantly evident. The ear does not process acoustical signals of speech segments in the same manner as the eye deciphers words. Even if the auditory system is capable of handling acoustical information about each speech segment at the normal rate of ten to fifteen phonemes per second, the fact remains that discrete acoustical equivalents of phonemes simply do not exist in normal speech. An alphabet letter, such as "d," retains its identity whether viewed alone, in a word, in a sentence, or in a book. The acoustical signal for the speech sound /d/, however, depends heavily on the vowel that follows it. Essentially the same can be said for the acoustical basis of all phonemes. Perception of speech depends on the context of sounds in which it occurs (Liberman and others, 1967).

As listeners, we are completely unaware of how varied the acoustical basis of speech perception really is. Listen to the first /d/ in "*d*eed" and "*d*ude." If you can hear any difference at all in those two sounds, it will be slight. The acoustical difference in them, however, is great. Conversely, very slight acoustical differences, as in spectrograph patterns of formants of /dɔ/ and /gɔ/, provide a clear basis for hearing the difference between "*d*awn" and "*g*one" (Lane, 1965).

How can it be that we perceive phonemes with the same clarity and certainty that we perceive alphabet letters, even though the acoustical basis for speech perception can vary radically? Some sort of decoding system must be used that permits us to extract invariant relationships that we hear as phonemes from the widely varied acoustical signals. Liberman and his colleagues at Haskins Laboratories (1967) have proposed as an explanation a *motor theory of speech perception.* They maintain that the decoding process for speech recognition consists of running the encoding process of speech production backward.

Essentially, they argue that both speech production and perception go along at such rapid rates that the nervous system could cope with neither on the basis of processing one sound at a time. Instead, successive phonemic segments are encoded and decoded in parallel. For encoding, phones are taken apart into articulatory features needed to produce them. These features are then overlapped so that as any one sound is being produced, others coming up are being anticipated, as, for example, in lip-rounding of /hj/ in "*h*uge" in anticipation of the vowel /u/. The effect on the acoustical signal of overlapping articulatory events is to produce overlapped sounds of speech. If the lips, for example, are in position for one sound while the tongue is moving into position for the next, both lips and tongue will imprint their articulatory effect on the acoustical signal.

For the listener to decode speech requires that he recover from the sound he hears the articulatory events by which the sound was encoded in the first place. Presumably, invariant neural auditory patterns by which phonemes are detected are matched far down in the neuromotor system with the neural pattern of commands to the speech muscles. This says, in effect, that we perceive speech by empathizing with the manner in which it is produced.

The motor theory of speech perception has been a lively theory, both in research stimulated and controversy stirred. As an example, if the theory were true, how would it explain one's ability to recognize dialects that differ widely from the way one produces his own

Does Lane (1965), in his critical review of the motor theory, disagree with it in any major ways?

speech? Or how would it explain the evidence that children appear to acquire speech by matching articulatory gestures to perceptual categories rather than vice versa (Menyuk and Anderson, 1969)? Perhaps the motor theory is necessary and applicable only at the fast rates of normal speech. At slow rates, articulators need not overlap in their movements to produce sequences of sounds, so that the resulting acoustical signal, reflecting

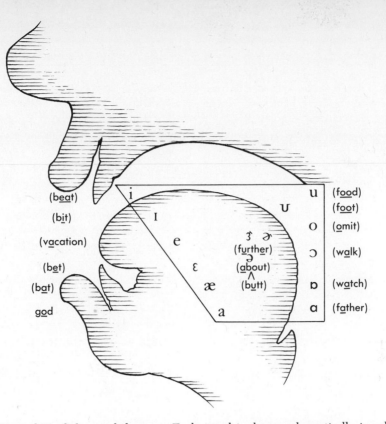

Fig. 3-7. Typical English vowel diagram. Each vowel is shown schematically in relation to the vertical and horizontal position of the arch of the tongue for its production.

articulator movements, corresponds more closely to phonemes perceived. How much of an explanation slow rate offers for exceptions to the motor theory has not been explored.

Completely aside from the scientific importance of an accurate understanding of how speech is produced and perceived, the issue is of considerable practical significance to the speech clinician. If speech is perceived by decoding how it was produced, then the most productive route to correcting defective speech would not be through ear training, the traditional approach in speech pathology. The fact that this approach does work, at least within limits, adds doubt to the adequacy of the motor theory as a complete account of speech perception. The evidence points to both an articulatory and an auditory basis for speech perception (Wickelgren, 1969).

Processes of speech production. Basically or practically, the physiologic processes of producing intelligible speech are fundamen-

tal. From the practical view of the clinician, defective speech is identified by the inability to speak intelligibly, which is tantamount to inability to produce proper physiologic movements of the speaking equipment. From the basic view of the speech scientist, motor physiology is undoubtedly fundamental to speech production, regardless of whether or not it is to speech perception.

The physiologic basis of speech is primary because it sets limits for all humans on sounds that can be produced (Peterson and Shoup, 1966b). Everyone's vocal tract is more or less similar, which means that everyone is capable of producing about the same range of sounds. An obvious requirement for a speech system of any language is that it utilize sounds that all speakers can produce. If, for example, a language contained phonemes that depended for distinctive differences on production of extremely high pitches of which only a few persons were capable, then only those few

Table 3-3. Typical English consonant chart

Manner of articulation	Place of articulation						
	Bilabial	Labio-dental	Dental	Alveolar	Palatal	Velar	Glottal
Nasal	m (*man*)			n (ma*n*)		ŋ (si*ng*)	
Plosive	p (*p*at) b (*b*at)			t (*t*oe) d (*d*oe)		k (*c*at) g (ta*g*)	ʔ (*uh uh*)
Fricative	hw (*wh*at) w (*w*att)	f (*f*at) v (*v*at)	θ (*th*in) ð (*th*at)	s (bu*s*) z (buz*z*)	ʃ (ru*sh*) ʒ (rou*ge*)		h (*h*at)
Affricate					tʃ (*church*) dʒ (*judge*)		
Glide				l (*l*et)	r (*r*at) j (*y*et)		

would be able to speak that language. When the range of sounds that the speech apparatus can produce is compared with the range that the auditory system can receive, it is apparent that we can hear a vastly wider variety of sounds than we can produce. Without doubt, the nature of speech is limited in the mouth of the speaker more than in the ear of the listener.

Articulatory-resonatory processes: physiologic phonetics. The goal of physiologic phonetics is to describe movements of the speech apparatus that produce various human sounds. On the surface, this task is straightforward. Any physiologic change in the vocal tract produces a corresponding change in the acoustical signal. Complications arise when one attempts to correlate these physiologic, acoustical, and phonetic events with perception of phonemes that are real only psychologically and linguistically. They are not real acoustically, phonetically, or physiologically. Still, they come close to standing in a one-to-one relation with physiologic movements. These movements produce phones heard as phonemes.

Traditionally, the relation between pho-

nemes and the physiology of their production is presented in the form of *vowel diagram* and *consonant chart.* The shape of the vowel diagram in Fig. 3-7 is intended to suggest the shape of the oral cavity. It shows the vowel sounds produced when the tongue is moved vertically or horizontally to various positions in the cavity. Because vowels are tones that depend on resonance for distinctive qualities, what the diagram presents is a suggestion of resonator shapes that produce different vowels.

Unlike vowel diagrams, consonant charts such as in Table 3-3 often bear no resemblance to physiologic mechanisms to which they refer. They specify the *place* in the vocal tract where the consonant is produced. For example, since /m/ and /b/ obviously involve both lips, a *bilabial* place of articulation is specified. They also specify the physiologic *manner* utilized at the place of articulation to produce the consonant (/s/ is produced by friction, hence fricative; /p/ by explosion, hence plosive).

The vowel diagram and consonant chart are so dissimilar as to suggest that vowels involve different parts of the vocal tract than consonants. Furthermore, they say practically nothing about those parts of the vocal tract that are not focal physiologic features for a particular sound. For example, /m/ is classified as a voiced, bilabial, nasal consonant. This classification indicates that the breath stream is voiced, the place of articulation is the lips, and the manner requires directing the airstream through the nose. Unspecified are a variety of other physiologic adjustments that are less directly relevant to production of /m/ but that are nonetheless involved. Produce /m/ while you move the tongue around in your mouth, while you lift a heavy object, while yawning, while inhaling instead of exhaling. You may have managed to continue to produce a recognizable /m/, but the quality of the sound probably changed.

The point is that speech is orchestrated physiologically, just as a symphony is orchestrated musically. Even though you may be aware only of instruments that play the melodic line, contribution of those instruments could be altered radically by other instruments that provide harmonic support. If each were playing its part of a different piece, the result would be cacophony. Obviously, a musical score must contain more than the melody. Similarly, a physiologic account of speech must contain more than a description of just those most noticeable adjustments of the vocal tract for a particular sound.

Fig. 3-8 shows a comprehensive attempt by Peterson and Shoup (1966b) to describe the full physiologic orchestration for any speech sound that could be produced in any natural language. Notice that in the primary parameters of their model the same physiologic dimensions have been displayed that have typically been presented separately in vowel diagrams and consonant charts. Note, too, that the secondary parameters contain an extensive account of additional physiologic factors that contribute to generating the breath stream and to modulating it with articulatory-resonatory processes.

Distinctive features. We have been flirting with a notion in this discussion that now will be confronted directly. Several years ago, Jakobson, Fant, and Halle (1952) proposed the idea that speech sounds are distinguished from each other by distinctive features. The dozen features they proposed were meant to denote linguistic discriminations. Presumably, these features could be identified physiologically and acoustically as well. The essential point of the concept is that it attempts to describe all speech sounds of any language with a relatively few easily distinguishable features, any one of which is normally maintained during production of several phonemes. For example, whether a sound is produced with voiced or voiceless breath stream is an easily recognized distinction. In fact, it is a feature so impervious to distortion that nearly half of our consonantal distinctions depend on it (for example, voiceless /p/ versus voiced /b/, /s/ versus /z/, /t/ versus /d/).

This idea of distinctive features is relevant to this discussion in several ways. A fundamental point is that any sound system must depend on distinctive features that all normal listeners can learn to discriminate with ease and that all normal speakers can learn to produce with ease. Sounds that require special ability to hear or produce would be of little communicative value for the less talented masses with average hearing and speaking ability. Another aspect of distinctive features of importance is that although each sound is a blend of many features, only one feature need change to alter the phoneme. In other words, once a physiologic adjustment is set for a feature—for example, the soft palate is raised to direct sound through the mouth instead of the nose—that adjustment is normally maintained for several phonemes while other features, such as place and manner of articulation, are being altered to produce distinctive differences. These parallel adjustments are called *coarticulation* (Daniloff, 1973).

Here, then, is a basis for parallel processing of neural signals for production of speech that is central to the motor theory of speech perception. If only a few of several distinctive features need be changed from phoneme to phoneme, neural instructions for forthcoming features can be transmitted while the adjustments for other features are in progress. The net effect is an articulatory rate that can be

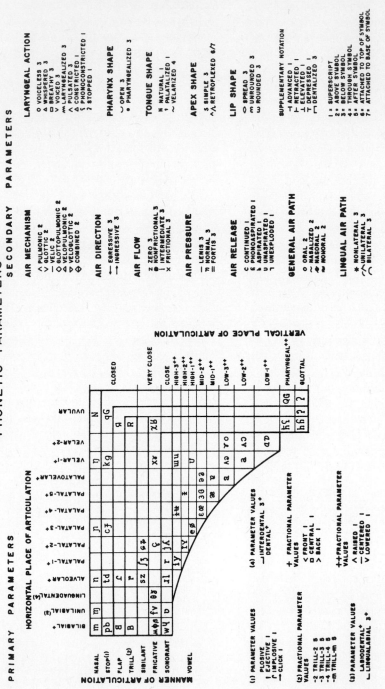

Fig. 3-8. Physiologic dimensions of speech. A system of marking primary and secondary phonetic parameters is provided by which the physiology of each speech sound can be described. Also, prosodic parameters to be measured are specified. (From Peterson, G., and Shoup, J., A physiological theory of phonetics, *J. Speech Hearing Res.,* **9,** 45[1966].)

much faster than would be possible if each feature had to be readjusted for each phoneme.

Phonemic targets: descriptive phonetics. By now, phonetics and phonemics must seem to embrace some of the more twisted and convoluted relations known to man. The fact that we can casually encode and decode speech attests to our remarkable linguistic facility, not to the ease of the task. That nature often disguises her most profound secrets in the cloak of apparent simplicity can be an illusion. If one does not look beyond the ease of articulation, for instance, explanations are unavailable for such questions as why speech sounds develop in a relatively predictable sequence, or why articulation defects involve some sounds more than others.

These questions become manageable when the intricacies of the structure behind the facade are probed. For instance, implicit in the abstract concept of distinctive features is the probability that some features are easier to discriminate than others. Since low back vowels are difficult to discriminate for acoustical reasons, many listeners do not hear a difference between such words as "four/for," "ore/or," "hoarse/horse." On the other hand, some consonants are difficult to discriminate for physiologic reasons. The dis-

tinctive features for production of such sounds as /s/, /r/, and /l/ involve subtle shapes of the tongue that do not have tactile contacts for guidance. Knowledge of contrasting features used in the sound system of a language opens doors to understanding how phonemic distinctions are learned and utilized for speech.

For the speech pathologist, the more exact his knowledge of sounds that should be produced, the more certain will be his efforts to correct defective articulation. The most observable and measurable information he has available is in acoustical and physiologic form. Sounds of speech arrive at the ear as acoustical waves that were generated and modulated in the vocal tract of the speaker as physiologic movements. If these movements could be controlled, the acoustical output could be controlled. The presumption, though, is that we know the movements necessary to yield the acoustical signal that is desired. Here we encounter again the imponderables of correlating physiologic and acoustical realities with the psychologic and linguistic realities of phonemes.

How much is known about transformation from physiologic to acoustical phonetics? A considerable amount is known, yet far from enough to say that the transformation is well

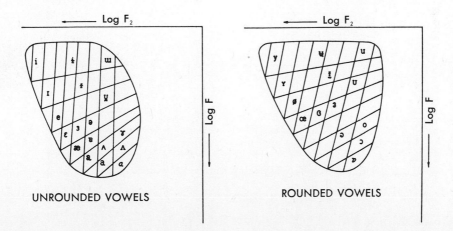

Fig. 3-9. Acoustical diagrams of vowels. Logarithms of formants 1 and 2 of lip-rounded vowels are shown to the right, of unrounded vowels to the left. By plotting logarithms of formant frequencies, the relations between F_1 and F_2 and the vowels are largely independent of differences among speakers. (From Peterson, G., and Shoup, J., The elements of an acoustic phonetic theory. *J. Speech Hearing Res.,* **9,** 96 [1966].)

understood. With vowels, the correlation is sufficient that by using the logarithm of only their first and second formant frequencies (F_1 and F_2), the resonator adjustments to produce them can be plotted, as shown in Fig. 3-9. Not only does this acoustical plot correspond to the traditional physiologic vowel diagram, but it also remains approximately constant for speakers of different age, sex, and size of vocal cavity. This is not to say that the formants for any given vowel are the same for all speakers—only that the relation between F_1 and F_2 holds relatively constant among speakers, a relation to which the listener apparently responds in vowel recognition (Peterson, 1961; Tiffany, 1959; Joos, 1948). Fig. 3-10 gives a clearer idea of how the physiology and acoustics of vowel production are correlated in a single speaker (Ladefoged, 1962).

This relatively uncomplicated relation between formant frequencies and vowel perception applies only for steady-state vowels produced in isolation in slow speech. At normal speaking rates, these *syllabic* sounds are produced as the sonorous element of the syllable, as the peak of the *breath pulse* (not to be confused with glottal pulse) that produces the syllable. Syllabic sounds (vowels and semivowels) are started, controlled, and checked by transitional movements of nonsyllabic consonant sounds (Stetson, 1951; Heffner, 1950). In normal speech that flows at about six or seven syllables per second, vowels are uttered almost as rapidly as consonants. They, too, must be encoded and decoded in the complex parallel processes suggested in the motor theory of speech perception. Thus the acoustical signal at no point corresponds directly to perception of the sound being produced. Rather, at any instant, merged influence of preceding and following sounds are also present (Liberman and others, 1967).

Transitions to and from vowel formants, syllabic targets toward which nonsyllabic movements seem to be aimed, generally carry the vital information for consonant perception. For example, first formant transitions are the same whether the vowel begins with /d/ or /g/. These F_1 transitions typically are cues for perception of manner of production

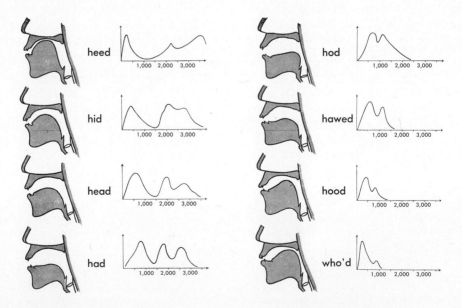

Fig. 3-10. Resonator shapes for vowel spectra. Vocal tract adjustments based on x-ray data taken during production of the vowel in each of the words listed. (From Ladefoged, P., *Elements of Acoustic Phonetics.* Chicago: The University of Chicago Press [1962]. Copyright 1962 by Peter Ladefoged.)

of consonants and for whether they are produced with voiced or voiceless breath stream. Since both /d/ and /g/ are produced in the plosive manner with voicing, their F_1 transitions are similar. Second formant transitions, on the other hand, are probably most important to perception of place of articulation. This involves distinctive features that determine discrimination of consonants produced in the same manner and with the same type of breath stream as are /d/ and /g/. Accordingly, differences between these consonants can be seen in F_2 transitions to the vowel (Liberman and others, 1967).

Unfortunately, these relations become considerably more complex as the sound moves from initial to medial or final position in a syllable, as syllables are strung together in context, as articulatory rate increases, and as the number of physiologic features are considered. Recall, for instance, the numerous physiologic parameters described by Peterson and Shoup (1966b). These authors note that since a change in any one would alter the sound, they have also attempted to describe acoustical correlates of each physiologic dimension—a sizable task (1966a).

Perhaps the most revealing index of the state of knowledge of physiologic, acoustical, and descriptive phonetics is seen in Fig. 3-11, an advertisement of Bell Telephone Laboratories. Bell has devised a computer model of the speaking system on which can be simulated physiologic adjustments of the vocal tract that will produce acoustical patterns that not only look much like human speech but sound much like it too—within limits.

How have Mermelstein (1967) and Schroeder (1967) managed to determine vocal tract shape from acoustical measurements?

A blessing of being human is that we come equipped to master the untold intricacies of speech with hardly a second thought. Though vistas may be opened for the clinician when the acoustics and physiology of speech are better known, the fact remains that the subjective processes of listening and speaking,

intuitive as they are, provide the most exact basis for articulation of acceptable speech. By sharpening skills of listening, the speech pathologist can develop a keen ear for phonemic targets of his language. By sharpening awareness of the "feel" of speech, many of the physiologic movements can be detected and controlled. In a word, the speech pathologist is endowed with the equipment that is needed to determine explicitly the articulatory behavior for which he holds responsibility.

Phonatory processes

As with articulation-resonance, the focus here will be on identifying as clearly as possible the phonatory behavior of importance to the speech pathologist. Whereas *phonation* will refer in the traditional sense to the generation of *voice*, *phonatory processes* will be used generically to identify the behavior for control of the breath stream, whether voiced or voiceless.

Voiced sounds are perceived by three dimensions: *pitch*, *loudness*, and *quality*. These perceptual dimensions serve a variety of functions, some of direct concern to the speech pathologist and some not. Pitch and loudness are major components of *stress* and of *prosody*. Too, each phoneme has a unique set of qualities. A speaker who cannot manage these linguistic functions of voice will therefore probably be in need of a speech pathologist's service.

Detection of impairment of many nonlinguistic functions of voice is much more nebulous. A person's identity is revealed vocally about as readily as it is visually, regardless of vocal adequacy. So are emotions, personality, even state of health. Virtually the only nonlinguistic aspects of voice that may require attention arise in those occasional instances when men's voices sound like women's, and women's like men's, and when the voice is judged as esthetically unpleasant (Perkins, 1971a).

Production vis-à-vis perception of voice. Major issues of vocal production are with identifying and assessing the adequacy of those processes of phonation that contribute

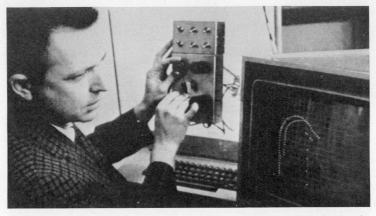

C. H. Coker adjusts controls which change the outline of the "vocal tract" simulated on the oscilloscope. At the same time, he hears the sound corresponding to the displayed shape. Desired vocal-tract shapes (representing sounds) can be stored in the computer memory.

Bell Laboratories' computerized vocal-tract model. (Head outline added.) The various parts can be positioned to imitate any speech sound. The model displays tract length versus cross-sectional area. It is based on anatomical measurements of the vocal tract made by a number of acousticians.

A feature of the model is that it reproduces the transition sounds between word fragments. The nonsense word eedah, for example, consists of ee plus d plus ah. But the d is not the same as in, say, eedee. That is, the d is noticeably affected by context. Coker handles this by storing dynamic properties of the vocal articulators (the tongue, lips and jaw). The program automatically incorporates these properties in assembling word fragments.

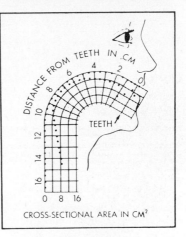

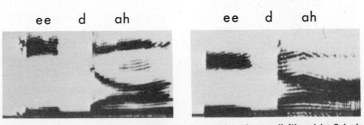

Comparison of nonsense word "eedah," pronounced by a human (left) and by Coker's program. These speech spectrographic patterns represent time (horizontal scale), frequency (vertical), and intensity (line density). The dark bars are called "formants" and are characteristic of speech sounds. The technique for making these diagrams was conceived and developed in the early 40's at Bell Telephone Laboratories.

Fig. 3-11. A computer that talks. (An advertisement of Bell Telephone Laboratories. Copyright 1968, Bell Telephone Laboratories, Inc.)

to perceived pitch, loudness, and quality. Let us begin by identifying the dimensions of vocal behavior that can be made explicit. Six are independent elements that can be controlled separately: *vocal pitch, vocal loudness, voicing, vocal constriction, vocal mode,* and *vocal focus.* Two are dependent and interact necessarily with all other elements: *vocal effort* and *vocal smoothness* (Perkins, 1971a,b).

Production of vocal pitch. When you listen to vocal pitch, you are responding for the most part to the rate at which the larynx is releasing glottal pulses into the vocal tract. It can range, depending on the speaker, from 50 to 500 Hz (McKinney, 1965). This glottal pulse rate is the foundation for harmonic structure of vocal tone, which is the reason it is called the *fundamental frequency.*

The important point for our consideration here is that pitch is a unidimensional parameter for production as well as perception. Perceptually, pitch can be quantified on a ratio scale (Chapter 2) for which the unit of measurement is the *mel.* Since the mel is a subjective unit of pitch, it does not correspond completely with the acoustical measure of frequency. The higher the frequency, the greater the increases must be for them to be heard as increases in pitch (Licklider, 1951). Nonetheless, frequency and pitch are related directly even though not linearly. In other words, when frequency increases, any pitch change heard will be an increase, not a decrease. This means that fundamental frequency, too, has a direct effect on pitch. Thus, fundamental frequency of voice can be regulated by the speaker as he listens to feedback of the pitch of his voice.

Production of vocal loudness. As with pitch, so with loudness we find a unidimensional parameter for production as well as perception. Again, although the relation is direct, it is not linear; subjective perception of loudness measured in *sones* on a ratio scale is not a linear dimension in relation to physical intensity of a sound. Subjective loudness varies with a number of conditions in addition to intensity. For instance, sounds at very high or very low frequencies require far more intensity than they do at 1,500 Hz to be heard as equally loud (Licklider, 1951). The fact remains, though, that a speaker can, by listening to loudness of his voice, control its intensity.

Production of vocal quality. Whereas pitch can be regulated along a unidimensional continuum from high to low, and loudness from soft to loud, no such easy solution is available for control of vocal quality. This characteristic has been a trial for speech pathologists. No one seems able to agree with anyone else on a description of what is meant by "voice quality," although the term generally refers to that aspect of quality that identifies the individual speaker. Confusion has proliferated over the years until we are now mired in a terminologic swamp. Nine texts in this field contain forty-three different terms for quality.

For much of this terminology we are indebted to voice teachers and elocutionists who, as specialists, have remarkable skill in achieving desired vocal production. Although they have described their subjective sensations accurately, they have tended to confuse psychologic perception with physiologic reality. Most of these voice professionals are not scientists. They are inclined to describe subjective vocal experience, such as where they feel the tone is being produced, with certainty that what they feel is the physiologic truth of the matter—hence such terms as "throaty," "nasal," "pectoral," "head," and "chest."

Most voice scientists, untutored in subtleties of vocal behavior, are apt to discount these subjective sensations as physiologic nonsense. They prefer acoustical and physiologic observations that can be measured. Both vocalists and scientists have a point, and the speech pathologist needs both: he needs scientific rigor, and he needs to know the subjective sensations by which vocal production can be guided.

Why is quality such a culprit? The basic reason is that its production is multidimensional, not unidimensional as are pitch and loudness. The majority of physiologic movements involved are below the level of direct awareness. Whereas glottal vibration rate stands in a direct (though not linear) relation to pitch, and intensity of glottal pulses to loudness, what production process stands in direct relation to perceived quality? None.

This is not to say that physiologic adjustments do not affect quality. To the contrary, it is influenced by the size and shape of the entire vocal tract, by the coupling effects of resonators as they interact with each other and with the larynx, and by the opening and closing rates of the glottis as it generates pulses to activate resonators. These and other physiologic processes contribute to quality in a variety of ways. Quality is a product of all of them. It cannot be assigned exclusively to any one of them.

That quality does not lie along a continuum probably contributes greatly to the abundance of terms that have mushroomed around it. Many represent efforts to generate opposite ends of a continuum: "tense-lax," "good-bad," "light-heavy," "thin-rich," etc.,

etc., etc. Each pair captures a segment of vocal quality, but none encapsulates the whole of it as "fundamental frequency" does pitch or "intensity" does loudness. Actually, the most exact system for specifying quality is the phonetic alphabet. Each phonetic symbol represents a different linguistic quality, so that whatever is meant by "voice quality" refers to some aspect of this attribute other than what is used for linguistic purposes.

Phonetic components of quality seem to be embedded acoustically for the most part in *frequency distribution of energy* (especially of the first two formants), and physiologically in pharyngeal, oral, and nasal areas of the vocal tract energized by either a voiced or voiceless breath stream. This suggests that the many nonlinguistic functions of "voice quality" must be carried acoustically by frequencies at which energy is distributed outside of the first two formants, as shown in Fig. 3-12. These functions may also be in phase relations among vibrating partials—as

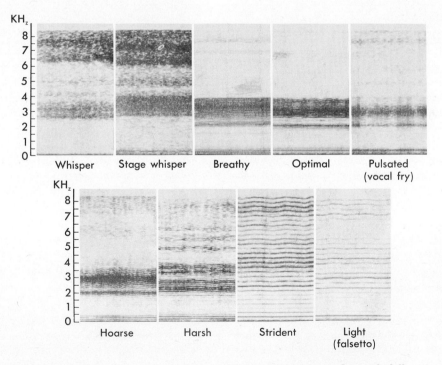

Fig. 3-12. Spectrograms of the same vowel produced by the same speaker with different vocal qualities. (From Perkins, W., Vocal function: a behavioral analysis. In Travis, L., [Ed.], *The Handbook of Speech Pathology and Audiology.* New York: Appleton-Century-Crofts [1971].)

well as in the rates at which energy in each glottal pulse is damped by resonators. This acoustical information is available from the wave form but not from a spectral analysis.

Conceiving of quality as the sound produced when all vocal dimensions are controlled simultaneously makes a manageable solution possible. With this approach, the question for the speech pathologist becomes: "What is the minimal set of behavioral dimensions that must be regulated to permit a speaker to achieve optimal quality for normal speech?" An adequate answer would provide a basis for solving a speaker's problems of vocal production. Furthermore, an adequate answer would require explicit vocal behavior that could be readily obtained, identified, and controlled.

Four independent dimensions, in addition to pitch and loudness, have emerged as basic to production of vocal quality: *voicing, vocal constriction, vocal mode,* and *vocal focus.* These behavioral dimensions should not be confused with their acoustical and physiologic correlates (Perkins, 1971a).

Voicing is regulated along a subjective continuum extending from the voicelessness of breathing, through whispering and various degrees of breathy production, to fully voiced tones that permit greatest vocal loudness. Physiologically, this continuum ranges from an adjustment with vocal cords abducted, permitting airflow through the glottis without vibration; through adducted adjustments that permit various combinations of airflow and vibration; to fully adducted adjustments in which all airflow is converted to glottal pulses by cord vibrations. Acoustically, the voicing continuum ranges from friction of voiceless airflow to the orderly arrangement of energy in the harmonic series of voiced tones. Because the fundamental vibratory portion of a vocal sound is analogous to alternating current, it is sometimes called the *ac* component. Similarly, continuous airflow is called the *dc* component by analogy to direct current. Thus voicing refers to behavioral management of the ac/dc balance of airflow.

Vocal constriction is the behavior by which the feeling of openness of the throat is regulated along a scale from open to closed. The open end is identified by the feeling of expansion at the peak of a yawn, the closed end by the feeling of constriction at the peak of a swallow. This term was chosen to describe *feeling* in the throat; it is not intended as a physiologic account of what actually happens. Physiologically, this continuum ranges from valvular constriction of true and false vocal folds, with the laryngeal inlet squeezed shut to prevent any air movement or sound, to the open condition, in which laryngeal and resonator adjustment facilitates rapid cord closure with each glottal cycle. For that matter, sensations of openness or closedness may prove to be correlated with inefficient resonator adjustments that impede glottal pulses much as West and Ansberry (1968) suggest.

Acoustically, the continuum ranges from the noise and weak intensity of constricted sounds to the focused intensity of unconstricted harmonic tones. If pressure waves from inefficiently tuned resonators reflected back to the glottis just as the vocal folds were being blown open by subglottal pressure, the two pressures would tend to cancel each other. Voice produced would be weak. To be heard, a speaker would be inclined to strain for greater loudness, thereby creating the condition of tension and tightness to which the closed feeling of constriction refers. Vocal power is impeded by constriction; as it increases, so does vocal inefficiency.

Vocal mode is the behavior by which the basic type of vocal adjustment is regulated. It differs as a dimension from pitch, loudness, voicing, constriction, and focus. It is basic to quality, but it does not involve a continuum. Rather, it is comprised of discrete classes, or *modes,* of vocalization within which the other independent dimensions function. Interactions among constriction, pitch, and loudness can be seen in relation to vocal mode (Fig. 3-13). The concept of modes is essentially the same as that of vocal *registers,* a term borrowed from the pipe organ and confused by an opaque mixture of pronouncements and observations of singers, elocutionists, laryngologists, and speech pathologists. Vocal mode is proposed as being more descriptive

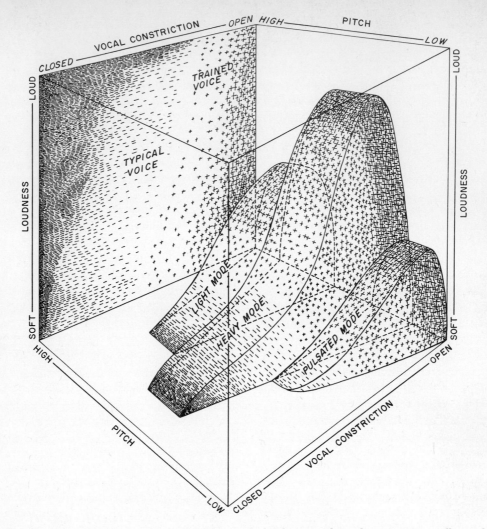

Fig. 3-13. Interactions among vocal mode, pitch, loudness, and vocal constriction. Effects of constriction in typical and trained voices are shown on the back wall and in each "shoe-shaped" vocal mode. (From Perkins, W., Vocal function: assessment and therapy. In Travis, L., [Ed.], *The Handbook of Speech Pathology and Audiology.* New York: Appleton-Century-Crofts [1971].)

of behavior. The mode permitting highest pitches is *light voice (falsetto)*, the most useful middle-pitch range is produced in *heavy voice (chest)*, and the lowest and most rarely used range involves *pulsated voice (glottal fry, or vocal fry)*. These modes can be identified in untrained voices, particularly of males, by the "break" between them (Mc-Glone and Brown, 1969).

Each mode has a distinctive quality and limits within which all other dimensions can be regulated. The name of each mode describes its quality. Heavy voice is used prob-ably by most men, women, and children because it provides the most socially useful pitch, loudness, and voicing ranges. Unfortunately, it also permits greatest vocal effort and constriction, the ingredients of vocal

---

Why do Hollien and his associates (1966) think that vocal fry (pulsated voice) is a separate register (mode)?

---

abuse. Although in trained voices other modes than these may be found that allow transit from lowest to highest pitches without a "break," such special modes are of more concern to voice coaches than speech pathologists (Vennard, 1967).

Physiologically, light voice is produced when the vocalis muscles are stretched, thinned, and used mainly to control pitch. Heavy voice is produced when the vocalis muscles are thicker and are used more to control loudness (Vennard, Hirano, and Ohala, 1970). Pulsated voice is produced by short, relaxed cords that close quickly and remain closed for a relatively long portion of each glottal cycle. Acoustically (Fig. 3-12), light voice permits the highest fundamental frequencies and has weak harmonic structure. Heavy voice permits the widest range of fundamental frequencies and intensities and the strongest harmonic structure. Pulsated voice permits only very low fundamental frequencies with complete decay of energy in each glottal pulse (Perkins, 1971b).

Vocal focus is the sensation associated with the placement of the tone in the head. It is the feeling of the location of the focal point of the tone. Although the singer, especially in controlling high pitches, is concerned with horizontal focus toward the front or back of the head, the speaker's concern, and ours, is mainly with vertical focus. At the low end of the focus continuum, the tone feels as though it is being squeezed out of the throat. At the high end, the tone seems to float in the head as though it were disconnected from the throat. Focus, like pitch, can be measured on a scale from low to high, but focus and pitch are distinctly separate dimensions of vocal production. Focus of the tone can be moved up or down without changing pitch. Similarly, pitch can be moved up or down without changing focus.

Vocal focus is the fundamental dimension by which professional vocalists, whether actors, announcers, or singers, align their voices (Vennard, 1967). In fact, in an electromyographic study of intrinsic and extrinsic laryngeal muscles used in singing, Vennard and Hirano (1971) used focus (defined as in this text) as the identifying characteristic for the normal singing voice. Interestingly, they found less muscular exertion for this normal voice with optimal focus than for any other type of phonation except breathy production —support for the concept that efficient production yields maximum output with minimal effort.

Vocal effort is a dependent dimension because, as the power supply for phonation, it necessarily interacts with independent vocal elements for control. It is the behavior by which respiratory force is scaled from low to high subglottal pressure. The low-pressure end of the continuum is typified by the effort required for quiet exhalation, the high-pressure end by that involved in lifting a heavy object. That changes in subglottal pressure are perceived as changes in vocal effort have been shown in physiologic investigations (Ladefoged, 1963; Ladefoged and McKinney, 1963; Netsell, 1973).

All aspects of speaking require vocal effort in some amount to produce the breath stream. Although vocal effort can be controlled independently for nonspeech activities, for phonation it depends on the extent to which other vocal elements require effort. When exerted beyond optimal requirements, it spills over unproductively into other dimensions. Greater effort than is needed for optimal loudness, for example, may show up in raised pitch, excessive breathiness, or, worse yet, unwanted vocally abusive constriction responses (Perkins, 1971b).

Vocal smoothness, also a dependent dimension, provides evidence of interaction among the other dimensions. It can be described along a continuum from smooth to rough and can be heard in any of the production dimensions, especially pitch. Roughness of pitch, called *pitch perturbation* and *jitter* in acoustical studies, has been found to result from various aspects of normal phonation, but it is mainly a sign of laryngeal pathology (Beckett, 1969; Perkins, 1975; Lieberman, 1961, 1963; Koike, 1967; Coleman and Wendahl, 1967).

Speech-flow processes: suprasegmental analysis

Whereas an articulatory analysis is a segmental analysis in which phonemic targets for speech production are identified, analysis of speech as it flows from phone to phone, syllable to syllable, phrase to phrase, and sentence to sentence is *suprasegmental*. Behavioral dimensions of speech-flow include *sequence, duration, rate, rhythm,* and *fluency*. Let us look first at how temporal effects of these characteristics are perceived, and then at how they are produced.

Temporal effects in speech perception

Sequence. Determination of phonemic sequence in speech depends on ability to determine temporal order. This ability is dependent on the time required by the nervous system to process acoustical stimuli of speech into phonemic segments. Arrangement of sounds in proper linguistic sequence is essential to acceptable pronunciation.

Duration. Phonetic duration of sounds contributes mainly to syllable stress in words and also to perception of phonemes. For example, the longer a vowel is held, the more stress the syllable containing it will carry, as when stress falls on the first in contrast with the second syllable of the word "object." Not only does stress determine whether this word functions as noun or verb, but it also determines the vowel produced in the first syllable: with stress, the vowel is "ah" (/a/), without stress, "uh" (/ə/). Likewise, duration of the vowel can determine perception of ambiguous consonants following it: "hat" is heard when the vowel is short, "had" when it is long, provided the final consonants are indistinct. As with so much of speech, phonetic duration is perceived in psychologic time that does not necessarily match acoustical time (Huggins, 1969).

Except for stressed vowels and silences longer than 0.3 second, relative durations of phonetic elements required for intelligible speech are quite inflexible. The only point of much phonemic flexibility is in duration of vowels in stressed syllables: they can be clipped as in "Walter Winchell" style, or prolonged as in a drawl. Similar latitude is permitted silent intervals longer than 0.3 second that are heard as pauses (as distinct from phonetic elements). Purposeful or not, they can be of almost any length. If purposeful they serve the syntactic functions of juncture in sentences, or they may serve for dramatic

effect. If they occur other than between clauses, they will be heard as unexpected hesitations, presumably indicating that the speaker has paused to collect his thoughts (Scott, 1965; Diehl, White, and Burk, 1959).

Rate. The rate of speech can be measured in several units; phonemes, syllables, and words are most frequently used. These rates reflect phonetic duration of silence as well as sound. Except for the tendency of articulation to be slurred and the control of speech-flow to disintegrate when maximum rate is exceeded, rate can be freely responsive to the nature of the communicative situation and to the psychologic condition of the speaker (Black, 1961; Scott, 1965).

How did Fairbanks (1966) manage to compress and expand speech without changing the pitch of the speaker's voice?

Phonetic and syllabic rate can be *expanded* or *compressed* considerably, if relative duration of phonetic elements is preserved. Effects on comprehension of expanding speech by prolonging vowels can be seen in song. That any comprehension is preserved is remarkable, considering how much the normal relations of vowel/consonant durations are distorted in singing. Much more research has been devoted to compressing speech than to expanding it. By keeping pitch and relative duration of phonetic elements reasonably normal, Fairbanks (1966) found that comprehension loss was slight when message time was compressed by 50%, thereby doubling an original speaking rate from 141 words per minute (wpm) to 282 wpm. Nonetheless, 50% compressed speech is far more difficult to understand (Zemlin, Daniloff, and Shriner, 1968). When compression was increased to 60% (353 wpm), comprehension dropped by one half.

Word rate, by contrast with phonetic and syllabic rate, permits wide variation in length of pauses between words. Comprehension and speech quality were unaffected in an experiment in which the speaking rate was artificially altered from 126 to 172 wpm merely by shortening or lengthening pauses (Diehl,

White, and Burk, 1959). Because a speaker has so much freedom to use pauses of any length between words, measures of word rate offer little assurance that they reflect a speaker's articulatory rate. A person could utter rapidly articulated words separated by long pauses and produce a very slow word rate but an extremely rapid phonetic and syllabic rate.

Rhythm. In speech, *rhythm* is the timing pattern of phonetic elements. When this timing is applied to syllables and words as they are organized into phrases, we have what can be considered as *language rhythm*—what we usually think of as the rhythm of speech. It provides cadence and is most pronounced in poetry. But *segmental rhythm* of phonetic units that make up syllables can also be described. This type of rhythm is closely related to fluency. It also contributes to differentiation of meaning of words, as for example in the two phrases: "ten scows" and "tense cows."

Neither type of rhythm plays a major role in the linguistic organization of speech; yet rhythm is a universal characteristic of speech. Perhaps it is pervasive for the same reason that it exists in all complex activities. It may reflect the natural tendency to organize motor behavior into patterned movements. Random muscular contractions are all but impossible to control. When they are grouped for speech, they are made manageable as syllables and phrases (Netsell, 1973).

Fluency. The suprasegmental dimension of fluency is perhaps the most subtle, yet vital, aspect of speech flow for the speech pathologist. It has to do with how smoothly sounds, syllables, words, and phrases are joined together. The issue of fluency rarely affects intelligibility, except perhaps to improve it with inadvertent repetitions of segments of the message. Probably the speaker does not live who is not *disfluent* at times, whether by repetition of phrases, syllables, words, or sounds. Who has not said "uh," the all-American sound of minds slipping into neutral in the midst of a statement? Possibly because comprehension is not endangered when larger units of speech are produced disflu-

ently, and because repetitions of words and hesitations between them are so typical of speakers as they "back and fill" their way through an idea, society is most tolerant of fluency lapses of this type. Conversely, intolerance is great for disfluency on sounds and syllables. Whatever the reason, the fact remains that society is much more severe in its judgment of the speaker who struggles to speak a word than of one who struggles to find it. What the former does is considered stuttering, whereas the latter is normal.

Temporal effects in speech production
Speech-flow constraints. Speech-flow behavior that is achieved in normal speech must lie within the capacity of the vast majority of speakers. What are physiologic limits that constrain the temporal dimensions? Sequential limits are bounded by permissible sound combinations (for example, /zsŋrf/ never occurs in English). On the other hand, one can construct an infinite number of utterances with a finite number of speech sound sequences. Another restriction is that speech not flow so fast that the sequence of phones cannot be detected, but few speakers can approach this limit for normal listeners.

Duration of voiced sounds is constrained only on the side of brevity by glottal pulse length and auditory ability to resolve time. The vocal tract must be energized with at least one glottal pulse before the quality of the sound can be detected, an event that could be just a millisecond (msec) or two in duration. At least two pulses are essential to detect pitch, an event requiring 2 to 20 msec. Curiously, 2 msec is the minimum time that two sounds must be separated to detect that more than one has been heard; 20 msec is the minimum needed to determine the order in which two sounds have been heard (Hirsh, 1959, 1966, 1967; Hirsh and Sherrick, 1961). Considering normal speech performance, physiologic constraints on duration impose few practical limits.

Rate, on the other hand, is limited sharply by the physiologic capacity to move articulators: in syllabic movements per second, the tongue tip could manage 8.2, the jaw 7.3, the

How do these rates compare with those reported by Fairbanks and Spriestersbach (1950) for oral structures?

back of the tongue 7.1, the velum and lower lip 6.7 (Hudgins and Stetson, 1937). These speeds come much closer to matching syllabic than phonetic rates; phonemes normally flow about fourteen per second. Again, the problem is how high-speed speech can be produced with low-speed equipment.

Whether or not rhythm has physiologic constraints is a moot question. Since everything in nature seems to have rhythm, speech being no exception, it undoubtedly has a physiologic basis. Abercrombie (1965) maintains that rhythm of speech is determined by interaction of rhythms of two respiratory pulse systems. One is the rapidly recurring *breath-pulse* that Stetson identified years ago as the basic motor unit of the syllable around which speech is produced. The second system consists, presumably, of less frequent pulselike chest movements that coincide periodically with breath-pulses to produce *stress-pulses*. The fact that all words are composed of syllables and that stress may fall on different words in a sentence makes Abercrombie's explanation of why different languages have different rhythms intriguing: both pulse systems operate when any language is spoken, but languages coordinate interaction of these pulses differently, English being stress-timed, and French, syllable-timed.

Finally we come to fluency, a dimension that seems to be a barometer for the entire speech system. Its limits are apparently set by adequacy of performance of the other dimensions of speech. "Perfect" fluency is possible only when all aspects of speech function "perfectly." Semantically, when one must search for an idea or the right word to express it, fluency is disrupted. Syntactically, when a thought is pursued to a grammatical "dead end," fluency is disrupted. Morphemically, when use of the wrong verb form, for example, is corrected, fluency is disrupted. Phonemically, when a mispronunciation is corrected, fluency is disrupted. Prosodically, when a stress or inflection is altered to correct a nuance of meaning, fluency is disrupted. All these disfluencies represent corrections of performance based on feedback of linguistic output. All these disfluencies are normal and acceptable.

But, when rate of speech shortens phonetic duration requirements so much that rate exceeds ability to control articulatory movements, the resulting disfluency is apt to seem abnormal and unacceptable. As the speaker utilizes various levels of linguistic feedback to correct utterance of an idea, so, too, he uses speech sound initiation feedback to correct movements of his articulators. Exactly how these phonetic movements are monitored, though, is still a puzzle despite extensive studies of effects on speech of *delayed auditory feedback* (Lee, 1950; Fairbanks, 1955; Fairbanks and Guttman, 1958; Chase and others, 1961). These studies consistently show that when a speaker's voice is delayed (with special equipment) in reaching his ear, speech tends to become disorganized: pitch and loudness increase, articulatory errors occur, and stutterlike behavior appears. These disruptions are maximal in adults when the delay is about 200 msec.

MacKay (1968) has come closest to a definitive exploration of how speech production is monitored by ear. He has shown that, by and large, children have slower maximum speaking rates than do adults; children also require longer auditory delays for maximum disruption of speech. The obvious connection is that maximally disruptive auditory delay increases as speech rate decreases. But this obvious connection is wrong. Adults are still disrupted most at 200 msec delay, regardless of how much they slow down. What proves to be the important limit for fluency is maximal speech rate. Irrespective of age, the slower the maximum rate, the longer the delay required for maximum disruption, and the greater the tendency for delay to produce a stuttering effect. On the other hand, when the rate is reduced voluntarily, the tendency that delay has to disrupt speech is reduced. Thus whatever factors limit maximum speech rate are linked to articulatory disfluencies.

The answers—résumé

1. What are the linguistic and psychologic dimensions of language processes?

In broadest outline, speech is composed of cognitive language processes and explicit speaking processes. Semantically, language utilizes consensually validated symbols, words, that denote objective meaning of the referent and connote subjective meaning of the associated concept. Acquisition and modification of word meaning is an aspect of language that psychology, with its principles of learning, can explain with reasonable success.

Grammatically, language is a formal system for signaling relations, basically between a subject idea and a predicate idea. The structure of language is built with a few dozen phonemic speech sound units that can change word meaning, and morphemic units with which meaningful words are constructed. Words are arranged according to syntactic rules to signal the fundamental relation between subject and predicate complete with discriminative modifications.

A psychologic explanation of grammar with known principles of learning is a relatively dubious venture. How to account for all cultures' having a language, for the basic similarity in structure and functions of all natural languages, for the exclusive ability of all normal children to learn immensely involved rules of the language they hear, for the human ability to generate novel innovative, statements, for the ability to transform essentially the same idea into any number of grammatical statements or to translate it into any language—these are thorny issues before which behavioral explanations falter. The speech pathologist can modify behavior that he can identify explicitly, but the essence of language is learned with acquisition of covert linguistic rules that can be observed only in speaking and writing effects.

2. What are the behavioral dimensions of speaking processes?

The surface structure of language is revealed through speaking processes. Explicit as phonetic behavior is, its relation to phonemic units of language is still puzzling and obscure. The speaking processes can be observed, measured, and controlled in three broad dimensions: phonatory processes of breath stream control, articulatory-resonatory processes of sound modulation, and speech-flow processes of phonetic movements from sound to sound.

Phonatory processes have to do with physiologic adjustments by which a voiced or voiceless breath stream is controlled for sounds that the vocal tract modulates by articulation-resonance. Vocal production of pitch, loudness, and quality that will meet all the linguistic and nonlinguistic functions of voice can be described in terms of six independent dimensions (pitch, loudness, voicing, vocal constriction, vocal focus, and vocal mode) and two dependent dimensions (vocal effort and vocal smoothness).

Articulatory-resonatory processes have to do with physiologic adjustments of the vocal tract that modulate acoustical characteristics of sound that the listener perceives as phonemes. Phonemic targets guide the speaker as he moves his articulators from one position to the next for production of distinctively different sounds.

Speech-flow processes can be observed and regulated in terms of sequence, duration, rate, rhythm, and fluency. Since sequence of sounds determines phonemic order, and hence pronunciation of words, it permits little freedom for variation from speech standards of the community. Except for duration of stressed vowels, duration of other phonetic segments of sound and silence contributes to perception of phonemes, so that a speaker's control of phonetic duration is prescribed by articulatory requirements for intelligible speech. Since rate of speech is not directly responsible for any aspect of intelligibility, it permits wide flexibility, even though it is sharply limited physiologically by the rate at which oral articulators can move. Rhythm is the timing pattern of phonetic elements. When applied to phonetic units that make up syllables, it is segmental rhythm. For syllables and words as they are organized into phrases, it is language rhythm. Fluency of speech carries no linguistic burden; yet it is a barometer for the entire speech system. Disfluencies that are for correction or planning of semantic, syntactic, morphemic, phonemic, or prosodic aspects of one's utterance are usually normal and acceptable. Disfluencies that reflect inability to control articulatory movements are deemed abnormal and unacceptable.

REFERENCES

Abercrombie, D., *Studies in Phonetics and Linguistics.* London: Oxford University Press (1965).

Allen, H., and others, *New Dimensions in English.* New York: McCormick-Mathers Publishing Co., Inc. (1966).

Beckett, R., Pitch perturbation as a function of subjective vocal constriction. *Folia Phoniatrica,* **21,** 416-425 (1969).

Black, J., Relationships among fundamental frequency, vocal sound pressure, and rate of speaking. *Language and Speech,* **4,** 196-199 (1961).

Braine, M., On learning the grammatical order of words. *Psychol. Rev.,* **70,** 323-348 (1963).

Brown, R., and Berko, J., Word association and the acquisition of grammar. *Child Developm.,* **31,** 1-14 (1960).

Brown, R., and Lenneberg, E., A study in language and cognition. *J. abnorm. soc. Psychol.,* **49,** 454-462 (1954).

Cairns, C., and Williams, F., Language. In Minifie, F., Hixon, T., and Williams, F. (Eds.), *Normal Aspects of Speech, Hearing, and Language.* Englewood Cliffs, N.J.: Prentice-Hall, Inc. (1973).

Chase, R., and others, A developmental study of changes in behavior under delayed auditory feedback. *J. genet. Psychol.,* **99,** 101-112 (1961).

Cherry, C., *On Human Communication.* New York: John Wiley & Sons, Inc. (1957).

Chomsky, N., *Syntactic Structures.* The Hague: Mouton Publishers (1957).

Chomsky, N., Verbal behavior. *Language,* **35,** 26-58 (1959).

Chomsky, N., *Language and Mind.* New York: Harcourt, Brace & World (1968).

Coleman, R., and Wendahl, R., Vocal roughness and stimulus duration. *Speech Monogr.,* **34,** 85-92 (1967).

Daniloff, R., Normal articulation processes. In Minifie, F., Hixon, T., and Williams, F. (Ed.), *Normal Aspects of Speech, Hearing, and Language.* Englewood Cliffs, N.J.: Prentice-Hall, Inc. (1973).

Darley, F., *Diagnosis and Appraisal of Communication Disorders.* Englewood Cliffs, N.J.: Prentice-Hall, Inc. (1964).

Denes, P., and Pinson, E., *The Speech Chain.* Murray Hill, N.J.: Bell Telephone Laboratories (1963).

Diehl, C., White, R., and Burk, K., Rate and communication. *Speech Monogr.,* **26,** 229-232 (1959).

Fairbanks, G., Systematic research in experimental phonetics. 1. A theory of the speech mechanism as a servosystem. *J. Speech Hearing Dis.,* **19,** 133-139 (1954).

Fairbanks, G., Selective vocal effects of delayed auditory feedback. *J. Speech Hearing Dis.,* **20,** 333-346 (1955).

Fairbanks, G., Experimental phonetics: selected articles. Urbana: University of Illinois Press (1966).

Fairbanks, G., and Guttman, N., Effects of delayed auditory feedback upon articulation. *J. Speech Hearing Res.,* **1,** 12-22 (1958).

Fairbanks, G., and Spriestersbach, D., A study of minor organic deviations in "functional" disorders of articulation. 1. Rate of movement of oral structures. *J. Speech Hearing Dis.,* **15,** 60-69 (1950).

Geschwind, N., Neurological foundations of language. In Myklebust, H. (Ed.), *Progress in Learning Disabilities* (Vol. 1). New York: Grune & Stratton (1968).

Gleason, H., *An Introduction to Descriptive Linguistics.* New York: Holt, Rinehart & Winston, Inc. (1961).

Gould, J., *Honey Bee Recruitment: the Dance-Language Controversy.* Science, **189,** 685-693 (1975).

Guilford, J., *The Nature of Human Intelligence.* New York: McGraw-Hill Book Co. (1967).

Heffner, R., *General Phonetics.* Madison: University of Wisconsin Press (1950).

Hirsch, I., Auditory perception of temporal order. *J. acoust. Soc. Am.,* **31,** 759-767 (1959).

Hirsh, I., Audition in relation to perception of speech. In Carterette, E. (Ed.), *Brain Function,* III. Speech, language, and communication, UCLA Forum in Medical Sciences No. 4. Los Angeles, University of California Press (1966).

Hirsh, I., Information processing in input channels for speech and language: the significance of serial order of stimuli. In Millikan, C., and Darley, F. (Ed.), *Brain Mechanisms Underlying Speech and Language.* New York: Grune & Stratton, Inc. (1967).

Hirsh, I., and Sherrick, C., Perceived order in different sense modalities. *J. expe. Psychol.*, **62**, 423-432 (1961).

Hollien, H., and others, On the nature of vocal fry. *J. Speech Hearing Res.*, **9**, 245-247 (1966).

Hudgins, C., and Stetson, R., Relative speed of articulatory movements. Arch. Neeanderl. Phonét. Expéri., **13**, 85-94 (1937).

Huggins, A., Just-noticeable differences for phoneme duration in natural speech (abstract). *J. acoust. Soc. Am.*, **46**, 115 (1969).

Jakobson, R., Fant, G., and Halle, M., *Preliminaries to Speech Analysis*. Technical Report No. 13. Cambridge: Acoustics Laboratory, Massachusetts Institute of Technology (1952).

Johnson, N., Linguistic models and functional units of language behavior. In Rosenberg, S. (Ed.), *Directions in Psycholinguistics*. New York: The Macmillan Co. (1965).

Joos, M., Acoustic phonetics. *Language Monogr.*, vol. 24 (1948).

Koike, Y., Experimental studies on vocal attack. *Pract. Otolog. Kyoto*, **60**, 663-668 (1967).

Kolers, P., Bilingualism and information processing. *Scient. Am.*, **218**, 78-86 (1968).

Kolers, P., It loses something in the translation. *Psychology Today*, **2**, 32-35 (1969).

Krauss, R., Language as a symbolic process in communication. *Am. Scient.*, **56**, 265-278 (1968).

Ladefoged, P., Elements of acoustic phonetics. Chicago: University of Chicago Press (1962).

Ladefoged, P., Some physiologic parameters in speech. *Language and Speech*, **6**, 109-119 (1963).

Ladefoged, P., and McKinney, N., Loudness, sound pressure, and subglottal pressure in speech. *J. acoust. Soc. Am.*, **35**, 454-460 (1963).

Lane, H., The motor theory of speech perception: a critical review. *Psychol. Rev.*, **72**, 275-309 (1965)

Langer, S., *Philosophy in a New Key*. New York: Mentor Books (1951).

Lee, B., Effects of delayed speech feedback. *J. acoust. Soc. Am.*, **22**, 824-826 (1950).

Liberman, A., and others, Perception of the speech code. *Psychol. Rev.*, **74**, 431-461 (1967).

Licklider, J., Basic correlates of the auditory stimulus. In Stevens, S. (Ed.), *Handbook of Experimental Psychology*. New York: John Wiley & Sons, Inc. (1951).

Lieberman, P., Perturbations in vocal pitch. *J. acoust. Soc. Am.*, **33**, 597-603 (1961).

Lieberman, P., Some acoustic measures of the fundamental periodicity of normal and pathologic larynges. *J. acoust. Soc. Am.*, **35**, 344-353 (1963).

Lilly, J., *Man and Dolphin*. Worlds of science. New York: Pyramid Publications, Inc. (1962).

Luria, A., *Human Brain and Psychological Processes*. New York: Harper & Row, Publishers (1966).

Luria, A., *The Working Brain*. New York: Basic Books, Inc. (1973).

MacKay, D., Metamorphosis of a critical interval: age-linked changes in the delay in auditory feedback that produces maximal disruption of speech. *J. acoust. Soc. Am.*, **43**, 811-821 (1968).

Matthews, J., Communication disorders in the mentally retarded. In Travis, L. (Ed.), *Handbook of Speech Pathology and Audiology*. New York: Appleton-Century-Crofts (1971).

McGlone, R., and Brown, W., Identification of "shift" between vocal registers. *J. acoust. Soc. Am.*, **46**, 1033-1036 (1969).

McKinney, N., *Laryngeal Frequency Analysis for Linguistic Research*. Communication Sciences Laboratory Report No. 14. Ann Arbor, University of Michigan (1965).

Menyuk, P., and Anderson, S., Children's identification and reproduction of /w/, /r/, and /l/. *J. Speech Hearing Res.*, **12**, 39-52 (1969).

Mermelstein, P., Determination of the vocal-tract shape from measured formant frequencies. *J. acoust. Soc. Am.*, **41**, 1283-1294 (1967).

Miller, G., Information and memory. *Scient. Am.*, **195**, 42-46 (1956).

Miller, G., Some psychological studies of grammar. *Am. Psychol.*, **17**, 748-762 (1962).

Mowrer, O., The psychologist looks at language. *Am. Psychol.*, **9**, 660-694 (1954).

Netsell, R., Speech physiology. In Minifie, F., Hixon, T., and Williams, F. (Eds.), *Normal Aspects of Speech, Hearing, and Language*. Englewood Cliffs, N.J.: Prentice-Hall, Inc. (1973).

O'Connor, J., Recent work in English phonetics. In Saporta, S. (Ed.), *Psycholinguistics*. New York: Holt, Rinehart & Winston, Inc. (1961).

Osgood, C., *Method and Theory in Experimental Psychology*. New York: Oxford Book Co., Inc. (1953).

Osgood, C., Suci, G., and Tannenbaum, P., *The measurement of Meaning*. Urbana: University of Illinois Press (1957).

Perkins, W., Vocal function: a behavioral analysis. In Travis, L. (Ed.), *Handbook of Speech Pathology and Audiology*. New York: Appleton-Century-Crofts (1971a).

Perkins, W., Vocal function: assessment and therapy. In Travis, L. (Ed.), *Handbook of Speech Pathology and Audiology*. New York, Appleton-Century-Crofts (1971b).

Perkins, W., Normal vocal tone generation; detection, diagnosis, and management of abnormal vocal tone generation. In Tower, D. (Ed.), *The Nervous System*. (Vol. 3): *Human Communication and Its Disorders*. New York: Raven Press (1975).

Perkins, W., and Curlee, R., Causality in speech pathology. *J. Speech Hearing Dis.*, **34**, 231-238 (1969).

Peterson, G., Parameters of vowel quality. *J. Speech Hearing Res.*, **4**, 10-29 (1961).

Peterson, G., and Fairbanks, G., Speech and hearing science. *Asha*, **5**, 539-543 (1963).

Peterson, G., and Shoup, J., The elements of an acoustic phonetic theory. *J. Speech Hearing Res.*, **9**, 68-99 (1966a).

Peterson, G., and Shoup, J., A physiological theory of phonetics. *J. Speech Hearing Res.*, **9**, 5-67 (1966b).

Premack, D., The education of Sarah. *Psychology Today*, **4**, 54-58 (1970).

Reddy, D., Computer recognition of connected speech. *J. acoust. Soc. Am.*, **42**, 329-347 (1967).

Robb, J., The hidden philosophical agenda: a commentary on humanistic psychology. *J. Am. Acad. Relig.*, **37**, (1) (1969).

Royce, J., *The Encapsulated Man*. Princeton, N.J.: Van Nostrand Reinhold Co. (1964).

Saporta, S., Psycholinguistics: a book of readings. New York: Holt, Rinehart & Winston, Inc. (1961).

Saporta, S., and others, Grammatical models and language learning. In Rosenberg, S. (Ed.), *Directions in Psycholinguistics*. New York: The Macmillan Co. (1965).

Schiefelbusch, R., Language studies of mentally retarded children. *J. Speech Hearing Dis.*, Monograph Supplement No. 10 (1963).

Schroeder, M., Determination of the geometry of the human vocal tract by acoustic measurements. *J. acoust. Soc. Am.*, **41**, 1002-1010 (1967).

Scott, R., *Temporal Effects in Speech Analysis and Synthesis*. Communication Sciences Laboratory Report No. 15. Ann Arbor: University of Michigan (1965).

Shannon, C., and Weaver, W., *The Mathematical Theory of Communication*. Urbana: University of Illinois Press (1964).

Skinner, B., *Verbal Behavior*. New York: Appleton-Century-Crofts (1957).

Smith, W., Messages of vertebrate communications. *Science*, **165**, 145-150 (1969).

Spreen, O., Language functions in mental retardation: a review. I. Language development, types of retardation, and intelligence level. *Am. J. ment. Defic.*, **69**, 482-494 (1965a).

Spreen, O., Language functions in mental retardation: a review. II. Language in higher level performance. *Am. J. ment. Defic.*, **70**, 351-362 (1965b).

Staats, A., *Learning, Language, and Cognition*. New York: Holt, Rinehart & Winston, Inc. (1968).

Stetson, R., *Motor Phonetics*. Amsterdam: North-Holland Publishing Co. (1951).

Sullivan, H., *The Interpersonal Theory of Psychiatry*. New York: W. W. Norton & Co., Inc. (1953).

Tiffany, W., Nonrandom sources of variation in vowel quality. *J. Speech Hearing Res.*, **2**, 305-317 (1959).

Vennard, W., *Singing: the Mechanism and the Technic*. New York: Carl Fischer, Inc. (1967).

Vennard, W., and Hirano, M. Varieties of voice production. *NATS Bull.*, **27**, 26-32 (1971).

Vennard, W., Hirano, M., and Ohala, J., Chest, head, and falsetto. *NATS Bull.*, **27**, 30-37 (1970).

Von Frisch, K., *Bees, Their Vision, Chemical Senses, and Language*. Ithaca, N.Y.: Cornell University Press (1950).

Wenner, A., Wells, P., and Johnson, D., Honey bee recruitment to food sources: olfaction or language? *Science*, **164**, 84-86 (1969).

West, R., and Ansberry, M., *The rehabilitation of Speech*. New York: Harper & Row, Publishers (1968).

Whorf, B., *Language, Thought, and Reality*. Cambridge: The M.I.T. Press (1956).

Wickelgren, W., Auditory or articulatory coding in verbal short-term memory. *Psychol. Rev.*, **76**, 232-235 (1969).

Wiener, N., *Cybernetics*. New York: John Wiley & Sons, Inc. (1948).

Winitz, H., The development of speech and language in the normal child. In Rieber, R., and Brubaker, R. (Eds.), *Speech Pathology*. Amsterdam: North-Holland Publishing Co. (1966).

Williams, W., and Cairns, H., Linguistic performance. In Minifie, F., Hixon, T., and Williams, F. (Eds.), *Normal Aspects of Speech, Hearing, and Language*. Englewood Cliffs, N.J.: Prentice-Hall, Inc. (1973).

Zemlin, W., Daniloff, R., and Shriner, T., The difficulty of listening to time-compressed speech. *J. Speech Hearing Res.*, **11**, 875-881 (1968).

Chapter 4

Development of speech

Questions

1. What are the origins of speech?
2. How does voice develop?
3. How does language develop?
4. How does articulation develop?
5. What factors contribute to speech development?

ORIGINS OF SPEECH

The puzzlements of speech and language are abundant. As Sapir (1921) pointed out years ago, language, unlike walking, is not instinctual. It does not develop normally without benefit of socialization within a culture. Yet, it is universal; over 3,000 languages are known (Fig. 4-1). No tribe has been found that does not have a fully developed language. A tribe may be primitive, but its system for speaking never is (Hoijer, 1966). The lowliest headhunter can have a more richly elaborated and perfected formal arrangement for symbolizing his ideas—crude as they may be—and for relating them one to the other than the most sophisticated literary

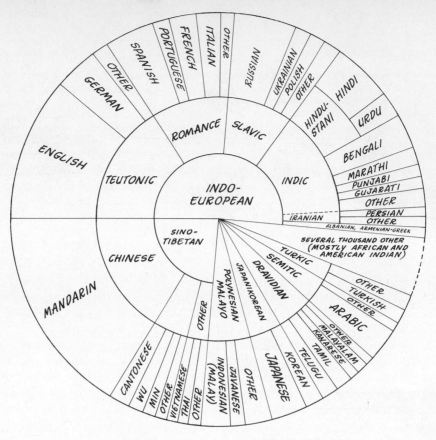

Fig. 4-1. Major languages of the world.

critic or atomic scientist. Sapir concluded from the universality and diversity of languages that they comprise probably the oldest, most ancient heritage of the human race.

What are the origins of language? The linguistic landscape was so littered with speculative answers at the turn of the century that the Linguistic Society of Paris barred further discussion of the question. Characteristics of these ill-begotten notions can be detected in the "ding-dong" theory, the "bow-wow" theory,* and similar explanations of the origins of speech. Perhaps a de-

finitive answer will never be found. Still, we are creatures of evolution, and the question prevails: "Why don't animals speak?" The usual answer—"Because they have nothing to say"—is clearly wrong. Animals have much to say, and they have elaborate signal systems for saying it, as any astute observer can attest—but they do not speak. Evidence of precursors of language should be available in our nearest zoologic brethren on the phylogenetic scale. It would be instructive, especially for speech pathologists with their responsibility for defective communication, to have some idea of the rudimentary skills from which speech and language evolved. An understanding of our linguistic origins would provide a frame of reference for assessing severely handicapped persons whose abilities are below the scales available for measuring speech.

---

*These theories posit a direct connection between the symbol and its referent: the "ding-dong" theory (dating back to Plato) says that speech resonates nature; hence, the first time man saw a cat, a bell rang in his mind and he said *cat*. The "bow-wow" theory is an inelegant nickname for the onomatopoetic theory, which says that words developed as echoes of the sounds of nature.

Compare this idea with that of Premack and Schwartz (1966), who conceive of the possibility of a phylogenetic scale of language development, with each species fitting into such a crude scale at some level of grammatical complexity. Then, following the old dictum, "Ontogeny recapitulates phylogeny," the human child's course of language development could be plotted along this phylogenetic scale.

Man's brain: a symbolic transformer

Suzanne Langer (1951) reasoned that evolution of a symbolic communication system could not be explained on the grounds that man "discovered" his need for speech. Aside from the logical trap of assuming his discovery of need for an ability about which he knew nothing, she pointed out that if man's purpose had been to meet his biologic needs, a more inappropriate skill than language could not have been found. With symbolic communication have come taboos and inhibitions of socialization. Rather than facilitating satisfaction of biologic needs, sex and elimination being prime examples, these functions are inhibited. Animals have greater freedom of biologic expression than does man with his elaborate speech system.

Clearly, the universality of speech attests to its serving some basic function for man. If not biologic needs, then what? Langer's answer has not been demonstrated conclusively, but it has the rightness of elegant simplicity: man's brain is a symbol-producing mechanism; the nature of its function is to transform sensory experience into ideational symbols. This answer is remarkably similar to that being offered by psycholinguists two decades later. They now agree that language does not depend on being intelligent or having a large brain; it depends on having a brain that makes human types of cognition possible. In short, language depends on being human.

This process of symbolic transformation of experience that Langer describes is carried on constantly. According to this view, we have access to knowledge of the world after it has been filtered through ideational processes. (More direct access apparently requires such mystical forms of experiencing

as are found in eastern religions, Zen Buddhism being a popular example.) Her point is that speech is but one manifestation of this continuous symbolizing process, others being art, music, ritual, religion, and the like. Give man his symbol-producing brain and his proclivity to live socially in tribes, and inevitably his symbols will become organized into a communication system in which particular symbols will have particular meanings within the culture—a tidy explanation of why language is universal yet widely divergent in form from culture to culture.

Again, Langer's idea foreshadows the current conception that language has a base structure of cognitive processes with which meaning is given to experience. Man is the only creature, according to this view, who can generate an overt expression in speech of this deep semantic structure. A growing body of evidence indicates, however, that man can no longer be considered an exclusive user of language symbols for communication. The Gardeners' chimpanzee, Washoe, if he used all of his 130 signs, could generate over 3 million four-word sentences. More remarkably, honeybees routinely use 40 million dance "sentences" symbolically to communicate information about distance, direction, type, quality, and odor of pollen. Lest we be carried away with these newly discovered language abilities of lower animals, let us reaffirm man's superiority over his nearest competitors. With a 10,000-word vocabulary he can generate 10^{22} seven-word sentences, not to mention the longer and shorter sentences of which he is capable (Gould, 1975).

None of these arguments and none of the evidence demonstrate conclusively how language evolved, or even that it did evolve. Yet we are in much the same position as the prizefighter in a *New Yorker* cartoon some years ago, who, looking at his gorilla-like opponent, said: "I won't fight 'til I hear him talk." Only man speaks. The question is why he alone in the animal kingdom is so blessed. We must assume that he has developed over the ages an innate capacity to acquire speech. How he came to develop this capacity has been explored by Lieberman (1973).

As Lenneberg (1967) concluded after weighing evidence from anatomy, physiology, genetics, embryology, neurology, linguistics, and psychology, the processes by which natural languages come about are deeply rooted in man's unique biology. He arrives at this innate capacity through biologic evolution—natural selection has provided a single direction for change: toward an increased ability to symbolize and organize experience. Still, it is speech as a vehicle of language that is unique to man. Yet speech may have evolved independently of language, and its peculiarities may not be as profound as we once believed (Cutting and Kavanagh, 1975; Mattingly, 1975).

How speech does not develop

The need myth. Before we attempt to understand how a child does learn speech, we had best lay some myths to rest. The first misconception is that children must be motivated to learn to speak. It is a manifestation of the myth that the child discovers that he must develop speech to communicate his needs more effectively—according to this notion he acquires it for utility purposes. Parents of late talkers are often admonished: "Make him ask for what he wants, and then he'll learn to talk." Translated, this is another way of saying: "Motivate him."

Sensible as the idea may seem that a child who does not need to speak never will, it has no evidence to support it. In fact, both evidence (circumstantial as it is) and reason point in the opposite direction. For one thing, a 1- to 2-year-old toddler would have to discover that he has some cravings that he cannot persuade his mother to satisfy by communicating his wants with gesturing, yelling, and crying. Add to this unlikely discovery the fact that he deciphers his parent's language code by age 2, and the concept of "motivating" speech acquisition looks more like the road to frustration than to language learning. Lenneberg (1966), however, has offered the most crushing argument. If a child acquired speech because he "needs" it, parents of every normal child throughout the world would have to conspire to motivate their children to respond to some indeterminate need for speech and then to discover the key to the adult language code—all within a few months between ages 1 and 2!

The babbling myth. Another common misconception is that speech develops progressively from reflexive crying through babbling and jargon to echolalia and first words. Granted, these different stages in a child's developing vocal performance can be detected and described. To the casual listener, the child may sound as if he is improving with practice. Actually, the only aspect of speech imitated during babbling that improves much with practice is the melody, the intonation patterns. Neither practice, imitation, nor babbling have much to do with the beginnings of meaningful speech.

How does McNeill (1966) explain the origin of speech? Does he agree with Brown and Bellugi (1964) about the role of imitation in speech acquisition?

In the first place, as Church (1961) has pointed out, babbled sounds that children spend endless hours practicing are essentially the same the world over. This is to say that the sounds (not the melodic patterns) babbled by a London infant and a Peking infant will bear far more resemblance to each other than to adult Chinese or English speech. These preverbal utterances follow a highly stereotyped course of development (and contrary to popular opinion, do not include all sounds of any language a child might learn). The speech sounds that parents use do not appear to be imitated much in babbling; what is imitated is the melody of the language.

Whether a child practices babbling little or lots seems to have slight bearing on acquisition of speech. It would make about as much sense to say that speech is selectively reinforced babbling as to say that writing is selectively reinforced scribbling. If learning a language were dependent on first perfecting recognizable utterances of words, then any number of animals—all the way from mynah birds to Siamese cats—could be taught to "talk." We need not suppose, though, that a dog who could say "ground sirloin" would be any closer to human speech than one who merely barked for his dinner.

The reinforcement myth. In 1965, George Miller wrote a warning to those who would study language:

If the hypothetical constructs that are needed seem too complex and arbitrary, too improbable and mentalistic, then you had better forego the study of language. For language is just that—complex, arbitrary, improbable, mentalistic—and no amount of wishful theorizing will make it anything else.

He wrote this warning for the benefit of those who would attempt to explain language learning by selective reinforcement of increasingly complex linguistic responses. Viewed as a problem in reinforcement, language learning has been a tribulation because the unit of behavior to be reinforced has persistently eluded detection. Skinner even invented a new set of linguistic units that describe functions of language in an effort to account for how it is learned by reinforcement (Chapter

---

How do Skinner's (1957) mands and tacts, for example, differ from linquistic categories such as phonemes, words, and sentences?

---

3). He, like many other psychologists, attempted to explain why speech progresses from unpatterned sounds of babbling to recognizable words to meaningful phrases and sentences.

This sequence of development is so regular that it is tempting to think of the child busily polishing phonemes with which he makes morphemes and words into the completed structure of mature language. Reinforcement would be the tool with which the supply of phonemes, morphemes, words, phrases, and sentences is shaped, presumably, and stored in memory.

This is the conception of how language is learned that generative grammarians have doubted. They believe that it leaves too many vital realities of speech acquisition unexplained. For example, how can an infant by age 1 year give evidence with first words that he is well on the way to learning the vastly complex linguistic code used by his parents if he must first learn phonemes and morphemes before even coming to words?

Furthermore, how can the year-old infant have selected, from the buzzing confusion of sounds he hears, just those which will make recognizable words, especially if he has to produce these sounds with reasonable accuracy before they can be reinforced, and especially if the babblings that parents reinforce are just as likely to be linguistically useless as to have eventual value as speech sounds? And why, with far less experience to guide him in what to learn than have adults, will his ability to decipher intricate rules of language be much greater than it will ever be again after he passes puberty? And why can one language be learned naturally just as easily as another, even though they vary immensely in number of sounds, morphemes, and words that must be mastered? And how can he possibly learn so much about language when his parents would not know what to reinforce if they tried to teach him? And how can he imitate language accurately when the speech he hears consists in large part of fragmented sentences, words, and false starts? And how, within a period of about 24 months, whether he will become a Jivaro headhunter or a Wall Street tycoon, can he learn to use accurately the rules of grammar that most adults cannot even explain?

Were these questions insufficient to sink an account of speech acquisition by reinforcement of overt speaking responses, the coup de grace would be Miller's (1965) torpedo. If a child learned speech by building a repertoire of reinforced sounds, words, and sentences on which to draw when he speaks, then he would at the very least have to hear, if not practice, these combinations that he might use. Miller calculates that by conservative estimate at least 10^{20} sentences twenty words long (about the length of this sentence) could be produced. Obviously, a child is capable of longer and shorter sentences, but if they were the extent of his linguistic storehouse, he would need approximately 1,000 times the estimated age of the earth just to listen to them, let alone produce them for reinforcement!

VOCAL DEVELOPMENT

Having completed funeral services for some major misconceptions about speech development, let us turn to how speech apparently does develop. Utterance of intelligible words marks the confluence of the developing processes of symbolic thinking (which culminate in meaningful language) with the meaningless flow of sound-making (which serves no discernible purpose for the months since birth, other than the sheer joy of babbling). To keep these streams of development in the sequence in which their effects can be observed in the growing child, we must begin with earliest forms of sound-making.

In the first year or two of a child's life, before use of meaningful speech becomes predominant, most utterances cannot be described properly as speech. They form a stream of sound that is an indiscriminate blend of babbling, burping, crying, yawning, belching, yelling, hiccoughing, chortling, or whatever. The term that comes closest to capturing the common thread that can be heard in all of this noisemaking is vocalization. So much of what the child does is vocal play with tones and noises that we can best characterize the course of this activity as vocal development.

The course of vocal development

Two different types of utterances can be heard during vocal development: sounds of distress and sounds of contentment. An infant during his first few days will sound as if he is protesting arrival in the world—he will utter mainly monosyllabic cries. Lenneberg (1967) points up lack of articulatory distinctions during crying with the remark: "In essence, the infant simply blows his horn without operating the keys." Irwin (1947a,b, 1948, 1949), who has devoted much of his life to studying infant speech, can detect in these early cries about eight sounds that will later be used for speech. Still, one should not think of these as speech sounds (they have no linguistic significance), nor should one think

that the more they are uttered, the more they will be perfected and ready for speech use when first words arrive. For that matter, many infant sounds will be either unrecognizable or useless for intelligible speech. The fact that 90% of recognizable sounds will be

---

Compare Jakobson and Halle's (1056) distinction between babbling and language with Irwin's description of infant speech. Is Irwin discussing phonemes (speech sounds) of language or phones (any sound, linguistic or otherwise)?

---

five vowels (mostly /æ/ as in "flat") in this early crying does not mean that these sounds function yet as vowels of speech.

Articulatory distinctions. What is more important to note than specific phones that can be recognized phonemically is the developing capacity to make these different sounds. As the infant's distress cries after birth give way to contented cooings and babblings that will continue for more than a couple of years, he will progress from about eight recognizable phones during his first 2 months to all adult vowels and all but two consonants by age 2½. At this point, he is able to make almost all phonetic differences that he will need eventually for the forty-odd phonemes of mature speech (Winitz, 1969). Note, though, that all that is demonstrated is the ability to produce most sounds. Until used in speech to make differences in meaning, they will not function phonemically in a linguistic system.

Irwin's (1949) work has shown that the development of the ability to make these sound distinctions follows a regular course. If the rate of development were plotted, it would appear as a parabolic curve. Because this curve decelerates with age, the older the child, the slower is the rate at which he increases his ability to make articulatory distinctions. Irwin has also found that during the first year, boys and girls progress at the same rate, but thereafter girls surpass boys. Boys, however, not to be outdone, use the fewer sounds that they do make with greater frequency than girls. This frequency of use is another measure of vocal development. As babies grow, they use the sounds they produce with increasing frequency. With this measure, differences associated with environmental influences can be detected. Infants from the homes of workers, for instance, do considerably less sound-making than do those with a parent in a profession.

Prosodic patterns. The consensus of observers of vocal development is that what children imitate most in babbling is their parents' intonation patterns. The newly arrived infant apparently responds to the most salient features in the maelstrom of foreign sounds in which he grows: the melody of speech. Development of intonation recognition continues at least into elementary school (Corlew, 1968). Observers frequently link intonational patterns with expression of emotion. Chase (1966) makes the point that this early link supports the observation that the infant has "a disproportionate capability for communicating information about affective states, to be supplemented at a later stage in development by proportional capability for the communication of more objective categories of experience, such as the operations of logical thought." In other words, he can voice how he feels before he can say what he thinks.

Products of vocal development

Out of this period of vocal development will come three skills: (1) a crude but effective communication system to relieve discomfort that will develop in connection with crying; (2) a system for expressing emotion that will develop in connection with intonation; and (3) a system of coordinations among mechanisms of breathing, vocalizing, articulating, and hearing that will develop with cooing and babbling and will be basic to perfecting later articulatory control of speech sounds.

This third skill, which we will consider in the next section, is the most vital as far as speech and language are concerned; neither of the others contributes much in American English. Crying functions as a signal of distress that needs urgent attention. It grows out of pressing vegetative needs. The com-

munication system that evolves from it is largely for emergency purposes. By its very nature it circumvents the time-consuming process of formulating a message in the logical discursive form required for language. It also avoids the additional delay of stringing words together in sense-making, meaningful speech. True, crying is soon differentiated after birth into a variety of distress signals that mothers are adept at recognizing. But effective as these signals (and the gestures that develop with them) are for urgent communication, they appear to be intimately related to conditions that oppose the calm contentment in which babbling and language processes flourish.

What role does Bolinger (1964) maintain that intonation plays in tone languages? Is English a tone language?

The most important groundwork for articulation of intelligible speech is laid in the infant's experimentation with oral-aural coordinations. He must get the feel of sound-making: control of breathing must be coordinated with control of the larynx, throat, tongue, soft palate, jaw, and lips. From first utterance at birth he is experimenting with coordinations of all these operations. The earliest are probably innate; they must be available reflexively for vegetative functions of sucking, swallowing, breathing, and the like. With the advent of cooing and gurgling, experimentation begins in earnest. The ability to babble an increasing number of different sounds attests to growing mastery of different coordinations. But as Lenneberg (1967) cautions: "Attainment of good control over the motor acts necessary for fluent speech is not the milestone at which language has its first beginnings."

LANGUAGE DEVELOPMENT
The infant: nature's linguistic cryptographer

Human infants apparently begin life as cryptographers innately equipped biologically to "crack" society's communication code within a few years. No other hypothesis offered so far comes close to explaining a baby's extraordinary capacity to decipher speech. When, near his first birthday, he speaks his first meaningful word, he gives evidence of having "broken" the semantic and phonemic codes. His first word has meaning. It clearly expresses an idea. It might, for example, be "moo," which, because it is night and no cows are in sight, is taken to refer to the moon in the sky. Although it is an elaborate statement, an adult can translate it into mature linguistic form: "That object up there is a moon." The child's first word and the adult translation are roughly equivalent semantically. Moreover, that an adult can single out meaningful words from meaningless babbling demonstrates the baby's skill at putting together sounds necessary to make the word recognizable. Obviously, mastery of the phonemic code is under way.

Mastery of these two codes, however, will not mark the infant's tremendous achievement during the next 2½ years. By age 1½, he will put words together in his first grammatical speech. During the 24 months after that, he will decipher the rules of grammar. The scope of this accomplishment is staggering. We could understand how he could, with diligent practice and keen ear, learn when and how to use the three dozen plus phonemes in the *phonologic* system—children normally accomplish this feat by 5 to 7 years of age. Or were the task further mastery of the semantic code, this, too, could fit within bounds of our understanding of the learning process—children normally expand their vocabularies from about 200 words at age 2 years to 2,500 words at age 6 years. For that matter, we normally spend much of life enlarging vocabulary and developing more semantically sophisticated ideas.

The grammar code. Mastery of rules of grammar is an achievement of another order of magnitude. What the infant does is to progress from no apparent knowledge of these rules to basic command of them within the brief span of 2 years. These are the rules of *phonology* and *morphology*, which govern how we build words from *phonemes* and *morphemes*, and the rules of *syntax*, which

govern how we arrange words into phrases and sentences. Once grasped, any sentence in the language can be generated. Were the child obliged to learn separately each sentence he might speak, his period of learning would literally extend to eternity: he can construct an infinite number of sentences to express ideas. Rather than follow infinity as it stretches to eternity, all normal infants somehow discover the incredibly economical solution of acquiring rules of grammar.

That language is achieved by breaking the syntactic and morphophonemic codes is abundantly apparent. How these grammatical rules are acquired, however, is one of life's great mysteries. To say that they are "learned" leaves too much unexplained, at least for generative grammarians. How can a 2-year-old baby learn rules that his parents do not understand well enough to make explicit? How many adults, for example, could explain why the first of the following string of words sounds like a sentence (even though it makes no sense) while the second string, containing the same words, is nothing but a grammatical jumble:

1. Colorful red fantasies awaken quietly
2. Quietly awaken fantasies red colorful

Adults know intuitively that the first string obeys the rules of a sentence and the second does not, but most parents could not state the rules to themselves vaguely, let alone to their baby clearly. "Well," you can say, "all good parents teach by example." True, but listen to a recording sometime of your best effort to be grammatical during conversation and see for yourself what your *best* example is like. Unless you are a paragon of grammatical virtue, you will be horrified by the frequency of your blunders; you will back up, fill in, start over, and stop in midsentence. How could a child who does not know the rules ever learn them from this type of example? In short, how can a child learn by imitation and reinforcement a model of language that he rarely hears?

Learning theorists such as Staats (1968) may have the answer. At present, though, their answers do not prevail as strongly as do the psycholinguists' questions (Chapter 3).

Such arguments of theirs as we have seen have led to the account we will explore of how language develops.

The course of language development

Inheritance of an innate cognitive capacity to learn the rules of any natural language seems reasonably certain. That maturation brings this cognitive capacity to a state of language readiness before 2 years of age and maintains it until puberty also seems likely. Uncertainty prevails, however, as to exactly what this universal readiness to learn rules of language entails. Some hold that the infant arrives preprogrammed with his language

---

Compare the opinions of Fodor (1966), Jenkins (1966), Lenneberg (1967), McNeill (1966), and Skinner (1957) about readiness of the infant for speech. Do any of them believe that speech is learned? Do any of them believe that speech is inherited?

---

rules intact. Others think that he is innately prepared to learn these rules, whereas still others recognize the possibility that he is intrinsically equipped to learn principles by which he will learn rules of language. Chomsky (1968), for example, makes the assumption that language universals are part of each child's innate linguistic competence; as such, they are not learned. What is learned is the specific manifestation of this competence in the particular language that the child will speak. The sum of this conception of language is that every normal man, woman, and child has an internal grammer (his

---

Compare Chomsky's (1968) idea of deep and surface structure with Penfield and Roberts' (1959) observation that brain-damaged persons may have a clear idea of what they want to say, and yet be unable to find the words to say it.

---

language competence) that serves as his theory of language. This theory gives him a basis for relating ideas to the sounds of speech in an infinite number of possible sentences: deep structure determines semantic content of thought, whereas surface structure determines phonetic form of utterance (Chapter 3).

Language development as theory construction. We now have a framework within which to fit an account of language development. Basically, the problem is how to explain the typical child's progression from no language at birth to one-word utterances at 1 year to fully developed sentences at 3½ years of age. This problem has two prongs: in the first place, we must answer why he changes toward an increasingly complex grammar, and and in the second, how he knows what changes to make that will move him closer to a mature language.

Why change? When the child produces his first one-word utterances, they must seem to him at the time grammatically sufficient for expressing his ideas to his satisfaction. His one-word pronouncements function as complete sentences. The fact that adults can translate them into full-blown, formally accurate, grammatical sentences supports this point.

Still, his first attempts to speak miss the mark of adult speech almost completely. Is his frustration at failing to match his model the prime reason why he moves on to new, more complex systems of grammar? Probably not. If we accept the reasonable assumption that Lenneberg (1967) makes on the basis of his biologic studies, we would say that language is an aspect of a fundamental, biologically determined process. Like all such processes, it grows. The course of development is typically characterized by a series of states of disequilibrium. The child is more or less continually faced with the need to regain balance as maturation persistently disrupts his solutions. Only with maturity can a stable performance be achieved that will not be disrupted subsequently by more growth.

The period of language readiness that begins around 2 years of age and declines with cerebral maturation at puberty would appear to be a manifestation of development of the biologic foundations of language. The course of all development is toward differentiation of function. The course of cognitive development is toward differentiation of perceptions and ideas. The course of language develop-

deep → semantic content
surface → phonetic form

ment moves toward systems capable of inter-relating and expressing these refined differences. As the child matures and becomes increasingly able to make finer distinctions in his thinking, he must also become increasingly able to express these developing nuances of meaning in his speech. Obviously, one-word sentences will not long serve the expressive needs of a child whose maturing mind is discovering the marvelously complex wonders of the world he has entered.

Which direction to change? How does the child know in which direction to change to achieve a language sufficiently complex to express his ideas and yet be identical in grammatical structure to that of the adults in his society? The answer seems to be that he approaches the riddle of language much as a scientist inquires about reality: he constructs a theory about the way he thinks it works. His trail of linguistic development is strewn with abandoned theories. We need not assume that every discovery he makes is "correct"; he may take wrong turns and end up temporarily in blind alleys. What we must assume, though, is that he has some innate restriction on the form of the grammar that he is equipped to discover. Without this assumption, presumably we could not explain how he "knows" that he is in a blind alley (Jenkins, 1966). On the other hand, if privileges of occurrence of parts of speech are as stable as some hold them to be, this presumption may not be accurate (Staats, 1968). What the child may learn as linguistic rules are the patterns of occurrence of aspects of speech that rarely vary, even when adults speak their usual ungrammatical utterances (Chapter 3).

No normal child pursues theories at random, or if he does, he soon abandons the pursuit. At birth he cannot know which language he is going to learn. To acquire knowledge of a language, especially at an age when he has neither intelligence nor experience to formulate immensely complex and abstract principles, he must have some type of restriction operating that limits the grammar he does learn to that of a natural human language. The marvel of being a human infant

is that, knowing nothing of these imponderables, he develops almost perfect working mastery of the grammatical principles of his native tongue by the age of 5 years, although refinements will continue until puberty (Chomsky, 1968; Fodor, 1966).

Development of grammar. So much for inferences about why language develops as it does; from them three points are self-evident: (1) to speak a language requires knowledge of its grammar; (2) some of this knowledge of language structure is probably innate; and (3) some information about the language must be learned from observation (Fodor, 1966). Let us look, now, at the pattern of development a child tends to follow as he tests and rejects theory after theory of how he thinks ideas are related to each other in sentences.

Syntactic development. Sometime before 18 months, the toddler watching a woman approaching his house may announce her arrival with "Mama." This one-word "sentence" refers grossly to the whole class of mamalike people who wear dresses and perhaps have long hair or other distinguishing apurtenances. An infant may develop a vocabulary of up to fifty single-word "sentences" before he moves on to putting words together sometime between 18 and 24 months. Neither castigation nor coaxing will hasten the day when he begins to combine words he may have been using singly. This he does suddenly and spontaneously, as if he had discovered a new two-word sentence principle that permits him to abandon his one-word principle. Having made this discovery, he will develop it rapidly within a few months. For instance, "Mama" may expand first to "Mama come," then to "Mama come home," and by 3½ to 4 years of age, it will have blossomed into such an expression as "Mama is coming home," if indeed, it is his mother. If it is not, he will make the necessary distinction and say, perhaps, "A lady is coming to our house" (McNeill, 1966; Lenneberg, 1967).

What the child is doing at all levels of language development is differentiating his idea and its expression. At the semantic level, he differentiates "mama" from a name for all women to the name for his mother—a specific woman. At the morphologic level, he corrects the inaccurate verb form in "mama come" to the accurately differentiated form "coming." At the phonologic level he differentiates his speech sounds toward increasingly precise and intelligible utterances. And most importantly, at the syntactic level he is differentiating relations among his ideas as he joins words into phrases. Fig. 4-2 shows how the grammatical categories grow out of and become differentiated expressions of the idea underlying the sentence.

Transformational development. A feature of language that has come into focus with the work of Chomsky and his collaborators is the ability to transform a basic idea into a variety of expressions. Think of the number of ways, for example, that the underlying idea can be expressed in the statement: "The boy watched a cat chase a bird." The following list does not exhaust the possibilities:

The boy watches the bird being chased by a cat.
While the boy watches, the bird is being chased by a cat.
The chasing of a bird by a cat is watched by the boy.
Why does the boy watch while the cat chases a bird?

A transformation does not affect the semantic meaning of the base structure of a sentence, but only the surface structure of its expression. Whether the deep idea is stated in active form, passive form, past tense, or as a question, it remains the same.

Study of the child's developing transformational ability has hardly begun. Probably rudimentary evidence of this ability will be found at the earliest stages of language recognition. What we know now, though, is that the child begins to use these transformations to produce speech relatively late in his linguistic career.

What evidence of development of transformational ability have Ervin (1964) and Menyuk (1963, 1964) found?

Appearance of questions illustrates how transformations can develop. At first, after the child can put two or more words together, he merely puts *no* at the beginning of the string and uses a rising inflection to indicate his question. About 10 months later, he will use a grammatically accurate transformation; a question that earlier might have been "No kitty stand up?" will now be "Why can't the kitty stand up?"

Similarly, the past tense is signaled at first by such verbs as "went," "was," and "were." Later, he will learn to use the past-tense morpheme *ed*, but it will tend to generalize to all verbs, producing such anomalies as "wented," "gaved," "knowed," and the like. In fact, this tendency for *ed* to slop over where it does not belong probably accounts for the all-time classic example of bad grammar: "If I'd a knowed that youed a want to

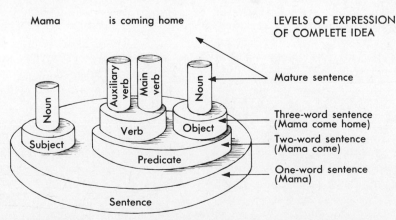

Fig. 4-2. Differentiation of a mature sentence from a one-word sentence.

goed, I'd a seed that youed a haded a way to wented." Curiously, use of the morpheme *s* to distinguish plural from singular verbs is among the slower transformations to develop. Still, it is usually established by 3 years of age. For that matter, basic mastery of grammar generally, and transformations specifically, are well accomplished by the fourth birthday.

Understanding, expression, and inner speech. A child's understanding may precede his ability to express himself grammatically by approximately 2 months—a sizable lead considering the speed with which his linguistic competence develops (Lenneberg, 1967). Presumably, understanding is related to thinking and uses of inner speech. Inner speech will, in mature form, provide a private, almost grammarless, type of thinking that can be disguised by what one actually says. The adult can make fine semantic distinctions in what he wishes to denote or imply. He can transform base structures of sophisticated ideas to obtain grammatical surface structures. He can apply phonologic representations to these surface structures to obtain an intelligible flow of speech sounds that express these ideas. Obviously, he has ample opportunity to obscure what he really means.

Are Myklebust's (1957) distinctions among the terms "inner language," "receptive language," and "expressive language" comparable to those made by Vigotsky (1961) or McNeill (1966)?

Young children in the throes of mastering language are not yet equipped to be devious. From the mouths of babes comes "straight talk." Their speech appears to be a direct expression of deep structure without benefit of semantic differentiation or of grammatical transformation. The infant has a small but growing repertoire of speech sounds, words, and primitive grammatical rules with which to express himself. When he speaks, he seems to apply his phonologic representation to the semantic base structure without benefit of grammatical rules that he is not yet mature enough to generate. If he is to speak,

he is hardly able not to say what he thinks. Differences between immature and fully developed language go far beyond vocabulary size, sound development, and even sentence length. As Hass and Wepman (1969) point out, a child's speech may be egocentric because his deep structure or transformational abilities are inadequate, or because he does not know proper surface structure forms by which to express his ideas.

Products of language development

What is the "payoff" from language development? It takes many forms: greater ability to symbolize experience, greater ability to communicate ideas, greater ability to think abstractly, greater ability to control one's world—the list could be extended interminably. A not-so-obvious thread that runs through these advantages is the child's growing ability to cope with larger and larger amounts of information in more and more economical ways (Chapter 3).

The child's ability to deal with information is the subject of Miller's (1967) delightful article "The Magical Number, Seven, Plus or Minus Two: Some Limits On Our Capacity for Processing Information."

For instance, let us say that each alphabet letter is worth one unit of information. If asked to remember the following fourteen letters, one would be extraordinary to succeed after one glance:

i o e o a p c n s n t n t l

Here is about twice too much information for the average person to recall, at least if he uses the uneconomical system of trying to remember the string letter by letter. If, however, one were to reorganize the same fourteen letters into a more familiar sequence—*Constantinople*—he would be able to remember all of them at a glance without reducing their information value. Moreover, he would be using such an efficient system for organizing them that he could remember five or six more unrelated words of equal length or longer.

Were a child to retain the primitive grammar of his one-word sentences, he would not only need a vast vocabulary of words to express his expanding ideas, but he would be limited to utterances of about seven words in length—his memory could not handle more. If, instead of having to remember a series of unrelated words, he had a system for organizing them into sentences, then all that he would need to recall would be the idea of the sentence. Not only would he now have easy access to all words in the sentence and all sounds in the words, he could even hold several ideas in mind with which to generate additional sentences. Mastery of transformational principles of grammar, complex as they may be, gives the child a system for generating an infinite number of different sentences with a minimum of rules. A fully developed language "pays off" by providing an incredibly economical device for processing and storing in the memory large quantities of information on which discrete judgments and appropriate action can be based (McNeill, 1966).

ARTICULATORY DEVELOPMENT

Development of articulation is a product of vocal development, but even more of linguistic development. Before articulatory ability is of value for anything more than the pleasure of vocal gymnastics, the child must know the words he wishes to say. This knowledge comes with language development. All of speech is directed by and functions in the service of underlying ideas. Since an infant has only the undeveloped base structure of his language available, his primitive "grammar" may provide only one-word sentences with which he can express himself. The sounds he uses are his interpretation of how he thinks this one word should be uttered.

Later, when language matures, sounds will be selected in terms of grammatical transformations and semantic choices: semantically, words chosen must reflect his idea accurately; syntactically, words must be selected to make a grammatical sentence; and morphologically, the form of each root word, its prefixes, and its suffixes must be grammatically proper. All these rules determine the words to be spoken. The remaining prob-

lem is to speak them intelligibly. Accordingly, we will turn to development of the *phonologic* system of language, the system by which articulatory production of contrasting differences in phones makes distinctive phonemic differences.

How does this definition of speech development compare with Winitz's (1966) discussion of articulation errors as sometimes reflecting a deviant phonemic system?

The course of articulatory development

Unlike language, which bursts into full bloom within 2 years, articulation develops rather slowly over a 4- or 5-year period. Articulatory-resonatory skills do not appear to be learned so much by rule as by specific instance. In fact, phonetic rules are hard to find, possibly because standards of pronunciation vary so much from region to region and from time to time. Sounds of speech are per-

Compare Templin's (1966) finding that children slow in perfecting articulation of speech sounds are also below average in their use of morphologic rules with Fry's (1966) observation about the difference between learning grammar and phonology.

fected by the tedious process of gradually correcting pronunciation of each word used in one's speaking vocabulary.

Contrasts guide development

Ease of production. Although binding rules are not available to guide phonologic development, the course of acquiring about forty-five phonemes is nonetheless influenced heavily by two factors: the ease with which distinctive contrasts can be produced and controlled, and the utility value of phonemic contrasts. One might wonder whether ease of *hearing* contrasts among sounds might not also be a factor. Apparently it is not, judging from early acquisition of sounds such as "p," "b," "d," "k," and "g" that, acoustically, vary widely from one phonetic context to another. On the other hand, such acoustically stable sounds as "r," "s," and "l" are notorious among speech clinicians for being defective. They should not be difficult to hear, but

Consider arguments of various authorities, such as Van Riper and Irwin (1958), about why these sounds are more defective than others. Compare these arguments with Fry's (1966) explanation of why the phonologic system develops as it does.

they are troublesome to produce with certainty—their basis for distinct contrasts is missing. The tongue or lips have definite places to make contact for "p," "b," "d," "k," and "g," whereas for "r," "s," and "l" delicate tongue adjustments must be made without benefit of a reference point of contact.

Utility value. The utility factor may play the major role in determining sequence of phoneme development for most children. By utility factor is meant use of a phoneme in a child's recognition or production of speech. Unless he hears and uses words with various sound sequences, he can hardly be expected to imitate them. As an example, many words that are likely to appear in a youngster's vocabulary contain /ʃ/: "*sh*e," "wa*sh*," "*sh*oe." This sound, as would be expected, is acquired fairly early. Its counterpart, /ʒ/, rarely found except in such adult words as "lei*s*ure" and "mea*s*ure," is among the last to be mastered, even though it differs from /ʃ/ mainly by being voiced rather than voiceless.

The utility function is aided considerably when sounds occur in *minimal pairs,* that is, when the difference between them determines the difference between two words. The contrast between /s/ and /ʃ/ makes the difference between hearing "*s*ee" and "*sh*e." If the child hears and uses these words often, he is likely to learn soon the difference between these two sounds. He may be considerably slower, however, about using these sounds correctly in a word like "lisp." If he lisps when he says the word "lisp," a change of /s/ to /ʃ/ does not change the meaning— "lisp" by an other sibilant still means "lisp."

Early prosodic features. At the beginning of life the infant produces and responds to gross whole patterns—little is differentiated perceptually or motorically. What he first hears of speech is a continuous flow of tones and noises. Presumably, the earliest feature of this flow in which contrasts can be recognized is the melody. For instance, the intonation of a question contrasts sharply with that of an exclamation, or even of a simple declarative statement. In English, these melodic differences reveal information about a speaker's intent and emotions. More importantly for speech development, these differences mark the beginning of the child's system of *prosody,* by which he will later be able to place stress on accented syllables—an ability that will become important as he acquires polysyllabic words in which he must locate stress on the proper syllables to make the words understandable (Lenneberg, 1967).

Auditory discrimination. Long before an infant speaks his first true word, he has been working on his system for deciphering the mysterious stream of jabber he hears when people talk. The fact that he can recognize the meaning of what is spoken before he himself can speak reveals the ability to recognize at least gross differences in sounds on which meaning hinges before he can produce these differences. This ability is often called *auditory discrimination.* Less is known about how this capacity to recognize differences develops than about development of capacity to produce speech sounds.

Phone contrasts. Early speech attempts are characterized by primitive phonemes, each containing a wide variety of phones. Most phones contrasted at first to make recognizable words are vowels. For instance, the infant's different pronunciation of "mama" and "daddy" may involve only the difference between the vowel combinations *ahah* for "mama" and *ahee* for "daddy." Not only are the contrasts he starts with gross, but they also tend to shift as he discards crude approximations of mature pronunciation for more refined versions. Still, by the thread of such tenuous differences hangs the delight of proud parents.

Much of the work on the articulatory contrasts by which the distinctive features of speech are recognized can be attributed to Jakobson and his collaborators (1951). Is this a concept widely accepted by linguists?

Developmental sequence. If the sequence of phoneme differentiation is determined largely by utility and ease of production, we should find many small variations among individuals with an overall pattern that is similar for most children. No two children are likely to use identical words at identical stages of development; yet types of words used at any stage are apt to be at least grossly similar. Likewise, sounds that are easy or difficult for one child to produce would probably present about the same production problem to most other children.

The picture of speech-sound development acquired from research fits this expectation. Since vowels and diphthongs are easy to produce and occur frequently, they are contrasted early and are usually completely mastered by 3 years of age. The exact sequence of acquisition varies. Consonantal development also accords roughly with expectation, as can be seen in Table 4-1. Those consonants that develop earliest are produced with relatively unambiguous articulatory adjustments and occur frequently. Those which develop latest occur infrequently and are complex to produce. Templin's (1957) findings, as well as

Table 4-1. Ages at which consonants are articulated accurately by 75% of children tested*

Age (years)	Consonants
3	m, n, ng, p, f, h, w
3.5	y
4	k, b, d, g, r
4.5	s, sh, ch
6	t, th, v, l
7	th, z, zh, j

* Based on Templin, M., *Certain Language Skills in Children: Their Development and Interrelationships.* Institute of Child Welfare Monograph 26. Minneapolis: University of Minnesota (1957).

What does Winitz (1969) say about the evidence gathered on speech and sound development? Are developmental norms phonemic or phonetic? What is the difference?

those of other developmental studies (Poole, 1934; Metraux, 1950), suggest an overall sequence, but they must be taken with the caution that any child may vary widely from this developmental pattern.

Products of articulatory development

We need not dwell long on the multitude of benefits that being able to speak bestows on us. Try being silent for one full day, and the merits will become rapidly and abundantly apparent. Not so apparent, perhaps, is the central role that speech as an auditory phenomenon plays in the acquisition and recognition of language. Obviously, articulation is learned by ear, but so is language. When language must be learned by eye, as with deaf persons, the innate processes that otherwise make normal acquisition so speedily effective fail. Even normal children in homes where the written word is valued highly never acquire language first visually—it is always by sound and then by sight (Fry, 1966).

Development of a phonologic system provides a device for recognizing spoken language. An American child is not born with a pigeonhole for each of the forty-odd phonemes he will use when mature or will hear from the beginning. He starts his linguistic career with a small but complete phonologic system. His first system may have less than a dozen slots into which he will sort all of the sounds that he hears. If he is using, for example, a simple ten-phoneme system to decode utterances encoded by speakers using a forty-five–phoneme system, he will grossly oversimplify his interpretation of what he hears. As he expands the number of phonemic categories, he will be able to differentiate speech into an increasingly larger number of recognizable words. Yet, as any first-grade teacher who has attempted to teach phonics can attest, the child does not realize that words are composed of individual sounds. Word recognition and articulation develop by differentiation of sequences of sounds in words and phrases.

DETERMINANTS OF SPEECH
Biologic determinants

The most profound determinants of speech are the biologic systems that limit thinking and speaking behavior of which man is capable. Sounds that we can produce are deter-

---

Lenneberg (1967) lays an embryologic, genetic, anatomic, and physiologic foundation for the premise that speech is rooted in man's unique biology. Do other psycholinguists agree with him?

---

mined by our vocal equipment. Similarly, we symbolize experience and organize verbal symbols in species-specific ways for linguistic expression. They are not the ways of any other animal. They result in our acquisition of a natural language. We can translate these languages from one to another, but we cannot translate cat-talk, bird-talk, porpoise-talk, or pig-talk—and no lower animal can translate human-talk. Speech is determined by biologic potentialities.

Vocal tract determinants. The design of man's vocal tract does not differ greatly from that of some of his neighbors on the phylogenetic scale. Such differences as do exist point to two developments. One is the streamlining of air spaces around the larynx and twisting of vocal muscles in such a way as probably to increase control of pitch, loudness, and quality. The other is development of dental and palatal structures that provide clear points of contact for the tongue and lips that probably make articulation of different phonemes relatively easy (Fink and Kirschner, 1959; Schultz, 1958; Sonesson, 1960). Too, man can adjust his pharynx for vowels in ways that his primate neighbors cannot (Lieberman, Klatt, and Wilson, 1969). Although these differences hardly seem to be major determinants of the ability to speak, they do account in some measure for the fact that the sounds we make are distinctively human (Lenneberg, 1967). Maturation

of these vocal tract structures and of their neurologic coordination is, of course, vital to development of speech. At birth, laryngeal coordinations of an infant's cry exhibit remarkable maturity. To this well-developed laryngeal ability is later added pharyngeal and oral maturity (Bosma, Truby, and Lind, 1965).

Auditory determinants. We can have no doubt that speech and language are better and more easily learned by ear than by eye. The reason for this phenomenon is not altogether apparent. Abundantly apparent is the necessity of being able to hear speech, at least minimally, if the sound system of the culture is to be acquired. Since even proficient lip-readers miss half the phonemes of the speech they are reading, it is inconceivable that a child could imitate all speech sounds accurately if he is guided only by what he sees and feels. That deaf-speech can be intelligible at all is remarkable, and frequently it is very adequate.

Judging from results obtained with severely hard-of-hearing children at the Nuffield Hearing and Speech Centre in London, the argument need not be that a child must hear what the normal child hears to develop normal speech. Children at this center have achieved surprisingly natural speech by being exposed to amplified sound from an early age. Such cues as they have are sufficient to develop a nearly normal phonologic system for recognizing speech; auditory signals are also sufficient to link with cues of touch and movement for guiding intelligible production of sounds. But if total deafness strikes earlier than about 4 years of age, such hearing as the child had will probably not be sufficient to prevent development of voice and speech that sounds like that of the congenitally deaf.

Turning to less apparent relationships of hearing to language development, a basic difference must be recognized between normal children who *learn* language and deaf children who are *taught* it. This difference is enormous. Whereas the normal child develops his conception through experience, the deaf child is instructed formally in rules of grammar with which he has limited experience. He must learn his native language in much the same way that we would learn a second language in school. That this approach is no match for the method a normal-hearing child uses can be seen from the following of Lenneberg's (1967) excerpts. These samples were taken after various amounts of formal instruction:

After 1 year of instruction:
  "A boy is stoling candy."
After 2 years of instruction:
  "We buy a card Valentine her mother."
After 3 years of instruction:
  "He forget to close the door."
After 5 years of instruction:
  "He was stolen many candy on the shelf and he ate it more and more."

You can see that, even after twice as much time as a normal child takes to master grammar, formal instruction of the deaf child has not improved his performance greatly. His sentences grow longer, he uses more parts of speech, but his idea of how a proper sentence is constructed remains faulty. Telling the child rules of grammar and expecting him to use them from the beginning does not seem to help much. These deaf children do, however, gradually improve sentences as they continue in school. Moreover, those who learn fastest are those who have had some exposure to language before deafness descended. Even as short an exposure to hearing speech as 1 year lays some foundation on which later language training can be based (Lenneberg, 1966; Hirsh, 1966).

The question remains: "To what extent is audition a determinant of language development?" The answer is clouded. If a child has only an innate capacity to learn language by ear, then hearing is a major determinant; we would expect considerable difficulty in learning it visually. But the difficulty the deaf child has can be explained in other ways. He may be past his peak years for language acquisition when training begins. If so, he would profit more if instruction began when speech is normally learned. Combine with this possibility the probability that his exposure to language is limited. Until instruction begins in school, his only encounter with language

is intermittent mouth movement in the faces he sees and perhaps the meaningless scrawl on the printed page. Yet he can learn language, and it appears that he does so when he has had sufficient experience using it rather than formal instruction in how to use it. Even if hearing is not an absolute necessity, it certainly is a major convenience for acquisition of language.

Another line of evidence that points strongly to special human auditory abilities as being fundamental to speech has been reviewed by Cutting and Eimas (1975). They make a persuasive case for the infant's being equipped at birth to recognize speech as a special type of signal that automatically activates special processing mechanisms. They doubt that a child could learn speech naturally without such equipment.

Neurologic determinants

Neuromuscular control. Although speech and general motor control usually develop together, one is probably not a function of the other; too many exceptions can be found in which one develops normally and the other does not. Moreover, control of the speech apparatus matures much earlier than does that of skeletal structures. Manual coordination, although improving between the ages of 2 and 5 years, is still immature during this period when speech control is all but fully established—even babbling requires precise coordinations among swift tongue, lip, throat, vocal cord, and respiratory movements.

Timing seems to be the key to the extraordinary feat of speaking. Speech is uttered normally at about the rate of six syllables per second. Since each syllable contains an average of 2.4 phones, we articulate, roughly, fourteen speech sounds per second—the problem of timing such a fast rate thus begins to become apparent. Over 100 muscles from the floor of the belly to the roof of the mouth must be coordinated. Intelligible speech depends on precise transitions from one phone to another, and these transitions depend on differences in muscular adjustment. To speak, "transition orders" must be issued to speech muscles fourteen times per second. During 1 minute of discourse, timing of 10,000 to 15,000 neuromuscular events must be coordinated!

An explanation that fits known facts is that speech articulation is only a manifestation of a basic neurophysiologic rhythm. With this rhythm, periodic neuromuscular adjustments occur at the rate of about six per second—which, perhaps not so coincidentally, is also the average rate of syllable utterance. This "timing rhythm" sets a cadence for articulation. Just as music is organized around a basic beat—the 4/4 time of the march, the 3/4 time of the waltz—so articulation appears to be organized around the six-per-second time of a neurophysiologic beat. Again, possibly not coincidentally, speech articulation does not develop much prior to establishment of this dominant rhythm around age 2 years (Lenneberg, 1966, 1967).

Neurologic design. None of the determinants presented so far contributes much to our understanding of why language develops. The size of man's brain relative to the size of his body, the *brain-weight index,* would seem to be an obvious possibility. But this lead comes to naught: the index decreases steadily from birth to maturity (Lenneberg, 1967). Another possibility is that new associational pathways have evolved in man's brain that provide the basis for ability to name objects. These new connections presumably permit interactions among visual, somesthetic, and auditory systems in man that are limited or nonexistent in lower animals. These pathways constitute virtually the only anatomic feature in serious contention as a determinant of language—and it is intended to explain only the capacity to symbolize experience; it offers little explanation for the ability to organize symbols grammatically (Geschwind, 1964).

Neurologic maturation. Lenneberg's (1967) argument is that language capacity cannot be attributed to specific structures of the brain, but rather to the way they function. We know that language and brain processes follow parallel courses of development, and thus we surmise that language is a consequence of biologic maturation. Man's brain develops much more slowly than does that of any other

animal, and its pattern of development is different. It will increase 350% in weight by 2 years of age and will increase only 35% during the next 10 years. By age 14 full weight will be achieved and no further increases will occur. Although the total number of neurons may not increase, they will grow, and distances and interconnections among them will increase. Along with structural growth, biochemical and neurophysiologic changes contribute to cerebral maturation. In Fig. 4-3 these growth dimensions are summarized in the percentage scores of brain maturation. Shown is the level of maturation at which various skills appear. Note that whether a child is normal or retarded, language does not begin until he has reached about 60% of adult value. Note, too, that the whole maturational schedule, not just speech, is "slowed down" with retardation. These observations, plus ineffectiveness of intensive training to alter this rate of development significantly, suggest maturation as the basis for man's capacity to learn language.

Man more than any other animal develops "brainedness" and "sidedness": so-called handedness, footedness, eyedness. Lenneberg (1967) argues that neither preference for use of one side of the body nor dominance of one hemisphere of the brain over the other is present at birth. They emerge early in development and are complete by puberty. Language readiness and dominance begin before age 2, when the first word is spoken and cerebral maturity is about 60% complete. They increase sharply during the next 2 years while grammar is being mastered and brain maturity is still progressing rapidly. They taper off but continue until puberty, at which time capacity for language acquisition has declined, the brain has matured, and cerebral lateralization has been irreversibly established.

Considerable doubt has been cast recently, however, on this proposed relation of laterality to speech acquisition. Instead of acquiring lateralization as he develops, the infant appears to be born with it. Furthermore, it does not seem to progress with age but rather decreases (Palermo, 1975). That lan-

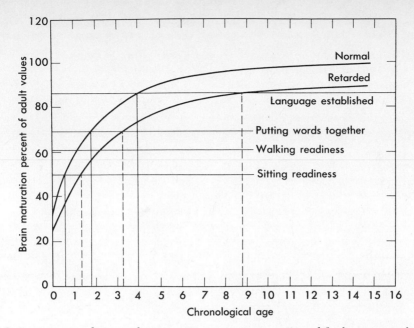

Fig. 4-3. Language readiness milestones. Brain maturation required for language is the same whether a child is retarded or normal. Retardation delays attainment of maturational levels and correlated language development. (From Lenneberg, E., *Biological Foundations of Language*. New York: John Wiley & Sons, Inc. [1967]).

guage acquisition parallels cerebral maturation remains a reasonable certainty. That the connection is establishment of cerebral dominance now seems unlikely.

Intellectual determinants

Intelligence as measured with standard tests does not correlate well with language capacity. Broadly speaking, if a child has sufficient intelligence to acquire language at all, he acquires it fully. Only in the very low ranges is any correlation apparent, and even idiots and imbeciles often have rudimentary understanding of verbal commands and a few words that they can speak (Lenneberg, 1967).

Memory. Of considerably more interest is the development of memory. It is the aspect of intelligence that is known to be vital for acquisition of language. The length of the verbal utterance that we can produce or com-

prehend is limited by memory span. What we can observe as the child strings more and more words together is an effect of growing memory.

Viewed in terms of one type of evidence, at least three different memory capacities appear to be involved in linguistic performance. Memory for phonologic production appears largest, for grammatical comprehension next largest, and grammatical production smallest. If evidence were available, we might even find different memories for remaining linguistic abilities: phonologic comprehension, semantic comprehension, and semantic production. In any event, existing evidence points to the greater ease of remembering how words are pronounced than how they are combined grammatically in sentences. It also points to the greater ease of comprehension than of production.

Viewed another way, we come face to face with the magical number seven. This number, immortalized for psychologists by George Miller's (1967) essay, recurs to haunt, tantalize, and persecute those who would understand language. Why just seven colors

---

What does McNeill (1966) have to say about evidence regarding memory produced by Ervin (1964) in comparison with that from the work of Fraser, Bellugi, and Brown (1963)?

of the rainbow? Why just seven notes of the musical scale? Why just seven-point rating scales? For that matter, why just seven days in the week? The magic of this number grows with the evidence that we can hold about seven items in our span of immediate memory at any one time, that we can judge absolute differences among categories only up

---

To top off the magic, how about Lenneberg's (1967) neurologic and articulatory rhythms of six or seven beats per second? Are these rhythms an example of coincidence or of cause and effect?

---

to about seven, and that our span of attention can encompass only about six or seven items at a glance. The temptation is great to suspect that all these sixes and sevens are but different aspects of a single underlying process.

As obviously related as span of immediate memory, span of attention, and span of category judgment appear to be, Miller has shown that they impose very different kinds of limits on the ability to process and communicate information. The advent of the mathematical theory of communication

---

The relation between memory and our ability to handle information is also discussed in another of Miller's (1967) essays, "Information and Memory."

---

opened the door to recognition of differences in these limits (Chapter 3). Our memories function as piggybanks that we can fill with coins of different informational values. A memory filled comfortably with large-denomination symbols such as words, grammatical rules, and perhaps images is far richer than one stuffed with the pennies of letters and sounds.

What Miller discovered when he looked at information processing from the standpoint of communication theory was that memory span is limited by the number of items—the number of coins. The number of categories that can be judged is limited by the amount of information involved—the value of the coins. Furthermore, for attention span, he has shown that in complex patterns involving more than six or seven features, we

sacrifice accuracy of individual features in order to improve accuracy of overall judgment. For example, if asked to describe some detail of appearance of a person whom you have recognized, you will probably be fuzzy about the details but certain about the person.

The relevance of these considerations for speech acquisition may be basic. Differences in the way in which information is organized and processed may account for the differences between grammatical and phonologic memory, and between memory (for comprehension) and production. Too, the number of distinctive features by which one speech sound is contrasted with another invariably is a maximum of eight or nine. Attending to so many features would diminish accuracy with which any one feature is perceived, and yet would increase overall accuracy of detection of the speech sound as a phoneme.

Furthermore, the amount of information to be handled as the child grows may force the development of increasingly efficient linguistic strategies. Memory limits the number of symbolic units that we can hold at one time—not the amount of information in each size of unit. A word holds many times the information of a sound, a sentence many times that of a word. Yet our memories can accommodate about as many units of one size as of another. With efficient linguistic organization we can, as Descartes once said, "relieve the memory, diminish the sluggishness of our thinking, and definitely enlarge our mental capacity."

Environmental determinants

Earlier, we laid to rest some commonly held notions about environmental determinants of speech. A few relatives of these deceased explanations live and have a rightful place in this developmental account. We will honor the living.

Conditions for reinforcement. Infants who because of disease have been voiceless for prolonged periods prior to restoration of voice have been reported to resume babbling at a normal level of performance without benefit of selective reinforcement (Lenneberg, 1967). That vocal responses in infants can be differentiated by conditioning has been demonstrated, however (Routh, 1969). Intonation patterns of a normal child will "drift" toward his adult model during the period of babbling (Weisberg, 1963). To the extent that reinforcement explains this drift, Mowrer's (1952) autism theory seems reasonable. Briefly, his idea is that because mothers talk lovingly to their babes in the course of mothering them, the sound of the mother's voice becomes a signal of hope to the infant that things will get better. More technically, vocal sounds are conditioned to the tension reduction of being fed, diapered, and burped. The infant, as yet unable to distinguish where his mother "leaves off" and he begins—hence, unable to distinguish between her voice and his—signals hope to himself each time he babbles.

Mowrer's explanation is also a persuasive argument for why infants learn to listen to speech in the first place, if indeed listening to speech must be learned. Much as adults may enjoy hearing themselves talk, our noises may not be indigenously attractive to the infant. He may have to learn to like them if he is to pay much attention to speech. This

---

Douglass (1975) provides a warm and perceptive account of the mother-child relationship in which speech matures. She observes that development of the child's ability to communicate well verbally seems to parallel the satisfaction each finds in relating to the other.

---

conclusion is buttressed by evidence such as the following: Children raised in socially deprived orphanage settings are typically retarded in speech development at age 3. Children of deaf parents (who use little speech) follow a normal sequence of vocal development, and yet, unlike children of hearing parents, do not babble when adults speak. Children with sufficient hearing loss to not hear a mother's quiet, loving sounds, but enough hearing to be traumatized by her angry voice, have been reported to have not developed speech until the mother learned to voice her love loudly. Fortunately, these socially deprived children appear to approach normal speech development quickly if their environments are enriched early enough (Fry, 1966; Lenneberg, 1966).

Granted, articulation of phones can be altered by carefully ministered reinforcement: witness successful effects of speech therapy. Granted, nonsymbolic communication systems can be shaped by environmental consequences: witness systems of gestures, whines, and cries that an infant, and even cats and dogs, will develop under social influence. But none of the foregoing involves symbolism and language. Judging from contrasting experiences of deaf and normal children, environmental consequences do not contribute to speech acquisition. Preschool deaf children develop effective techniques for communication, none of which include speech. During this period, a normally hearing child will learn language. Why? Because his parents have forced him to it? Because they have selectively reinforced his correct responses that parents of deaf children did not know how to elicit? Possibly, but more likely acquisition of rules of semantics, syntactics, morphemics, or phonemics is not hastened much by reward, threat, or punishment of parents, teachers, or speech clinicians.

Conditions for imitation. The distinction here between "conditions for imitation" and "conditions for reinforcement" is largely a matter of emphasis. Although children must be born with innate capacity only for rules of natural languages, they still must learn rules for their specific language. This means that somehow the rules they hit on are reinforced. Apparently, this reinforcement comes from self-satisfaction of mastering more efficient grammatical structures for organizing ideas—extrinsic rewards seem not to influence linguistic progress. Until the final approximation is reached and mature language is acquired, none of the temporary developmental approximations are direct imitations of an adult model. It is as if the child turns to his model not so much to imitate it as to find clues for building his own linguistic structure. The fact that what he finally produces is a replica of the adult model attests to his inability to work out a unique solution that is successful (McNeill, 1966).

Expansions. Aside from providing a good model against which the child can test his evolving linguistic theories, is there no more that adults can do to facilitate speech development? Yes, but not much. Evidence for this answer is limited, and Brown (1964) and Slobin (1964) have provided most of it. They have observed that parents often repeat what a child has said as if to check whether they understand the statement correctly—imitation in reverse, in which parent echoes child. Frequently, they give the imitation a slight twist; they *expand* the child's utterance. The expansion adds one or two missing linguistic features that serve to clarify the intent. As an example, suppose that a 2-year-old announces: "Donna cry." The mother, hearing her baby awakening, responds: "Donna is crying?" The 2-year-old nods his head. The mother has not only confirmed his meaning, but she has also expanded his grammar on the assumption that he can understand the expansion even if he cannot produce it.

Expanded imitations seem to be about the only instructional device to which the child will respond. This is not to say that expansions will significantly accelerate language development, but to the extent that it can be accelerated, this approach seems to be effective. Although children imitate adult speech only about 10% of the time, and although only about 15% of these imitations involve responses to adult expansions, what is interesting is that half of these responses will

themselves be expansions. That is, the child's second utterance after a parental expansion has a 50% chance of being an expanded version of his first utterance. If our 2-year-old has responded with more than a nod to his mother's expansion, "Donna is crying?" he might have replied, "Donna crying," this reply itself being an expanded version of his first statement, "Donna cry."

The possible importance of expansions is also suggested by Brown's (1964) tentative finding that whereas middle-class parents expand around 30% of their children's statements, lower-class parents do so far less often—and the rate of speech and language development among lower-class children is strikingly slower. If expansions do affect de-

---

Cazden (1966) has reviewed various environmental factors that operate in subcultural language. To what extent does he attribute subcultural differences to the environment?

---

velopmental rate, the lower-class child may be retarded because he must work out rules of grammar with less parental help than the middle-class child. Too, the parent who expands his child's statements does so presumably to understand him. The parent must therefore feel that the child has something to say worthy of attention. Whether interest, affection, or expansion is responsible, the attentive parent's effect on development is to be desired.

The answers—résumé

1. What are the origins of speech?

The best educated guess is that man's unique ability to speak is rooted in biologic development. He has evolved a brain that symbolically transforms experience, as can be seen in the increasing tendency for animals higher on the phylogenetic scale to exhibit symbolic behavior. Although use of symbols is not unique to man, his innate capacity to learn a natural language is. He does not learn speech only because he "needs" it to communicate or because of a happy concatenation of behavioral events selectively reinforced. The basis for innate capacity to learn speech is probably related to the unique functional design of man's brain and to its maturational characteristics.

2. How does voice develop?

Vocal development begins with an indiscriminate flow of burps, cries, yawns, squalls, chortles, and the like—sounds of distress and contentment. Several phones occur that the infant will use later when he talks, but they are not yet speech sounds. As his cries of distress after birth give way to cooing and babbling, the child will, by 3 years of age, be capable of producing most of the forty-odd articulatory distinctions he will need for mature speech. The number of sounds that he will actually use in early speech attempts, however, will be only a fraction of those of which he is capable. Although accurate articulatory imitation of adult speech may not arrive until the child is in his seventh year, prosodic imitation is apt to be mastered before speech begins. Three skills will come from vocal development: a crude communication system with which urgent needs can be expressed, a system for expressing emotion, and coordination of the speech apparatus for rapid articulation.

3. How does language develop?

The course of language development parallels that of cognitive development toward differentiation of perception and ideas. As the child matures and becomes increasingly able to make finer distinctions in thinking, he must also become increasingly able to express these delineated ideas in speech. Before the first word appears, soon after his first birthday, his ability to understand speech will be well under way. The first word will be a semantically crude but complete "sentence." Before his second birthday, he will have a vocabulary of about fifty single-word "sentences." Soon, he will discover the "two-word principle," and, by the time he is 4 years old, he will be constructing fully developed, grammatically accurate sentences.

4. How does articulation develop?

Mastery of speaking skill may stretch normally into the seventh year. It will be guided by contrasts among sounds. The earliest contrasts the infant will make will be of prosodic features. The more difficult articulatory distinctions among about forty-five phonemes of American English will be affected mainly by the ease with which sounds can be produced and by the utility value of differences among them.

5. What factors contribute to speech development?

To the extent that speech development in man can be distinguished from that in animals, it probably reflects vocal equipment more capable of being controlled for pitch, loudness, and quality; vocal tract design that permits rapid, flexible articulation; and neurologic equipment that permits recognition and coordination of sounds into patterns that are used for speech. Man's unique biologic evolution, which has prepared him to acquire a natural language by ear, probably involves functional and maturational characteristics of his brain. A threefold increase in brain weight matches the burst of language acquisition around 2 years of age. By puberty, when full brain weight has been achieved, the period of readiness for language learning will have passed. Normal intelligence is apparently not a requirement for language development, although memory is an important ability. The efficiency with which we organize information for storage, more than memory per se, is probably crucial. Another factor is exposure to the language to be learned. We may be born with the innate capacity to acquire a natural language, but an infant must listen for some time to the one that he will speak before he will learn to use it with ease. Probably the primary factor that equips man to articulate sound involves his neurologic mechanism for coordinating and controlling speech muscles. The rapid rate, intricate complexity, and fantastic precision of speech coordinations that are available when general motor coordinations are still grossly immature point to unique biologic preparation to speak.

REFERENCES

Bolinger, D., *Intonation as a Universal*. In Proceedings of the 9th International Congress of Linguists, Cambridge, Mass., 1962. Utrecht: Het Spectrum (1964), pp. 833-848.

Bosma, J., Truby, H., and Lind, J., Upper respiratory actions of the infant. Proceedings of the Conference: Communicative Problems in Cleft Palate, *Asha Reports*, **1**, 35-49 (1965).

Brown, R., The acquisition of language. In Riach, D., and Weinstein, E. (Eds.), Disorders of communication. *Res. Publ. Asso. Nerv. Ment. Dis.*, **42**, 56-61 (1964).

Brown, R., and Bellugi, V., Three processes in the child's acquisition of syntax. In Lenneberg, E. (Ed.), *New Directions in the Study of Language*, Cambridge, Mass.: The M.I.T. Press (1964).

Cazden, D., Subcultural differences in child language: an interdisciplinary review. *Merrill-Palmer Quart. Behav. Developm.*, **12**, 185-219 (1966).

Chase, R., Evolutionary aspects of language development and function. In Smith, F., and Miller, G. (Eds.), *The Genesis of Language*. Cambridge, Mass.: The M.I.T. Press (1966).

Chomsky, N., Language and the mind. *Psychology Today*, **1**, 48-51, 66-69 (1968).

Church, J., *Language and the Discovery of Reality*. New York: Random House, Inc. (1961).

Corlew, M., A developmental study of intonation recognition. *J. Speech Hearing Res.*, **11**, 825-832 (1968).

Cutting, J., and Eimas, P., Phonetic feature analyzers and the processing of speech in infants. In Kavanagh, J., and Cutting, J. (Eds.), *The Role of Speech in Language*. Cambridge, Mass.: The M.I.T. Press (1975).

Cutting, J., and Kavanagh, J., On the relationship of speech to language. *Asha*, **17**, 500-506 (1975).

Douglass, L., How a child learns to talk. *Reiss-Davis Clin. Bull.*, **12**, 90-96 (1975).

Ervin, S., Imitation and structural change in children's language. In Lenneberg, E. (Ed.), *The New Directions in the Study of Language*. Cambridge, Mass.: The M.I.T. Press (1964).

Fink, R., and Kirschner, F., Observations on the acoustical and mechanical properties of the vocal folds. *Folia Phoniatrica*, **11**, 167-172 (1959).

Fodor, J., How to learn to talk: some simple ways. In Smith, F., and Miller, G. (Eds.), *The Genesis of Language*. Cambridge, Mass.: The M.I.T. Press (1966).

Fraser, C., Bellugi, V., and Brown, R., Control of grammar in imitation, comprehension, and production. *J. verb. Learning verb. Behav.*, **2**, 121-135 (1963).

Fry, D., The development of the phonological system in the normal and the deaf child. In Smith, F., and Miller, G. (Eds.), *The Genesis of Language*. Cambridge, Mass.: The M.I.T. Press (1966).

Geschwind, N., The development of the brain and the evolution of language. *Monograph Series on Languages and Linguistics*, No. 17 (April, 1964).

Gould, J., Honey bee recruitment: the dance-language controversy. *Science*, **189**, 685-693 (1975).

Hass, W., and Wepman, J., Surface structure, deep structure, and transformations: a model for syntactic development. *J. Speech Hearing Dis.*, **34**, 303-311 (1969).

Hirsch, I., Teaching the deaf child to speak. In Smith, F., and Miller, G. (Eds.), *The Genesis of Language*. Cambridge, Mass.: The M.I.T. Press (1966).

Hoijer, H., The problem of primitive languages. In Carterette, E. (ed.), *Brain Function. III. Speech, Language, and Communication*. U.C.L.A. Forum in Medical Sciences No. 4. Los Angeles: University of California Press (1966).

Irwin, O., Infant speech: consonantal sounds according to manner of articulation. *J. Speech Dis.*, **12**, 402-404 (1947a).

Irwin, O., Infant speech: consonantal sounds according to place of articulation. *J. Speech Dis.*, **12**, 397-401 (1947b).

Irwin, O., Infant speech: development of vowel sounds. *J. Speech Hearing Dis.*, **13**, 31-34 (1948).

Irwin, O., Infant speech. *Scient. Am.*, **181**, 22-25 (1949).

Jakobson, R., Fant, G., and Halle, M., *Preliminaries to Speech Analysis*. Cambridge, Mass.: The M.I.T. Press (1951).

Jakobson, R., and Halle, M., *Fundamentals of Language*. The Hague: Mouton Publishers (1956).

Jenkins, J., Reflections on the conference. In Smith, F., and Miller, G. (Eds.), *The Genesis of Language*. Cambridge, Mass.: The M.I.T. Press (1966).

Langer, S., *Philosophy in a New Key*. New York: Mentor Books (1951).

Lenneberg, E., The natural history of language. In Smith, F., and Miller, G. (Eds.), *The Genesis of Language*. Cambridge, Mass.: The M.I.T. Press (1966).

Lenneberg, E., *Biological Foundations of Language*. New York: John Wiley & Sons, Inc. (1967).

Lieberman, P., *On the Origins of Language: An Introduction to the Evolution of Human Speech*. New York: Macmillan Publishing Co. (1975).

Lieberman, P., Klatt, D., and Wilson, W., Vocal tract limitations on the vowel repertoires of rhesus monkey and other nonhuman primates. *Science*, **164**, 1185-1187 (1969).

Mattingly, I., The human aspect of speech. In Kavanagh, J., and Cutting, J. (Eds.), *The Role of Speech in Language*. Cambridge, Mass.: The M.I.T. Press (1975).

McNeill, D., Developmental psycholinguistics. In Smith, F., and Miller, G. (Eds.), *The Genesis of Language*, Cambridge, Mass.: The M.I.T. Press, (1966).

Menyuk, P., A preliminary evaluation of grammatical capacity in children. *J. verb. Learning verb. Behav.*, **2**, 429-439 (1963).

Menyuk, P., Alternation of rules in children's grammar. *J. verb. Learning verb. Behav.*, **3**, 480-488 (1964).

Metraux, R., Speech profiles of the preschool child 18 to 54 months. *J. Speech Hearing Dis.*, **15**, 37-53 (1950).

Miller, G., Some preliminaries to psycholinguistics. *Am. Psychologist*, **20**, 15-20 (1965).

Miller, G., *The Psychology of Communication*. New York: Basic Books, Inc. (1967).

Mowrer, O., Speech development in the young child. I. The autism theory of speech development and some clinical applications. *J. Speech Hearing Dis.*, **17**, 263-268 (1952).

Myklebust, H., Aphasia in children—language development and language pathology. In Travis, L. (Ed.), *Handbook of Speech Pathology*. New York: Appleton-Century-Crofts (1957).

Palermo, D., Developmental aspects of speech perception: problems for a motor theory. In Kavanagh, J., and Cutting, J. (Eds.), *The Role of Speech in Language*. Cambridge, Mass.: The M.I.T. Press (1975).

Penfield, W., and Roberts, L., *Speech and Brain Mechanisms*. Princeton, N.J.: Princeton University Press (1959).

Poole, I., Genetic development of articulation of consonant sounds in speech. *Element. Eng. Rev.*, **11**, 159-161 (1934).

Premack, D., and Schwartz, A., Preparations for discussing behaviorism with chimpanzee. In Smith, F., and Miller, G. (Eds.), *The Genesis of Language*. Cambridge, Mass.: The M.I.T. Press (1966).

Routh, D., Conditioning of vocal response differentiation in infants. *Developm. Psychol.*, **1**, 219-226 (1969).

Sapir, E., *Language*. New York: Harcourt, Brace, & World, Inc. (1921).

Schultz, A., Palatine ridges. In Hofer, H., Schultz, A., and Starck, D. (Eds.), *Primatologia: Handbook of Primatology* (Vol. III, Part I). Basel: S. Karger AG (1958).

Skinner, B., *Verbal Behavior*. New York: Appleton-Century-Crofts (1957).

Slobin, D., Imitation and the acquisition of syntax. Paper presented at the Second Research Planning Conference of Project Literacy (1964).

Sonesson, B., On the anatomy and vibratory pattern of the human vocal folds; with special reference to a photo-electrical method for studying the vibratory movements. *Acta Otolaryng.*, Suppl. 156 (1960).

Staats, A., *Learning, Language, and Cognition*. New York: Holt, Rinehart & Winston, Inc. (1968).

Templin, M., Certain language skills in children, their development and interrelationships. Institute of Child Welfare Monograph Series 26. Minneapolis: University of Minnesota (1957).

Templin, M., The study of articulation and language development during the early school years. In Smith, F., and Miller, G. (Eds.), *The Genesis of Language*. Cambridge, Mass.: The M.I.T. Press (1966).

Van Riper, C., and Irwin, J., *Voice and Articulation*. Englewood Cliffs, N.J.: Prentice-Hall, Inc. (1958).

Vigotsky, L., Thought and speech. In Saporta, S. (Ed.), *Psycholinguistics*. New York: Holt, Rinehart & Winston, Inc. (1961).

Weisberg, P., Social and nonsocial conditioning of infant vocalizations. *Child Developm.*, **34**, 377-388 (1963).

Winitz, H., The development of speech and language in the normal child. In Rieber, R., and Brubaker, R. (Eds.), *Speech Pathology*. Amsterdam: North-Holland Publishing Co. (1966).

Winitz, H., *Articulatory Acquisition and Behavior*. New York: Appleton-Century-Crofts (1969).

Disabilities of speech

Part II deals with knowledge from related professions about conditions that disable normal functions of the speech mechanism. The concern here is with disruptive effects of these disabilities on speech during development and after it is acquired.

Chapter 5

Neurologic disabilities

Questions

1. What neurologic disabilities affect speech?
2. What is the etiology of neurologic disabilities?
3. What is the speech pathologist's responsibility in the treatment of neurologic
   disabilities?

NATURE OF NEUROLOGIC DISABILITIES THAT AFFECT SPEECH
Brain functions of speech

How do we go about making sense of damage to a mechanism with 10 billion parts interconnected in more ways, literally, than there are atoms in all of creation, and that is packaged in a container smaller than a football? As Livingston (1967) pointed out, "We can be certain of two things: none of our direct ancestors died before reaching reproductive age, and all of them succeeded in reproducing something." We stand as biologic heirs of a highly sophisticated apparatus for goal-seeking behavior. The most sophisticated legacy of all is speech. It is the culmination of successful biologic mechanisms inherent in the chassis of our surviving ancestors. It is a capacity that has been hammered out on the anvil of evolution in the compelling test of survival. It is an inheritance with parts that date back beyond the most ancient kingdom, beyond civilization, beyond the time when our ancestors slithered from the primeval sea. The mechanisms we now utilize for speech have been safeguarded across these billions of years at molecular, cellular, and behavioral levels of organization. Clearly, we are launched for our journey through life with much of our neurologic organization for speech provided as a legacy of evolution. Our innate capacity for language has been encoded for genetic transmission. That even a single protein molecule can store many times this much information is apparent when we realize that if all of its possible DNA code combinations were synthesized, the resulting mass of amino acids would exceed the weight of the universe (Lehninger, 1967).

Double codes of the brain. A compelling assumption is that our image of the world, the seat of intellect and speech, is represented in a brain code preserved somehow in neural circuitry. This representation is probably constituted of biochemical and bioelectrical activity in glial cells and neurons. The code itself, however, completely eludes us. What is known is analogous to knowing the chemical properties of ink and paper on which a message is written in an unknown language.

Yet various cerebral areas can be identified as vital for certain speech and cognitive abilities. Even though the overall picture can only be sketched in gross outline, it carries an implication worth noting. The brain must use at least two codes to establish and preserve the internal image of the outside world. The image from which we retrieve memories from yesterday, a month ago, or perhaps an untapped memory from a lifetime back must be encoded and preserved in some form of static organization that is all but impervious to the violent disruption of head injury, convulsions, shock treatment, deep anesthesia, and so on. This code is used for long-term memory storage. Where this permanently encoded information for any given memory is stored is anyone's guess.

What seems clear is that the other code, the dynamic code of patterns of neural transmission, the code of short-term memory, must be used to lay down permanent memory traces. To do this utilizes the organization of neural circuitry, which means that different operations of speech and thought probably use different networks interwoven through different regions of the brain. Thus we should expect to find specific cortical areas more involved in certain information-processing operations of language and intellect than in others (Sperry, 1967).

Cerebral hemisphere functions. From studies of the effects of head injuries, electrical stimulation of the cortex, surgical ablation, and aphasia and especially from systematic studies of the effects of disconnecting the two sides of the brain at various levels (in split-brain operations done on animals for experimental purposes and on humans for medical purposes), a gross outline can be sketched of how the right and left hemispheres of the brain are involved in speech, language, and thought. Although the idea is widely held that cerebral dominance is a unique characteristic of man and is slowly established in correlation with brain maturation and the acquisition of language, the facts show otherwise. Brain asymmetry is found in animals, and in man it is present in infancy. Thus establishment of dominance does not seem to be a cause of language acquisition, but the specialized functions of the two hemispheres are certainly strongly related to speech.

What is especially clear is that the experiencing, learning, and remembering mechanisms of the two hemispheres, when surgically separated, operate almost completely independently of each other. What one hemisphere knows can be unknown to the other. Sperry (1967) has shown, for example, that both cerebral hemispheres, in man as well as in animals, have short-term and long-term memory mechanisms for vision and somesthesis that can operate altogether separately from each other.

Normally, of course, they do not. If they did, the right hand would literally not know what the left hand is doing. But in split-brain subjects the separation is vividly evident for the processing of what Guilford (1967) calls *figural information* (direct sensory experience of concrete objects). In fact, with figural information, whether visual, somesthetic, or probably even auditory, Sperry's evidence suggests that the different cognitive operations can be applied to various levels of discrimination in either hemisphere. In other words, both hemispheres are apparently equipped to learn and to function intelligently without the other, although normally they work together.

With symbolic and semantic information (that is, with speech) the picture is quite different. In split-brain subjects, the minor hemisphere is almost mute and agraphic. It cannot speak. It cannot read. It cannot write. With prompting, it can manage to speak and comprehend a few simple familiar words, but mainly it is limited to responses such as pointing, signaling, and drawing. Careful nonverbal testing is required to demonstrate that the minor hemisphere is not as stupid as it appears superficially.

That the minor hemisphere probably has latent capacity for handling language up to puberty, when cerebral maturation is completed, can be seen in those persons who, as young children, had their dominant left hemispheres removed and still proceeded to develop normal speech (Lenneberg, 1969; Dreifuss, 1975). The minor hemisphere also seems to develop linguistic functions when the corpus callosum, which interconnects the hemispheres, is damaged in infancy. This has led Sperry to the conclusion that in man the corpus callosum functions normally to prevent learning, especially of language, in both hemispheres. By contrast, the corpus callosum in lower animals appears to foster bilateral learning. Why this difference and how it works is not known, nor is it known how important the difference is for the existence of speech in man and its absence in his phylogenetic neighbors.

Whereas the minor hemisphere is somewhat superior in managing spatial relations, the dominant hemisphere, when disconnected from its nondominant counterpart, continues to perform its reading, writing, speaking, listening, and mathematical functions as if nothing had happened. Neurologists have for years been describing damage in the dominant hemisphere in relation to symptoms of aphasia. The evidence leaves little doubt that speech is a function of these discrete portions of the dominant hemisphere. Yet none of the evidence supports a notion that words, as such, are stored in permanent memory. Clearly, the neurologic mechanisms for storing, retrieving, and processing speech information are in the dominant side of the brain, but the nature of the units of speech that are stored, retrieved, and processed remains a puzzle (Sperry, 1967).

Sperry

Goal-directed organization. Perhaps the answer, or part of it, lies in the interdependence among mechanisms for motor, perceptual, and cognitive learning. How a motor response is represented in the brain is an old question. Is it represented by memory of the muscles involved or the movement desired? Neuroscientists now suspect that neither of these representations is the answer. A more likely answer is that once one has decided on appropriate goal-directed behavior, the motor response is organized cortically in terms of expected effect. That the frontal lobes are crucially involved in goal-directed functioning of higher intellectual activities has been shown by Luria (1966, 1970). When motor signals are sent to muscles, corollary signals are also sent to the sensory system in preparation for perceiving these expected effects of movement.

Luria

Research has shown, too, that animals in which the motor cortex has been removed can still direct movement from visual perception areas left intact. Details of achieving a desired response, such as articulating a stream of meaningful sounds, are left apparently to the cerebellum and subcortical centers. The job of these lower motor centers is to translate the intended movement into muscle coordinations that will produce a response that matches the desired perceptual result (Sperry, 1967). The foregoing merely restates the theme, introduced in Chapter 3, that the speaking process functions as a servosystem in which output is compared with input to achieve an intended result—a process that gives assurance that what is said and done is what one intends to say and do.

Hollien's (1975) recent servosystem model of neural control of speech (Fig. 5-1) is attractive on two counts. One is that it applies the biofeedback principle of cybernetics to unify a conception of how the brain operates. The other is that it relates functional mechanisms of speech to each other in a way that does not require shaky assumptions about where they are actually located anatomically. For example, the speech decoding mechanism shown in the central processing unit

probably involves Wernicke's area, but it may also include Broca's area and portions of the brain stem. Although we are not yet able to say with great precision which structures carry out some of the operations shown, we know enough to piece together the picture shown in Fig. 5-1 with reasonable certainty.

Localizing speech, language, and cognitive functions. If Guilford's (1967) concept is correct, brain mechanisms for speech would be needed to store discriminations of different types of information made at different conceptual levels. These mechanisms of learn-

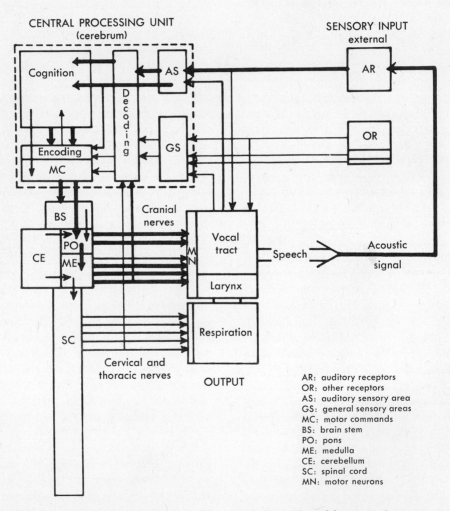

Fig. 5-1. Servosystem model of the neural control of speech and language functions. (From Hollien, H., Neural control of the speech mechanism. In Tower, D. B. [Ed.], *The Nervous System.* [Vol. 3] *Human Communication and Its Disorders.* New York: Raven Press [1975], p. 488.)

ing would be responsible for short-term and long-term memory. To use this stored infor-- mation, brain mechanisms would be needed that can recall discriminations and process them logically, creatively, and meaningfully. These mechanisms would transport informa- tion through the neural network from the various storage locations.

How are brain mechanisms designed to function in ways peculiarly related to speech? The teaching of classic neuroanatomy has emphasized the associated fiber connections that have been thought to link widespread areas of the cerebrum. This classic view is, apparently, more valid for the brains of men than of monkeys. Man does have some con- nections among his association areas. These connections, which permit transfer of infor- mation among sensory modalities, are not found even in primates. Here, then, is a design feature that separates, linguistically, the "haves" from the "have-nots."

Geschwind (1968), from his investigations of man's brain, has proposed that the area of the angular gyrus is crucial for speech be- cause it is an association cortex for association cortices. It is an area, found only in man, in which association fibers are interconnected from three sensory modalities vital for speech: audition, vision, and somesthesis. The angular gyrus lies along the borders of the areas for these three modalities. More- over, it is the region of the human brain that, in comparison with primate brains, has enlarged the most. It is also a region in which neural cells mature late in childhood development—another correlation with speech development that tempts one to sus- pect cause and effect.

This area of the angular gyrus that Gesch- wind (1968) described was found to be crucial for language formulation in the earlier work of Penfield and Roberts (1959). Their con- clusions were based on two techniques for studying patients for whom neurosurgical operations were necessary. Those in whom portions of the brain were excised were in- vestigated for subsequent speech effects. For others, speech effects of electrical stimula- tion of the cortex were observed. These pa-

tients had segments of their skull removed under local anesthesia, but they were con- scious when points on their brains were stimulated in the areas shown in Fig. 5-2.

Patients stimulated in *voice control* areas in either hemisphere would lie on the operat- ing table, helplessly producing long-drawn vowel sounds (interrupted only long enough to catch a breath) until the current stopped. This area has been removed in either hemi- sphere without permanent loss of voice. Similarly, the *supplementary motor area* has been excised in either hemisphere without permanent effects, except for temporary *aphasia* (impairment of language) when this area is removed on the dominant side. Such vocalization cannot, apparently, be elicited by stimulation in lower animals.

The two most important sectors found for ideational speech were the *posterior speech area (Wernicke's area)* and the *anterior speech area (Broca's area)* in the dominant hemisphere. Stimulation of either region blocked attempts to find the word to express an idea, but excision of the posterior area resulted in profound and permanent aphasia, whereas patients eventually recovered from aphasic effects of damage to the anterior area. It is this posterior speech area that is located in the region of the angular gyrus. This is the area that is closely concerned with auditory organization of ideational language, with uti- lization of grammatical rules that allow mean- ingful expression of ideas through selection and ordering of words. Broca's area, on the other hand, is a way station between Wer- nicke's area and speech musculature areas of the cortex. It is concerned with motor organization of speech (Chase, 1972).

Because cortex surrounding these ide- ational speech areas could be removed with- out producing aphasia, the conclusion was that information is transferred from one corti- cal area to another through subcortical con- nections. This conclusion fits with the view of the cortex as a recently evolved extension of the old brain. As such, the cortex plays the role of subcontractor to the thalamus; cortical elaborations are sent back to the thalamus for coordination with other activities of the brain.

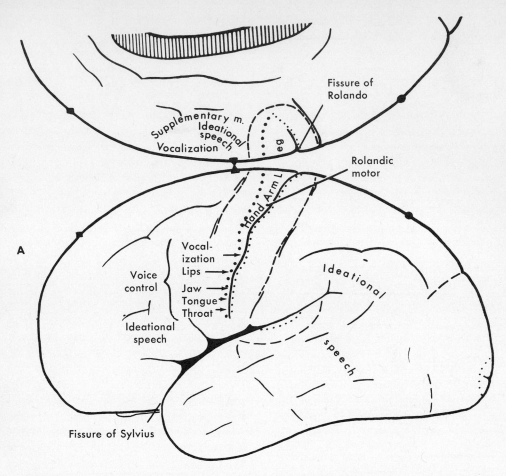

Fig. 5-2. Areas of the dominant cerebral hemisphere that control speech. Emphasized on the left, **A**, are areas that control voice and articulatory movements. Organization of these movements for ideational speech is controlled in the three areas shown on the right, **B**. Evidence for location and function of these areas comes from electrical stimulation and surgical excision of the cortex. (From Penfield, W., and Roberts, L., *Speech and Brain-Mechanisms*. Princeton, N.J.: Princeton University Press [1959]. Reprinted by permission.)

Support for this idea comes from more recent work that shows a thalamic role in language that differs from its role in general cortical activity. Like the cerebrum, the left thalamus seems more related to language than the right. It apparently plays this role by its involvement in arousal and attention, and its interaction with memory mechanisms (Pribram, 1971; Eisenson, 1975; Ojemann, 1975; and Darley and colleagues, 1975).

Penfield and Roberts (1959) also reported on the brain mechanisms for memory. They observed that when a region of the temporal lobe adjacent to the posterior speech area was stimulated, the patient might reexperience a stream of consciousness in which he remembered the details of an earlier event as vividly as if he were living it again. They noted, however, that perceptual memory of experiences is not the same as memory of concepts or words. For example, they observed that a patient could, by stimulation, recall a specific butterfly, but when asked to name an outline drawing of one while the electrode was on any speech area, he would be unable to find the word he wanted. He might say: "Moth. No. That's not right. I know the name, but I just can't think of it."

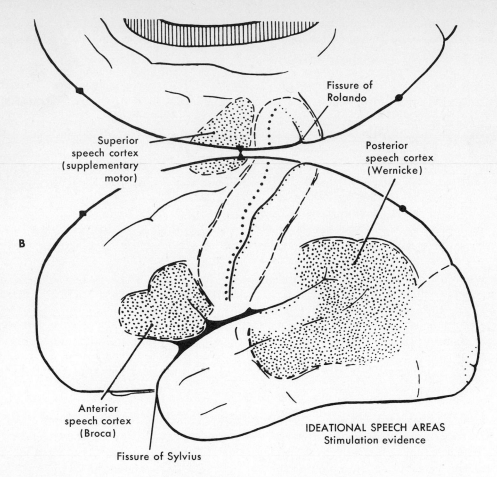

Fissure of
Rolando

Superior
speech cortex
(supplementary
motor)

Posterior
speech cortex
(Wernicke)

B

Anterior
speech cortex
(Broca)

IDEATIONAL SPEECH AREAS
Stimulation evidence

Fissure of Sylvius

Fig. 5-2, cont'd. For legend see opposite page.

When the electrode was lifted, he would say: "Butterfly! I knew what it was all along." From this type of response, Penfield and Roberts concluded that the brain mechanism for storing perceptual memories is separate from that for selecting an idea, which is separate from that for expressing the idea in language. Cortical speech areas are somehow involved in word selection but apparently are not necessary for selection of an idea, which they conceived as being the responsibility of the *centrencephalic system*, located in the brain stem and especially in the thalamus (Fig. 5-2).

Motor control of speech. Like a grand piano, the neuromuscular system can be used for performance ranging from exquisite precision to gross clumsiness. The *lower motor neuron*, with its synaptic connections in the spinal cord, corresponds to the piano key; the muscle fiber, to which the lower motor neuron attaches, corresponds to the hammer that strikes the piano string. Just as the piano key and hammer form a functional unit, so do the lower motor neuron and muscle fiber. Strike the piano key with sufficient force, and the hammer will strike the string; the harder the key is struck, the louder will be the sound. Fire the lower motor neuron, and the muscle will contract; the faster the firing to a fiber, and the more fibers innervated simultaneously, the stronger will be the muscular contraction. Whether or not firing will occur is determined by whether the sum of facilitatory influences from higher motor centers is greater than the sum of inhibitory influences. These influences are weighed at the synapses of lower motor neurons.

The neuromuscular system, like the grand piano, permits skilled performance only when properly tuned. The piano is tuned by adjusting tension in the strings, whereas the neuromuscular system is tuned by adjusting tension in the muscles. Muscle tone is maintained by the balance of tension between opposing muscles. When the biceps, for example, contracts to flex the arm, it is opposed by the triceps (the biceps, as the prime mover, is called the *agonist;* the triceps is called the *antagonist*). The more the antagonist resists relaxing as the agonist contracts, the greater is the muscle tone—that is, the less slack there is in the system. Muscles are tuned reflexively by the *gamma system* (French, 1960; Jung and Hassler, 1960). This sytem regulates the background of muscle tone against which all movements are made. Tone is low when relaxed, and high when alert—an arrangement that permits fitting one's quickness of response to his estimation of the situation.

The lower motor neuron keyboard, like its musical counterpart, has no control over the uses to which it is put. As a novice can bang dissonance from the piano, so can old motor centers in lower levels of the brain control the spinal keyboard to produce gross reflexive responses. Unlike the grand piano, however, that usually sits idle, awaiting the touch of an artist, the lower motor neuron keyboard is in constant use. The higher the neural level, the more priority it has for control of this keyboard, and the more skillful the performance. But when the cortical level, for example, relinquishes control, as in sleep, intoxication, an emotional outburst, or injury, the next level down that is ready to function then gains control. As long as an organism remains alive, some level will be ready to function—and the lower that level, the cruder will be its function. From this discussion, it should be apparent that higher centers must inhibit lower ones in order to control lower motor neurons and produce skilled responses (Paillard, 1960; Denny-Brown, 1960).

Upper motor neuron control systems. The *pyramidal* and *extrapyramidal motor systems* are the two upper motor neuron systems that play speech tunes on the lower motor neuron keyboard. The pyramidal system is "wired in parallel," unlike the extrapyramidal system that is "wired in series." This type of wiring permits the new pyramidal system that mediates purposeful volitional movement, to dominate the old extrapyramidal system that mediates various reflexive responses, as in postural adjustments and emotional expression.

The pyramidal system is designed to provide discrete control for skilled movement. Its topography is arranged so clearly that stimulation of specific cortical motor areas consistently produces movements in specific muscles (Paillard, 1960). Those parts of the body that require finest control have the largest supply of pyramidal motor neurons and, incidentally, of sensory neurons to feed back information about muscle contraction and movement.

Speech can occur under any condition in which humans survive. Whether en route to the moon, swimming, parachuting, jumping, eating, or in an emotional state of ecstasy, man still talks. Obviously, we are built to coordinate the motor activities of speech with just about any reflexive activity of which we are capable. The pyramidal system, with its nonstop motor traffic from cortex to lower motor neuron, is an express route for fine coordination of speech. Alone, however, the pyramidal system produces only isolated segments of movement. For these movements to be smoothly integrated, pyramidal activity must be harmonized with that of the extrapyramidal system that, like the mail train, stops at every motor station from the cortex to the spinal cord to pick up neural

---

Geschwind (1975) describes the anatomic organization of the language areas and motor systems of the brain as they relate to apraxia. Importance of the corpus callosum and extrapyramidal connections with Wernicke's area is stressed.

---

information for reflexive adjustments (Paillard, 1960; Jung and Hassler, 1960).

The cerebellum and self-adjustment. In any *servosystem,* and the nervous system is a supreme example of a self-regulating mechanism, the intended performance is compared with actual performance to improve accuracy. At target practice, for instance, if one misses the bull's-eye, he checks to determine which way to correct his aim for the next shot. The correction depends on detecting a discrepancy between intent and *feedback* information about the performance. In such self-adjusting mechanisms as computers, detection of performance error and correction for it is accomplished in devices called comparators.

The cerebellum has been described as the comparator of the nervous system. It is informed in advance of the movement intended. This plan is sent ahead several milliseconds before the act is begun, presumably to prepare the cerebellum for a check on adequacy of the performance when proprioceptive feedback about the movement arrives from muscles, tendons, and joints. It checks response against command and sends modified impulses back to the motor centers and, indirectly, out to the muscles. This corrective modification serves to smooth the response by coordinating contraction of the agonistic muscles producing the desired movement, and of the antagonistic muscles opposing it (Paillard, 1960; Snider, 1958; Teuber, 1967; MacKay, 1968).

The reticular formation: traffic control center. The reticular activating system directs motor traffic. It can amplify or inhibit motor activity ranging from voluntary movement at the cortical level to the lowly "knee-jerk" reflex at the spinal level. It is the system that must function properly for movements to be smooth and polished. By its connections with cortical motor centers, basal ganglia, and other brain-stem motor centers, cerebellar centers, and sensory pathways— that is, by its connections with the pyramidal, extrapyramidal, and sensory systems—the reticular system is centrally located to stitch all of the separate activities of the nervous system into an integrated whole. It awakens the brain and keeps it alert; it monitors the stimuli that flood our senses, accepting those of importance to us and rejecting the rest; and it directs neural traffic, focusing and refining our motor responses to the problem at hand. In fact, it is probably basic to thinking, to attention, to selection of ideas, and to reasoning about them (French, 1957, 1960). The reticular activating system, then, seems to be at the neurologic hub of speech.

You can see, then, that the question of localization of function in the brain swings on two hinges: where the products of information are stored, and the location of neural pathways over which the information travels when it is retrieved and processed. To say which of these functions is involved in the brain areas known to be of importance to speech would be pure conjecture.

The practical significance of this knowledge, however, is considerable. Has a brain-damaged person with aphasia, for instance, lost his speech because the injured area stored vital information that has been permanently destroyed? Or is he unable to speak because the area contains neural circuits over which speech information must travel in the course of being retrieved and processed? Is a child mentally retarded and his speech impaired because the neural circuitry for making discriminations is damaged, because the biochemical processes for storing discriminations is deficient, because the information retrieval mechanism is disabled, or because the circuitry for high-level mental operations is defective? No one knows for sure. Clearly, though, to have lost a memory forever is one thing; to still have it but be unable to recall it is quite another. Yet another is to still have it, be able to recall it, but be unable to use it in constructing meaningful grammatical statements. Still another is to never have made the discrimination and stored the information in the first place.

Neural signals can be transmitted over so many alternate circuits that knowledge of damage in one area offers less than exact certainty of speech consequences. Like a driver in a large city who reaches his destination despite detours for road repairs, neural signals have multiple paths available. Only when bridges, major intersections, or dead-end streets to a specific address are closed or when freeways are clogged is a driver's trip seriously disrupted. The nervous system, too, has bridges (such as the corpus callosum), major intersections (such as the thalamus), dead-end streets (lower motor neurons), and freeways (the pyramidal motor tract); the effects of damage to these types of structures are reasonably predictable. But the bulk of the brain is comprised of associational paths that permit all but endless switching from one route to another. Without some rudimentary grasp of how various parts of the nervous system are organized into a functional whole, we could drown in details of exceptions to most rules about the effects of neurologic damage.

Brain maturation effects. The variety of behavioral effects of brain damage in a particular location is even greater when mature and immature nervous systems are compared. With neurologic maturation goes development of relatively stable patterns of neural firing. These patterns appear to underlie all aspects of organized behavior, such as memory, perception, and all facets of speech and language (Hebb, 1949, 1963). The more stable these networks of neural functioning become, the more immutable they become. In effect, the brain becomes less plastic, less flexible, less adaptable to insult the more it matures. A young nervous system, when injured, is better able to develop new patterns than an old system. Knowledge of location and the extent of neural damage must be interpreted against knowledge of development of neural functioning if we are to appreciate the effects of brain injury and the possibilities of recovery (Chase, 1972).

The brain and behavior are separate domains. Efforts to link them are improving, but knowing details of brain injury does not yet permit precise prediction of exact behavioral consequences, or vice versa. Yet both domains taken separately can be described reasonably well. The neurologist, neurosurgeon, neurophysiologist, and neuroanatomist can state conditions of the nervous system with some accuracy. Their knowledge

is the province of this chapter. The speech pathologist and psycholinguist can describe normal and defective speech. Details of their analyses will be emphasized in Part III. Let us examine the relation between these two bodies of knowledge to determine as best we can how neurologic disabilities affect communicative behavior.

A model of neurologic disabilities and speech disorders

Several years ago, Wepman and his associates (1960) devised a model to show how language is functionally related to the central nervous system. Though only one of many efforts to relate neural and speech defects, this conceptual design helps to clarify the essence of the functional relationship between a very complex mechanism, the brain, and an equally complex activity, speech, around which a remarkably perplexing set of terms has arisen.

This model, shown in expanded form in Fig. 5-3, will be used as a framework for our discussion, not because it is necessarily the most definitive concept, but because it simplifies without being simplistic. Moreover, it dovetails neatly with other sophisticated conceptions, such as Hebb's (1963), of how the brain is organized. He holds that it is comprised of semiautonomous systems that carry out input, integrative, and output functions. The entire brain may be involved in functions of each system, but these functions are essentially independent of one another.

Input transmission disorders

Sensation without meaning: agnosia. A disorder in the transmission of any sensory input is best identified as *agnosia.* The term is descriptive of the condition: "a," without; "gnosia," knowing or cognition. Agnosia is a disorder in which sensation is experienced but without meaning, as the click of a telegraph key would be meaningless for one who does not know Morse code.

This disorder is specific to the sensory modality disabled. A patient with *auditory agnosia* would be unable to recognize speech heard but might have no difficulty reading.

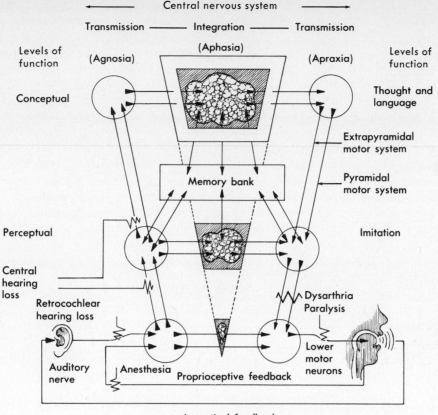

Fig. 5-3. Levels of function in the nervous system in relation to speech functions and disorders. Wepman's diagram is expanded to include peripheral input and output disabilities. (From Wepman, J., *J. Speech Hearing Dis.*, **25**,326 [1960].)

With impaired speech recognition, he would be unable to monitor and guide his own speech by listening to himself. Conversely, one with *visual agnosia* could perform normally in conversation but be unable to recognize what he reads. *Tactile agnosia*, on the other hand, is of little consequence to speech but would be of vital importance to the blind. To be unable to recognize objects touched would preclude being able to read braille. Since agnosia describes cognitive inability to recognize sensation, it implies damage high enough in the central nervous system to permit sensory information to reach the brain. When the damage is so close to the sensory receptor that little if any information is transmitted, the more appropriate term is

deafness, blindness, or, in the case of touch, *anesthesia*. Whether a patient experiences meaningless sensations or no sensation at all over the external auditory feedback channel or the internal tactual and kinesthetic channels, ability to control accuracy of speaking behavior will be impaired.

Integrative disorders

Aphasia. The term for language disorders related to central integrative disabilities is *aphasia* (from Greek, meaning "without speech"). This term has been the subject of more writing, more disagreement, and more confusion than most others in speech pathology. What it designates is disruption of the integrative process after a stimulus is free

Do Wepman and associates (1960), Schuell, Jenkins, and Jimenez-Pabon (1964), and Darley (1967) agree on characteristics of aphasia? Do they use the same terms to mean the same things? You can read the historical background for this problem in the chapter by Schuell and Jenkins (1961).

---

of its input modality (Schuell, Jenkins, and Jimenez-Pabon, 1964; Wepman and others, 1960). Unlike agnosia, aphasia is no respector of sensory channel: speech heard and speech read are equally disturbed.

The other distinguishing feature of aphasia involves disruption of language processes. To define aphasia, Brown (1968) described four components of a central language process:

1. A vocabulary of meaningful symbols
2. A grammar (linguistic rules for assembling symbols)
3. A long-enough memory for symbols to permit processing them
4. An ability to utilize linguistic rules for decoding (sorting out speech signals from noise) and for encoding (selecting appropriate linguistic units)

Aphasia is an impairment of any combination of these components. Much of the confusion in terminology has arisen over what to call the combinations.

Because impairment may fall anywhere within this central language process (CLP), Wepman and associates (1960) recognized three types of aphasia. The patient who cannot find language to give meaning to any stimulus, irrespective of modality, has *pragmatic aphasia*. (In Sperry's [1968] split-brain subject, this would correspond to the non-dominant hemisphere's knowing what an object is but, disconnected from the dominant language hemisphere, being unable to verbalize this knowledge.) Pragmatic aphasia is a breakdown in the decoding operation of CLP component 4. It resembles agnosia but differs in two important respects: it is not specific to a particular sensory modality, and nonverbal recognition is still possible. A second type, *semantic aphasia*, involves inability to select words to express meaning; it is essentially a vocabulary retrieval problem of CLP components 1 and 4. This is the type

of aphasic lapse that anyone who cannot find the right word experiences in mild form. The third type, *syntactic aphasia*, is primarily a breakdown in CLP components 2 and 3. Patients of this type, either because they cannot remember linguistic rules or because they cannot retain symbols in mind long enough to complete a grammatical sentence, exhibit faulty syntax. More recently Wepman and Jones (1966) have added *jargon aphasia*, failure to understand speech and to speak intelligibly (involving disability of at least CLP component 4), and *global aphasia*, complete loss of language that could reflect breakdown in various degrees of all four CLP components.

Neat as these distinctions would be, in reality they rarely are found in isolation. An auditory agnosia may occur with some form of receptive aphasia. Expressive aphasia may occur in conjunction with some receptive impairment, and may be indistinguishable from an accompanying apraxia. Because these language disorders take so many bewildering forms, they have been described in many ways by many authorities. In adults, *nonfluent aphasia*, *motor aphasia*, *expressive aphasia*, *verbal aphasia*, and *anterior aphasia*, are roughly equivalent to *Broca's aphasia*, or *Wepman's syntactic aphasia*. By the same token, *receptive aphasia*, *sensory aphasia*, *posterior aphasia*, and *fluent aphasia* identify essentially the same language disorder as *Wernicke's aphasia*, or *pragmatic aphasia* (Schuell, Jenkins, and Jimenez-Pabon, 1964; Weisenberg and McBride, 1935; Darley, 1967; Wepman and others, 1960; Eisenson, 1971; Goodglass and Kaplan, 1972).

Childhood aphasia. As for aphasia in childhood, it necessarily involves defective auditory processes for decoding speech (Myklebust, 1971; Chase, 1972). Speaking of these children as "developmentally aphasic," Eisenson (1968) characterizes their disability by five features:

1. Perceptual dysfunction in one or more (but not all) sensory modalities
2. Auditory dysfunction beyond that attributable to audiometrically measurable loss

3. Intellectual inefficiency beyond that attributable to measurable levels of intelligence
4. All but complete verbal impairment semantically, syntactically, and phonologically
5. Perseveration, inconsistent response, and emotional lability under stress

Eisenson attributes retarded speech development to defective memory storage and recall capacity for spoken language (but not necessarily for other sounds), defective discrimination of speech in context, and defective processing and sequencing of speech signals at normal speaking rates.

Output transmission disorders

Speech effects of disabilities of the output transmission system take two major forms: apraxia, difficulty in motor formulation of articulated language, and dysarthria, incoordination in execution of the speech act.

When motor aphasia is not aphasia: apraxia. Apraxia describes a disorder that has existed under many labels. Broca's effort in 1861 to differentiate it from aphasia, by calling it *aphemie,* was soon muddied by Trousseau, who, in 1864, confused the issue by renaming it *aphasie.* Since then, it has been called Broca's aphasia, motor aphasia, subcortical motor aphasia, predominantly expressive aphasia, Marie's anarthria, verbal aphasia, phonetic disintegration of speech, cortical dysarthria, and apraxic dysarthria. What this blizzard of terms is intended to denote is a modality-bound impairment of motor expression of language. The impairment is not a problem of aphasia, since the central language processes are intact. The patient can select words he wants, the correct grammatical structure for his idea, and the proper sequence of phonemes. The deficit is specific to the output transmission channel; for speech, it is called *oral verbal apraxia,* and for writing, *motor agraphia.*

Such patients have speech replete with inconsistent articulatory substitutions, omissions, and distortions as they grope for correct positioning of articulators. Errors spiral out of control as they struggle to correct

clumsy articulatory movements, especially in polysyllabic words. These patients initiate speech disfluently, with repetitions of sounds, syllables, and words, and their speech prosody is disturbed as they attempt to compensate for mistakes. Still, they may have no problem in auditory comprehension or written expression. Patients with oral verbal apraxia often learn to tiptoe through speech; wary, unsure of how phonemes are produced, they approach sounds cautiously and, rather slowly and monotonously, move the articulators with exaggerated deliberation from position to position (Darley, 1964; La Pointe, 1975).

Neuromuscular speech disorders: dysarthria. Dysarthria, by contrast, is a problem characterized by weakness, paralysis, or incoordination of the speech apparatus itself. Actually, we should probably use a plural term, "dysarthrias," because specific manifestations vary with the wide range of neurologic disabilities underlying this disorder. Neural lesions can range all the way from lower motor neuron paralyses, through extrapyramidal *hyperkinesias* (excessive motor function) or *hypokinesias* (decreased motor function), to cerebellar incoordinations. These disabilities can differentially disturb any of the speech production processes: respiration, phonation, articulation, resonation, or prosody (Darley, 1967). *Flaccid* (flabby) and *spastic* (spasm) dysarthrias, for example, are characterized by rather consistent articulatory errors, whereas *ataxic* (incoordinated) and *hyperkinetic* dysarthrias typically show inconsistent misarticulations.

Work done at the Mayo Clinic (Darley, Aronson, and Brown, 1969a,b) has delineated these five types of dysarthria. What the Mayo investigators suspected was that a phonetically trained ear could, on the basis of listening to differences in dysarthric speech, determine the type of neurologic disability, sometimes even before it could be diagnosed neurologically (Grewel, 1957). From such quaint descriptions of dysarthric speech as "slobbery" or "mush in the mouth," they have refined distinctive speech and voice characteristics of different dysarthric groups that, in turn, mirror different kinds of abnormal neuromuscular functioning. Table 5-1 shows how they related what they heard to types of dysarthria and to neurologic defects. Only a sample is provided of the thirty-eight speech and voice factors that were analyzed for distinctive patterns.

An insult to the motor system that strikes prenatally or during early growing years can disturb patterns of development profoundly, often in ways extending far beyond direct effects of the disability. Normal processes and tactics for acquiring the usual collection of human skills, for shaping personality, and for intellectual growth can be skewed badly, if not seriously retarded. In the mature person, the same neurologic insult can produce considerably more discrete effects on existing abilities. Still, the young nervous system is far more plastic and capable of developing new patterns to cope with damage than is the older, more mature system, in which neural functioning is stabilized. Of brain damage, it is not enough to know "where" and "how much"; "when" weighs heavily, too.

Cerebral palsy: childhood dysarthria. As all good rules have exceptions, so do all good

organizational schemes. We will now violate ours. You may be puzzled as to why *cerebral palsy*, a much publicized problem, has not been mentioned up to this point. Has this handicap, like infantile paralysis, been eliminated so that it no longer needs to be considered? Hardly. It is as much with us as ever, and three in every thousand of our population are estimated to be cerebral palsied; one such person is born every 53 minutes. Of the more than 500,000 cerebral-palsied persons in the United States, only one third are under 21 years of age (McDonald and Chance, 1964).

The problem of discussing this dramatically crippling condition is one of relating it to all the other neurologic disabilities. Like a camel with its head in the organizational tent, it encompasses a bit of everything. Although it is basically a problem of childhood, two thirds of those afflicted are now adults. Cerebral palsy, although primarily a motor transmission defect, can include an associated defect of sensory input, as well as intellectual and behavioral disturbances; it is not limited to dysarthrias but can include apraxias, aphasias, and agnosias. Although mainly a birth injury defect, it can be caused by genetic

Table 5-1. Dysarthric characteristics of neuromotor disabilities

Characteristic speech-voice factors	Type of disorder	Type of disease
Strain-strangle, harsh voice Hypernasality Imprecise consonants Monotony	Spastic dysarthria	Pseudobulbar palsy Amyotrophic lateral sclerosis
Hypernasality Breathy voice Imprecise consonants Monopitch	Flaccid dysarthria	Bulbar palsy
Excess and equal stress Irregular articulatory breakdown Harsh voice	Ataxic dysarthria *incoordinated*	Cerebellar disease
Monopitch Monoloudness Reduced stress Imprecise consonants	Hypokinetic dysarthria	Parkinsonism
Irregular articulatory breakdown Harsh voice Monopitch Vowels distorted	Hyperkinetic dysarthria	Dystonia Choreoathetosis

factors or by prenatal and postnatal disease, infection, or trauma. Practically, cerebral palsy is a microcosm of the whole world of neurologic disabilities.

A clinical entity known for many years as *Little's disease* and as *spastic paralysis,* cerebral palsy designates not a disease but a motor system disability and associated defects in young children. Its primary symptoms reflect motor damage: paralysis, weakness, and incoordination. Note that these are also the symptoms of dysarthria, but whereas dysarthria designates only speech muscle disablement, cerebral palsy can apply to any musculature, especially of arms and legs. Associated symptoms can run the gamut of those handicaps that any child might have: defective speech, impaired hearing, impaired vision, orthopedic defects, convulsions, perceptual difficulties, retarded intellectual development, dental anomalies, and emotional problems. Cerebral-palsied persons are generally, but not always, multiply handicapped.

These disorders can be so mild as to be unnoticed or so severe that the cerebral palsied are never able to care for themselves. Doubly handicapped by being afflicted as children, they must build their lives around their limitations. The need to learn may be reduced because of overprotection. Discrimination of what is to be learned may be disturbed because of perceptual impairment. Ability to perfect motor skills may be difficult because of primary neuromuscular disability. Even rewards for learning may be weakened if the need to learn is reduced in the first place. Still, many of these children who, a few years ago, were said to be in the "farthest corner" have reached adulthood and have carved useful and satisfying slots for themselves in society (Wright, 1960).

Cerebral palsy is classified by neurologic characteristics two ways: by motor disability and by topography of limbs afflicted. Topographically, disability can involve primarily one limb (*monoplegia*), both lower limbs (*paraplegia*), half of the body (*hemiplegia*), three limbs (*triplegia*), or all four limbs (*quadriplegia*). In terms of type of motor dis-

ability, a point to bear in mind is that all types have one thing in common: reflexive behavior is released that normally is suppressed and integrated by higher levels of neural control. Some of this reflexive behavior is so basic and primordial that we are usually not aware that it functions in automatic coordination of movement. Readily apparent in an infant who, while being held upside down, is suddenly dropped a few inches, or, more commonly, in the righting movements of a cat tossed unceremoniously out the door, this behavior may be a mani-

---

Does Mysak (1968) view evaluation of the condition of a cerebral-palsied person's reflexes of fundamental or secondary importance to the treatment of his speech problems?

---

festation of spinal reflexes, brain-stem reflexes, midbrain reflexes, or more complex equilibrium reactions mediated at the level of the basal ganglia, cerebellum, and cortex. As Travis (1931) observed years ago, the lower neural centers continue to serve their basic reflexive functions, but as the infant develops, higher centers assume a directive and regulatory control over them.

Although the most prevalent system of classification has followed Phelps' (1950) categories of *flaccid paralysis, spasticity, athetosis, ataxia, tremor,* and *rigidity,* Crothers and Paine (1959) make the convincing point that in children these distinctions are difficult if not impossible to determine. They prefer as more useful a division of cases into two major types of cerebral palsy: *spastic* and *extrapyramidal.* These types include the majority of cases, but rare types in which the predominant feature is *rigidity, tremor, ataxia,* or *atonia* can be found.

Spastic cerebral palsy is considered to be predominantly a consequence of pyramidal motor system disability that provides innervation to discrete muscle groups. Since spastic effects can be limited to any limb or combination of limbs, they can be classified topographically. Clinical signs of spasticity include the "clasp knife" type of muscular hypertonus, hyperreflexia and exaggerated postural reflexes, positive Babinski reflex, loss of voluntary control of fine movements, and spread of associated movements.

In extrapyramidal cerebral palsies, named for the motor system predominantly involved, the major clinical features include incoordination, delayed postural development, abnormal muscle tone that is likely to be hypotonic in infancy and hypertonic in later life, and, of special interest, dysarthric speech caused largely by poor respiratory control. Not only are extrapyramidal characteristics not limited topographically to spe-

---

Do McDonald and Chance (1964) accept the point of view that different types of cerebral palsy can be associated with anatomic sites of brain lesions?

---

cific muscle groups, they overlap and shift in predominant form with age (a major reason why Crothers and Paine prefer a broader classification system). Thus *athetosis* (involuntary writhing movements that accompany purposeful or postural movement), *chorea* (involuntary irregular spasmodic contractions that accompany purposeful activity), *dystonia* (involuntary rhythmic twisting distortions of the trunk), and *ballismus* (coarse involuntary jerking of an extremity) may be seen together, but athetosis is the predominant feature.

The dysarthric speech effects of different types of cerebral palsy described in Table 5-1 can be as much a consequence of interference of this multiple handicap with development as a consequence of specific disablement of muscular control. Respiratory anomalies, for example, are characteristic. Shallow, irregular breathing, vegetative breathing, and simultaneous inhalatory and exhalatory movements of "reversed" breathing predominate. None is effective for speech purposes. Hardy (1961) points out that ability to develop sufficient intraoral breath pressure for articulation is one indicator of a child's physiologic readiness for speech.

Among other ways that cerebral palsy can interfere with development, some are directly and some are indirectly related to

speech acquisition. Persistence of infantile suckle-swallow reflexes during the speech-learning period interferes with development of highly differentiated articulatory and phonatory movements. On the other hand, many speech disorders of these children can be attributed more to mental retardation, severe hearing loss, or psychologic immaturity than to dysarthria. If a child requires institutional care, that type of environment is conducive to retardation. Even if raised at home, this handicap invites overprotection or rejection, with the attendant effects on development (Mysak, 1971a).

Because the disablements of cerebral palsy are so pervasive, hope for these children is more than usually dependent on early intervention. Parents need special preparation. The children need special feeding training, special head and thoracic balance training, and special breathing training months before speech begins. During speech acquisition special types of intervention will be needed, all the way from surgical alleviation of a disabling condition, to the use of bioengineering devices for nonverbal alternatives to oral communication, to special techniques for facilitating development of speech and language (Mysak, 1971b).

Adult dysarthrias. A rather large group of disturbances in adults, adolescents, and older children can affect various portions of the motor transmission system with dysarthric results, some of which are shown in Table 5-1. More extensive descriptions of dysarthric speech characteristics are available in reports of work at the Mayo Clinic (Darley, Aronson, and Brown, 1969a,b). These disabling effects, tending to be more discrete than in children, can be best grasped by presenting them in relation to location of disability in the nervous system.

Among the disabilities involving the extrapyramidal system are *Sydenham's chorea,* occurring mainly in children but also in adolescents and adults; *Huntington's chorea,* which will be discussed later as a presenile psychosis; and *parkinsonism* and *dystonia.* Parkinsonism, also called *paralysis agitans,* is a progressive condition that usually begins after age 40. It is marked by a masklike facial expression, a persistent "pill-rolling" hand tremor, muscular rigidity, and slow movement. *Dystonia* is a rare chronic disease in which involuntary irregular clonic spasms contort the body forward and sideways grotesquely. (at trunk level!)

Pyramidal system disabilities affect upper motor neurons that connect right and left extremities only with contralateral cerebral hemispheres but that connect speech structures bilaterally with both hemispheres. Because of this arrangement, paralysis of a limb may be the only evidence of damage to the cortical motor area in one hemisphere, for example, after a stroke. Years later, perhaps, a stroke in the motor area of the other hemisphere may paralyze the opposite limb but additionally involve muscles of speech and swallowing. The reason, of course, that the speech mechanism is affected after the second but not the first stroke is that upper motor neuron paths from both hemispheres had to be injured before dysarthric symptoms appeared.

Pseudobulbar palsy is the upper motor neuron clinical syndrome most often encountered that affects speech. It is characterized by bilateral lesions, often caused by arteriosclerosis, of the cortical motor fibers that supply the lower motor neurons to muscles of the throat and mouth. The "pseudo" portion of the term designates symptoms of paralysis of these muscles for swallowing, chewing, and speaking that appear similar to those of *bulbar palsy* in which *lower* motor neurons in the bulb-shaped brain stem are damaged.

Lower motor neuron lesions that affect speech are often deadly. Because these low-level neural fibers are the sole paths by which muscles receive innervation, when they are destroyed the muscle fiber supplied is paralyzed, becomes flaccid, and atrophies. Whereas upper motor neuron lesions leave deep reflexes intact (if not exaggerated), even these reflexes are weakened with lower motor neuron disablement. When muscles

served are those of head and neck, not only speech is disrupted but sometimes also swallowing, chewing, and breathing—without which life is in jeopardy.

Motor neuron disease is a term for any disease of motor neurons; those affecting speech include progressive bulbar palsy, progressive muscular atrophy, acute ascending paralysis, and, one of the most common (and fatal) forms, amyotrophic lateral sclerosis. *Progressive bulbar palsy* specifically involves motor nerves of the brain stem to face, tongue, pharynx, and palate. Dysarthria is the prelude to death, since this paralysis progresses to the point of immobilizing the biologic functions of these structures. *Progressive muscular atrophy* is marked by weakening and wasting of muscles throughout the body, whereas *acute ascending paralysis* (also called *Landry's paralysis*) begins in the feet and ascends rapidly until fatal. Neither is specific to speech structures but usually involves them. Similarly, *amyotrophic lateral sclerosis*, marked by hardening of motor portions of the spinal cord, progresses within 3 years to the medulla in the brain stem, at which time it is inevitably fatal.

With the exception of respiratory muscles, the speech apparatus is served by peripheral sensory and lower motor neurons that leave the protective central nervous system housing through the cranium: hence the name *cranial nerves.* Of the twelve seen in Fig. 5-4, we will look only at the seven directly involved in speech and hearing.

The *trigeminal* nerve (cranial nerve V) carries sensation from face and mouth and carries motor signals to muscles of mastication. Brain tumors in the area of the brain stem near its origin commonly disable it. Loss of sensation in the face and mouth accompanies lesions of its sensory components. Paralysis of portions of tongue and jaw muscles with deviation to the paralyzed side marks damage to the motor segment of the fifth cranial nerve. The soft palate can also be affected, although specific contributions of different cranial nerves to palatal action are not clear.

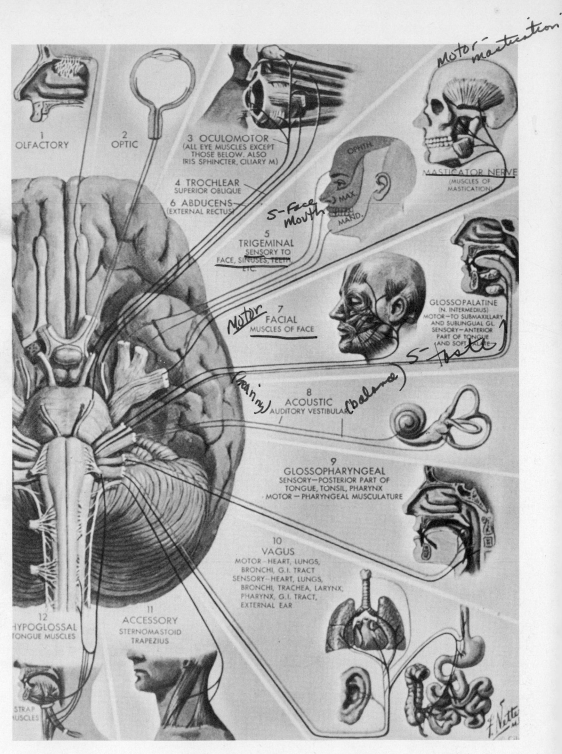

Fig. 5-4. Cranial nerves. Nerves V, VII, VIII, IX, X, XI, and XII carry sensory and motor signals for control of the speech mechanism. (From Netter, F. H., *The Ciba Collection of Medical Illustrations*. [Vol. 1] New York: CIBA Pharmaceutical Products, Inc. [1953].)

The *facial nerve* (cranial nerve VII) is mainly a motor nerve to muscles of the face, although it sends some branches to other muscles in the head and carries a sensory component, such as for taste, in the front of the tongue. When the facial nerve is injured, usually by a lesion, the side of the face supplied becomes paralyzed, an impairment called *Bell's palsy*. Involvement can extend to the entire side of the face, to a corner of the mouth, or to an eyelid that droops (ptosis).

The *acoustical* nerve (cranial nerve VIII) is a sensory nerve that combines two parts: the *vestibular* branch carrying sense of balance and the *cochlear* branch carrying auditory information. Menière's disease, producing *vertigo* (dizziness) and progressive deafness in the middle and later years, is the chief affliction of the eighth nerve. Tumors, such as *acoustical neurinoma*, also attack it but more infrequently and without vertigo as a primary complaint.

A mixed sensory and motor nerve, the *glossopharyngeal* (cranial nerve IX) serves throat and tongue. Its most important disease is *glossopharyngeal neuralgia*, which consists of bursts of sharp, severe pain in the throat and ear precipitated by swallowing.

Vagus (cranial nerve X) means "wandering," and that describes the course of this nerve; it even wanders as far as the abdomen. With motor and sensory fibers, it serves larynx, pharynx, and soft palate. Diseases that affect it include *poliomyelitis* and *diphtheria*. Depending on branches afflicted, tenth nerve pathology can result in paralysis of soft palate, pharyngeal constrictor muscles, or larynx. Because the *recurrent* branch to the larynx wanders close to the thyroid gland, a major cause of laryngeal paralysis is surgical accident during operation on the thyroid gland.

The *accessory* nerve (cranial nerve XI) is a motor nerve that serves a few muscles of the soft palate, neck, and chest. Since it has no specific disease associated with it, when the accessory nerve is afflicted, the condition is described as *neuritis*. Strictly speaking, this term means "neural inflammation"; actually, the pathology is more often a tumor.

The *hypoglossal* nerve (cranial nerve XII) is primarily a lingual motor nerve with some sensory fibers. Lesions paralyze the tongue, causing it to protrude to the affected side.

ETIOLOGY OF NEUROLOGIC DISABILITIES
Congenital neuropathologies

Congenital injuries. Children with cerebral palsy, developmental aphasia, and probably autism (Chapter 10) generally suffer neural insult early in the course of their existence. Congenital neural damage can occur *prenatally* (between conception and onset of labor), *paranatally* (during and immediately after birth), and *postnatally* (during infancy).

About 30% of cerebral-palsied children suffer prenatal insults resulting either from hereditary factors or from difficulties arising during gestation. Genetic factors can be responsible for metabolic disturbances such as diabetes and for Rh factor incompatibility of the blood of the mother and fetus, from

---

Students who would like a bit more detail about neuropathologies are referred to such a reference as Forster's *Clinical Neurology* (1973); those who would like considerably more, to appropriate sections of Cecil and Loeb's *Textbook of Medicine* (1959); and those who would like a definitive statement, to Grinker, Bucy, and Sahs' *Neurology* (1960).

---

which the brain-damaging condition of kernicterus can arise. Gestational difficulties can be attributed to a wide range of maternal conditions. Malnourishment, x-ray overexposure, injury of fetal brain tissue, predisposition to miscarriage, and infections (especially during the early months of pregnancy, and especially rubella) can harmfully alter the chemistry of the fetal environment. Too, a variety of circumstances can produce fetal anoxia: for example, kinked umbilical cord, placenta (in which fetal oxygen and carbon dioxide are exchanged) disturbed by bleeding, infarcts (tissue death caused by obstructed circulation), and reduced oxygen level during a coma after severe maternal injury. In truth, the unborn infant as it passes from a single- to a trillion-cell organism can encounter a multitude of hostile environments (McDonald and Chance, 1964).

The most perilous trip in life is entry into the world after passage through the birth canal. During this paranatal period, the fetus is forcefully dislodged from the stillness of an existence cushioned in amniotic fluid, bumped and shoved against the mother's bony pelvic girdle, propelled headfirst down the birth canal to emerge gasping for breath, his life as a parasite ended and as an independent being started. If all goes well, he will have only a few bruises to show for the experience.

The majority of infants who will be cerebral palsied suffer brain damage during this trip. Their passage may be too long, and they suffocate. It may be too precipitous, or too premature, or they may be delivered by cesarean section. The cerebral blood vessels may rupture, or the adjustment from intrauterine to atmospheric pressure may not be made quickly enough. The baby's brain may be injured by traumatic pounding against the pelvis or by obstetric forceps. His umbilical cord may be obstructed. His respiratory centers may be depressed by excessive maternal anesthesia to ease delivery pains. His respiratory tract may be blocked with plugs of mucus. Either condition can obstruct an adequate supply of oxygen to his brain after birth.

The *neonatal* (newborn) period does not end the tribulations that can result in cerebral palsy. About 10% of the cerebral palsied suffer brain damage during the postnatal period. Brain injury may result from trauma (skull fractures and head wounds), infection (encephalitis, meningitis, and brain abscesses), cerebral hemorrhage (congenital aneurysm [blood vessel "blowout"] and cerebrovascular thrombosis [blood clot]), anoxia (carbon monoxide, strangulation, and high altitudes), or enlarged brain tumors.

Congenital anomalies. Children born with congenital anomalies are often mentally retarded and multiply handicapped, some to the extent that they require care in institutions. Prime examples are *microcephalic* children, who are born with small skulls and brains, and *hydrocephalic* children, whose skulls have enlarged from pressure of cerebrospinal fluid that has not been permitted normal drainage from the head.

Mongolism, the familiar name for *Down's syndrome*, and *cretinism* present some similar symptoms but dissimilar etiologies and prognoses. Children with these diseases are alike in poor birth weight, short neck, and slow response to stimuli. Mongoloids, with characteristic mongolian appearance, protruding tongue, and in-turned little fingers, are usually affectionate but may be uneducable. The etiology of the disease is associated with a chromosomal deviation related to the mother's age; mongoloids are usually produced prematurely by women near the end of their reproductive years. Cretins, by contrast, are usually full-term babies whose disability stems from poor development or absence of the thyroid gland. Their prognosis is good if they are treated early for thyroid deficiency.

Three other chromosomal abnormalities associated with mental retardation are *cri du chat (cat's cry) syndrome*, *Klinefelter's syndrome*, and *Turner's syndrome*. Cri du chat syndrome is named for its most striking clinical feature: a high-pitched cry resembling a cat's mewing. Children with this syndrome, who are usually microcephalic, may reach a trainable level of retardation, but their speech is likely to be unintelligible. Klinefelter's syndrome occurs only in males, and its counterpart, Turner's syndrome, only in females. Psychologic and sexual dysfunctions along with mild retardation are characteristic (Gearheart and Litton, 1975).

Two conditions inherited as mendelian recessive traits are *phenylketonuria* and, rarer, *galactosemia*. Children with phenylketonuria have defective metabolism. They lack a necessary enzyme, and thus protein accumulates (especially from consumption of large quantities of milk) and forms a brain-damaging toxic reaction. Similarly, children with galactosemia accumulate toxic amounts of galactose that permanently damage brain and liver.

Other congenital metabolic diseases include *Tay-Sachs disease* and *Wilson's disorder* ease—also known as *progressive lenticular degeneration, tetanoid chorea*, and *pseudosclerosis*. Wilson's disease is a progressive disease, usually of infancy, in which abnormal copper metabolism leads to degeneration of the brain, particularly of the corpus striatum, a major extrapyramidal motor center. Athetoid movements follow rigidity, and in those children who live long enough to talk, speech is generally dysarthric. With recent medical advances, hope for children with Wilson's disease is improving, and some of the severe speech and voice problems are proving reversible (Darley, 1969). Tay-Sachs disease is found mostly in Jewish children. These children appear normal at birth, but lipids begin accumulating in the nervous system by 6 months of age. Subsequent deterioration of hearing, vision, motor, and mental functions is progressive (Gearheart and Litton, 1975).

Infections

Brain infections in children can result in *chorea, meningitis*, and *encephalitis*, among other conditions. Chorea comes in more than fifty forms, the one most related to children being *Sydenham's chorea*, better known as St. Vitus' dance (in honor of the patron saint of dancers; in fact, "chorea" is the Greek word for dancing, but choreic movements are jerky, not rhythmic). Rarely seen in infants, they may first appear, especially in girls between ages 5 and 15 years, in connection with measles and rheumatic fever. Fragmentary movements often are seen in lips, tongue, and fingers before they increase and spread to extremities. Speech is frequently involved during the several months that the disease usually lasts.

In meningitis, the meningeal covering of the brain and spinal cord can become infected at most any age or location. Thus, aside from fever and headache, no characteristic symptoms can be described. *Spinal meningitis* attacks the spinal cord and can result in paralysis, whereas *encephalitis* sometimes called "sleeping sickness," is presumed to result from viral infection. It refers to inflammation of the brain, increased pressure from edema being especially injurious. Because different areas can become infected —generally the basal ganglia are involved —symptoms vary. They usually include drowsiness and lethargy and can include choreoathetotic types of movement. Neural infection can also arise from spread of localized abscesses such as occur in the middle ear or sinuses.

Tumors

1/10 of tumors in nervous system

Nearly one tenth of all tumors occur in the nervous system. Of these, 80% are in the brain and 10% in the spinal cord. Tumors effect their damage largely by occupying space, thereby increasing pressure; symptoms depend largely on location. Tumors increase pressure mainly by blocking flow of blood or cerebrospinal fluid and, to a lesser extent, by infiltrating neural tissue, thus increasing its mass. They can be benign as are *meningiomas* that develop from fibrous tissue in the meningeal covering of the nervous system. Gliomas *malignant* constitute 45% of brain tumors, however, and are generally malignant growths that arise directly from brain tissue. They do not tend to *metastasize* (spread), but prognosis is poor. Another 20% of *neoplasms* (new growths) in the brain are metastatic tumors that have spread from growths in other parts of the body. When a tumor blocks a drainage channel for cerebrospinal fluid in young children, it can cause sufficient pressure to produce a hydrocephalically expanded head. On the other hand, impairment can range through seizures to hardly noticeable mild focal symptoms.

Epilepsy

1/200 - incidence

Epilepsy is an affliction of adults as well as young children. Not only is its incidence high in the population (at least one person in two hundred has it) but it can be caused, literally, by every known disease of the nervous system. The term "epilepsy" does not connote cause, only the fact that a patient has seizures. As knowledge has advanced, the proportion of patients said to have *idiopathic* (unknown origin) *epilepsy* has shrunk, whereas the proportion said to have *symp-*

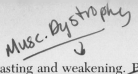

tomatic or *acquired epilepsy* that can be attributed to other factors has grown. Among the most frequent causes of focal epilepsy are lesions that involve brain atrophy and cerebral tumors. In idiopathic epilepsy chances of normal intelligence are good. In acquired epilepsy, seizures are produced by conditions that can impair mental and motor performance.

A seizure can be so mild as to pass unnoticed, or it can be of demoniacal fury. Epileptics often experience an aura, a premonition, of a *grand mal* seizure to come. These convulsions, usually found in acquired epilepsy, are severe: respiration is suspended, the patient loses consciousness, and his body becomes rigid. *Petit mal* does not mean, strictly, what its name implies; it refers to a type of seizure (usually of genetic origin), not to its small size. Loss of consciousness is the primary symptom. It comes without warning, lasts only a few seconds, leaves no trace, and may recur many times daily.

West (1958) likened stuttering to *pyknolepsy*, a childhood condition akin to petit mal epilepsy. Can you find support for this similarity in medical descriptions of pyknolepsy?

Demyelinating diseases

Schilder's disease, generally found in children under 10 years of age, involves progressive erosion of myelin (insulation on nerve fibers) in the interior of first one and then the other cerebral hemisphere. Early symptoms are hemiplegia; later, quadriplegia and dementia appear, and eventually, death.

The major demyelinating disease among adults is *multiple sclerosis.* It occurs primarily between ages 20 and 40. For unknown reasons, lesions appear at random in the white myelin insulation of neurons throughout the nervous system. As the disease progresses, ataxia ensues and speech becomes dysarthric.

Muscular diseases

Several muscular diseases can affect speech during developmental years. Probably best known is *muscular dystrophy*, a progressive wasting and weakening. Primarily of hereditary origin, it afflicts males three times as frequently as females, attacks the torso, and gradually extends to extremities. By contrast, *myotonia congenita* is a mild hereditary muscular disability in which, when movement is initiated, muscles remain contracted for several seconds. The condition lasts for life but is not progressive. On the other hand, *amyotonia congenita*, first seen in early months of life, is characterized by such underdevelopment of muscles that most children so afflicted die within 5 years, usually of pneumonia.

The adult muscular disease that most directly affects speech is *myasthenia gravis*. It is marked by progressive weakening with use of specific muscles, frequently of the jaws, tongue, face, larynx, and pharynx. The muscles do not atrophy; rather, they fatigue quickly. The condition results from a biochemical lesion where the motor nerve joins the muscle.

Progressive muscular dystrophy, by contrast, is a hereditary degenerative disease of young male adults, as well as of children, in which skeletal muscles and those of the extremities waste away. A similar disease, *myotonic dystrophy*, is a hereditary disease of middle-aged adult males in which facial muscles as well as those of the extremities atrophy.

Cerebrovascular disturbance

A notorious leveler of men, *cerebrovascular accident* (in neurologic jargon, CVA; in layman's terms, stroke) is the third most common cause of death in elderly persons. The term describes the condition: "cerebro" locates damage in the cerebrum; "vascular" denotes blood supply as being impaired; and "accident" specifies that because of head injury occurring for no directly apparent reason, a blood vessel accidentally plugs up, is cut, or "blows out."

Cerebrovascular accidents come in two main forms: *ischemic lesions* and *hemorrhagic lesions*. Ischemic lesions, the type usually referred to as "stroke," restrict arterial blood supply to portions of the cerebrum. If ischemia is followed by *infarct*, in which neural tissue, deprived of blood, dies and is replaced with scar tissue, brain damage in that area becomes permanent. Hemorrhagic lesions, on the other hand, follow rupture of an aneurysm (usually in a weakened artery) or severing of arteries, veins, or capillaries by physical trauma.

Effects of a CVA depend on several factors: area, extent, and permanence of damage. Almost any symptom of brain injury can be a consequence of some combination of these factors. This type of disability is the major basis for aphasia; it can also produce dysarthria, paralysis of various extremities, and impairment of mental efficiency and emotional stability. Much initial trauma from a CVA results from edema in the cranium. As pressure subsides and normal neural function is restored, many initial symptoms diminish.

Trauma

Traumatic injury to the nervous system is closely related to vascular impairment because damage to blood supply can cause more havoc to the brain than direct injury of neural tissue. Trauma can be classified by location: head injuries, spinal cord injuries, and peripheral nerve injuries. *Head injuries* can be *open* or *closed*, depending on whether or not the scalp is punctured. With either type, intracranial hemorrhage and amnesia are common. The duration of amnesia is generally proportional to amount of permanent brain damage. *Spinal cord injuries*, often the result of bullet or knife wounds, are also common to traffic accidents with characteristic "whiplash" injury that bruises and stretches the cord. Spastic paraplegia often results. *Peripheral nerve injuries*, unlike central nervous system insults, do permit recovery (central neurons will not regenerate, whereas peripheral neurons will).

Mental disturbance

One third of patients first admitted to a mental hospital suffer brain pathology. Memory, judgment, comprehension, learning, emotional response, personal appearance, movement, and, our major concern, speech can be impaired. These impairments can be behavioral manifestations of brain tumors, infection, metabolic disturbances, and head injuries.

More consistently associated with mental disorders are degenerative diseases that give the appearance of senile psychosis yet occur in patients who have not yet reached senility. These diseases are the so-called *presenile psychoses*. This group includes *Huntington's chorea*, *Alzheimer's disease*, and *Pick's disease*. Huntington's chorea is genetically transmitted to half of the children of a parent who carries it. Unfortunately, since it does not appear until years after parents have had their families, carriers of this rare disease are not detected in advance. It attacks the extrapyramidal system, producing dysarthria along with athetosis and mental deterioration. *Alzheimer's disease* and *Pick's disease*, with onset between the ages of 40 and 60 years, are similar in the relentless progression of effects of cerebral atrophy, from language disturbance, to psychosis, and often death. *Korsakoff's psychosis*, too, generally occurs prior to senility, but it is the sequel to alcoholic impairment of the brain.

Psychoses of the aged are often accompanied by brain damage. *Arteriosclerosis* (hardening of arteries), for instance, can injure brain tissue by impairing circulation. In *senile dementia*, with age of onset around 75, the brain degenerates, but the extent of damage is not necessarily proportional to symptoms exhibited.

THE SPEECH PATHOLOGIST'S RESPONSIBILITY IN THE TREATMENT OF NEUROLOGIC DISABILITIES

Obviously, the speech pathologist holds no direct clinical responsibility for disturbances of the nervous system. He has three indirect responsibilities, however: (1) to understand the relation between neural and speech functions; (2) to assist in the diagnosis of neurologic impairment by accurate appraisal of communicative behavior; and (3) to further knowledge of brain mechanisms underlying speech, and to apply this knowledge to minimize the effects of neurologic disability on speech and language.

Understanding the brain mechanisms of speech

The better we understand how the brain operates, the better we will understand the limits it imposes on speech and the better will be possibilities of developing effective remedial procedures for disorders of communication. The importance of this understanding applies not only to such problems as aphasia and cerebral palsy that are "obviously" related to neuropathology; it applies equally to so-called "functional" problems. Were we to understand, for example, how the nervous system manages timing of neural events for speech, we might discover new keys to treatment of stuttering.

From the practical standpoint of the clinician, knowledge of brain mechanisms is imperative if he is to participate in successful programs of therapy. Speech problems do not exist, nor can speech pathologists function, in isolation. Neural impairment is associated with so many communicative disorders that the neurologist must often be involved; his language and his concepts must be understood. With multiply handicapped persons, work on speech must be coordinated with other therapies. Indeed, its remediation may be impossible without the aid of other specialists. Clearly, the speech pathologist is responsible for solid knowledge about the nervous system and its disabilities.

Assisting in neurologic diagnosis

The speech pathologist has important information to contribute to neurologic diagnosis when speech is defective. Neural impairment can sometimes be detected by a trained ear before neurologic evaluation reveals disease. Such early warning is of considerable importance, but it requires exact knowledge of what to listen for and careful examination of speech to detect it.

Furthering knowledge of brain mechanisms of speech

Perhaps, in the final analysis, furthering knowledge of the neurology of speech is the most important responsibility of the speech pathologist. Being an applied behavioral scientist, he is uniquely qualified to investigate the brain mechanisms of speech. As a scientist, he has necessary research skills to further knowledge. As a scientist interested in speech, he is concerned with the most complex yet in many ways most neurologically revealing behavior that man exhibits. As a scientist interested in applying knowledge to understand breakdowns in speech, he is privy to the window that has so far let in the most light on brain mechanisms of oral language: speech effects of neural damage. As a clinical scientist, he holds prime responsibility for determining the special problems of speech, language, and even nonverbal communication posed by neurologic handicaps. He is equally responsible for devising strategies to meet these needs, which may range from major feats of bioengineering to minor adaptations of standard clinical procedures.

The answers—résumé

1. What neurologic disabilities affect speech?

Speech effects of neurologic disabilities depend largely on the location of the impairment. If the input transmission system is disabled, disorders of sensation or perception can result. If the transmission process is disabled, loss of sensory information ensues (for audition, this would be hearing loss or deafness); in higher levels of input processing, if ability to assign meaning to sensation is hampered, an agnosia specific to the disabled sensory modality is likely.

If central integrative processes are impaired, the disability affects all input and output modalities for language, the most frequent disorder being aphasia, an impairment of ability to apply rules of language in listening or speaking, reading or writing. Other related disorders include confused language and generalized intellectual impairment.

Where the output transmission system is disabled, the result can be specific to either speech or writing. If motor patterning for articulation is impaired, the problem will be apraxia, an inability to articulate sounds smoothly and easily. If the speech muscles are weakened, paralyzed, or incoordinated by disability of the motor transmission function (by pyramidal, extrapyramidal, or lower motor neuron impairment), the problem will be dysarthria.

2. What is the etiology of neurologic disabilities?

Causes of neurologic disabilities range across a wide spectrum of impairments: hereditary malformations, prenatal injuries, metabolic and toxic disturbances, tumors, traumas, epilepsies, infectious diseases, demyelinating diseases, muscular diseases, and vascular impairments. Some of these conditions occur before, some during, and some following birth, some in childhood, some in adults, some in the aged, and some at any time. Whether they strike before or after speech is acquired will bear heavily on effects of the disability. Some affect input, some output, some the integrative system, and some can strike anywhere in the nervous system. Location of impairment is a major determinant of behavioral effects.

3. What is the speech pathologist's responsibility in the treatment of neurologic disabilities?

The speech pathologist holds no direct responsibility for treatment of neurologic impairments, but he holds three indirect responsibilities for them. He must understand the brain mechanisms of speech in order to work effectively with other specialists. He holds the responsibility to contribute to neurologic diagnosis by developing skill in detecting how patients with different neurologic characteristics typically sound. Finally, he has a responsibility to further knowledge of the brain mechanisms of speech and to apply it in developing special methods of meeting the communicative needs of the neurologically handicapped.

REFERENCES

Brown, J., A model for control and peripheral behavior in aphasia. Paper read at the Academy of Aphasia, Rochester, Minn. (1968).

Cecil, R., and Loeb, R., *A Textbook of Medicine.* Philadelphia: W. B. Saunders Co. (1959).

Chase, R., Neurological aspects of language disorders in children. In Irwin, J., and Marge, M. (Eds.), *Principles of Childhood Language Disabilities.* New York: Appleton-Century-Crofts (1972).

Crothers, B., and Paine, R., *The Natural History of Cerebral Palsy.* Cambridge, Mass.: Harvard University Press (1959).

Darley, F., *Diagnosis and Appraisal of Communication Disorders.* Englewood Cliffs, N.J.: Prentice-Hall, Inc. (1964).

Darley, F., Lacunae and research approaches to them. (Vol. 4). In Millikan, C., and Darley, F., *Brain Mechanisms Underlying Speech and Language,* New York: Grune & Stratton, Inc. (1967).

Darley, F., Differential speech and language characteristics in patients with apraxia of speech, aphasia, confusion, and diffuse intellectual changes. In *Special Intensive Short Course,* American Speech and Hearing Association Convention (1968).

Darley, F., Personal communication (1969).

Darley, F., Aronson, A., and Brown, J., Clusters of deviant speech dimensions in the dysarthrias. *J. Speech Hearing Res.,* **12,** 462-496 (1969a).

Darley, F., Aronson, A., and Brown, J., Differential diagnostic patterns of dysarthria. *J. Speech Hearing Res.,* **12,** 246-269 (1969b).

Darley, F., Brown, J., and Swenson, W., Language changes after neurosurgery for Parkinsonism. *Brain and Language*, **2**, 65-69 (1975).

Denny-Brown, D., Motor mechanisms—introduction: the general principles of motor integration. In Field, J., Magoun, H., and Hall, V. (Eds.), *Handbook of Physiology*. (Section I) *Neurophysiology*. (Vol. II) Washington: American Physiological Society (1960).

Dreifuss, F., The pathology of central communicative disorders in children. In Tower, D. (Editor-in-chief), *The Nervous System*. (Vol. 3) *Human Communication and Its Disorders*. New York: Raven Press (1975).

Eisenson, J., Developmental aphasia (dyslogia): a postulation of a unitary concept of the disorder. *Cortex*, **4**, 184-200 (1968).

Eisenson, J., Aphasia in adults: basic considerations. In Travis, L. (Ed.), *Handbook of Speech Pathology and Audiology*. New York: Appleton-Century-Crofts (1971).

Eisenson, J., Language rehabilitation of aphasic adults: a review of some issues as to the state of the art. In Tower, D. (Editor-in-chief), *The Nervous System*. (Vol. 3) *Human Communication and Its Disorders*. New York: Raven Press (1975).

Forster, F., *Clinical Neurology*. (3d ed.) St. Louis: The C. V. Mosby Co. (1973).

French, I., The reticular formation. *Scient. Am.*, **196** (5) (1957).

French, I., The reticular formation. In Field, J., Magoun, H., and Hall, V. (Eds.), *Handbook of Physiology*. (Section I) *Neurophysiology* (Vol. 2) Washington: American Physiological Society (1960).

Gearheart, B., and Litton, F., *The Trainable Retarded: a Foundations Approach*. St. Louis: The C. V. Mosby Co. (1975).

Geschwind, N., Neurological foundations of language. In Myklebust, H. (Ed.), *Progress in Learning Disabilities*. (Vol. 1) New York: Grune & Stratton, Inc. (1968).

Geschwind, N., The apraxias: neural mechanisms of disorders of learned movement. *Am. Scient.*, **63**, 188-195 (1975).

Goodglass, H., and Kaplan, E., *Boston Diagnostic Aphasia Examination*. Philadelphia: Lea & Febiger (1972).

Grewel, F., Classification of dysarthrias. *Acta Psychiatr. Neurolo. Scand.*, **32**, 325-337 (1957).

Grinker, R., Bucy, P., and Sahs, A., *Neurology*. Springfield, Ill.: Charles C Thomas, Publisher (1960).

Guilford, J., *The Nature of Human Intelligence*. New York: McGraw-Hill Book Co. (1967).

Hardy, J., Intraoral breath pressure in cerebral palsy. *J. Speech Hearing Dis.*, **26**, 309-319 (1961).

Hebb, D., *The Organization of Behavior*. New York: John Wiley & Sons, Inc. (1949).

Hebb, D., The semiautonomous process: its nature and nurture. *Am. Psychol.*, **18**, 16-27 (1963).

Hollien, H., Neural control of the speech mechanism. In Tower, D. (Editor-in-chief), *The Nervous System*. (Vol. 3) *Human Communication and Its Disorders*. New York: Raven Press (1975).

Jung, R., and Hassler, R., The extrapyramidal motor system. In Field, J., Magoun, H., and Hall, V. (Eds.), *Handbook of Physiology*. (Section I) *Neurophysiology*. (Vol. 2) Washington: American Physiological Society (1960).

Kimura, D., Cerebral dominance for speech. In Tower, D. (Editor-in-chief), *The Nervous System*. (Vol. 3) *Human Communication and Its Disorders*. New York: Raven Press (1975).

LaPointe, L., Neurologic abnormalities affecting speech. In Tower, D. (Editor-in-chief), *The Nervous System*. (Vol. 3) *Human Communication and Its Disorders*. New York: Raven Press (1975).

Lehninger, A., Molecular biology: the theme of confrontation. In Quarton, G., Melnechuk, T., and Schmitt, F. (Eds.), *The Neurosciences*. New York: Rockefeller University Press (1967).

Lenneberg, E., On explaining language. *Science*, **164**, 635-643 (1969).

Livingston, R., Introduction: brain circuitry relating to complex behavior. In Quarton, G., Melnechuk, T., and Schmitt, F. (Eds.), *The Neurosciences*. New York: Rockefeller University Press (1967).

Luria, A., *Higher Cortical Functions in Man*. New York: Basic Books, Inc. (1966).

Luria, A., *Traumatic Aphasia: Its Syndromes, Psychology and Treatment*. The Hague: Mouton (1970).

MacKay, D., Neural communications: experiment and theory. *Science*, **159**, 335-353 (1968).

McDonald, E., and Chance, B., *Cerebral Palsy*. Englewood Cliffs, N.J.: Prentice-Hall, Inc. (1964).

Myklebust, H., Childhood aphasia: an evolving concept. In Travis, L. (Ed.), *Handbook of Speech Pathology and Audiology*. New York: Appleton-Century-Crofts (1971).

Mysak, E., *Neuroevolutional Approach to Cerebral Palsy and Speech*. New York: Teachers College, Columbia University (1968).

Mysak, E., Cerebral palsy speech syndromes. In Travis, L. (Ed.), *Handbook of Speech Pathology and Audiology*. New York: Appleton-Century-Crofts (1971a).

Mysak, E., Cerebral palsy speech habilitation. In Travis, L. (Ed.), *Handbook of Speech Pathology and Audiology*. New York: Appleton-Century-Crofts (1971b).

Ojemann, G., The thalamus and language. *Brain & Language*, **1**, 1 (1975).

Paillard, J., The patterning of skilled movements. In Field, J., Magoun, H., and Hall, V. (Eds.), *Handbook of Physiology*. (Section I) *Neurophysiology*.

(Vol. 2) Washington: American Physiological Society (1960).

Penfield, W., and Roberts, L., *Speech and Brain Mechanisms*. Princeton, N.J.: Princeton University Press (1959).

Phelps, W., *Etiology and Diagnostic Classification of Cerebral Palsy*. In Proceedings of the Cerebral Palsy Institute. New York: Association for Aid of Crippled Children (1950).

Pribram, K., *Languages of the Brain*. Englewood Cliffs, N.J.: Prentice-Hall, Inc. (1971).

Schuell, H., and Jenkins, J., The nature of language deficit in aphasia. In Saporta, S. (Ed.), *Psycholinguistics*. New York: Holt, Rinehart & Winston, Inc. (1961).

Schuell, H., Jenkins, J., and Jimenez-Pabon, E., *Aphasia in Adults*. New York: Harper & Row, Publishers (1964).

Snider, R., The cerebellum. *Scient. Am.*, **199**, August. (1958).

Sperry, R., Hemisphere deconnection and unity in conscious awareness. *Am. Psychol.*, **23**, 723-733 (1968).

Sperry, R., Split-brain approach to learning problems. In Quarton, G., Melnechuk, T., and Schmitt, F. (Eds.), *The Neurosciences*. New York: Rockefeller University Press (1967).

Teuber, H., Lacunae and research approaches to them. (Vol. 1) In Millikan, C., and Darley, F. (Eds.), *Brain Mechanisms Underlying Speech and Language*. New York: Grune & Stratton, Inc. (1967).

Travis, L., *Speech Pathology*. New York: Appleton-Century-Crofts (1931).

Weisenberg, T., and McBride, K., *Aphasia: a Clinical and Psychological Study*. New York: Commonwealth Fund (1935). (Reprint available: New York: Hafner Publishing Co., Inc.)

Wepman, J., and Jones, L., Studies in aphasia: a psycholinguistic method and case study. In Carterette, E. (Ed.), *Brain function*. (Vol. 3) *Speech, Language and Communication*. U.C.L.A. Forum in Medical Sciences (No. 4) Los Angeles: University of California Press (1966).

Wepman, J., and others, Studies in aphasia: background and theoretical formulations. *J. Speech Hearing Dis.*, **25**, 323-332 (1960).

West, R., An agnostic's speculations about stuttering. In Eisenson, J. (Ed.), *Stuttering: a symposium*. New York: Harper & Row, Publishers (1958).

Wood, N., *Delayed Speech and Language Development*. Englewood Cliffs, N.J.: Prentice-Hall, Inc. (1964).

Wright, B., *Physical Disability—a Psychological Approach*. New York: Harper & Row, Publishers (1960).

Chapter 6

Peripheral sensory disabilities

Questions

1. What is the nature of peripheral sensory disabilities that affect speech?
2. What are the speech effects of peripheral sensory disabilities?
3. What is the speech pathologist's responsibility in the treatment of peripheral sensory disabilities?

NATURE AND SPEECH EFFECTS OF PERIPHERAL SENSORY DISABILITIES

Separation of sensory from neurologic disabilities is arbitrary. Its justification is the preservation of focus. Our discussion of neurologic impairments was concerned with input-output transmission and integrative difficulties. Here we will focus on the speech effects of peripheral auditory and somesthetic disabilities as they affect early stages of input transmission of information important to speech.

Nature and speech effects of auditory disabilities

Over 10% of speech defects can be attributed to impaired hearing (National Advisory Neurological Diseases and Stroke Council, 1969). Four main types of hearing loss, once called *conductive deafness, nerve deafness, central deafness,* and *perceptive deafness,* are now more commonly identified as *conductive hearing loss, sensorineural hearing loss, retrocochlear hearing loss,* and *central hearing loss.* Symptoms of the last three types of losses are difficult to differentiate, a condition reflected in the overlapped meaning of the terms. Because these differentiations are of more importance to the diagnostic localization of auditory lesions than to the determination of speech effects, we will consider retrocochlear and central types of hearing loss together.

Before looking at the nature, causes, and speech effects of these types of hearing problems, let us be clear about the meaning of various forms of the word *deafness.* It can be used generically, as it has been here, to mean any amount of hearing loss. When contrasted with the terms *deafened* and *hard of hear-*

Do Goodhill and Guggenheim (1971) use this classification system for hearing impairment? How do they use the terms *anacusis, dysacusis,* and *hypacusis*? What types of deafness do Davis and Silverman (1970) describe?

---

ing, deaf refers to a hearing loss that meets two conditions: it occurs prior to speech acquisition, and it is so severe that the child is unable to understand and learn speech naturally by hearing. *Deafened* differs from *deaf* only by applying to severe loss of hearing after speech has been learned. The two conditions are equal insofar as inability to hear speech is concerned, but the deaf face the problem of acquiring language, the deafened the problem of conserving what they have. *Hard of hearing,* on the other hand, identifies an auditory abnormality in which sufficient sensitivity remains to permit oral communication (West and Ansberry, 1968.)

Conductive hearing loss

Causes. A common and remediable type of hearing loss is a *conductive* impairment. It depends on some abnormality in the mechanical system (shown in Fig. 6-1) for transmitting acoustical waves to the cochlea (inner ear). The external ear can be plugged with wax, peas, or chewing gum. The tympanic membrane (eardrum) can be perforated or missing. The middle ear can be filled with fluid, pus, or scarlike adhesions, as in otitis media. Transmission of vibration by the ossicular chain (the bony linkage between eardrum and cochlea) may be impaired by conditions ranging from arthritic fixation of the joints to necrosis of the incus (the middle bone in the linkage). The stapes may be pathologically fixated in the oval window, as in otosclerosis, or the round window may be blocked. All these etiologic conditions can be treated, with varying success, medically or surgically (Goodhill and Guggenheim, 1971).

Nature of hearing disability. Conductive impairment never results in total loss of hearing, and the partial loss never exceeds 60 to 65 decibels (dB), as measured by *pure tone* *audiometry* (a type of hearing test in which pure tones of known intensity and frequency are presented serially through earphones and vibrators to determine the threshold of hearing). It is to bone-conducted sound that man is indebted for this limit. No matter how blocked the route that air-conducted sound normally follows to the inner ear, sound as loud as conversational speech will vibrate the skull and be transmitted to the *basilar membrane* (Fig. 6-2).

Thus a diagnostic clue for conductive impairment is an *air-bone gap*—pure tone hearing as tested by bone conduction, which is considerably better than by air conduction. Another clue is a "flat" hearing loss in which all frequencies are more or less uniformly impaired and can be readily improved by amplification of sound. Persons with this type of loss are considered good candidates for hearing aids. Still another clue is that hearing for speech is not seriously impaired. Also, *speech reception thresholds* (measured by presenting selected words rather than pure tones) correlate well with middle-frequency pure tone thresholds, and when speech is loud enough for them to hear, the *speech discrimination* ability of persons with this type of hearing loss is normal.

Speech effects. Conductive impairments are responsible only for the auditory conditions of hard-of-hearing persons, never for that of the deaf or deafened. Accordingly, conductive losses are not likely to seriously impede a child's acquisition of language or his ability to use it once acquired. Of course, people so afflicted may have to listen especially attentively and may miss much that is said. Too, their voices may not be as loud as is needed for a speaking situation, an effect (easily demonstrated by speaking to a friend with your ears plugged) attributable to hearing one's own speech by bone conduction as louder than it sounds to a listener, who hears only by air conduction. Even so, this disability does not severely cripple the development or maintenance of speech.

Sensorineural hearing loss. Traditionally, sensorineural hearing loss, the most frequent type of impairment, is attributed to a lesion

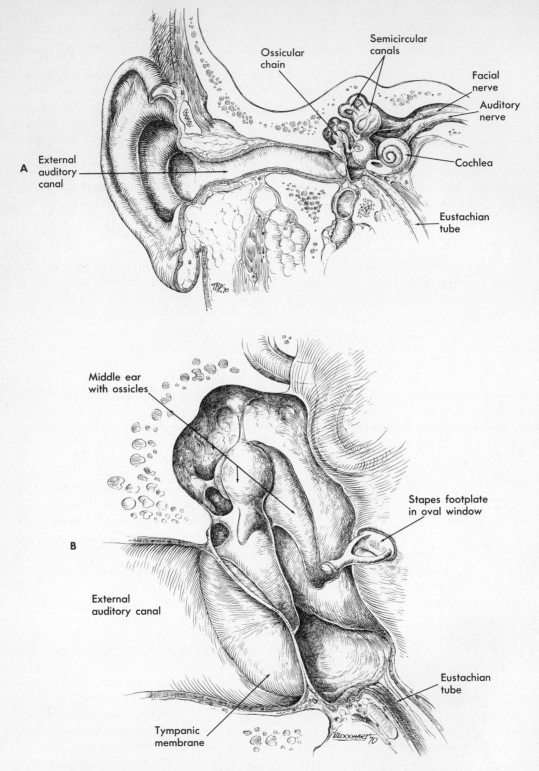

Fig. 6-1. Peripheral auditory mechanism. **B** shows the ossicular chain by which vibrations are transmitted mechanically to the inner ear.

in the peripheral cochleoneural system (Carhart, 1967). This term identifies lesions either in the cochlea or in the eighth cranial nerve. Because auditory nerve impairment is more specifically identified as retrocochlear hearing loss, we will avoid overlap and concentrate here on disability in that part of the sensory apparatus that encodes sound waves into neural signals—the cochlea. Unlike conductive losses, sensorineural deafness can be complete. Worse still, no treatment yet exists that will improve a damaged cochlea. The best foreseeable hope is in prevention.

Causes. Functions of the *organ of Corti* (the sensitive neural receiving apparatus in the cochlea) can be disabled temporarily by fatigue or injury or permanently by degeneration of the sensory cells or auditory nerve.

Such consequences are of major concern to industries that must protect their employees from damaging noise. Many youth, however, who listen to rock music at traumatically high loudness levels are apparently not persuaded of the danger to their hearing. Temporary damage results mainly from short-term exposure to loud sounds. With prolonged exposure, or when the sound is so loud as to be traumatic, temporary effects become permanent. In fact, progressive hair cell degeneration with consequent high-tone hearing loss, which so typically occurs in old age as to be called *presbycusis* (as good Presbyterians know, their name derives from their board of elders), may be less a price of aging than of living in a noisy civilization. Tests of Mabaan tribesmen in the African

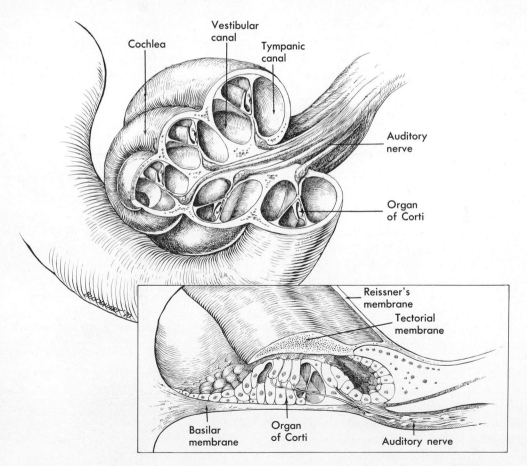

Fig. 6-2. Inner ear with semicircular canals of the cochlea. The organ of Corti is stimulated by undulations of the basilar membrane as waves of hydraulic pressure pass through the fluid-filled canals.

Sudan, who ordinarily hear sounds no louder than a bird call, seem to show hearing as keen in natives of 75 years of age as of 15.

Lesions from which degeneration of the organ of Corti stem can be hereditary, but most are acquired—some before, some during, and some soon after birth, as well as some in childhood and adulthood. Though rare, hereditary lesions range from *cochlear aplasia,* in which the infant is born without an organ of Corti, to *hereditodegenerative hypacuses,* in which degeneration begins any time from infancy to late in adult life, apparently for genetic reasons.

Causes of acquired lesions associated with pregnancy and birth may be toxic factors that can result from doses of such ototoxic drugs as quinine or streptomycin; maternal infections such as German measles (rubella) or congenital syphilis; Rh incompatability between mother and fetus resulting in erythroblastotic kernicterus; anoxia; and occasionally trauma to the inner ear. Note that many of these conditions are also among the causes of brain damage, especially resulting in cerebral palsy. One reason that brain-damaging factors also affect the cochlea is that auditory nerve fibers, when injured, do not regenerate. As they degenerate, so eventually do their ends, the hair cells in the organ of Corti, a form of *retrograde degeneration.* In childhood and later, the lesions may result from viral infections, mumps, bacterial diseases, ototoxic drugs, or intracranial tumors. Only in adults are the lesions caused by *Menière's disease,* which begins with sensations of dizziness and *tinnitus* (noises in the ear) as fluid pressure in the inner ear increases abnormally until hearing is permanently affected by deterioration of the organ of Corti (Davis and Silverman, 1970; Sataloff, 1966).

Nature of hearing disability. Loss of hearing with sensorineural impairment can range from the mildest loss to profound deafness. In contrast with conductive dysfunctions, air-conduction and bone-conduction tests show equal threshold losses, and hearing for speech is variably affected, as is ability to profit from amplification. Furthermore,

hearing for high frequencies is more consistently disabled than for low frequencies, and for some reason tones around 4,000 Hz are particularly vulnerable. Loudness often increases abruptly with increases in sound intensity. Unfortunately, such increases do not improve hearing for speech; rather, they tend to impair intelligibility. This phenomenon, called *recruitment,* explains the annoyance of those hard-of-hearing persons who, complaining that they can barely hear reasonably loud speech, complain even more that the speaker is shouting when he increases loudness only slightly (Davis, 1951; Sataloff, 1966; Graham, 1967).

Speech effects. Of hearing disabilities of the ear, sensorineural impairments are the most damaging to speech. Most damaged of all is the child born deaf or severely hard of hearing. Not hearing speech, his natural talent for learning his native tongue by ear remains untapped (Chapter 4). Though he may be able to learn language later through formal instruction in a school for the deaf, it will not come easily, as with the normal child. It will be acquired laboriously, if at all. Once learned, it will be spoken much like a foreign language, which, of course, is essentially how it was learned. The child will have little sense of the structure of his language, and his articulation and voice will betray an accent that identifies him as being from the land of the deaf.

What of the child born hard of hearing? Certainly his chances of hearing enough speech (no matter how distorted) to decipher the linguistic code are much better than if he hears none at all. His voice, too, is not likely to betray the telltale sounds of deafness if he has at least some hearing. His articulation, however, may suffer. Although vowels and consonants that depend on low frequencies for intelligibility are not apt to be affected, those consonants characterized by high frequencies, such as the friction sounds /s/ and /sh/, may be difficult to learn to differentiate with sensorineural high-frequency disability.

The effect on speaking skills of even the deafened, whose auditory impairment has occurred after speech acquisition, is another matter. Assuming that they had mastered speech, they know the linguistic rules, the sounds to be articulated, and the sound and feel of a normal voice. These three bodies of knowledge are not isolated; they are inter-related. Knowing the syntactic structure of language enables one to predict with con-siderable accuracy the words in a sentence, even when some are garbled. Knowing words provides knowledge of sounds and vocal stress with which they are pronounced. And because vocal pitch can be deduced as the common denominator of frequencies con-taining energy in a complex speech sound, only segments of speech need be heard to determine vocal pitch.

At the risk of laboring the obvious, the point is that speech is highly redundant. With mere fragments, one can decipher the whole statement; the safety factor for com-

What are the physical properties of acoustical signals that are the basic correlates of speech perception? Licklider (1951), Licklider and Miller (1951), Graham (1967), and Hirsh (1967) will be helpful in answering this question.

prehension is surprisingly large as it is, too, for speech production. Speech effects of an acquired hearing loss are therefore difficult to predict. A severe high-frequency loss, for example, may have no apparent conse-quences for articulation of high-frequency sounds. Likewise, a listener may compre-hend far more than his hearing would pre-sumably permit.

Retrocochlear and central hearing loss. Many auditory test refinements have been developed by audiologists to aid otologists, neurologists, and neurosurgeons in diagnos-

Sophisticated tests of hearing to aid in differential diagnosis of these types of hearing disabilities are described by such authorities as Newby (1964), O'Neill and Oyer (1966), Glorig (1965), Davis and Silverman (1970), and Northern and Downs (1974).

ing the locations of lesions in the auditory system. The practical consideration for the speech pathologist is whether hearing impair-ment affects acuity for all sounds or is limited to speech sounds. If, as in conductive hear-ing loss, acuity for pure tones as well as speech is decreased, the therapeutic problem is to raise acuity by amplification (hearing aid), medication, or surgery. If the ability to discriminate speech sounds, however, is more affected than acuity, then amplification will tend to increase speech distortion—the hearing aid is not a panacea for all types of hearing problems. Generally, the farther the damage goes into the auditory transmission system, the greater is the distorting effect on speech and the less evidence there is of effect on acuity for pure tones. This difference in effect is called *phonemic regression* because hearing ability for speech regresses from what it is for pure tones.

Thus no phonemic regression is seen in conductive impairment. Evidence of it begins to appear in sensorineural impairment be-cause even the earliest stages of neural pro-cessing involve complex integrative activities. Much the same evidence of it can be seen in *retrocochlear* hearing loss, in which the lesion affects the auditory nerve carrying sensation (as it was encoded in the cochlea) to the first synaptic nucleus in the brain. Lesions in the auditory paths beyond the first synapse are said to cause *central* hearing loss. With it, acuity for pure tones is unimpaired; pho-nemic regression prevails; the person hears sound but does not understand speech, es-pecially when it is spoken at normal rates. As you can see from the preceding chapter, this problem has already been discussed; it is identified by the speech pathologist as *audi-tory verbal agnosia.* One potential point of confusion remains to be cleared, however. The term "central" in "central hearing loss" refers to lesions in the auditory transmission system that produce a modality-bound ag-nosia. This meaning should be distinguished from that of "central" in "central integrative mechanism," which, when disabled, pro-duces a modality-free aphasia.

Special considerations for hearing reha-bilitation. Those persons facing permanent loss of hearing will often need more than a hearing aid to help understand and use speech. Two such types of help are auditory training and speech reading. Sanders (1971) and Northern and Downs (1974) offer detailed discussions of these topics.

Auditory training is intended to make the most of residual hearing. It is applicable both to children who have no speech and to adults whose speech is still normal but whose hearing has waned. A necessary preliminary step to this training is an accurate assessment of the auditory ability for speech. The best hearing available may be with amplification, as would be expected were the dysfunction conductive, or even were it sensorineural if the high-frequency drop in acuity is not too sharp, the recruitment increase in loudness not too abrupt, or phonemic regression not too predominant.

Amplification will not necessarily ensure maximal benefit from residual hearing. Hearing problems often come in mixed form: conductive and sensorineural dysfunctions can occur together, central and sensorineural combinations are not uncommon, and all three types may prevail. The characteristics of one can nullify gains available from help for another. A conductive hearing loss can generally be aided with amplification, for instance. If accompanied by a steep high-frequency sensorineural loss complete with considerable recruitment, then sufficient amplification to balance loudness at high frequencies with that at low frequencies will encounter the complications of recruitment. Worse yet, if central impairment is also involved, amplification may distort rather than improve speech comprehension.

Utilizing what is deemed to be optimal conditions for residual hearing, the objective of auditory training with children who have not learned to talk is to help them to recognize and appreciate sounds of speech. Obviously, the child must make gross discriminations between sounds that are speech and those that are not. Equally obviously, he must make fine discriminations among phonemes if he is to understand and use speech. Less obviously, perhaps, he must find satisfaction in hearing speech if he is to want anything to do with it. A normal infant is

Mowrer (1952) describes a suggestion that he made to the mother of a hard-of-hearing child that led to speech development. What did he recommend?

bathed in the soft, tender sounds of a mother's love. These sounds a severely hard-of-hearing child will not hear. If he hears any human sounds, they will probably be loud and angry—hardly conducive to enjoyment of speech.

Those with adventitious hearing loss, for whom talking is second nature, will find two purposes in auditory training: help in conserving the speaking skills that they already have, and help in listening sharply to sounds of speech that, with normal hearing, they have not had to be aware. For speech conservation, they have what remains of sounds along with feel (touch and kinesthesis) of speech to guide them. For listening, they have sounds and also sight from which to detect cues that will permit comprehension. The process of obtaining information about a speaker's message by observing him visually is called *speech reading* or, less descriptively, *lip reading* (West and Ansberry, 1968).

Nature of speech effects of somesthetic disabilities

By comparison with the rich literature on audition, the literature concerned with the *somesthetic* (bodily) senses, especially as they relate to speech, is impoverished. Only in recent years have these senses become the focus of research. They are nonetheless of fundamental importance. Clearly, a mature speaker has the ability to make his speech mechanism produce most of the sounds he intends without close attention to the process. Presumably, he relies heavily for this performance on *touch* (sense of cutaneous pressure) and *kinesthesis* (an ambiguous term defined for speech pathologists by Shelton [1972] as "awareness of position and movement of the speech mechanism"). These sensations arise within the body, unlike auditory sensations that arise externally. This distinction is reflected in the description of audition as an *exteroceptive* sense and of body information as *proprioceptive.*

Control of speech by "feel." Technically, we are concerned with somesthetic mechanisms. Practically, our interest is in the "feel" of speech. We are indebted to the Greeks for the word to describe this interest—"haptic," derived from a term meaning "to lay hold of." The *haptic system* includes more than sensations of touch and kinesthesis; it includes the neural processes by which one perceives his body in relation to objects and space. It is this perceptual system by which we are literally in touch with our environment. Unlike specialized sense organs that passively receive stimulation (such as the eyes and ears), sense organs of the haptic system are ubiquitous and active. They are everywhere in the body—in most of its parts and on all of its surfaces. What's more, they are embedded in the motor organs. Equipment for "feeling" includes equipment for "doing." Stimulation of greatest importance comes from proprioceptors when they are moving. Detection of forms of objects by "feeling" them in the mouth (*oral form recognition*, less accurately called *oral stereognosis*), for instance, relies on the ability to move objects around with the tongue, lips, and jaw (Shelton, 1972). Perhaps it is for this reason that these tests of oral stereognosis appear to be related to speaking ability (Rutherford and McCall, 1967; Baker, 1967; Moser and colleagues, 1967; McDonald and Aungst, 1967). Speech occurs only when the speaking apparatus is in motion; sound cannot be produced without movement (Gibson, 1967).

Nowhere can knowledge of one bodily part in relation to others be more vital to performance than for speech. Take the tongue and larynx as cases in point. Both are attached to the *hyoid*, a small horseshoe-shaped "floating" bone suspended like the Golden Gate Bridge by a muscular sling stretching from the chin to the base of the skull. To the hyoid bone is anchored the tongue, which is adjusted for each speech sound. The tip, the edges, and the base must sometimes make as many movements as thirty per second, and each movement must hit the target at which it is aimed with extraordinary accuracy. If it misses by even a fraction of an inch, the wrong sound can be produced. While the tongue flies through its trajectories, so does the jaw, the throat, and the soft palate—and some of the muscles that move these structures also move the hyoid bone that moves the base of the tongue.

Dissuade yourself of any thought that the complexity of structural interrelations for speech production has been tapped. Not only is the tongue anchored to the hyoid bone above, but the larynx is suspended from it below, an arrangement that probably increases the complexity of speech adjustments by several orders of magnitude. Movements in the larynx must be accurate within hundreths of an inch; yet they can occur as rapidly as several hundred times per second. Each adjustment for each movement in any of these structures involves balancing a multitude of vectors of force. Change a single vector and the entire balance must be reestablished. This rebalancing process during speech goes on continuously at remarkable rates. Intricate as this arrangement must seem, it is still a grossly oversimplified description of the problem that the haptic system must solve during speech.

A few pioneer investigators are building a body of information about oral sensory functions in relation to speaking (McCroskey, 1958; Ringel and Steer, 1963; Ringel and Ewanoski, 1965; Ringel, Saxman, and Brooks, 1967; Ringel and Fletcher, 1967; Rutherford and McCall, 1967; Shelton, Arndt, and Hetherington, 1967). In an excellent review of the current state of knowledge, Shelton (1972) indicates certainty of at least moderate correlation between oral sensations and articulatory proficiency. He also finds evidence that the front of the mouth is better equipped than the back with sensory capacity for articulation. Perhaps his point of greatest practical importance is that kinesthetic awareness of articulation is at best only partial. Sensory information from muscle spindles and tendons, unlike kinesthetic information from joints, reaches only the cerebellum for automatic coordination. It does not travel on to the cortex to contribute to awareness or volitional control of speech movements. Because no physiologic mechanism for kinesthesis seems to exist in unjointed structures (and most speech structures, such as tongue, lips, and palate, are unjointed), awareness of articulatory movement and position is notably limited, especially deep in the vocal tract.

The paradox is how speaking, the epitome of skilled movement that must require exquisite sensory feedback of oral motor functions, is learned and controlled when kinesthetic information is apparently unavailable. Perhaps the answer lies in Gibson's (1967) contention that "kinesthesis is perceptual without being sensory." Kinesthesis and touch do not differ in the types of receptors employed. Their difference may lie, instead, in patterns of mechanical stimulation. Touch is perceived as deformation of the skin, whereas movement is perceived as angular change around a joint, but these differences are in perception, not sensation. Gibson points out a variety of means of perceiving movement: "articular" kinesthesis for movements of joints, "vestibular" kinesthesis for movements of the skull, "cutaneous" kinesthesis for movements of touch on the skin, "visual" kinesthesis for movements of the eyes, and even "auditory" kinesthesis for binaural sound localization. Maybe to his list we will have to add "speech" kinesthesis for movements of jointless speech structures.

Somesthetic disabilities. Little is known about somesthetic disabilities, especially as they affect speech. Theoretically and from existing knowledge, the "feel" of speech must be vital for normal performance. That we could speak at all were it not for tactual and kinesthetic senses is all but inconceivable. Between this surmise on one side and established evidence of speech effects of somesthetic disabilities on the other is a yawning chasm of ignorance that only a few have begun to explore.

Much of what is known has been learned from studying two patients at the Clinical Center of the National Institutes of Health.

One girl was first seen at 15 years of age, the other at 5. Both were unable to acquire intelligible articulation, yet neither had difficulty understanding speech. Both had trouble with biting, chewing, and drooling, yet neither was impaired in infantile sucking, swallowing, and breathing functions. Neither was able to move the tongue or jaw or to phonate with much volitional control. Both were impaired in oral sensation and perception, failing completely in tests of oral stereognosis. Yet in all other respects—intellectually, neurologically, socially—they seemed normal, and they came from families free of these problems (Bosma, Grossman, and Kavanaugh, 1967; Rootes and MacNeilage, 1967).

From such work as has been done, three risky observations about somesthetic disabilities appear relevant. First, these problems seem to involve impairment of the sensory transmission system rather than of somesthetic receptors. Second, these problems closely resemble motor dysfunctions that are sometimes diagnosed as oral apraxias (Bloomer, 1967). Third, these problems apparently are congenital rather than acquired.

That somesthetic disabilities do not appear to be a consequence of impairment of sensory receptors is not surprising. These receptors are so omnipresent and, seemingly, so unspecialized that they may be all but impervious to damage. On the other hand, the cause, nature, or location of a neural lesion that would account for this unusual syndrome of impaired oral function is practically unknown. The most sensible explanation is that the disability stems from a lesion fairly high in the somesthetic transmission pathway (Chase, 1967).

Because somesthetic disabilities are congenital, they may be doubly linked to motor speech dysfunctions. As Chase (1967) points out, defective somesthetic functions could impair motor speech performance in either of two ways. One way is that the motor control system must "know" what the muscles of speech are doing before appropriate neural signals for smooth articulation can be dispatched. Impairment of this feedback function, however, should affect speech at any age. The other way would be particularly disruptive if the somesthetic impairment occurred before articulatory patterns were stabilized. Were the child unable to establish the reference pattern for sounds he was attempting to articulate, he would have no basis for determining from feedback whether he had produced what he intended or not. Whereas the speechless congenitally deaf child is deprived of hearing the target sounds at which he should aim, the congenitally somesthetically impaired child is deprived of the feel of what he should be doing. Accordingly, his articulatory performance could appear as confused and aimlessly directed as if he had an oral motor apraxia.

Additional consideration should be given to normal development of oral function if one is to appreciate the interaction between motor production and oral sensation that is affected by somesthetic disability. Bosma (1967) has shown that earliest suckling actions of the infant do not slowly evolve into mature patterns of mastication, nor do infant cries bear much relevance to mature vocalization and speech. Whereas infant suckle involves a total undifferentiated reflex oral response, mature feeding action depends on independent differentiated response of tongue, lips, jaw, and the like. Similarly, infant cry is a trembling, tense reflexive performance that varies little from one cry to the next. Mature vocalization that evolves into speech, by contrast, depends on discrete control of location, speed, and amount of movement of articulators. Of importance here, differentiated control of oral structures for speech or feeding becomes possible only as the somesthetic apparatus in the head and neck matures.

SPEECH PATHOLOGIST'S RESPONSIBILITY IN TREATMENT OF PERIPHERAL SENSORY DISABILITIES

So much is known about behavioral characteristics of hearing that the speech patholo-gist's next of kin, the audiologist, has made this subject his field of study. Furthermore, his ability to assess hearing is of such importance to medical diagnosis that he is one of the very few nonmedical specialists who can be reimbursed directly under Medicare. By contrast, so little is known about any aspect of somesthesis, behavioral or medical, that we hardly know how to define these senses, let alone determine lines of responsibility for them. The speech pathologist's role in problems of hearing and somesthesis can be clarified better by considering these areas separately.

Responsibility for treating hearing disabilities

For ethical, legal, and practical reasons the speech pathologist's first responsibility on discovering a problem of hearing is to refer the person to a physician for an otologic examination. This responsibility holds even if the speech pathologist is also an audiologist, as many are. Although the otologist will probably want an audiologic evaluation to aid in his diagnosis, still it is a medical responsibility to determine the status of the hearing mechanism.

Practically, determination of whether or not the hearing condition can be improved medically or surgically is basic to any program of habilitation or rehabilitation. Furthermore, the speech pathologist must know whether the auditory disability is temporary, permanent, or progressive. If the impairment can be expected to remain stable for many years, the therapeutic goals will be different from those that would apply if the prognosis were for progressive deterioration or for eventual recovery.

Once the medical picture is clear, the speech pathologist's responsibility shifts to consultation with the audiologist to determine optimal conditions for utilizing residual hearing—possibly a hearing aid is needed. He should consult, too, with teachers, family, and employers to determine sources of failure and optimal possibilities for success (West and Ansberry, 1968).

Responsibility for treating somesthetic disabilities

The speech pathologist has a unique opportunity to detect what apparently are rare instances of somesthetic impairment. Medical recognition of these disabilities, and testing procedures for them, are in their infancy. These problems are easily confused with motor coordination difficulties. Because children so afflicted will have severe voice and articulation problems, parents may seek help for speech first. The speech pathologist who is alert to the syndrome of impaired oral sensation (severe speech and feeding problems in a child normal in all other respects) may have to be particularly diligent to find specialists, medical and otherwise, who are knowledgeable about disabilities of oral sensation and perception. With effective remedial procedures for such handicaps yet to be developed, his reward for diligence is more apt to be from furthering knowledge than from applying it to improved treatment.

The answers—résumé

1. What is the nature of peripheral sensory disabilities that affect speech?

Hearing can be disabled by impairment of the mechanical transmission apparatus of the middle ear. This type of conductive dysfunction, which produces only partial loss of hearing, can generally be improved by medical or surgical treatment. Sensorineural dysfunction of the inner ear is likely to be permanent if not progressive; it can result in total deafness. Unfortunately, no means of improving it is known. Retrocochlear and central impairments involve neural lesions in the auditory transmission pathway that can distort speech perception severely.

Somesthetic disability appears to occur high in the neural transmission paths, not in the sensory receptors. It may be congenital, and it is easily confused with neuromuscular disorders of coordination. A person whose somesthetic senses are impaired will have severe problems of voice and articulation as well as of feeding, but he can be normal in all other respects.

2. What are the speech effects of peripheral sensory disabilities?

Except for possible decreased loudness of the speaker's voice, conductive deafness is not apt to be a serious problem for speech. Sensorineural, retrocochlear, and central hearing losses are another matter. Singly or together, they can blot out or distort speech so completely that a child cannot learn it naturally, or, if deafness is acquired later, they can make auditory comprehension of speech difficult if not impossible.

With impairment of oral sensation, language comprehension and expression in writing can apparently develop adequately. Development of speaking processes, however, is grossly disturbed, probably because the "feel" of normal speech cannot be established as a guide for articulation.

3. What is the speech pathologist's responsibility in the treatment of peripheral sensory disabilities?

Ethical, legal, and practical considerations dictate that all hearing problems be examined medically before undertaking any program of therapy. Diagnosis of the type of loss and a prognosis are of paramount importance in devising an effective program of treatment for speech. The responsibility for oral sensory disabilities is similar to that for hearing, but with so little knowledge, the problem is more difficult to recognize and to manage therapeutically.

REFERENCES

Baker, D., The amount of information in the oral identification of forms by normal speakers and selected speech-defective groups. In Bosma, J. (Ed.), *Symposium on Oral Sensation and Perception.* Springfield, Ill.: Charles C Thomas, Publisher (1967).

Bloomer, H., Oral manifestations of dysdiadokokinesis, with oral astereognosia. In Bosma, J. (Ed.), *Symposium on Oral Sensation and Perception.* Springfield, Ill.: Charles C Thomas, Publisher (1967).

Bosma, J., Human infant oral function. In Bosma, J. (Ed.), *Symposium on Oral Sensation and Perception.* Springfield, Ill.: Charles C Thomas, Publisher (1967).

Bosma, J., Grossman, R., and Kavanagh, J., A syndrome of impairment of oral perception. In Bosma, J. (Ed.), *Symposium on Oral Sensation and Perception.* Springfield, Ill.: Charles C Thomas, Publisher (1967).

Carhart, R., Summarization of symposium (Vol. 2) In Graham, B. (Ed.), *Sensorineural Hearing Processes and Disorders.* Boston: Little, Brown & Co.

Chase, R., Abnormalities in motor control secondary to congenital sensory deficits. In Bosma, J. (Ed.), *Symposium on Oral Sensation and Perception.* Springfield, Ill.: Charles C Thomas, Publisher (1967).

Davis, H., Psychophysiology of hearing and deafness. In Stevens, S. (Ed.), *Handbook of Experimental Psychology.* New York: John Wiley & Sons, Inc. (1951).

Davis, H., and Silverman, R., *Hearing and Deafness.* New York: Holt, Rinehart & Winston, Inc. (1970).

Gibson, J., The mouth as an organ for laying hold on the environment. In Bosma, J. (Ed.), *Symposium on Oral Sensation and Perception.* Springfield, Ill.: Charles C Thomas, Publisher (1967).

Glorig, A., *Audiometry: Principles and Practices.* Baltimore: The Williams & Wilkins Co. (1965).

Goodhill, V., and Guggenheim, P., Pathology, diagnosis, and therapy of deafness. In Travis, L. (Ed.), *Handbook of Speech Pathology and Audiology.* New York: Appleton-Century-Crofts (1971).

Graham, B. (Ed.), *Sensorineural Hearing Processes and Disorders.* Boston: Little, Brown & Co. (1967).

Hirsh, I., Information processing in input channels for speech and language: the significance of serial order of stimuli. In Millikan, C., and Darley, F. (Eds.), *Brain Mechanisms Underlying Speech and Language.* New York: Grune & Stratton, Inc. (1967).

Licklider, J., Basic correlates of the auditory stimulus. In Stevens, S. (Ed.), *Handbook of Experimental Psychology.* New York: John Wiley and Sons, Inc. (1951).

Licklider, J., and Miller, G., The perception of speech. In Stevens, S. (Ed.), *Handbook of Experimental Psychology.* New York: John Wiley & Sons, Inc. (1951).

McCroskey, R., *Some Effects of Anesthetizing the Articulators Under Conditions of Normal and Delayed Side-Tone.* Project NM 001 104 500 Report No. 65. United States Naval School of Aviation Medicine, Naval Air Station, Pensacola, Florida (1958).

McDonald, E., and Aungst, L., Studies in oral sensorimotor function. In Bosma, J. (Ed.), *Symposium on Oral Sensation and Perception.* Springfield, Ill.: Charles C Thomas, Publisher (1967).

Moser, H., La Gourgue, J., and Class, L., Studies of oral stereognosis in normal, blind and deaf subjects. In Bosma, J. (Ed.), *Symposium on Oral Sensation and Perception.* Springfield, Ill.: Charles C Thomas, Publisher (1967).

Mowrer, O., Speech development in the young child. I. The autism theory of speech development and some clinical applications. *Speech Hearing Dis.,* **17,** 263-268 (1952).

National Advisory Neurological Diseases and Stroke Council, *Human Communication and Its Disorders.* Bethesda, Md.: National Institute of Neurological Diseases and Stroke (1969).

Newby, H., *Audiology.* New York: Appleton-Century-Crofts (1964).

Northern, J., and Downs, M., *Hearing in children.* Baltimore: The Williams & Wilkins Co. (1974).

O'Neill, J., and Oyer, H., *Applied Audiometry.* New York: Dodd, Mead & Co. (1966).

Ringel, R., and Ewanowski, S., Oral perception. I. Two-point discrimination. *J. Speech Hearing Res.,* **8,** 389-398 (1965).

Ringel, R., and Fletcher, H., Oral perception. III. Texture discrimination. *J. Speech Hearing Res.,* **10,** 642-649 (1967).

Ringel, R., Saxman, J., and Brooks, A., Oral perception. II. Mandibular kinesthesia. *J. Speech Hearing Res.,* **10,** 637-641 (1967).

Ringel, R., and Steer, M., Some effects of tactile and auditory alterations on speech output. *J. Speech Hearing Res.,* **6,** 369-378 (1963).

Rootes, T., and MacNeilage, P., Some speech perception and production tests of a patient with impairment in somesthetic perception and motor function. In Bosma, J, (Ed.), *Symposium on Oral Sensation and Perception.* Springfield, Ill.: Charles C Thomas, Publisher (1967).

Rutherford, D., and McCall, G., Testing oral sensation and perception in persons with dysarthria. In Bosma, J. (Ed.), *Symposium on Oral Sensation and Perception.* Springfield, Ill.: Charles C Thomas, Publisher (1967).

Sanders, D., *Aural Rehabilitation.* Englewood Cliffs, N.J.: Prentice-Hall, Inc. (1971).

Sataloff, J., *Hearing Loss.* Philadelphia: J. B. Lippincott Co. (1966).

Shelton, R., Oral sensory function in speech production. In Bzoch, K. (Ed.), *Communicative Disorders Related to Cleft Lip and Palate.* Boston: Little, Brown & Co. (1972).

Shelton, R., Arndt, W., and Hetherington, J., Testing oral stereognosis. In Bosma, J. (Ed.), *Symposium on Oral Sensation and Perception.* Springfield, Ill.: Charles C Thomas, Publisher (1967).

West, R., and Ansberry, M., *The Rehabilitation of Speech.* New York: Harper & Row, Publishers (1968).

Chapter 7

Laryngeal and lower respiratory disabilities

Questions

1. What are the nature and etiology of laryngeal and bronchopulmonary disabilities?
2. What are the speech effects of laryngeal and bronchopulmonary disabilities?
3. What is the speech pathologist's responsibility in the treatment of laryngeal and bronchopulmonary disabilities?

NATURE AND ETIOLOGY OF LARYNGEAL DISABILITIES

Speech can be affected by five types of laryngeal conditions:

1. Those which disrupt synchrony and smooth approximation of the cords (lesions can increase the mass of the af-

fected cord, and asymmetric arytenoid approximation affects vibratory phase by forcing one cord to move farther than the other for closure)

2. Those which limit adduction or abduction of the cords (laryngeal paralysis can immobilize vocal folds in either para-

median or intermediate positions, and interarytenoid growths can prevent adduction)

3. Those which alter contractile ability of the cords (tensor paralysis, myasthenia laryngis, and myasthenia gravis impair laryngeal resistance to air pressure)

4. Those in which endocrine imbalances alter anatomy or physiology of the larynx (mutational changes in males and virilization of female voices affect control of pitch)

5. Those in which essential tissue is destroyed (laryngectomy and injury may require the substitution of alaryngeal speech)

Let us now examine the nature of these laryngeal disabilities.

Lesions of laryngeal tissues

Laryngeal lesions, which are most often responsible for disabling vocal cord movement, occur mainly as *neoplasms* (new growths) or *inflammation* (Ryan and colleagues, 1970).

Inflammation

Laryngitis. Inflammation of the larynx may be a consequence of disease processes ending in *acute* or *chronic laryngitis.* The common cold and other upper respiratory infections are prime contributors to acute conditions marked by *edema* (swelling) of the vocal cords and *hyperemia* (engorgement with blood) of the mucous membranes. Chronic laryngitis can reflect chronic upper respiratory infection with its postnasal drip. Depending on its severity and duration, it may involve only superficial layers of mucous membrane, or it may include hyperemia, edema, and *fibrosis* (formation of fibrous tissue).

Acute laryngotracheobronchitis. Now that diphtheria is no longer a serious public health problem, *acute laryngotracheobronchitis* has replaced it as the prime cause of severe inflammation in small children, especially in little boys under 3 years of age. With this disease, vocal effects are the least concern. For a day or two the child may appear to have a common cold, but then, with frightening speed, severe inflammation that obstructs the air passage may strike within hours. Without prompt intervention, death from suffocation may occur.

Laryngeal abuse. A prime cause of inflammation is intermittent or persistent vocal abuse. Too much yelling and screaming, smoking and drinking, singing, talking over background noise, or straining to make oneself heard are typical examples of conditions conducive to laryngeal inflammation.

Neoplasms

Benign tumors. Benign tumors are neither malignant nor necessarily consequent to vocal abuse. Since they are generally not expected to vanish with vocal rehabilitation, treatment is by surgical removal, with voice therapy as a possible follow-up procedure. The etiology of benign tumors is often unknown. Their effect on voice is determined largely by the type and location of the disability. As seen in Fig. 7-1, neoplasms can hang by a stalk from a vocal fold or be broadly based in the mucous membrane. Commonly, but not necessarily, they are found along the free margin of a vocal cord. If spread along the glottal edge, a tumor will interfere with the mass of the cord, the tightness of closure, and the vibratory pattern during phonation. On the other hand, if based away from the cord edge, it may produce little or no vocal effect. If it hangs from a stalk, its effects can be erratic. As a suspended bag of fluid, it may interfere only when blown into the glottis by air current during phonation. A person with this type of growth may exhibit a clear voice that suddenly goes hoarse and just as suddenly clears again.

The only method of differentiating benign tumors from each other is histologically by cellular makeup; they cannot be distinguished by gross appearance. Histology is not a major issue for us, but since you will encounter these terms, we will at least strive for a nodding acquaintance with them. *Polyps* are the most frequently found benign growths and are considered by some to be a consequence of vocal abuse (Brodnitz, 1969b). They are covered with epithelium and contain connective tissue, mucus, and serous glands. Next are *fibromas*, consisting

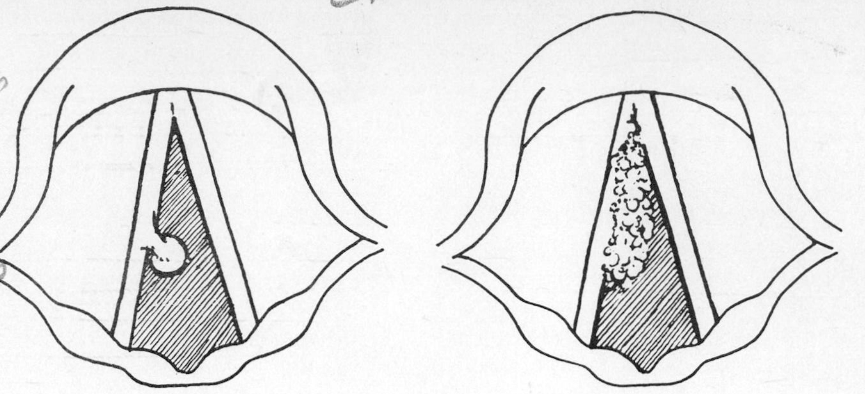

[handwritten top margin: Benign · Organic · Malign · Carcinoma]

[handwritten left margin list: polyps / papillomas / fibromas / cysts / angiomas / lipomas]

Fig. 7-1. Broad-based and stem-based vocal fold neoplasms. The polyp on the left hangs by a stalk, whereas the papilloma on the right extends along much of the cord. (From Ryan, R., von Leden, H., Ogura, J. H., Biller, H. F., and Pratt, L. L., *Synopsis of Ear, Nose, and Throat Diseases.* St. Louis: The C. V. Mosby Co. [1970].)

of fibrous tissue. *Papillomas*, grapelike epithelial clusters along the vocal margin, are probably related to hormonal changes and occur mainly in children from birth to puberty; they are not caused by vocal trauma. *Cysts* (encapsulated bags filled with fluid), *angiomas* (full of blood or lymph vessel tissue), and rarely *lipomas* (full of fatty tissue) are among other benign tumors to be found.

Malignant tumors. Fortunately, malignant laryngeal neoplasms are rare in children. Unfortunately, they are relatively common among older adults, especially in those over 50, and especially in men—ten times as many men have cancer of the larynx as women. Most laryngeal malignancies are *carcinomas* originating from epithelium of the mucosal lining. Rarely, they are *sarcomas* arising from connective tissue of muscles, tendons, and cartilages.

If cancer of the vocal cords is detected and treated early, the prognosis is second only to that for cancer of the skin. But chances of recovery slip rapidly away with each month's delay in treatment. Hoarseness is usually the only warning. With *intrinsic* laryngeal malignancies located on the cords, this warning comes early. Coupled with late *metastasis* (spread of disease), early warning provides a good chance for recovery of a laryngeal structure that will function adequately. With *extrinsic* laryngeal malignancies, however, the prospect of partial or total *laryngectomy* (surgical removal of the larynx) looms large. Located off the vibrating cords, these tumors do not produce hoarseness as a warning, and they tend to metastasize early. By time of detection, they are often at an advanced stage.

Functional disabilities. Some of the most common benign swellings on the vocal folds, such as vocal nodules, hematomas, and granulomas, are not true neoplasms but are consequences of one form or another of vocal abuse. They will be considered as a functional disability—a special type of benign tumor.

Vocal nodules. The most common of the functional swellings are vocal nodules, sometimes called *screamer's nodes, singer's nodes, preacher's nodes,* or *teacher's nodes*—depending on who acquired them and how. These names describe the condition for acquiring them: abusive vocal use. Nodules are generally located at the juncture of the anterior and middle thirds of the vocal folds, the midpoint of the vibrating glottis, at which the folds slam together hardest (Fig. 7-2). They can develop on one or both cords. That they are generally associated with high pitches and screaming points to tense vocal muscles as a major culprit in the trauma. If the muscles were relatively relaxed (compliant) and slammed together, the blows would be cushioned, but with tension, mucosal edges are pounded between hard muscles.

[handwritten left margin, vertical: (common) carcinoma – epithelium · (10:1 men) cancer of larynx]

[handwritten bottom margin: intrinsic laryng. malignancy → hoarseness → metastas— / extrinsic " " → metastasis → laryngecto—]

front
nodules
hematomas
contact ulcer
myasthenia laryngis - feature

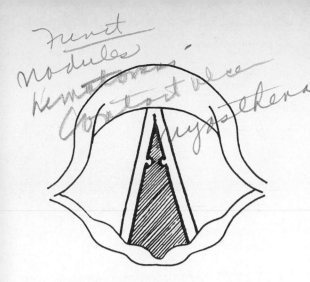

Fig. 7-2. Vocal nodules. Location at juncture of anterior and middle third of the vocal cord is typical. (From Ryan, R., von Leden, H., Ogura, J. H., Biller, H. F., and Pratt, L. L., *Synopsis of Ear, Nose, and Throat Diseases*. St. Louis: The C. V. Mosby Co. [1970].)

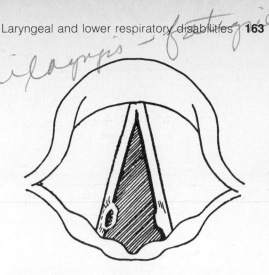

Fig. 7-3. Contact ulcer. Posterior location over vocal process of arytenoid cartilage is typical. (From Ryan, R., von Leden, H., Ogura, J. H., Biller, H. F., and Pratt, L. L., *Synopsis of Ear, Nose, and Throat Diseases*. St. Louis: The C. V. Mosby Co. [1970].)

Does this explanation differ from Arnold's (1962a) analysis of why vocal nodules develop?

Nodules start as edematous lesions, like a bruise. While in the formative stage, they can be reversed with vocal rehabilitation. This is the stage at which laryngologists sometimes recommend vocal rest. If abuse continues, nodules develop scar tissue, become fibrous as in a callus, and become resistant to cure by voice therapy. Then surgical removal is required, followed by supportive voice therapy to head off recurrence.

2) *Hematomas.* A hematoma occurs for much the same reason as a vocal nodule, but the tissue reaction is hemorrhage. Typically found in elastic tissue connecting the mucous membrane with underlying ligaments or muscles, hematomas, like nodules, will in time show fibrotic changes that will require their removal. Like nodules, they have much the same prognosis and need much the same treatment, especially for vocal rest to afford opportunity for complete absorption.

3) *Contact ulcers.* The name "contact ulcer" describes the presumed cause of the lesion: ulceration of mucous membrane by grinding, hammering contact of cartilaginous vocal processes (Fig. 7-3). Visual inspection by *direct*

or *indirect laryngoscopy* reveals a break in the surface epithelium over a vocal process. The mucous membrane surrounding the ulceration becomes swollen in an attempt to wall off the lesion—hence the craterlike appearance. Granulation tissue forms at the base of the crater. With continued irritation and infection, the lesion spreads, and granulated layer builds on granulated layer, producing a protruding granuloma from the ulcer.

Apparently, forceful adduction of the tips of the arytenoid processes is used to produce voice at excessively low pitches, especially by males who may be achieving a bit of pseudomasculinity. It is perhaps for this reason that contact ulcers are more prevalent among men than women. That it tends to be more a disorder of executives than laborers suggests that it may also have a psychosomatic component—its victims may be ulcer prone (Brodnitz, 1961). Voice rest, avoidance of ir-

---

Do von Leden and Moore (1960) explain contact ulcer the same as does Brodnitz (1961)?

---

ritants, and vocal reeducation are typical recommendations for treatment.

4) *Myasthenia laryngis.* Most persons who do not produce voice with exceptional ability

hypofunctional myasthenia laryngis — vocal fatig

have probably encountered mild forms of myasthenia laryngis, or vocal fatigue. A *hypofunctional* disorder, it is a consequence of prolonged *hyperfunction* (strained use of voice), but it is usually not considered a laryngeal disability until exaggerated (Brodnitz, 1965; Froeschels, 1943). It indicates weakness of one or several intrinsic laryngeal muscles or, more probably, faulty vocal habits with muscular imbalances that, to compensate, overload muscles not designed for so strenuous a task.

congenital webs — (rare)

traumatic webs (adhesion between VF)

Miscellaneous disabilities. Laryngeal lesions may come in a variety of other forms. They include the rare *congenital webs* of infants and young children. Also included are the more common *traumatic webs*, adhesions that form between the vocal folds after injury to the anterior portion of the larynx, sometimes by surgical stripping of polypoid thickening from both cords at the same time (Brodnitz, 1969b). They sometimes tend toward malignancy, as with *leukoplakia* and *hyperkeratosis* that show white, thickened patches and are often associated with smoking. They may be the result of fractures of the laryngeal skeleton, or they may be caused by injuries to the cartilaginous joints or to the extrinsic or intrinsic laryngeal muscles. They may be *granulomas*—granular ball-shaped lesions, usually on the glottal edges between the arytenoids, that generally follow traumatic insertion of a bronchoscope or a tracheal tube for anesthesia. Location of trauma is determined by placement of the tube through the glottis. Voice rest or surgery, more than vocal reeducation, is indicated in such cases. Our purpose is served if you know that such disabilities exist and can find your way to more detailed information about them, such as Luchsinger and Arnold (1965) and Cooper (1973) provide.

Paralyses of laryngeal muscles

Laryngeal paralyses affect vocal fold adduction-abduction functions that will be considered here. A special word is in order about the perilous course followed by *recurrent laryngeal nerves* (one on the right side, the other on the left), since they carry a heavy

load (assisted by the *superior laryngeal nerves*) of motor information to laryngeal muscles. These impulses leave the midbrain over cranial nerve X, the *vagus* (the term means "wandering"), which wanders through the chest into the abdomen. From it, in the neck, branch the superior laryngeal nerve to the cricothyroid muscle and the more important recurrent laryngeal nerve that also wanders. To reach the larynx from the chest, the recurrent nerve on the right crosses under the subclavian artery, whereas the one on the left winds around the aorta close to the heart. They then ascend between trachea and esophagus close to lymph nodes and thyroid gland. Laryngeal paralysis can result from swelling of any of these structures, from neurotoxic effects of virus diseases that often heal spontaneously, and from surgery that imperils this vulnerable nerve even more. Of a variety of possible paralyses, we will look at two important groups (Luchsinger and Arnold, 1965).

Unilateral paralyses. In unilateral paralyses only one vocal cord is affected. The paralysis may be *incomplete*, usually involving damage in the recurrent laryngeal nerve, or *complete*, resulting from involvement of the vagus nerve. The paralyzed cord in incomplete paralysis is usually fixed near the midline in the *paramedian position*. Because the other cord can approximate the paralyzed cord normally, the voice may show few, if any, signs of disability. If the cord is completely paralyzed, it will be fixed in the *intermediate* or, rarely, the *lateral* position (Fig. 7-4). Since the healthy cord has considerable difficulty moving across the midline far enough to compensate, poor approximation and poor voice are typical. Injection of Teflon paste or diced cartilage into the paralyzed cord is sometimes used in selected cases to displace the free margin medially enough for reasonably adequate approximation (Arnold, 1955, 1962b; Luchsinger and Arnold, 1965).

Bilateral paralyses. Both vocal folds are paralyzed in bilateral paralyses. In the most common form, *bilateral abductor paralysis*, the cords are fixed near the midline, usually as a consequence of damage to both recur-

recurrent laryngeal nerve — motor info. to laryngeal mus

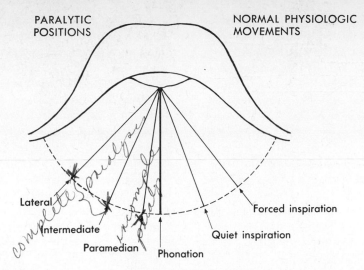

PARALYTIC
POSITIONS

NORMAL PHYSIOLOGIC
MOVEMENTS

Lateral

Intermediate

Paramedian

Phonation

Forced inspiration

Quiet inspiration

Fig. 7-4. Paralytic positions of vocal folds in comparison with normal physiologic movements. For phonation the normal cord must move past the midline to reach the position of the paralyzed cord.

rent laryngeal nerves during extensive thyroid surgery. Although adductor as well as abductor muscles are paralyzed, the intact superior laryngeal nerve continues to supply the cricothyroid muscle, which, without opposition from paralyzed abductors, can approximate the cords toward a midline position. Evidence of the paralysis may not be immediately apparent after surgery and may appear only gradually as a hoarse, weak voice. Not surprisingly, considering that the cords are fixed near the midline, breathing is more likely a problem than phonating. Unfortunately, unless a *tracheotomy* is performed to provide breath directly into the trachea through a *stoma* (hole) below the obstruction, anything done to the larynx to improve breathing will impair the voice. The lateral position *(bilateral adductor paralysis)* of the cords occurs less frequently than the median position, probably because it represents more extensive damage to the nerve supply. The lateral position poses little problem for breathing but effectively eliminates voice, a condition that can sometimes be improved by surgery.

Manifestations of systemic disease

The problem in considering manifestations of systemic disease will be to keep the discus-

sion within bounds. The larynx can be affected by diseases ranging from those of the neurologic through the muscular to the endocrine systems. Even such rarities as leprosy, scleroma, mycosis, and pemphigus can affect it (Luchsinger and Arnold, 1965). We will look at only endocrine and muscular system disorders in this chapter.

Endocrine disorders. To examine effects of each endocrine gland separately is a bit like trying to appreciate a symphony by isolating the sound of each instrument in the orchestra. Thyroids, parathyroids, gonads, and adrenals all interact under direction of the pituitary, which takes its orders from the hypothalamus in the brain.

Thyroid. Disturbances in the secretion of the thyroid glands that produce vocal disorders can occur as *hyperthyroidism,* but they are generally seen as *hypothyroidism.* The poorly understood laryngeal consequences seem to include muscular weakness and, possibly, clinical changes in the cords comparable to chronic laryngitis. On the other hand, a deficiency of thyroid hormone in early infancy can retard growth of the larynx, as well as of the rest of the body, and can result in *cretinism.* Later in childhood, or in adults, hypothyroidism can result in *myxedema,* with edema or muscular dystrophy in the larynx.

Parathyroids. Even less is known about laryngeal effects of defective parathyroid glands than of the thyroid behind which they are embedded. Insufficient secretion appears to cause overexcitability of muscles, if not tetany. Conversely, excessive secretion is associated with reduced excitability and muscular weakness.

Gonads. The gonads can produce virilizing or feminizing effects in the larynx. The excessive administration of drugs containing male androgenic hormones can virilize the young female larynx and produce perverse mutation, with pathologic growth to male dimensions and corresponding masculine pitch. The result would be a female basso. For older women at menopause, reduction in ovarian estrogens and hormone drug treatment can result in virilization (Damsté, 1967). The closest male counterpart is absence of mutation, with resultant eunuchoid voice that corresponds to the undeveloped child's voice. At puberty the boy's vocal cords lengthen about 10 mm, and pitch drops an octave; the girl's cords lengthen only 3 to 4 mm, and pitch descends about one-third octave (Luchsinger and Arnold, 1965). These vocal changes may occur gradually over several years or abruptly, seemingly overnight. Various degrees of mutation are possible, but none should be confused with light vocal mode (falsetto). This is not the mode that the child normally uses, but it is the mode with which a male whose larynx has grown normally avoids a mature voice after mutation.

Papers by Curry (1940, 1946, 1949) and Weiss (1950) contain much of the evidence about pubertal voice change.

Adrenals. The major condition associated with insufficient functioning of the adrenal cortex is Addison's disease. One of its characteristics is muscular weakness. As it progresses with advance of disease, so does vocal weakness until, heralding the advent of death, complete aphonia results.

Pituitary. The pituitary, being the master gland, is involved in all endocrine effects discussed. The condition affecting voice most typically associated with hyperfunction of the anterior pituitary is acromegaly, the disease that produces giants. A feature of this condition is thickening of cartilages, including those in the larynx. Extensive virilization of voice is often remarkable in women. Thickening can progress to such a degree that epiglottis and arytenoids all but block the laryngeal inlet.

Muscular disorder

Myasthenia gravis. The major disorder of the muscular system affecting voice is myasthenia gravis. It is characterized by rapid reduction in contractility of voluntary muscles. The striated muscles are excessively weak and easily fatigued; yet no demonstrable anatomic changes are apparent in either muscle or nervous system. The problem, which may be inherited in the case of infants, appears to result from a neuromuscular block that prevents stimulation of the muscle. The face droops, chewing and swallowing actions are weak, respiration is difficult, and fatigue from prolonged talking leads to temporary paralysis of afflicted muscles.

Manifestations of emotional disturbance

Vocal effects of emotional disturbance can be described as laryngeal hyperfunctions or hypofunctions (Brodnitz, 1965). We will follow that distinction.

Hypofunctional laryngeal disability— functional aphonia. The most characteristic emotionally based hypofunctional disability is traditionally called *hysterical aphonia* (or *dysphonia*, depending on whether functional loss of voice is total or partial). *Functional aphonia* (or *dysphonia*) is a preferred alternative to the pejorative word "hysterical" (Aronson, Peterson, and Litin, 1964; Brodnitz, 1969a). Use of voice for primitive purposes, such as laughing, coughing, crying, or even singing and swearing, is likely to be unimpaired. For purposive communication, the aphonic person behaves as if he has given up trying; all that is produced is a whisper. Characterized by the *la belle indifférence syndrome*, loss of voice seems to be of slight consequence to him (Brodnitz, 1965).

Hyperfunctional laryngeal disabilities. Two conditions can be described as hyperfunctional: *spastic dysphonia* and *ventricular dysphonia.* Whether they are of emotional origin is a matter of divided opinion and careful diagnosis (Arnold, 1959).

Spastic dysphonia. Spastic dysphonia has sometimes been described as stuttering with the vocal cords. Like stuttering, it varies with the communicative situation. When singing, talking to oneself, choral reading, or speaking to children or animals, no problem may be apparent. Arrival of an adult, preferably prestigious, can reduce the voice to a strained, squeezed, creaking, choking squawk. Its variability and symptomatic implications of

underlying personality disturbance have convinced the majority of voice specialists of its neurotic origins (Bloch, 1965). Others, however, find tentative evidence to support the idea that it is a symptom of a central nervous system lesion (Aronson and others, 1968; Robe, Brumlik and Moore, 1960). Regardless of etiology, it is a problem exceedingly resistant to effective treatment.

Compare the explanations for spastic dysphonia of Brodnitz (1965), Robe, Brumlik, and Moore (1960), and Aronson and his colleagues (1968). Do they agree? Do they prefer the same terms?

Ventricular dysphonia. Ventricular dysphonia also has several pseudonyms, the

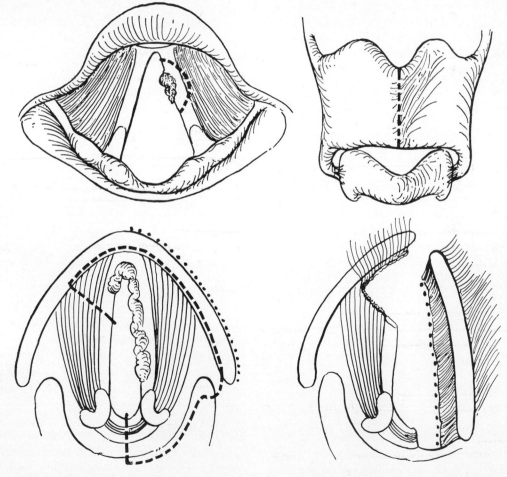

Fig. 7-5. Conservation surgery. Laryngofissure for removal of limited cordal carcinoma is shown above, subtotal laryngectomy and reconstruction below. (From von Leden, H., Conservation surgery of laryngeal carcinoma, *Intern. Surg.*, **45**, 264-265 [1966].)

most common being *dysphonia plicae ventricularis*. More frequently suspected than actually found, it illustrates the subversion of overlaid communicative functions by more primitive biologic protective needs. The ventricular bands are the false vocal folds, the middle valve in the larynx. When primitive valving action intrudes on normal phonation, ventricular dysphonia can be thought of as a form of regression of function—hence the speculation that it is symptomatic of emotional disturbance.

One set of classifications, however, differentiates six forms of ventricular dysphonia: (1) habitual origin, being the ultimate form of strained phonation; (2) emotional origin, in times of stress for neurotic individuals; (3) compensatory origin, for laryngeal paralysis; (4) cerebral origin, being a form of dysarthria; (5) cerebellar origin; and (6) vicarious origin, as compensation for defective vocal cords (Luchsinger and Arnold, 1965). Although probably excessive, these categories do suggest enough alternatives to an explanation of psychoneurosis to keep the door ajar for other possibilities.

Surgery of laryngeal cancer

Laryngeal surgery is undertaken with two considerations: preservation of health and life, and restoration of vocal function. Since life is rarely at stake in surgical excision of benign laryngeal lesions, normal vocal function is the paramount concern. With laryngeal malignancies, however, health outweighs voice; radical removal of the neoplasm with a safe margin of healthy tissue is the usual procedure. Whether *total laryngectomy* or *conservation surgery*, the tissue essential to vocal function is sacrificed, often to the extent that a form of *alaryngeal speech* (speech without a larynx) must be learned as a substitute for the normal voice (Brodnitz and Conley, 1967; von Leden, 1966).

Conservation surgery, undertaken to preserve as much of the larynx as possible, may extend from partial excision of one vocal cord to removal of three fifths of the larynx (Fig. 7-5). Of the various procedures described by von Leden (1966), the following are most

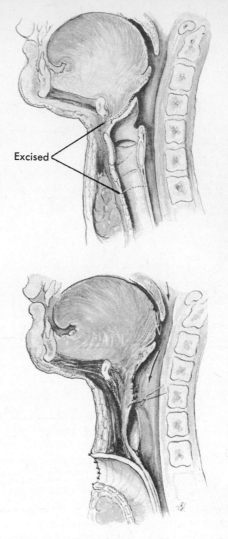

Fig. 7-6. Total laryngectomy. The normal arrangement, seen above, is altered by surgery as seen below. The severed trachea is sutured to a hole in the skin of the neck. Removal of the larynx leaves a hiatus in the pharynx shown being sutured. (From Snidecor, J., *Speech Rehabilitation of the Laryngectomized.* [2nd ed.] Springfield, Ill.: Charles C Thomas, Publisher [1969].)

likely to impair vocal production severely: *hemilaryngectomy* (removal of half of the larynx), *frontolateral laryngectomy* (removal of one entire vocal cord and an anterior section of thyroid cartilage), *subtotal laryngectomy* (removal of one whole cord and up to one third of the other), and *anterior partial laryngectomy* (removal of anterior section of

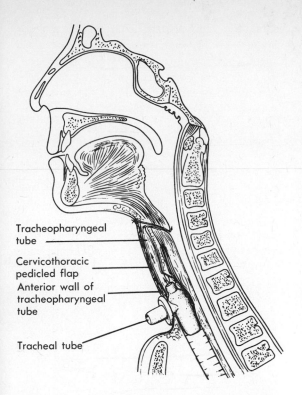

Fig. 7-7. Asai type of surgery to restore voice after laryngectomy. Occlusion of the tracheal tube forces air through the tracheopharyngeal tube into the pharynx for speech. (From Montgomery, W., and Toohill, R., Voice rehabilitation after laryngectomy, *Arch. Otolaryng.*, 88, 505 [1968].)

Labels on figure:
Tracheopharyngeal tube
Cervicothoracic pedicled flap
Anterior wall of tracheopharyngeal tube
Tracheal tube

thyroid cartilage and vocal cords). To restore the voice after conservation surgery, Brodnitz and Conley (1967) have devised a reconstructive technique for resurfacing the glottis.

Total laryngectomy, as shown in Fig. 7-6, involves excision of the entire larynx from the trachea to the base of the tongue, often including the hyoid bone (Levin, 1962). With this radical procedure, normal voice is eliminated. The most popular and successful forms of alaryngeal speech that can be substituted for the loss of voice are esophageal speech and speech with an artificial larynx (Chapter 13).

Of several surgical strategies to provide the laryngectomized patient with a pseudoglottis that can be activated by normal respiration, the *Asai technique* is one that can be successful when used with carefully selected patients. Devised by Asai in Japan, it has

been utilized by such American surgeons as Miller (1967, 1968) and Montgomery and Toohill (1968). It involves a three-stage operation, after removal of the larynx, to form a tube of skin extending from trachea to lower pharynx (Fig. 7-7). Air can then be directed through this dermal tube to activate a pseudoglottis at the base of the tongue (Asai, 1969). Speech is thereby possible soon after surgery (Chapter 13).

NATURE AND ETIOLOGY OF LOWER RESPIRATORY DISABILITIES

The plethora of pulmonary disabilities of the lower respiratory system is balanced by a dearth of speech consequences. The normal speaker's major problem is maintenance of steady alveolar pressure, a problem related to thoracic and abdominal musculature (Hixon, 1973). These structures may be accidentally injured or affected by neurologic disabilities, but they are not much prone to disease. Various pulmonary disabilities, on the other hand, affect *vital capacity*, the total usable supply of air available. Were our major concern the singer or professional speaker, the effects of these disabilities would loom larger—problems of sustaining long phrases would be of more consequence. As it is, most speakers could get by, if necessary, with reasonably short phrases and a small supply of air.

Bronchopulmonary obstructions

Any obstructions that develop within the bronchial tree will tend to exclude the obstructed section from participating in respiration and will deplete air supply. Naturally, any foreign substance that inadvertently gets by laryngeal valves guarding the lungs will offer some degree of obstruction from slight to total.

Bronchopulmonary diseases

Diseases that can obstruct the lungs range from *bronchogenic carcinoma* to *emphysema*, from *tuberculosis* to *pneumonia*, and from *bronchial asthma* to *vocal pseudoasthenia*. Of these conditions, emphysema and bronchial asthma are the most frequently encountered. Bronchial asthma works its effects by paroxysms of constriction and spasmodic contractions of the bronchial tubes. Emphysema, on the other hand, involves loss of respiratory efficiency caused by atrophy of the alveoli at the tips of the bronchial tree. Tuberculosis of the lungs forms tubercles in the tissues and usually leads to pneumonia, which produces congestion and obstructs the lungs with exuded fluids. As bronchogenic carcinoma progresses, the cancerous neoplasm blocks the diseased section of the bronchial tree. Finally, vocal pseudoasthenia, found in connection with hyperthyroidism and Addison's disease, involves reduced vital capacity and vocal weakness (Luchsinger and Arnold, 1965).

Tissue collapse or removal

A lung can be collapsed intentionally or unintentionally, or it can be removed. *Artificial pneumothorax* can be induced to collapse a lung for medical reasons, but *pneumothorax* is a condition analogous to a flat tire; just as a flat can occur unintentionally, so can pneumothorax. When the pleural lining, corresponding to the inner tube, is punctured by wound or abscess, the lung goes flat. Effects of this condition are akin to those of *atelectasis,* which may involve incomplete expansion of the lungs at birth, or collapse of an adult lung for complex reasons that have to do with surface tension on the air sacs. More drastic is surgical removal of a lobe of a lung *(lobectomy),* or of an entire lung *(pneumonectomy).*

SPEECH EFFECTS OF LARYNGEAL AND LOWER RESPIRATORY DISABILITIES

Practically, laryngeal and lower respiratory disabilities are important to speech pathology to the extent that they affect speech. These effects are most apparent in the voice, but they also appear in nonvocal forms. Such nonvocal effects are generally of less concern, so let us look at them only briefly.

Nonvocal effects

The nonvocal speech properties of phrasing, syllabic stress, and voiced-voiceless ar-

ticulatory adjustments, as well as the non-speech problems of swallowing, can be affected by disabilities of the larynx, of the bronchopulmonary structure, and of respiratory muscles. Disabilities that impair vital capacity impair the ability to spin long phrases. A similar effect is produced by the disabled ability to set the flow of air into vibration efficiently; breathy speech is wasteful of air (Hardy, 1968; Noll, 1968).

As for a speech syllable, it is characterized physiologically by a pulse of subglottal pressure (Netsell, 1973). Subglottal pressure, in turn, is a function of airflow and how much it is impeded in the vocal tract. Air that flows through the vocal tract with minimal interference by laryngeal valves, pharynx, tongue, and lips is air under minimal pressure. Conversely, the faster it flows, the greater will be the pressure built up against whatever obstruction is offered. Syllabic pulses involve rapid changes in pressure as speech flows quickly from stressed through unstressed syllables; this ability will therefore be affected by any respiratory or laryngeal condition that impairs quick pressure changes. All articulated speech sounds are to some degree voiced or voiceless. Accordingly, impaired ability to abduct and adduct the vocal cords rapidly would affect the ability to make necessary voiced-voiceless articulatory distinctions (Chapter 3).

As for the nonspeech problem of swallowing associated with neurologic impairment of the ability to obtain adequate vocal cord adduction, the speech pathologist can be of special assistance. As Diedrich (1969) points out, with skill in procedures that modify laryngeal activity (such as pushing techniques), patients can be freed from feeding tubes and returned to normal swallowing.

Vocal effects

The vocal effects of disabilities of the vocal tract are revealed in pitch, loudness, or quality of voice. Moore (1968a,b) provides an especially helpful analysis for understanding these effects. He starts with the traditional description of the generation of a train of glottal pulses: breath pressure overcomes

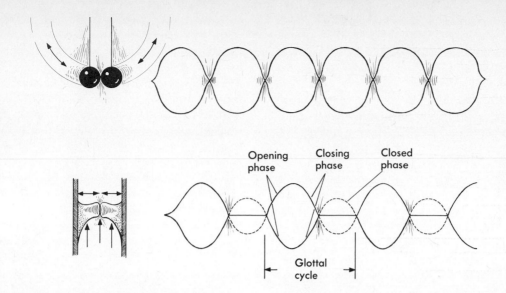

Fig. 7-8. Absorption of vibratory impact by compliant vocal folds in contrast with reflection of impact by resilient steel balls. (Based on a sketch by Moore, P., Otolaryngology and speech pathology, *Laryngoscope*, **18**, 7 [1968].)

vocal cord resistance; a pulse of pressure spurts through the glottal opening, reducing subglottal pressure; the cords snap closed. This process continues so long as air pressure and laryngeal resistance continue this interaction. He then points out two considerations necessary to complete the description. First, several factors affect movement of each vocal fold as it vibrates independently, and second, the two cords affect each other when they make contact during the closed phase of a vibratory cycle.

The paired vocal folds normally vibrate in *phase* (open and close together) and *synchrony* (vibrate at the same rate) because they are comparable in such factors as *mass*, *length, elasticity,* and *compliance.* * If they differed in any of these factors, they would vibrate at different rates. Each cord functions as an independent unit. The greater its length, the heavier is its mass; or the more

*Compliance is inversely related to elasticity. As elasticity increases, compliance decreases. The advantage of using "compliance" is that it offers a convenient term for identifying the characteristic of elasticity that controls duration of cord closure during a vibratory cycle. For more detailed descriptions of laryngeal functions for speech, see Broad (1973), Hirano (1975), and Perkins (1975).

its compliance (its softness and compressibility), the slower is its movement. Conversely, increased elasticity quickens movement. Thus, for vocal folds to vibrate in synchrony and in phase requires that they be equivalent in these factors affecting independent movement.

During normal phonation, however, closing movements of the folds during a vibratory cycle bring each fold to the midline at the same instant—they collide. During the collision (the period of glottal closure) the folds cease to function independently; while closed they operate together, as a unit. The duration of closure is determined by the compliance factor, as suggested in Fig. 7-8. Were mucosal texture and underlying laryngeal tissue so firm as to be noncompliant as, for example, two steel balls, the folds would bounce apart without compression, as in the upper diagram. They would move almost wholly independently, with no period of closure. Being compliant, they absorb the collision by compressing; the more compliant, the greater is the compression and the longer is the closure. This phenomenon is shown in the lower diagram of typical glottal cycles, the dotted curve suggesting dissipation of energy as each cord absorbs the impact of the other. Then, as breath pressure overcomes laryngeal resistance, the most compliant portion of the cord yields first, initiating complex undulations of the folds as the next vibratory cycle begins.

Pitch, loudness, and quality. With Moore's analysis, we can understand laryngeal factors that will affect pitch, loudness, and quality. Since pitch is determined mainly by glottal pulse rate, compliance (which affects the length of glottal closure) and mass, length, and elasticity (which affect the quickness of independent cord movement during opening and closing phases of vibration) are primary determinants. Since loudness is affected by the amount of energy released in each glottal pulse, factors affecting closure and synchronous vibration are important: closure permits buildup of subglottal pressure for an explosive glottal pulse; synchronous vibration of the two cords is essential if they are to collide and afford a period of closure. Quality is affected by vibratory symmetry. Asymmetric vibration results from cord differences in factors affecting both independent movement and closure. For example, if one fold is more compliant than the other, it would be forced to open sooner, be displaced farther, move slower, and be compressed more than its partner. Too, if the cords were positioned to require one to move farther than the other for contact, they could vibrate out of phase even if both moved independently in synchrony.

SPEECH PATHOLOGIST'S RESPONSIBILITY IN TREATMENT OF LARYNGEAL AND LOWER RESPIRATORY DISABILITIES
Responsibility for referral

The speech pathologist's most vital responsibility for the physical condition of a patient's vocal tract is to ensure that he is placed under competent medical care. Not equipped legally or by training to make professional judgments about laryngeal or bronchopulmonary disabilities, he may peer into a patient's throat with a laryngeal mirror for his own edification, but not to make an evaluation or recommendation about the physical status of the mechanism.

The speech pathologist can and should use his ears critically, however, He may be the first to detect an early sign of hoarseness. Not infrequently, people seek nonmedical professional advice first about the voice. The speech pathologist should know that persistent hoarseness, even mild sporadic hoarseness, can be the only early warning of serious disease. Zinn (1945) found it as the first symptom in 93% of 144 cases of laryngeal cancer, many of which were not diagnosed for a year. The speech pathologist should know that the hoarseness of a trifling case of laryngitis cannot be distinguished from the hoarseness of incipient cancer (Yanagihara, 1967). He should know that a patient's larynx, indeed his life, may hang by the thread of early detection of disease—that the safest course is to assume the worst until proved otherwise. He should know that to begin voice therapy without certain knowledge of the physical condition of the vocal apparatus is to risk damage in the name of therapy. He should know that astute medical judgment of the condition of the phonatory structures is the foundation on which effective vocal rehabilitation is built.

Responsibility for consultation and treatment

Informational traffic between the speech pathologist and the laryngologist flows both ways. The laryngologist needs information about vocal behavior, especially abusive vocal behavior. He also needs to reduce vocal abuse. This is the speech pathologist's area of responsibility; he is best prepared to appraise behavioral functioning of the vocal mechanism as it is affected by disabilities and as it is conducive to functional damage to the cords. Maintenance of the voice for oral communication is, next to life itself, of paramount importance. The speech pathologist serves as consultant in matters regarding pitch, loudness, and quality of voice as they function in the linguistic and nonlinguistic service of interpersonal communication.

The answers—résumé

1. What are the nature and etiology of laryngeal and lower respiratory disabilities?

The most common laryngeal disabilities stem from lesions of vocal cords, paralysis, manifestations of systemic disease (such as endocrine disorders), and hypofunctional and hyperfunctional manifestations of emotional disturbance. Voice is affected most severely by surgery for laryngeal cancer; it may range from conservative procedures to total laryngectomy, with which normal voice is eliminated. Bronchopulmonary disorders result mainly in depletion of the air supply because of an obstructing foreign substance in the bronchial tree, obstruction of lungs from disease, or collapse or removal of a lung. Depletion of vital capacity does not necessarily result in an inability to maintain subglottal pressure, but it does affect length of time that pressure can be maintained.

Causes of disabling laryngeal disorders are varied. Inflammation may stem from acute laryngotracheobronchitis to chronic laryngitis. Tumors may be benign or malignant growths. Vocal nodules, contact ulcers, and granulomas are generally the consequence of vocal abuse. Paralysis can result from swelling or surgery. Various laryngeal disabilities are produced by such systemic diseases as involve thyroid, parathyroid, gonad, adrenal, and pituitary glands. Laryngeal hypofunction of hysterical aphonia, or hyperfunction of spastic dysphonia and ventricular dysphonia, though usually considered manifestations of emotional disturbance, may be of neurologic origin.

Causes of bronchopulmonary disorders may be found in disease, physical obstruction, tissue collapse, or tissue removal. When the larynx fails in its task of excluding foreign substances from the lungs, obstruction results. A more common cause of obstruction is disease, mainly from atrophy of alveolar air sacs in emphysema or constriction of the bronchial tubes in asthma. Occasionally, a lung is collapsed or surgically removed.

2. What are the speech effects of laryngeal and lower respiratory disabilities?

Speech is affected by the laryngeal and bronchopulmonary apparatus as follows:
a. Ability to provide an air supply is essential, but only phrase length depends on vital capacity, which can be impaired by bronchopulmonary obstructions and disabled control of respiratory muscles.
b. Ability to maintain stable subglottal pressure from instant to instant and ability to vary it quickly are essential. Subglottal pressure is affected by disabilities of respiratory and laryngeal adjustments.
c. Ability to adduct vocal folds for phonation and abduct them for voiceless sounds is basic to control of voicing. Impairment of this ability can disable articulatory and phonatory skill.
d. Ability to stretch the vocalis muscle (thereby changing its mass, length, elasticity, and compliance) and to tense the vocal ligament (a function of tilting the

cricoid cartilage by contracting the cricothyroid muscle) affects regulation of pitch, loudness, and quality. Laryngeal conditions that alter control or synchrony and phase relations of vocal folds as they vibrate together affect voice.

3. What is the speech pathologist's responsibility in the treatment of laryngeal and lower respiratory disabilities?

   The speech pathologist has two basic responsibilities in treating disorders of the laryngeal and upper respiratory apparatus: referral and consultation. As a specialist in vocal behavior, he consults with physicians regarding adequacy of vocal production and refers patients to them for judgments about the physical status of the speech mechanism. Because he is trained to listen critically, he may be the first to detect hoarseness, the early warning sign of laryngeal pathology; he knows that a patient's larynx, and perhaps his life, may hinge on referral to a physician for early detection of disease.

REFERENCES

Arnold, G., Vocal rehabilitation of paralytic dysphonia. I. Cartilage injection into a paralyzed vocal cord. *Arch. Otolaryng.*, **62**, 1-17 (1955).

Arnold, G., Spastic dysphonia. *Logos*, **2**, 3-14 (1959).

Arnold, G., Vocal nodules and polyps: laryngeal tissue reaction to habitual hyperkinetic dysphonia. *J. Speech Hearing Dis.*, **27**, 205-217 (1962a).

Arnold, G., Vocal rehabilitation of paralytic dysphonia. IX. Technique of intracordal injection. *Arch. Otolaryng.*, **76**, 358-368 (1962b).

Aronson, A., Peterson, H., and Litin, E., Voice Symptomatology in functional dysphonia and aphonia. *J. Speech Hearing Dis.*, **29**, 367-380 (1964).

Aronson, A., and others, Spastic dysphonia. I, II. *J. Speech Hearing Dis.*, **33**, 203-231 (1968).

Asai, R., Personal communication (1969).

Bloch, P., Neuro-psychiatric aspects of spastic dysphonia. *Folia Phoniatrica*, **17**, 301-364 (1965).

Broad, D., Phonation. In Minifie, F., Hixon, T., and Williams, F. (Eds.), *Normal Aspects of Speech, Hearing, and Language.* Englewood Cliffs, N.J.: Prentice-Hall, Inc. (1973).

Brodnitz, F., Contact ulcer of the larynx. *Arch. Otolaryng.*, **74**, 70-80 (1961).

Brodnitz, F., *Vocal Rehabilitation.* Rochester, Minn.: American Academy of Ophthalmology and Otolaryngology (1965).

Brodnitz, F., Functional aphonia. *Ann. Otol. Rhinol. Laryng.*, **78**, 1244-1253 (1969a).

Brodnitz, F., Personal communication (1969b).

Brodnitz, F., and Conley, J., Vocal rehabilitation after reconstructive surgery for laryngeal cancer. *Folia Phoniatrica*, **19**, 89-97 (1967).

Cooper, M., *Modern Techniques of Vocal Rehabilitation.* Springfield, Ill.: Charles C Thomas, Publisher (1973).

Curry, E., An objective study of the pitch characteristics of the adolescent male voice. *Speech Monogr.*, **7**, 48-62 (1940).

Curry, E., Voice change in adolescent males. *Laryngologica*, **56**, 795-803 (1946).

Curry, E., Hoarseness and voice change in male adolescents. *J. Speech Hearing Dis.*, **14**, 23-25, (1949).

Damsté, P., Voice change in adult women caused by virilizing agents. *J. Speech Hearing Dis.*, **32**, 126-132 (1967).

Diedrich, W., Personal communication (1969).

Froeschels, E., Hygiene of the voice. *Arch. Otolaryng.*, **38**, 122-130 (1943).

Hardy, J., Respiratory physiology: implications of current research. *Asha*, **10**, 204-205 (1968).

Hirano, M., Phonosurgery, basic and clinical investigations. *Otologia* (Fukuoka) (Suppl. 1), **21**, 239-440 (1975).

Hixon, T., Respiratory function in speech. In Minifie,

F., Hixon, T., and Williams, F. (Eds.), *Normal Aspects of Speech, Hearing, and Language.* Englewood Cliffs, N.J.: Prentice-Hall, Inc. (1973).

Levin, N., Surgery of the larynx, trachea, and neck. In Levin, N. (Ed.), *Voice and Speech Disorders: Medical Aspects.* Springfield, Ill.: Charles C Thomas, Publisher (1962).

Luchsinger, R., and Arnold, G., *Voice-Speech-Language.* Belmont, Calif.: Wadsworth Publishing Co., Inc. (1965).

Miller, A., First experiences with the Asai technique for vocal rehabilitation after total laryngectomy. *Ann. Otol. Rhinol. Laryng.*, **76**, 829-833 (1967).

Miller, A., Further experiences with Asai technique of vocal rehabilitation after laryngectomy. *Trans. Am. Acad. Ophthalmol. Otolaryng.*, **72**, 779-781 (1968).

Montgomery, W., and Toohill, R., Voice rehabilitation after laryngectomy. *Arch. Otolaryng.*, **88**, 499-506 (1968).

Moore, P., Discussion of Lieberman's paper. *Ann. N.Y. Acad. Sci.*, **155**, 39-41 (1968a).

Moore, P., Otolaryngology and speech pathology. *Laryngoscope*, **78**, 1500-1509 (1968b).

Netsell, R., Speech physiology. In Minifie, F., Hixon, T., and Williams, F. (Eds.), *Normal Aspects of Speech, Hearing, and Language.* Englewood Cliffs, N.J.: Prentice-Hall, Inc. (1973).

Noll, J., Discussion of respiratory physiology: implications of current research. *Asha*, **10**, 205-206 (1968).

Perkins, W., Normal vocal tone generation: detection, diagnosis and management of abnormal vocal tone generation. In Tower, D. (Editor-in-chief), *The Nervous System.* (Vol. 3) *Human Communication and Its Disorders.* New York: Raven Press (1975).

Robe, E., Brumlik, J., and Moore, P., A study of spastic dysphonia: neurologic and electroencephalographic abnormalities. *Laryngoscope*, **70**, 219-245 (1960).

Ryan, R., von Leden, H., Ogura, J., Biller, H., and Pratt, L., *Synopsis of Ear, Nose, and Throat Diseases.* (3rd ed.) St. Louis: The C. V. Mosby Co. (1970).

Von Leden, H., Conservation surgery of laryngeal carcinoma. *Internat. Surg.*, **45**, 261-271 (1966).

Von Leden, H., and Moore, P., Contact ulcer of the larynx. *Arch. Otolaryng.*, **72**, 746-752 (1960).

Weiss, D., The pubertal change of the human voice. *Folia Phoniatrica*, **2**, 127-159 (1950).

Yanagihara, N., Significance of harmonic changes and noise components in hoarseness. *J. Speech Hearing Res.*, **10**, 531-541 (1967).

Zinn, W., The significance of hoarseness. *Trans. Am. laryng. rhinol. otol. Soc.*, pp. 133-134 (1945).

Chapter 8

Orofacial and upper respiratory disabilities

Questions

1. What are the nature and the etiology of orofacial and upper respiratory disabilities?
2. What are the speech effects of orofacial and upper respiratory disabilities?
3. What is the speech pathologist's responsibility in the treatment of orofacial and upper respiratory disabilities?

NATURE OF OROFACIAL AND UPPER RESPIRATORY DISABILITIES

The functional relation between a pathologic condition of the vocal tract, such as cleft palate, and defective speech is far from direct or obvious. Admittedly, knowledge of etiology or nature of an anatomic anomaly does not specify its effect on speech. Still,

Morris (1968) offers an excellent review of the etiologic bases of cleft palate speech characteristics.

to appreciate disabled speech functions requires knowledge of the *morphology* (structure) of abnormal parts of the speaking apparatus.

Oropharyngeal disabilities

Functions of the throat and mouth cavities for speech can be disabled by *velopharyngeal* defects (defects in the mechanism by which the velum, soft palate, and pharynx close the nasal from the oral cavity); by enlarged tonsils and adenoids or by their removal; and by defects of the tongue. Palatal and dental conditions are also involved, but we will consider them separately.

Velopharyngeal insufficiency. The problem most commonly associated with velopharyngeal disability is *cleft palate*. Clefts can appear in a variety of structures. Of these, velar clefts are the ones of concern in this consideration of ability to separate the throat from the nasal cavity. If the soft palate is cleft or is too short or too immobile to reach the posterior pharyngeal wall, *velopharyngeal competence* (ability to separate the nasal from the oral cavity) will be impaired (Blackfield and others, 1962).

Although some have speculated that velopharyngeal inadequacy in persons with cleft palate can be attributed in part to excessive pharyngeal depth, available evidence contradicts this possibility (Engman, Spriestersbach, and Moll, 1965; Ross, 1965). This is not to say that velopharyngeal incompetence is never caused by an abnormally deep pharyngeal wall that a normal palate cannot reach; it can be. The evidence merely indicates that persons with cleft palate are not different from normal in this respect (and a person with a normal palate can have an abnormally deep nasopharynx).

Tonsils and adenoids. The ring of lymphoid tissue of which tonsils and adenoids are a part can impair functions of the oropharyngeal cavity. Although *hypertrophied* (enlarged) palatine tonsils can reach sufficient size so that they almost block the oropharynx and thereby create a resonance as well as a breathing problem, their removal is often discouraged by surgeons and dentists on the grounds that they do contribute to velopharyngeal closure, especially when a prosthodontic appliance is used to close a cleft (Shelton, 1969).

The same is true with adenoids; their removal as well as their hypertrophy can create problems. The adenoids can maintain the functional balance of the nasopharynx, as they normally do during growth of the facial skeleton (Subtelny and Koepp-Baker, 1956). For instance, enlarged adenoids can compensate for a soft palate that is too short or too immobile to reach a pharyngeal wall of normal depth; or if the velum is normal, adenoids can compensate for an abnormally deep pharyngeal wall. Either way, velopharyngeal competence would depend on the presence of sufficient adenoidal tissue for the velum to make contact with it. Obviously, removal of adenoids that are serving this compensatory function will disable the mechanism for separating the nose from the throat. Routine surgical removal of adenoids can convert a child with normal speech into a child with hypernasal speech. Conversely, enlarged adenoids in a normal nasopharynx can occlude it so much that even when the velum is depressed the nasal cavity remains closed off from the throat. A child so afflicted would sound as if he had a perpetual "cold in the nose."

Lingual defects. Because the tongue is the most flexible structure for adjusting size and shape of throat and mouth, it is the organ of speech most vital to intelligible articulation of sounds. The tongue must move forward and backward to adjust resonance of the pharyngeal cavity; it must move up and down to adjust oral resonance; it must constrict, open, or block the vocal tract at any point; it must spread laterally or groove down the center; and its tip must protrude, raise, or lower. Disable any of these skills, and normal functions of the tongue for speech would be impaired (Bloomer, 1971).

Abnormalities that can disable the tongue involve its size, shape, or mobility. The tongue may be too large to function normally, it may be too small, it may be misshapen, or it may be immobile. The point to be stressed here is the nature of the structural abnormality, not its cause. The consequent functional disability is what affects speech, not the etiology of the abnormality. As an example, two children may produce defective sounds, and both may be unable to protrude the tongue between the teeth for this sound. The articulatory defect is more directly a function of the nature of the lingual disability than of its cause: paralysis, let us say, in one child, and tongue-tie in the other.

Nasopalatal disabilities

Nasal obstruction. The nose is a resonating cavity of fixed size. Normally, it contributes to speech by virtue of the size of the velopharyngeal opening by which it is coupled acoustically with the vocal tract. The normal contribution of the nose to resonance can be altered, however, by obstructing it. Obstruction may come in various forms, such as inflammation of the mucosal tissue, as in a head cold, or a deviated septum, which may result from injury. Normal nasal resonance can also be affected by clefts in the hard

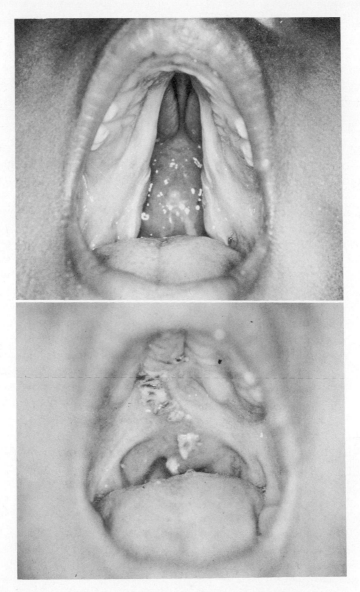

Fig. 8-1. Bilateral incomplete cleft before and after surgical closure. (Courtesy John Goin, M.D., Los Angeles.)

palate that separate the nose from the mouth.

Palatal clefts. Clefts in the hard palate can occur *unilaterally* or *bilaterally,* they can range from invisible *submucosal clefts* to *complete clefts* of the entire palate, and they can be found alone or in combination with clefts of the velum, lip, and alveolar dental arch. Clefts occur when the bones of the hard palate that grow toward the midline fail to unite with the center partition of the nose that grows downward from the base of the skull. If these bony processes fail to fuse on one side, the result is a *unilateral cleft* that opens one side of the nasal cavity directly to the oral cavity. If the midline *septum* and *vomer* of the nose fail to fuse with the palate on both sides, the result is a *bilateral cleft* (Fig. 8-1) that opens the entire nasal cavity to the mouth. With a perforation in the partition that normally separates the nose from the mouth, the ability to produce nonnasal sounds would be impaired.

A less obvious disability visually, but one that can play havoc with normal resonance, is the *submucous cleft*. In this condition the bones of the hard palate fail to unite to one extent or another, but the mucous membrane over the cleft is intact. Although the nasal cavity appears to be separated from the oral cavity, acoustically it is not; the mucous covering over the cleft acts much as a drumhead to transmit vibration from mouth to nose. Actually, a submucous cleft can be detected visually because the mucous lining is thin and lacks supporting musculature, and the indentation of the cleft can be seen. Also, a typical accompanying defect is a divided uvula or a soft palate that is short or cleft (Koepp-Baker, 1971a; Luchsinger and Arnold, 1965).

Dental-facial disabilities

Dental and facial abnormalities are grouped here because the major defect of these structures, a cleft in them, often involves the lip and upper dental arch together.

Facial abnormalities. Facial defects are troublesome, not so often because they affect speech, but mainly because of cosmetic effects. The social consequences of cosmetic impairment can be vitally important, but they will take us afield from our primary concern: speech. Lips can be immobilized by paralysis, by injury, and by stretching and shortening after unsuccessful cleft lip repair. The most profound disability would result from an unrepaired cleft of the lip, but modern treatment methods have all but eliminated this possibility, at least in the United States. Lip clefts are identified by the physician at birth and are repaired shortly afterward (Fig. 8-2). Whether or not normal lip function will be possible after surgical closure involves such factors as amount of lip tissue available and patterns of growth.

Dental abnormalities. The tongue and lips work in relation to the teeth, especially the upper incisors, to produce a sizable group of consonants (Bloomer, 1971). Dental abnormalities can affect production of these sounds. The forms that these abnormalities can take, among those with clefts and those without, are sufficiently different that we will discuss them separately.

Dental abnormalities associated with clefts. Persons born with a cleft of any type are likely to exhibit multiple dental abnormalities. Although these abnormalities include condition of the teeth per se (for example, their size and shape) and typical malocclusions, they also include missing teeth and supernumerary teeth that can be so misplaced as to grow out of the hard palate (Jordan, Kraus, and Neptune, 1966). Also, alveolar clefts of the upper dental arch as seen in Fig. 8-3 (the extent of the lip cleft is a good index of alveolar cleft at the same site) not only disturb patterns of dental and facial growth but also provide another source of air leakage from the mouth (Koepp-Baker, 1971a; Bloomer, 1971).

Malocclusion. Occlusion has to do with alignment of teeth in the upper and lower dental arches. Positioning of both the individual teeth and the jaws must be considered. As a result, two systems for classifying malocclusions have been developed, one for relationship of the jaws, the other for relationship of the teeth (Bloomer, 1971).

The first system for classifying malocclu-

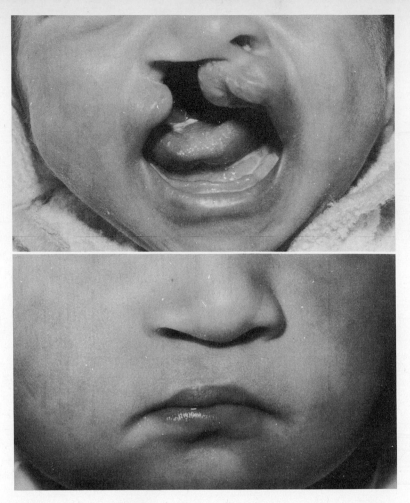

Fig. 8-2. Unilateral lip cleft before and after surgical closure. (Courtesy John Goin, M.D., Los Angeles.)

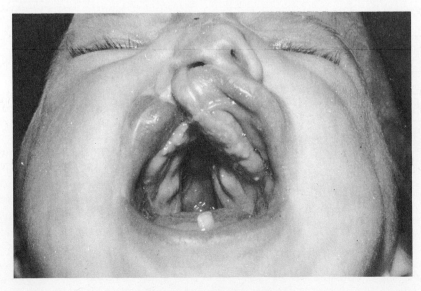

Fig. 8-3. Unilateral lip and alveolar cleft. (Courtesy John Goin, M.D., Los Angeles.)

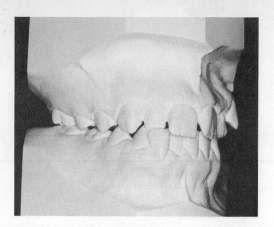

Fig. 8-4. Class I malocclusion. Molar occlusion is normal, whereas anterior occlusion is abnormal. (Courtesy Harry Dougherty, D.D.S., University of Southern California School of Dentistry.)

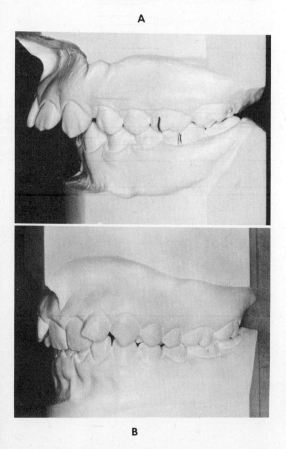

A

B

Fig. 8-5. Class II malocclusion. **A,** Division 1; **B,** division 2. (Courtesy Harry Dougherty, D.D.S., University of Southern California School of Dentistry.)

sion was devised by Angle in 1899. His three classes still provide the standard basis for describing the relationship of upper to lower jaw. Note that Angle's system does not describe relationship of upper and lower teeth. Following are his three classes of malocclusion:

Class I. Class I, shown in Fig. 8-4, describes any malocclusion in which jaw relationship is normal but teeth are positioned abnormally. A Class I description says nothing about how teeth are positioned abnormally. This term tells only that jaw positions are normal but that a malocclusion does exist. It is not a classification for normal occlusion.

Class II. Malocclusions involving a mandible that is retruded in relation to the maxillary dental arch fit Angle's Class II (Fig. 8-5). This is a condition in which the upper teeth protrude forward abnormally beyond the lower teeth. Again, this classification says nothing about tooth position, nor about whether the undershot lower jaw is too small or the overshot maxillary arch is too large. The mandible could be small and the maxilla normal, or the maxilla large and the mandible normal.

Class III. The prognathic mandible that protrudes beyond the upper jaw is described by Angle's Class III (Fig. 8-6). It is the opposite of Class II. Persons with this class of malocclusion may compensate by pro-

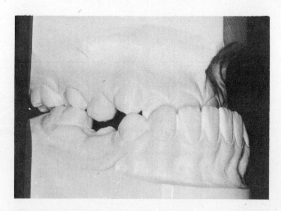

Fig. 8-6. Class III malocclusion. (Courtesy Harry Dougherty, D.D.S., University of Southern California School of Dentistry.)

ducing /f/ and /v/ with the upper lip against the lower teeth rather than vice versa. The acoustical result can sound normal, but the cosmetic appearance is abnormal: a speech problem that appears to exist in face-to-face conversation is not heard on the telephone.

Terms that have grown out of general usage for classifying improper positions of individual teeth include the following:

axiversion Inclination of the tooth along an improper axis.

distoversion Backward tilt of posterior teeth or tilt away from the midline of anterior teeth.

infraversion A condition in which tooth has not erupted far enough to reach the line of occlusion. Infraversion of the front teeth can produce an open bite, of the back teeth a closed bite.

labioversion Tilt of a tooth toward the lips or cheek.

linguoversion Tilt of a tooth toward the tongue.

mesioversion Forward tilt of posterior teeth or tilt toward the midline of anterior teeth. Mesioversion is the opposite position from distoversion.

supraversion Growth of a tooth past the normal line of occlusion. It is the opposite condition from infraversion and produces opposite effects.

torsiversion Rotation of a tooth along its long axis.

transversion A condition in which a tooth is in the wrong position in the dental arch.

ETIOLOGY OF OROFACIAL AND UPPER RESPIRATORY DISABILITIES
Congenital disabilities

Cleft lip and palate. Although clefts of the lip or palate occur on the average only once in every 750 births (Morris and Greulich, 1968), they are among the most expensive congenital malformations; they exact a high price in individual suffering and in the burden imposed on society. Their cause is still poorly understood, despite a vast amount of research. Attesting to the scope of interest is a multiprofessional organization, the American Cleft Palate Association, composed mainly of dental specialists, medical specialists, and specialists in communicative disorders, which has as its primary purpose the development of an understanding of this orofacial pathology.

In view of the extent of work accomplished, we must attribute much of the remaining uncertainty about the etiology of cleft conditions to the complexity of circumstances that produce them. This much is known. During the second month after conception, often before the prospective mother even knows she is pregnant, building blocks of the face, mouth, tongue, nose, and palate normally will have formed and grown together at the midline to separate the nasal from the oral cavity. If the *primary palate* (upper lip and gum ridge) fails to grow together, roughly during the sixth week, a unilateral or bilateral cleft of the lip will occur that can extend through the alveolar process. If the *secondary palate* (hard and soft palate) fails to grow together around the eighth week, a unilateral or bilateral cleft of the palate will occur (Hagerty, 1965).

The question of why these structures sometimes fail to unite remains. The difficulty in obtaining a clear answer can be appreciated by considering some of the factors involved. First, tissues of the primary and secondary palates must have sufficient growth potential to be able to reach each other at the midline. A disturbance, whether genetic or environmental, that impairs growth can prevent palatal structures from fusing. Several forms of evidence point to germ plasm defects that could retard palatal growth. For one thing, 10% to 25% of those born with a cleft will have other congenital anomalies (Lis, 1965); multiple dental abnormalities are typical of infants born with clefts (Jordan, Kraus, and Neptune, 1966). For another thing, 20% to 30% of children with clefts come from families with a history of clefts. Still, the chance that identical twins will both have clefts is only 40% (Morris and Greulich, 1968). Parental age seems to be another contributing factor, as may be the sex of the child (Hay, 1967; Greene, Vermillion, and Hay, 1965; Meskin, Pruzansky, and Gullen, 1968). The female, usually hardier than the male, seems more likely to have a cleft than does the male.

A second factor that probably contributes to palatal failure is that the pattern of de-

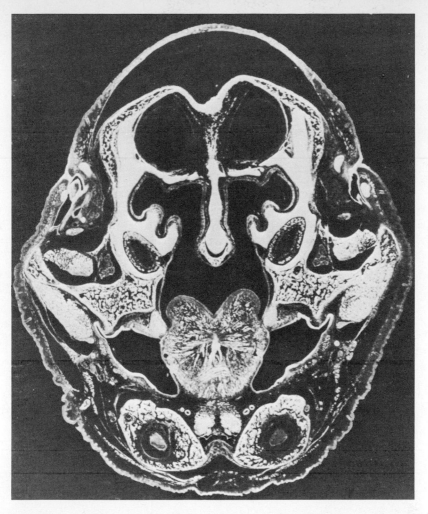

Fig. 8-7. Coronal x-ray film of a cleft palate in a 20-day rat fetus. (From cover photograph by Anthony Steffek, D.D.S., in *Science* [Vol. 160] June 7, 1968. Copyright 1968 by the American Association for the Advancement of Science.)

velopment involves dynamic interaction between tongue resistance and tissue growth strength. Shelves of the secondary palate that will form the roof of the mouth begin their movement not horizontally but vertically, straight downward. Whether pressure of the tongue is responsible for turning the direction of movement of these shelves to the horizontal is not certain, but it seems possible if not probable. In any event, as can be seen in Fig. 8-7, an x-ray film of a 20-day rat fetus with a cleft palate (the process of facial formation is remarkably similar in rat and human embryos), the tongue must be displaced by the palatal shelves before they can unite. If the tongue resists the shelf force too vigorously, failure of the palatal processes to fuse could result.

A third factor in fusion failures is synchrony of growth patterns. The problem is somewhat akin to that of the men on the flying trapezes: moving parts must be at the right place at the right time if the necessary connections are to occur. Unlike trapeze artists who, with a safety net, can rectify failures to connect, palatal growth apparently has no safety net. When the time passes during which the primary and secondary palatal parts would normally unite (second intrauterine month), late arrival of the struc-

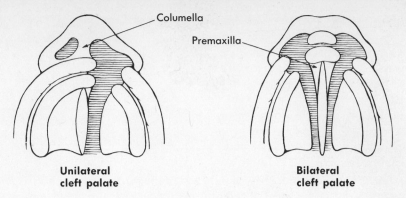

Fig. 8-8. Unilateral and bilateral complete clefts. The columella, shown intact on the left, is collapsed on the right. Also shown on the right is the wedge-shaped premaxilla separated from the maxillary bones on both sides of the bilateral cleft.

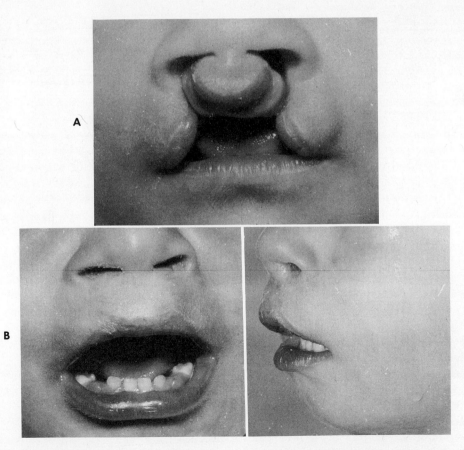

Fig. 8-9. Bilateral lip cleft before and after surgery. Although the philtrum (indentation in the center of the upper lip) is somewhat flattened (**B**), the columella (**C**) has been restored. The prolabium (vermilion border of the lip), separated by the cleft, is made continuous by surgery. (Courtesy John Goin, M.D., Los Angeles.)

tures leaves them too far apart to meet. The maxillary arch has widened, and if the primary palate is cleft, normal lip resistance to maxillary expansion will be reduced, thereby increasing the likelihood of excessive widening (Fraser, 1967).

Patterns of palatal growth can take so many forms that a coding scheme has been devised to identify over fifty possible combinations of clefts (McCabe, 1966). Let us review only the major forms already identified: *unilateral*, *bilateral*, *complete*, and *incomplete*. If unilateral, the palate has fused to the vertical nasal partition (septum and vomer) on one side but not on the other; if bilateral, it has failed to fuse to the nasal partition on both sides (Fig. 8-8). If complete, the cleft extends from the lip through the alveolar process, hard palate, and soft palate. If incomplete, the cleft may be limited to just the lip, the alveolar process, the hard palate, or the soft palate, or it may be limited to a combination of these structures.

The feature of these clefts that may be difficult to grasp involves the primary palate. We have talked of palatal structures growing together in the midline. As can be seen from Fig. 8-8, this is not quite true of clefts of the lip or of the alveolar process. The facial tissue unites just off the midline, with a column of tissue descending from the nose and containing, as shown in Fig. 8-9, the *philtrum* (the indented median portion of the lip), below which is the *prolabium* (the red portion of lip), the *columella nasi* (the fleshy anterior portion of the nasal septum), and the *premaxilla* (a wedge-shaped bone in the maxillary arch from which the upper incisors grow). Thus clefts of the lip or alveolar process occur on one side or the other, or on both sides, of this nasal column. One of the urgent reasons for early surgical repair of the lip is to prevent this isolated column of bone and lip from protruding out from the face.

Patterns of growth and clefts. For an appreciation of how patterns of growth can complicate disabilities stemming from congenital clefts of the lip or palate, a brief résumé of normal growth of the skull and face is needed. Most of what is known about

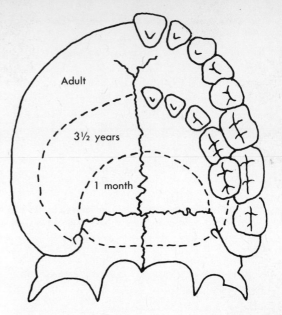

Fig. 8-10. Growth of palate and dental arch. The effects of growth shift the maxillary complex downward and forward. (From Zemlin, W. R., *Speech and Hearing Science: Anatomy and Physiology.* Englewood Cliffs, N.J.: Prentice-Hall, Inc. [1968].)

human skull growth comes from x-ray studies, a type of study fraught with complex problems of measurement. To gather useful data about growth, an investigator must be able to compare one x-ray film with another, so more than two dozen reference points and reference lines are used to provide a basis for comparison (Lundstrom, 1960; Zemlin, 1968). It is complicated by different forces and patterns of development. Cranial growth is related to the brain, which is 90% complete by age 10. The facial skeleton grows in relation to teeth and muscles such as the tongue, lips, and soft palate, and the growth continues until adulthood.

During the first year the cranium grows rapidly, but after that, growth of the facial skeleton is faster. As you can see in Fig. 8-10, the hard palate grows longer and wider, an increase that shifts the palate forward and downward. The maxillary process, and also the mandible, have spurts of growth related to dental eruption: around 5 years of age with first molars, around 11 years with

primary palate - upper lip + gum ridge
secondary palate - hard + soft palate

permanent incisors and cuspids, and at 16 with wisdom teeth. Growth in facial height, too, is linked to dental eruption. It is greatest during the first 6 months, when the incisors are developing, and then again when deciduous teeth are replaced by permanent dentition. The effect of this downward and forward growth of the face not only moves the palate farther down from the skull but also increases the height and depth of the nasopharynx.

It is now important to consider the effect of these different developmental patterns on velopharyngeal closure. Adenoid growth during childhood tends to offset the increased size of the nasopharynx. The net result is that increased nasopharyngeal size tends to be gradual from infancy to adulthood. Moreover, the soft palate grows longer fastest during the first 2 years, the same period in which the nasopharynx undergoes rapid growth. Subtelny (1957) determined that nasopharyngeal depth is normally about two-thirds the length of the soft palate. He also found that velar tissue can be reduced as much as 60% to 70% below this normal proportion and still achieve velopharyngeal closure, but likelihood of adequate closure decreases with higher percentages. Although some have speculated that persons with clefts have abnormal pharyngeal depth that complicates velopharyngeal closure, available evidence does not support this idea (Engman, Spriestersbach, and Moll, 1965; Ross, 1965). On the other hand, persons without clefts can have large nasopharyngeal dimensions, a short soft palate, or a short hard palate, and the result can be velopharyngeal incompetence (Blackfield and others, 1962).

Against this background of normal growth, let us consider the effects of lip and palatal clefts. Because muscle growth and function interacts with skeletal growth, even during embryonic life, a congenital cleft of any type will leave an indelible imprint on orofacial development, regardless of how soon the cleft is repaired following birth; the later the repair, the more pervasive the effects will be. With lip clefts, not only are maxillary arches free to spread laterally without resistance, but muscular coordinations for such lip actions as sucking are impaired. With palatal or velar clefts, tongue growth can be altered somewhat, but tongue function can be affected considerably. Extensive compensatory movements of the tongue and pharyngeal wall that pervert the muscular synergies needed for speech tend to develop for swallowing (Koepp-Baker, 1971a). Still, if a cleft palate is properly repaired, it can grow in what appears to be a normal manner (Subtelny, 1962). With repair, especially by surgical techniques, the growth situation is altered considerably. To appreciate how growth is affected requires some knowledge of remedial procedures.

Surgical treatment of clefts. Surgeons have long recognized that closure of a palatal cleft is of secondary importance to improvement of speech. One said: "There are three aims of such treatment: to make the patient speak well, eat well, and look well, in that order of importance" (Kilner, 1958). In the case of cleft lip repair, however, surgery is usually undertaken during the first 4 months after birth for the main purpose of restoring muscle alignment. At this stage, encouragement of proper growth and function of the lip is considered more important than cosmetic improvement. Appearance can be improved at a later date with secondary plastic operations (Fig. 8-9).

The margin for surgical error in lip closure increases with age. As the infant grows older, more lip tissue becomes available, and with this tissue the surgeon can achieve a normally loose, full lip. The effects of lip closure appear to depend on the type of cleft as well as on the age at the time of surgery. In fact, the flattened facial contour, no longer common in persons with repaired clefts thanks to improved procedures, is probably a consequence more of lip than of palatal repair. Visualize the maxillary arch as a cathedral arch pushed out from inside by the tongue, pushed in from the outside by lip and cheeks, and supported at the center by the premaxilla and the nasal partition (Fig. 8-11). If only the lip is cleft, even if bilaterally, the arch has sufficient support to be

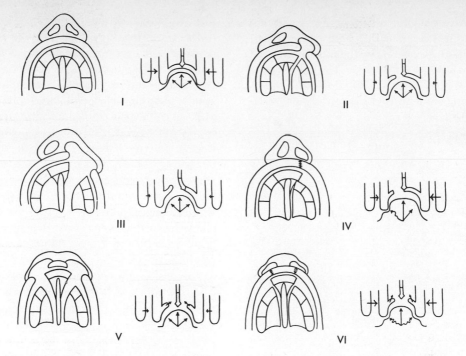

Fig. 8-11. Buttress forces in normal and cleft palates. Normal alignment is shown to be maintained by tongue and lip in I and by tongue in II and III. Medial displacement of alveolar processes from lip pressure after repair is shown in IV and VI. (From Hagerty, R., Embryology, anatomy, and growth of the orofacial complex. *Asha Reports*, **1**, 24-25 [1965].)

unaffected by excessive force of a tight repaired lip. If, however, the cleft extends into the palate, then so much support is lost that the dental arch on the cleft side will collapse inward under labial pressure after lip repair. Apparently a tight upper lip, with its effect of limiting anteroposterior maxillary growth, can be minimized if not avoided by delaying lip surgery a year or more. Although normal facial growth can be achieved with greater certainty by such a delay, the price paid in feeding difficulties and lip dysfunction may outweigh the gain (Hagerty, 1965).

Palatal surgery has made great strides in recent years; now clefts of the hard and soft palates can be repaired at an early age, with successful healing and speech results reported in as high as 90% of patients (Converse, 1965). Unfortunately, this high success rate may not be for permanent speech improvement, judging from a report from the National Institute of Dental Research (1967): growth spurts several years after surgery can lead to velopharyngeal incompetence and nasal speech.

When palatal surgery is undertaken, modern techniques are available to obtain a functional and anatomically restored soft palate along with mobile pharyngeal muscles (often needed to assist velopharyngeal closure). The operations fall into two general classes: *primary operations*, to close the palatal cleft and provide a functional velum, and *secondary operations*, to improve velopharyngeal closure.

Two types of surgical procedures are used widely for the primary operation. The *modified Langenbeck* technique (Fig. 8-12) involves lateral incisions to permit the palatal mucosa to be pulled together and sutured. The other major primary operation is the *Veau-Wardill-Kilner* procedure (Fig. 8-13). Surgeons are of the opinion that it permits greater palatal length than the Langenbeck method. Two supplementary procedures are sometimes used to help achieve closure of the hard palate. The *vomer flap* technique involves freeing a flap of nasal mucosa from the vomer and using it to help close clefts in the anterior hard palate. The other technique is *bone grafting*, in which a segment of bone from a rib or a shin is taken to help fill a cleft in the hard palate (Converse, 1965).

The secondary operations to improve velopharyngeal closure (performed by some surgeons in conjunction with primary operation) are divided into four groups: palatal lengthening, pharyngeal flap, pharyngoplasty, and pharyngeal implantation. The *palatal lengthening, or push-back,* procedure has been largely superseded by the pharyngeal flap technique. The push-back method, developed by Dorrance, provided palatal length but with a deficiency of muscle tissue, and velopharyngeal closure is more dependent on the latter than the former. The *pharyngeal flap* procedure not only attaches the soft palate to the nasopharynx but also adds muscle tissue to the velum. The flap can be raised either from the roof of the nasopharynx or from the posterior pharyngeal wall (Fig. 8-14). *Pharyngoplasty* can be applied to a velar problem by transplanting muscle to the pharyngeal wall to create a dynamic bulge high in the nasopharynx against which the velum can close. This technique can be used when a mobile soft palate, which can elevate during speech, fails to effect adequate velopharyngeal closure because the nasopharynx is too large.

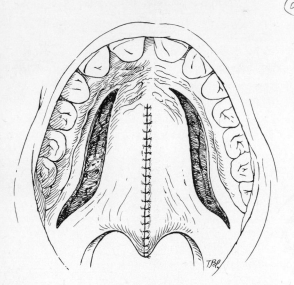

Fig. 8-12. Modified Langenbeck operation. Palatal mucous membrane is shown sutured after completed operation. The palate is not lengthened by this operation.

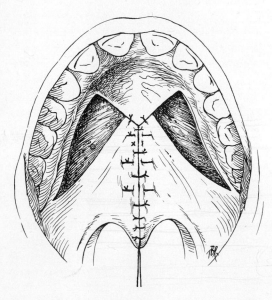

Fig. 8-13. Veau-Wardill-Kilner operation. This procedure, shown completed, provides tissue for a lengthened palate.

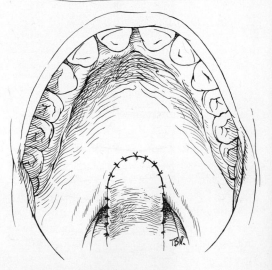

Fig. 8-14. Pharyngeal flap operation. In the completed surgery as shown, an inferiorly based flap for pharyngeal fixation of the soft palate is used. Superiorly based pharyngeal flap operations fixate the soft palate from above.

The same purpose is served by *pharyngeal implantation*, in which the posterior wall is enlarged with implantation of such inert substances as Teflon (Converse, 1965).

Dental treatment of clefts. Although lip clefts can be closed only with surgery, surgical closure of clefts of the palate, both hard and soft, is not always the treatment of choice. Insufficient tissue may be available to achieve closure that would provide a functional velum. Surgery may be postponed for several years to allow growth of sufficient tissue that would increase prospects of success. Meanwhile, the child has a cleft that interferes with vegetative as well as speech functions. For him, the dental specialty of *prosthodontics* can offer help.

A prosthetic speech aid, similar to a dental plate, can be built to meet three goals. First, it must obturate the palatal cleft; thus it is sometimes called an *obturator*, as shown in Fig. 8-15. The portion of the appliance

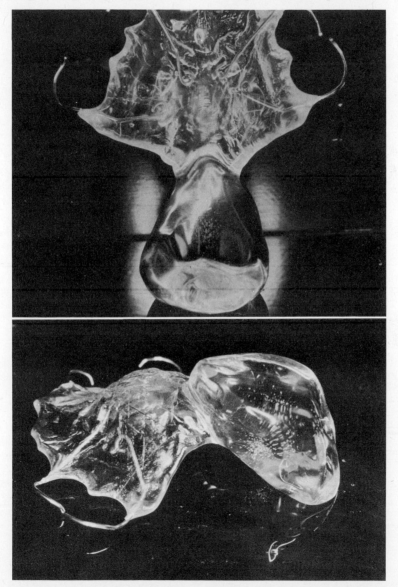

Fig. 8-15. Clear plastic obturator. Two views of a speech aid, showing the pharyngeal bulb and the palatal portion with its dental clasps. (Courtesy Irving Gault, D.D.S., Beverly Hills.)

that covers the cleft corresponds to the dental plate. Second, it must provide a surface against which muscles of the pharyngeal wall can squeeze to open and close the naso-pharyngeal valve. The plastic bulb of the appliance can be fitted for this purpose. Third, it must be anchored firmly and com-fortably to the teeth, and yet be removable for cleaning. At least a few good teeth are helpful for a speech aid, a requirement that sets the arrival time of deciduous teeth as the usual minimal age for fitting children with obturators. Of course, children who wear speech appliances must have them ad-justed to the changing dimensions of the nasopharynx and palate as their growth pro-gresses.

The other imperative dental specialty, regardless of whether the cleft is closed sur-gically or prosthetically, is *orthodontics*. We normally think of orthodontic treatment as being needed to align permanent teeth when they arrive. With cleft palate children, an even more important function is served by beginning treatment with deciduous denti-tion. Collapse of the maxillary arch can be prevented, and alignment of structures to permit proper development of bones and muscles of the skull can be achieved. The orthodontist is a vital ally of the surgeon in achieving normal cosmetic appearance and of the speech pathologist in achieving normal speech (Koepp-Baker, 1971b; Ross and Johnston, 1967).

Acquired disabilities

Paralysis. Functions of the various oro-facial structures can be disabled by paralysis. Because central neurologic disorders are dis-cussed in Chapter 5, we will comment only on peripheral nerve damage. Although the neural supply to the soft palate is not well understood, its paralysis results mainly from damage to cranial nerve X (the vagus), usually from diseases such as bulbar lesions, poliomyelitis, diphtheria, and influenza, from injury, or from surgical accidents.

Paralysis of the tongue is a consequence of injury to cranial nerve XII (the hypo-glossus), frequently as a result of lesions or

of radical neck surgery for advanced stages of cancer. Lingual paralysis can be uni-lateral or bilateral. If paralysis is unilateral, the functional consequences may be rela-tively slight; if it is bilateral, the tongue is immobilized and tends to atrophy.

Paralysis of lip and facial muscles (Bell's palsy) follows injury to cranial nerve VII (the facial). The cosmetic effect of unilateral facial paralysis, with half of the face immo-bilized and masklike, is likely to be more severe than the functional effect. With the less frequent bilateral paralysis, however, the whole face including the lips is immobilized, so that speech functions are disturbed (Luch-singer and Arnold, 1965).

Infection and lesions. We will begin at the top of the respiratory tract and work down-ward. Typical infections and lesions of the nasal cavity include *rhinitis* and *sinusitis* (in which mucosal tissue is inflamed), nasal polyps, and tumors, both benign and malig-nant. The nasopharynx is more apt to be afflicted in children and juveniles than in adults. Adenoids, when enlarged, are a sim-ple form of *hyperplasia* (excessive growth) of lymph tissue. Malignant tumors are often found in the same area; some of them metastasize early and are quite deadly. In the oropharynx, hyperplasia of faucial tonsils is the most common disease.

In the mouth, the soft tissues (lips, tongue, and cheek) can be afflicted by infec-tion and by benign and malignant tumors. Such inflammations as canker sores and fever blisters are of little functional consequence to speech. The more common benign tumors include fibromas and papillomas. Among malignant tumors, carcinoma is the most prevalent and typically is found in elderly men—again, the female proves hardier than the male. Unless tumors reach sizable pro-portion, they are not apt to disturb speech functions much.

As for dental structures, the consequence of importance for us is loss of teeth, espe-cially the upper incisors, which provide a cutting edge for many friction sounds. Den-tal infection may strike by two routes. One, via the pulp of the tooth, is from the inside

[Handwritten margin notes, left side:]
sp > Vagus Nerve (X)
facial nerve (VII)
tongue → hypoglossus (XII)
lip/facial

out and is usually a sequel to dental caries. The other route, involving *periodontal disease* such as *pyorrhea*, is from the outside in. Inflammatory and degenerative processes begin at the gingival margin (where the mucous membrane joins the tooth) and progressively erode away supporting structures until the tooth is lost for lack of anchorage in the jaw (Ash, 1966; Bhaskar, 1973; Gorlin and Boyle, 1966).

Injury. Although accidental injuries can account for damage to the face, lips, nose, and teeth, damage to other orofacial structures, especially the tongue, is more likely to be necessary for surgical reasons. Considering the amount of tongue loss after glossectomy, the extent to which speech can be recovered attests to a remarkable capacity for compensatory adjustment. The same is true of young children who, by sticking "live wires" in their mouths, literally fry their tongues so badly that the tips become necrotic and drop off. Surprisingly, these children are reported to have no resulting speech consequences (Luchsinger and Arnold, 1965; Brodnitz, 1960).

SPEECH EFFECTS OF OROFACIAL AND UPPER RESPIRATORY DISABILITIES

Speech is an exceedingly complex phenomenon in which respiratory, phonatory, and articulatory processes function as inseparably integrated components of the physiologic system for generating sounds. Understanding speech production requires knowledge of degree, direction, ordering, and timing of movements. Any structure in the system can be disabled in any of these ways, and the result can be defective speech. Although knowledge of these relations has grown impressively, it has been gathered largely by studying a few variables at a time. Consider, for instance, the number of factors that could explain reduced nasal air flow: improved velopharyngeal closure, reduced respiratory pressure, weak vocal production, use of glottal stops, nasal obstruction, or constriction of the nares (Spriestersbach, 1965; Subtelny and others, 1968). With the caution in mind that we have limited evidence about

interaction of all relevant parameters for any problem of speech, let us look at various effects of orofacial disabilities.

Moll (1968) has provided a thorough review of research on speech characteristics associated with cleft lip and palate.

Speech effects

Articulation-resonance

Nasality. The effect most typically associated with cleft palate speech is, of course, nasality. The articulatory feature used normally to make essential phonemic distinctions is obscured by the inability to produce nonnasal sounds. Nasality must be viewed, therefore, as more than an undesired resonance characteristic. It is an impairment of ability to make necessary articulatory distinctions. The cause-and-effect relationship between cleft and nasality seems so obvious as to be simple. Alas, it is not. Nasality exists only as a judgment made by a listener of what he hears. If the conditions under which such judgments are made are controlled carefully, and if the judges are trained to agree on

Bradford, Brooks, and Shelton (1964) and Spriestersbach (1955) studied judgments of nasality in cleft palate children. Why did they obtain different results?

what they will call "nasality," then highly reliable judgments can be achieved. Under clinical conditions and without special training, however, agreement is poor. In other words, if judges are left on their own to decide under clinical conditions whether or not speech is nasal, their opinions will vary widely, even though the judges may be experienced speech clinicians (Philips and Bzoch, 1969). For those who have listened to nasality with a critical ear, this observation will not be a revelation—nasality comes in so many confusing forms: "hooty" nasality, "twangy" nasality, and "cold-in-the-nose" denasality.

You may already foresee where this uncertainty will lead us. If nasality exists only as a subjective judgment, then the only way it could be objectified is by measuring the physiologic correlates by which it is produced or the acoustical correlates of the sound that is judged as nasal. But if we cannot agree on judgments of nasality, we would not improve that agreement by measuring objective physiologic or acoustical correlates of it. These objective correlates are reliable and meaningful only with judgments that are reliable and valid (Moll, 1964). In practical terms, such judgments are essential to therapeutic

---

Curtis (1968) has written an excellent discussion of the acoustics of nasality. Does Schwartz (1968) think that nasality can be measured in objective acoustical terms? Would Shelton and others (1967) agree with him?

---

modification of nasality (Chisum and others, 1969).

Results of acoustical and physiologic research on nasality vary considerably. How much of the sound of nasality is produced in the nose or in the mouth is problematic. More importantly for treatment, how much of hypernasality to attribute to a high back-tongue position and how much to velopharyngeal incompetence remains in some doubt. Although we do not know exactly how much velopharyngeal closure is necessary to prevent hearing nasality—it will undoubtedly prove to be less than a 4 mm gap (Björk, 1961; Subtelny, Koepp-Baker, and

---

Does Spriestersbach (1965) agree with McDonald and Koepp-Baker (1951) about the importance of lingual position to nasality?

Subtelny, 1961)—we do know that closure must be more complete with high vowels than with low ones (House and Stevens, 1956). Moreover, we have no doubt that the primary cause of nasality in cleft palate is inadequate velopharyngeal function (Hagerty and Hoffmeister, 1954).

Consonantal distortion. Clearly, the primary speech problem of nasal air escape in cleft palate conditions is distortion of consonants. Often, substitution of nasal for non-nasal consonants lingers as habit after the palate has been repaired (for example, /s/ may continue to be produced through the

nose despite an adequate palate). Thus, cause-and-effect relations are confused further among palatal clefts, velopharyngeal closure, misarticulations, and nasality (Bzoch, 1964b, 1965). Nonetheless, Spriestersbach's (1965) summary of articulation problems is appropriate:

1. Persons with clefts, especially children, are generally retarded in development of articulatory skills.

2. Certain types of sounds are more defective than others. Surprisingly, vowels are seldom in error, even though they are nasalized. Defectiveness of consonants depends on the manner in which they are produced. Nasal sounds are (as we might expect) least affected, affricates and fricatives suffer most, and in between are plosives and glides. Too, voiced consonants are less affected than their voiceless cognates, and single consonants are less affected than consonantal blends. In general, those speakers with marginal velopharyngeal competence are more likely to be able to compensate when the speaking task is simple than when it is complex.

3. Certain types of misarticulations are more likely to occur than others. Glottal stops (in which air is blocked by the vocal cords and then released explosively) are favorite substitutes for plosives. Pharyngeal fricatives are often substituted for oral fricatives. Both fricatives and plosives are produced with nasal air leakage. Although these substitutions are the ones most likely to occur, the most frequent type of misarticulation is omission of a sound altogether, or less obviously and more probably, slighting of the sound as a result of reduced oral pressure.

4. Despite the prevalence of characteristic articulatory errors, persons with clefts are variable in their articulatory errors, suggesting that they are dissatisfied with their performance. Proficiency varies, too, with the type of cleft and with the ability to build up air pressure in the mouth.

Effects of velopharyngeal incompetence. Having looked at characteristic speech effects of cleft palate, the question remains, "How does a cleft condition produce these effects?" The obvious part of the answer, "Because air escapes through the gap," applies equally to conditions of short or immobile soft palates. The critical diameter of opening necessary for acceptable speech is about 5 mm (Isshiki, Honjow, and Morimoto, 1968). Only with such small degrees of velopharyngeal incompetence is the size of the aperture revealed by nasal emission of air, however. If the palate fails to meet the back wall of the throat by more than this amount, nasal air escape will reflect other factors (such as amount of air pressure) as much as, if not more than, the size of velopharyngeal opening (Warren, 1967).

Moreover, the importance of velopharyngeal incompetence is not just that it permits nasal air leakage; it also reduces intraoral pressure. The very sounds that require the most intraoral pressure (plosive, fricative, and voiceless consonants) are the ones most likely to be misarticulated or, for lack of pressure, slighted or omitted altogether. Ability to achieve intraoral pressure is undoubtedly crucial to normal articulation (Hardy, 1965). In the final analysis, velopharyngeal incompetence is the key to defective articulation, as well as to the loss of intraoral pressure

---

Compare the work and arguments of Spriestersbach (1965) or Hardy and Arkebauer (1966) with that of Shelton, Brooks, and Youngstrom (1964, 1965). Do they agree on the predictive significance of intraoral pressure measures?

(Van Demark, 1966). To test this competence for speech, the easiest and most useful clinical index is a measure of articulatory accuracy (Shelton, Brooks, and Youngstrom, 1964, 1965). It is a better indication of velopharyngeal adequacy for speech than swallowing or blowing (which usually involve more forceful closure that may be aided by the back of the tongue) and possibly even than direct measures of nasal and oral air flow and pressure, although a sophisticated technique has been devised for displaying pressure-flow graphically in relation to velopharyngeal closure during speech (Netsell, 1969).

Effects of compensatory adjustments for velopharyngeal incompetence. When velo-pharyngeal closure is inadequate, a variety of compensatory adjustments to achieve closure may be attempted. Some persons develop movement of the posterior pharyngeal wall and some develop lateral pharyngeal wall movement; some increase breath pressure and some decrease it; some prolong duration of velopharyngeal closure and some shorten it; some speak slower and more carefully; some use the tongue to close the palate and some push it against the pharyngeal wall. Some constrict the nares to build oral pressure, some use pharyngeal fricatives, and some use glottal stops (Spriestersbach, 1965; Warren and Mackler, 1968; Hagerty and Hill, 1960). In certain situations, some of these compensatory adjustments improve speech intelligibility; in others they do not, but they become so automatic as to be permanent if they persist to adulthood (Shelton, 1969). More important, some forms of therapy lead to helpful adjustments, but compensations produced by other forms of treatment are detrimental.

For example, efforts to achieve closure by increasing the pharyngeal wall movement are beneficial, but Shelton and his associates (1969) were unable to achieve such movement with speech therapy. Some exercises, especially swallowing and to a lesser extent sucking, improve closure; others, such as the time-honored technique of blowing, are less than useless (Massengill and others, 1968). Blowing (and also sucking) exercises often position the tongue against palate and pharyngeal wall, a posture conducive to defective articulation and inadequate velopharyngeal closure. Similarly, when a person with inadequate closure imitates a clinician's voice, the result can easily involve undesirable compensatory tongue adjustments. This type of undesirable lingual retraction is more apt to occur with back than front vowels (Brooks, Shelton, and Youngstrom, 1965, 1966). On the other hand, the firmness of velopharyngeal closure and the height of the soft palate tend not to be as great for sounds with a low tongue position as for those with a high position (Hardy and Arkebauer, 1966; Bzoch, 1968).

Effects of cleft repair. We will be concerned here mainly with the effects of palatal cleft repairs. Palatal condition and velopharyngeal competence, far more than lip condition, are responsible for articulatory and resonatory problems. In addition to the importance of palatal closure is the major consideration for articulation of palatal arch alignment and dental occlusion. The palate can be repaired surgically or managed prosthetically. We will start with effects of surgical repair.

In general, postsurgical conditions fall into three categories (Koepp-Baker, 1971a,b). First is the condition in which the lip and alveolar process have been closed but the cleft in the hard or soft palate is still open. This situation, most often seen in children, leaves an individual with almost no ability to achieve intraoral breath pressure and normal articulation. Second is the condition in which the palate and velum have been wholly or partially closed, but dimensions (and resonating characteristics) of the palatal vault have been changed substantially and the soft palate is short and tense. In this situation the palate has been repaired without benefit of velopharyngeal closure. The speech effects may be as disastrous as in the first condition. Fortunately, improved surgical procedures are reducing the frequency of this type of result. Third is the condition to be desired. The hard and soft palates are closed, the palatal vault is nearly normal, and the velum permits adequate velopharyngeal competence for normal speech. Although the probability of better speech with early surgery seems likely (Hagerty, Hess, and Mylin, 1968), age at the time of surgery does not seem to be a major determinant of speech effects (Drexler, 1968).

The alternative to surgical repair is a prosthetic speech appliance. Success of an obturator depends in part on length of the soft palate, but not in the way that common sense would dictate. One would think that the longer the palate, the better the speech results. This is not the case. Long, immobile palates usually involve placement of the obturating bulb relatively low in the pharynx, thereby lessening closure of the lateral pharyngeal wall against it. Very short palates, on the other hand, permit high placement of the obturating bulb, which capitalizes on lateral and posterior wall movement (Fig. 8-16). Moreover, the bulb must be high enough to avoid interference with tongue movement and small enough to permit nasal drainage, nasal respiration, and articulation of nasal sounds (Subtelny, Sakuda, and Subtelny, 1966; Falter and Shelton, 1964). An obturator that is too large can convert "cleft palate speech" to "cold-in-the-head" speech. Further, Shelton and his associates (1968) postulate that a bulb large enough to assure closure is more critical for articulatory acquisition than for maintenance of adequate articulation once established.

Surgical and prosthetic repair can be equally effective. On the one hand, such secondary surgical operations as pharyngoplasty, pharyngeal implantation of Teflon, and pharyngeal flap have been demonstrated to produce what appears to be permanent improvement in speech (Bzoch, 1964a; Bluestone and others, 1968; Hess, Hagerty, and Mylin, 1968). On the other hand, equally good improvement has been achieved with speech appliances. In fact, Bzoch (1964a) and Byrne, Shelton, and Diedrich (1961) concluded that speech successes and failures obtained with obturators can be so similar to those obtained with surgery that a decision about physical management must rest on factors other than the treatment that can yield the best speech. Furthermore, some have recommended programs of treatment that capitalize on the merits of both approaches (Blakeley, 1964). For cerebral-palsied children with palatal paresis, however, Hardy and his colleagues (1969) have shown that prosthetic management is the procedure of choice.

Neither surgical nor prosthetic repair offers a panacea for articulation problems. Tongue adjustments that are learned to compensate for palatopharyngeal insufficiency, for example, do not necessarily disappear when the insufficiency is remedied. Some of these tongue adjustments interfere with normal articulation. Persistence of undesirable compensatory adjustments helps to preserve defective articulation, even after adequate velopharyngeal closure can be achieved (Brooks, Shelton, and Youngstrom, 1965, 1966). In fact, when children with successfully repaired clefts are compared with children who have had no problem with velopharyngeal closure, and yet have defective articulation, the speech of these two groups of children cannot be distinguished.

In other words, adequate velopharyngeal closure does not prevent a child from having an articulation problem, but it does help to prevent him from sounding as though he has a cleft palate problem (Van Demark and Van Demark, 1967).

Effects of lingual disabilities. Although a normal tongue can function abnormally in attempts to compensate for palatopharyngeal insufficiency and thereby contribute to misarticulations, the tongue can also contribute

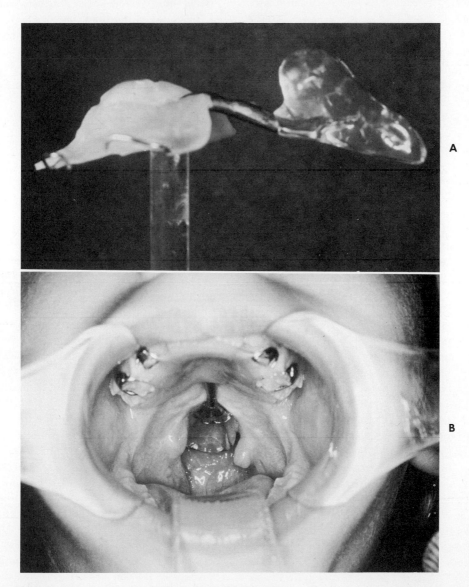

Fig. 8-16. Prosthetic speech aid. The obturator (**A**) is shown fitted into the nasopharynx and attached to the teeth (**B**). (Courtesy Irving Gault, D.D.S., Beverly Hills.)

by virtue of its own defectiveness. The most popular defect in the layman's eyes is tongue-tie, technically called *ankyloglossia*. For years, various speech and medical specialists have attempted to stem the tide of "clipping" tied tongues as a routine surgical solution for speech disorders.

They have perhaps been too successful in creating the prevailing clinical attitude of routinely ignoring relations among tongue mobility, lingual frenum size, and speech proficiency (Crawford, Adamson, and Ashbell, 1969). Certainly tongue-tie is not in the same class with cleft palate as a factor in defective articulation. Still, current evidence points to lingual mobility as a fruitful clinical consideration (Fletcher and Meldrum, 1968).

Occasionally the tongue is too large (*macroglossia*), too small (*microglossia*), too long, or partially or entirely missing (*aglossia*). Considering how vital it is for normal articulation, one can hardly envision anything approximating normal speech with a grossly abnormal tongue, but it is possible. Some persons, after a complete glossectomy to remove cancer of the tongue, have achieved reasonably intelligible speech by developing compensatory movements. Lips and teeth can substitute for tongue tip sounds, the floor of the mouth and the stump of the tongue can be raised toward the palate for midtongue sounds, and the palatal arches can be approximated for back tongue sounds (Bloomer, 1971). In one of the rare instances of *congenital lingual hypoplasia* (incomplete development of the tongue), the child acquired intelligible speech with only a few sibilant distortions without benefit of therapy (Weinberg and others, 1969).

The lingual problem most frequently of mutual concern to dentists and speech pathologists is often called "tongue thrust." It is also called by less appropriate terms such as *reverse swallowing* (strictly speaking, this would describe regurgitation), *visceral swallowing* (as if normal swallowing is not visceral), and *deviant swallowing* (a term shadowed by doubt as to how abnormal "deviant" swallowing really is). Generally, dental

effects of tongue thrust are of greater consequence than are speech effects. Teeth are shoved out of alignment and orthodontic improvement is disturbed more seriously and possibly more consistently than articulation is affected, although sibilant sound production is definitely not aided by this type of swallow pattern. Because it is evident in 50% of normal 8-year-olds, most of whom will outgrow it by age 12 years, Mason and Profitt (1974) doubt the necessity of special swallowing therapy prior to puberty.

These considerations have led some speech pathologists to question whether they should assume responsibility for this problem in the absence of a demonstrable speech defect. Others have heeded the call for help of distressed orthodontists and have attempted

---

Compare the discussions of Palmer (1962), Fletcher, Casteel, and Bradley (1961), and Subtelny, Mestre, and Subtelny (1964). Do they all think that tongue thrust is abnormal? That speech is affected? That most children outgrow it? That defective dental sounds will be corrected when the tongue thrust is corrected? That speech pathologists should be responsible for this problem?

---

to correct problems of tongue thrusting, irrespective of speech involvement. This group has been inclined to approach the problem in the manner of oral physical therapy. Their objective is to change the swallowing pattern and the balance of orofacial muscle pressures with what they call *myofunctional therapy* (Barrett and Hanson, 1974). When an articulatory problem exists, it, too, is included in their concern. Stansell's (1970) study has demonstrated, however, that a sigmatism training technique designed to keep the tongue away from the incisors is more effective in reducing dental overjet than is deglutition training.

Generally, tongue thrust swallow is described as a forward thrust of the tongue against the front teeth coupled with tight lip closure in a kind of sucking movement. By contrast, normal swallow involves a sweeping motion of the tongue against the palate, an action that does not require tight pursing of the lips. Because adults swallow up to 800 times a day and children up to 1,500, and because tongue thrusters push on their teeth longer and with at least twice normal pressure, the explanation for accompanying dental malformations seems obvious (Graber, 1966). What is less obvious is why this type of swallow also predisposes one to defective articulation. Apparently, from Stansell's evidence, tongue thrusters with defective sibilants apply more pressure on their incisors when speaking than when swallowing, possibly because the tongue pushes against the incisors more frequently during sibilant production than during swallowing.

Effects of dental and facial disabilities. Let us dispense with speech effects of facial disabilities first: they are likely to be slight. Cosmetic effects may be severe, but speech movements of the lips need not be precise, thus permitting normal sound production even with a tight, immobile lip (Bloomer, 1971).

The effect of dental abnormalities is small, too, by comparison with cleft palate. This is not to say that articulatory effects are non-existent (Snow, 1961). The extent to which they do occur depends largely on the compensatory adjustment used. With /s/, for instance, if the tongue tip is protruded or if the lips are used to compensate for missing upper incisors, the sound will probably be defective. If, however, the tip is kept below the lower incisors and the blade is arched toward the alveolar ride, /s/ is likely to sound normal.

Language. Children with cleft palates have been found retarded in development of both language comprehension and usage (Philips and Harrison, 1969). Although retarded in the size of their vocabulary and in the amount they speak, such children nonetheless appear to have acquired adequate syntactic abilities (Morris, 1962; Smith and McWilliams, 1968; Spriestersbach, Darley, and Morris, 1958). Philips and Harrison (1969) hypothesize that parental reaction to early defective speech impedes linguistic development.

Phonation. Some clinicians have suspected that cleft palate speakers are prone to voice problems other than hypernasality. What research evidence is available supports this suspicion, especially that they are prone to vocal quality defects that involve breathiness (Brooks and Shelton, 1963; Shelton, Hahn, and Morris, 1968). The presence of such defects is not surprising in view of the difficulty that a cleft condition, even when repaired, imposes on management of oral and nasal breath pressure. As Warren, Wood, and Bradley (1969) have shown, excessive respiratory effort and airflow accompany velopharyngeal insufficiency.

Hearing effects

Speech may be impaired by a conductive hearing loss, which sometimes occurs as an indirect effect of cleft palate. Such a hearing loss is not inevitable with a cleft condition, but it does occur with considerably greater frequency than in the normal population (Spriestersbach, 1965). Because it develops out of problems of drainage and infection of the middle ear that stem from involvement of the eustachian tube, and because such involvement can be present from birth with a congenital cleft, the hearing loss can occur during the speech acquisition years. If the loss is sufficiently severe or prolonged, speech and language development can be affected. The fact that these losses can often be reversed by appropriate medical treatment points up the importance of early observation of hearing in cleft palate children (Hayes, 1965).

What audiologic and otologic considerations do Prather and Kos (1968) associate with cleft palate?

Psychosocial effects

The other indirect speech effect of orofacial disabilities that we will consider is the most nebulous and yet the most personal: the psychosocial problems of these people. As Goodstein (1968) concludes after reviewing the empirical evidence, having an infant with a cleft palate arouses parental anxiety. Parents generally lack prior knowledge about the problem, and they are beset with imagined and real concerns for their child. This parental distress is understandable. Such parents are generally not poorly adjusted, but they are much in need of early counseling lest they overprotect or reject the child by their emotional reactions. That these consequences are typical is probably seen in the moderate intellectual and linguistic retardation of children with cleft palate.

Clinicians are often of the opinion that persons who have suffered the unfortunate accident of being born with cleft lip or palate must also suffer severe social and psychologic consequences. This opinion seems so obviously and logically justified that failure of the research evidence to support it is startling (Phipps, 1965; Clifford, 1967). Of course, the reason that severe psychosocial problems have not shown up more frequently may be that the tests in use are too insensitive or are not measuring important variables. That the clinical opinion would seem to have some justification is seen in the depressed language output of cleft palate persons. They may not talk much for reasons that have nothing to do with their orofacial difficulty, but such a conclusion seems farfetched. Here is another case in which the practicing clinician would do well to keep his power of observation alert and his prejudices in check lest he leap to ill-advised conclusions.

SPEECH PATHOLOGIST'S RESPONSIBILITY IN TREATMENT OF OROFACIAL AND UPPER RESPIRATORY DISABILITIES

The speech pathologist's responsibility for treating orofacial and upper respiratory impairments is to refer, consult, and develop special procedures for facilitating acquisition of intelligible speech. Cleft palate, the structural anomaly that impairs speech most, poses unique problems of velopharyngeal valving, nasal resonance, and management of intraoral pressure. Techniques for modifying articulation and voice in the speaker with normal orofacial structures must often be adapted to the need posed by velopharyngeal incompetence.

Unlike laryngeal pathologies, with their

Wells (1971) and Bzoch (1972) provide remedial procedures that are adapted to the needs of the child with cleft palate. Their texts present a comprehensive view of this problem from the standpoint of the speech pathologist.

early sign of hoarseness, vocal tract disabilities, other than palatal clefts and velopharyngeal insufficiencies, must become fairly gross before speech is affected. Thus the speech pathologist may be the last rather than the first to know about them. Nonetheless, he remains responsible for being alert to a patient's medical and dental needs that may require referral.

Cleft palate team

With no other structural abnormality is the speech pathologist's consultative advice valued more than with cleft palate. He is an indispensable member of the cleft palate team. With this group, his judgments can weigh as heavily as those of his dental and surgical colleagues. These teams can be found throughout the country. They have grown through recognition by various professional specialists that more effective treatment can be provided for children with cleft palate when all work in close cooperation than when all work alone. Frequently, teams will include psychologists, pediatricians, social workers, and other specialists, but the basic plans for treatment usually rest with a core team of surgeon, orthodontist, prosthodontist, and speech pathologist.

Probably the speech pathologist's judgment about cleft palate is esteemed because he has worked vigorously and successfully to build a reasonably solid body of knowledge about orofacial correlates of speech. He knows the speech effects of cleft palate better than anyone else. Certainly, his knowledge is neither complete nor perfect. Still, unlike some other areas of speech pathology, in which fact has not yet slain fantasy, many of the functional conditions of orofacial structures for adequate speech are more a matter of observational knowledge than of armchair speculation. Because all members of the cleft palate team share a common concern for achieving good speech, they turn to the speech pathologist for guidance in this matter. He has, then, a heavy responsibility to advise when further physical treatment is needed. This advice will rest on his judgment of how much he can accomplish if no palatal modification is made, if a limited modification can be achieved, or if a "normal" palate can be developed.

The answers—résumé

1. What are the nature and etiology of orofacial and upper respiratory disabilities?

Disabled functioning of the orofacial and upper respiratory structures that produce speech effects results from abnormalities that include velopharyngeal insufficiency; adenoids that are too small or too large for the nasopharynx; tonsils that block the oropharynx; a tongue that is too large, too small, or too immobile; clefts of the soft palate, hard palate, alveolar ridge, or lip; nasal obstructions; teeth that are misaligned or malformed; and tongue-thrust swallow. These abnormalities can be congenital consequences of genetic factors, especially when the primary palate fails to fuse, resulting in clefts of the lip and alveolar process. Hard and soft palate clefts are more likely consequences of defective embryologic patterns of growth. Many of the other abnormalities can also be congenital, but many can be acquired as a result of surgery, injury, paralysis, or disease.

2. What are the speech effects of orofacial and upper respiratory disabilities?

Disabled functioning of orofacial and upper respiratory structures affects articulation as the major consequence. Articulation can be impaired by velopharyngeal incompetence, undesirable compensatory adjustments of the tongue, unsuccessful cleft palate repair, and lingual, dental, and facial disabilities. In addition, hearing impairments can interfere somewhat with speech and language development. Whether a lip or palatal cleft is as psychologically or socially punishing as has been presumed is a matter for conjecture. Those children with clefts who are retarded in their development of expressive or receptive language skills and in the amount of speaking they do may be reflecting negative reactions to their problem, particularly on the part of their concerned parents.

3. What is the speech pathologist's responsibility in the treatment of orofacial and upper respiratory disabilities?

Although the speech pathologist assumes no direct responsibility for physical management of orofacial abnormalities, he does hold heavy responsibility for advising about probable speech effects of various types of surgical or prosthetic treatment. Because improved speech is the primary goal of cleft palate repair, the speech pathologist is a key member of the cleft palate team.

REFERENCES

Ash, J., Organs of special senses. In Anderson, W. (Ed.), *Pathology*, (5th ed., Vol. 2) St. Louis: The C. V. Mosby Co. (1966).

Barrett, R., and Hanson, M., *Oral Myofunctional Disorders*. St. Louis: The C. V. Mosby Co. (1974).

Bhaskar, S., *Synopsis of Oral Pathology*. (4th ed.) St. Louis: The C. V. Mosby Co. (1973).

Björk, L., Velopharyngeal function in connected speech. *Acta Radiolog.* Suppl. 202, (1961).

Blackfield, H., and others, Cinefluorographic evaluation of patients with velopharyngeal dysfunction in the absence of overt cleft palate. *Plast. reconstr. Surg.*, **30**, 441-451 (1962).

Blakeley, R., The complementary use of speech prostheses and pharyngeal flaps in palatal insufficiency. *Cleft Palate J.*, **1**, 194-198 (1964).

Bloomer, H., Speech defects associated with dental malocclusions and related abnormalities. In Travis, L. (Ed.), *Handbook of Speech Pathology and Audiology*. New York: Appleton-Century-Crofts (1971).

Bluestone, C., and others, Teflon injection pharyngoplasty. *Cleft Palate J.*, **5**, 19-22 (1968).

Bradford, L., Brooks, A., and Shelton, R., Clinical judgment of hypernasality in cleft palate children. *Cleft Palate J.*, **1**, 329-335 (1964).

Brodnitz, F., Speech after glossectomy. *Current Problems: Phoniatrics and Logopedics*, **1**, 68-71 (1960).

Brooks, A., and Shelton, R., Incidence of voice disorders other than nasality in cleft palate children. *Cleft Palate Bull.*, **13**, 63-64 (1963).

Brooks, A., Shelton, R., and Youngstrom, K., Compensatory tongue-palate-posterior pharyngeal wall relationships in cleft palate. *J. Speech Hearing Dis.*, **30**, 166-173 (1965).

Brooks, A., Shelton, R., and Youngstrom, K., Tongue-palate contact in persons with palate defects. *J. Speech Hearing Dis.*, **31**, 14-25 (1966).

Byrne, M., Shelton, R., and Diedrich, W., Articulatory skill, physical management, and classification of children with cleft palates. *J. Speech Hearing Dis.*, **26**, 326-333 (1961).

Bzoch, K., Clinical studies of the efficacy of speech appliances compared to pharyngeal flap surgery. *Cleft Palate J.*, **1**, 275-286 (1964a).

Bzoch, K., The effects of a specific pharyngeal flap operation upon the speech of forty cleft-palate persons. *J. Speech Hearing Dis.*, **29**, 111-120 (1964b).

Bzoch, K., Articulation proficiency and error patterns of preschool cleft palate and normal children. *Cleft Palate J.*, **2**, 340-349 (1965).

Bzoch, K., Variations in velopharyngeal valving: the factor of vowel changes. *Cleft Palate J.*, **5**, 211-218 (1968).

Bzoch, K., *Communicative Disorders Related to Cleft Lip and Palate*. Boston: Little, Brown & Co. (1972).

Chisum, L., and others, The relationship between remedial speech instruction activities and articulation change. *Cleft Palate J.*, **6**, 57-64 (1969).

Clifford, E., Connotative meaning of concepts related to cleft lip and palate. *Cleft Palate J.*, **4**, 165-173 (1967).

Converse, J., The techniques of cleft palate surgery. Proceedings of the Conference: Communicative Problems in Cleft Palate, *Asha Reports*, **1**, 55-82 (1965).

Crawford, H., Adamson, J., and Ashbell, T., Tongue-tie. *Cleft Palate J.*, **6**, 8-23 (1969).

Curtis, J., Acoustics of speech production and nasalization. In Spriestersbach, D., and Sherman, D. (Eds.), *Cleft Palate and Communication*. New York: Academic Press, Inc. (1968).

Drexler, A., Age of surgery for cleft palate patients and speech proficiency. *Cleft Palate J.*, **5**, 327-333 (1968).

Engman, L., Spriestersbach, D., and Moll, K., Cranial base angle and nasopharyngeal depth. *Cleft Palate J.*, **2**, 32-39 (1965).

Falter, L., and Shelton, R., Bulb fitting and placement in prosthetic treatment of cleft palate. *Cleft Palate J.*, **1**, 441-447 (1964).

Fletcher, S., Casteel, R., and Bradley, D., Tongue-thrust swallow, speech articulation and age. *J. Speech Hearing Dis.*, **26**, 201-208 (1961).

Fletcher, S., and Meldrum, J., Lingual function and relative length of the lingual frenulum. *J. Speech Hearing Res.*, **11**, 382-390 (1968).

Fraser, F., Cleft lip and cleft palate. *Science*, **158**, 1603-1606 (1967).

Goodstein, L., Psychosocial aspects of cleft palate. In Spriestersbach, D., and Sherman, D. (Eds.), *Cleft Palate and Communication*. New York: Academic Press, Inc. (1968).

Gorlin, R., and Boyle, P., Lips, mouth, teeth, salivary glands, and neck. In Anderson, W. (Ed.), *Pathology*. (6th ed., Vol. 2) St. Louis: The C. V. Mosby Co. (1971).

Graber, T., *Orthodontics: Principles and Practices*. Philadelphia: W. B. Saunders Co. (1972).

Greene, J., Vermillion, J., and Hay, S., Utilization of birth certificates in epidemiologic studies of cleft lip and palate. *Cleft Palate J.*, **2**, 141-156 (1965).

Hagerty, R., Embryology, anatomy, and growth of orofacial complex. Proceedings of the Conference: Communicative Problems in Cleft Palate, *Asha Reports*, **1**, 5-34 (1965).

Hagerty, R., Hess, D., and Mylin, W., Velar motility, velopharyngeal closure, and speech proficiency in cartilage pharyngoplasty: the effect of age at surgery. *Cleft Palate J.*, **5**, 317-326 (1968).

Hagerty, R., and Hill, M., Pharyngeal wall and palatal movement in postoperative cleft palates and normal palates. *J. Speech Hearing Res.*, **3**, 59-66 (1960).

Hagerty, R., and Hoffmeister, F., Velopharyngeal closure: an index of speech. *Plast. reconstr. Surg.*, **13**, 290-298 (1954).

Hardy, J., Air flow and air pressure studies. Proceedings of the Conference: Communicative Problems in Cleft Palate, *Asha Reports*, **1**, 141-152 (1965).

Hardy, J., and Arkebauer, H., Development of a test for velopharyngeal competence during speech. *Cleft Palate J.*, **3**, 6-21 (1966).

Hardy, J., and others, Management of velopharyngeal function in dysarthria. *J. Speech Hearing Dis.*, **34**, 123-136 (1969).

Hay, S., Incidence of clefts and parental age. *Cleft Palate J.*, **4**, 205-213 (1967).

Hayes, C., Audiological problems associated with cleft palate. Proceedings of the Conference: Communicative Problems in Cleft Palate, *Asha Reports*, **1**, 83-90 (1965).

Hess, D., Hagerty, R., and Mylin, W., Velar motility, velopharyngeal closure, and speech proficiency in cartilage pharyngoplasty: an eight-year study. *Cleft Palate J.*, **5**, 153-162 (1968).

House, A., and Stevens, K., Analog studies of the nasalization of vowels. *J. Speech Hearing Dis.*, **21**, 218-232 (1956).

Isshiki, N., Honjow, I., and Morimoto, M., Effects of velopharyngeal incompetence upon speech. *Cleft Palate J.*, **5**, 297-310 (1968).

Jordan, R., Kraus, B., and Neptune, C., Dental abnormalities associated with cleft lip and/or palate. *Cleft Palate J.*, **3**, 22-55 (1966).

Kilner, T., The management of the patient with cleft lip and/or palate. *Am. J. Surg.*, **95**, 204-210 (1958).

Koepp-Baker, H., Orofacial clefts: their forms and effects. In Travis, L. (Ed.), *Handbook of Speech*

Pathology and Audiology. New York: Appleton-Century-Crofts (1971a).

Koepp-Baker, H., The treatment of orofacial clefts: surgical, orthopedic, and prosthetic. In Travis, L. (Ed.), *Handbook of Speech Pathology and Audiology.* New York: Appleton-Century-Crofts (1971b).

Lis, E., Other concomitant conditions: other physical conditions. Proceedings of the Conference: Communicative Problems in Cleft Palate, *Asha Reports*, **1**, 91-102 (1965).

Luchsinger, R., and Arnold, G., *Voice-Speech-Language.* Belmont, Calif.: Wadsworth Publishing Co., Inc. (1965).

Lundstrom, A., *Introduction to Orthodontics.* New York: McGraw-Hill Book Co. (1960).

Mason, R., and Profitt, W., The tongue thrust controversy: background and recommendations. *J. Speech Hearing Dis.*, **39**, 115-132 (1974).

Massengill, R., and others, Therapeutic exercise and velopharyngeal gap. *Cleft Palate J.*, **5**, 44-47 (1968).

McCabe, P., A coding procedure for classification of cleft lip and cleft palate. *Cleft Palate J.*, **3**, 383-391 (1966).

McDonald, E., and Koepp-Baker, H., Cleft palate speech: an integration of research and clinical observation. *J. Speech Hearing Dis.*, **16**, 9-20 (1951).

Meskin, L., Pruzansky, S., and Gullen, W., An epidemiologic investigation of factors related to the extent of facial clefts. 1. Sex of patient. *Cleft Palate J.*, **5**, 23-29 (1968).

Moll, K., "Objective" measures of nasality. *Cleft Palate J.*, **1**, 371-374 (1964).

Moll, K., Speech characteristics of individuals with cleft lip and palate. In Spriestersbach, D., and Sherman, D. (Eds.), *Cleft Palate and Communication.* New York: Academic Press, Inc. (1968).

Morris, H., Communication skills of children with cleft lips and palates. *J. Speech Hearing Res.*, **5**, 79-90 (1962).

Morris, H., Etiological bases for speech problems. In Spriestersbach, D., and Sherman, D. (Eds.), *Cleft Palate and Communication.* New York: Academic Press, Inc. (1968).

Morris, A., and Greulich, R., Dental research: the past two decades. *Science*, **160**, 1081-1088 (1968).

National Institute of Dental Research, *Research news from NIDR*, October, No. 45 (1967).

Netsell, R., Evaluation of velopharyngeal dysfunction in dysarthria. *J. Speech Hearing Dis.*, **34**, 113-122 (1969).

Palmer, J., Tongue thrusting: a clinical hypothesis. *J. Speech Hearing Dis.*, **27**, 323-333 (1962).

Philips, B., and Bzoch, K., Reliability of judgments of articulation of cleft palate speakers. *Cleft Palate J.*, **6**, 24-34 (1969).

Philips, B., and Harrison, R., Language skills of preschool cleft palate children. *Cleft Palate J.*, **6**, 108-119 (1969).

Phipps, G., Psychosocial aspects of cleft palate. Proceedings of the Conference: Communicative Problems in Cleft Palate, *Asha Reports*, **1**, 103-110 (1965).

Prather, W., and Kos, C., Audiological and otological considerations. In Spriestersbach, D., and Sherman, D. (Eds.), *Cleft Palate and Communication.* New York: Academic Press, Inc. (1968).

Ross, R., Cranial base in children with lip and palate clefts. *Cleft Palate J.*, **2**, 157-166 (1965).

Ross, R., and Johnston, M., The effect of early orthodontic treatment on facial growth in cleft lip and palate. *Cleft Palate J.*, **4**, 157-164 (1967).

Schwartz, M., The acoustics of normal and nasal vowel production. *Cleft Palate J.*, **5**, 125-140 (1968).

Shelton, R., Personal communication (1969).

Shelton, R., Brooks, A., and Youngstrom, K., Articulation and patterns of palatopharyngeal closure. *J. Speech Hearing Dis.*, **29**, 390-408 (1964).

Shelton, R., Brooks, A., and Youngstrom, K., Clinical assessment of palatopharyngeal closure. *J. Speech Hearing Dis.*, **30**, 37-43 (1965).

Shelton, R., Hahn, E., and Morris, H., Diagnosis and therapy. In Spriestersbach, D., and Sherman, D. (Eds.), *Cleft Palate and Communication.* New York: Academic Press, Inc. (1968).

Shelton, R., and others, The relationship between nasality score values and oral and nasal sound pressure level. *J. Speech Hearing Res.*, **10**, 549-557 (1967).

Shelton, R., and others, Effect of prosthetic speech bulb reduction on articulation. *Cleft Palate J.*, **5**, 195-204 (1968).

Shelton, R., and others, Effect of articulation therapy on palatopharyngeal closure, movement of the pharyngeal wall, and tongue posture. *Cleft Palate J.*, **6**, 440-448 (1969).

Smith, R., and McWilliams, B., Psycholinguistic abilities of children with clefts. *Cleft Palate J.*, **5**, 238-249 (1968).

Snow, K., Articulation proficiency in relation to certain dental abnormalities. *J. Speech Hearing Dis.*, **26**, 209-212 (1961).

Spriestersbach, D., Assessing nasal quality in cleft palate speech of children. *J. Speech Hearing Dis.*, **20**, 266-270 (1955).

Spriestersbach, D., The effects of orofacial anomalies on the speech process. Proceedings of the Conference: Communicative Problems in Cleft Palate, *Asha Reports*, **1**, 111-128 (1965).

Spriestersbach, D., Darley, F., and Morris, H., Language skills in children with cleft palates. *J. Speech Hearing Res.*, **1**, 279-285 (1958).

Stansell, B., Effects of deglutition training and speech training on dental overjet, *J. South. Calif. Dent. Ass.*, **38**, 423-437 (1970).

Subtelny, D., A cephalometric study of the growth of the soft palate. *Plast. reconstr. Surg.*, **19**, 49-62 (1957).

Subtelny, D., A review of cleft palate growth studies reported in the past ten years. *Plast. reconstr. Surg.*, **30**, 56-67 (1962).

Subtelny, D., and Koepp-Baker, H., The significance of adenoid tissue in velopharyngeal function. *Plast. reconstr. Surg.*, **17**, 235-250 (1956).

Subtelny, J., Koepp-Baker, H., and Subtelny, D., Palatal function and cleft palate speech. *J. Speech Hearing Dis.*, **26**, 213-224 (1961).

Subtelny, J., Mestre, J., and Subtelny, D., Comparative study of normal and defective articulation of /s/ as related to malocclusion and deglutition. *J. Speech Hearing Dis.*, **29**, 269-285 (1964).

Subtelny, J., Sakuda, M., and Subtelny, D., Prosthetic treatment for palatopharyngeal incompetence: research and clinical implications. *Cleft Palate J.*, **3**, 130-158 (1966).

Subtelny, D., and others, Synchronous recording of speech with associated physiological and pressure-flow dynamics: instrumentation and procedure. *Cleft Palate J.*, **5**, 93-116 (1968).

Van Demark, D., A factor analysis of the speech of children with cleft palate. *Cleft Palate J.*, **3**, 159-170 (1966).

Van Demark, D., and Van Demark, A., Misarticulations of cleft palate children achieving velopharyngeal closure and children with functional speech problems. *Cleft Palate J.*, **4**, 31-37 (1967).

Warren, D., Nasal emission of air and velopharyngeal function. *Cleft Palate J.*, **4**, 148-156 (1967).

Warren, D., and Mackler, S., Duration of oral port constriction in normal and cleft palate speech. *J. Speech Hearing Res.*, **11**, 391-401 (1968).

Warren, D., Wood, M., and Bradley, D., Respiratory volumes in normal and cleft palate speech. *Cleft Palate J.*, **6**, 449-460 (1969).

Weinberg, B., A cephalometric study of normal and defective /s/ articulation and variations in incisor dentition. *J. Speech Hearing Res.*, **11**, 288-300 (1968).

Weinberg, B., and others, Severe hypoplasia of the tongue. *J. Speech Hearing Dis.*, **34**, 157-168 (1969).

Wells, C., *Cleft Palate and Its Associated Speech Disorders*. New York: McGraw-Hill Book Co. (1971).

Zemlin, W., *Speech and Hearing Science*. Englewood Cliffs, N.J.: Prentice-Hall, Inc. (1968).

Chapter 9

Learning and intellectual disabilities

Questions

1. What is the nature of learning and intellectual disabilities that affect speech?
2. What are the speech effects of learning and intellectual disabilities?
3. What is the speech pathologist's responsibility in the treatment of learning and intellectual disabilities?

NATURE OF DISABILITIES OF LEARNING AND INTELLIGENCE THAT AFFECT SPEECH

Our interest now will be in those conditions that disable a child's learning and intelligence so severely that he is *mentally retarded*. This term, as defined by the American Association on Mental Deficiency (AAMD) (Heber, 1959): "refers to subaverage general intellectual functioning which originates during the developmental period and is associated with impairment in one or more of the following: (1) maturation, (2) learning, and (3) social adjustment." Levels of retardation are shown in Table 9-1.

According to Guilford (1967), intellectual ability is more a function of learning than one might imagine. He has so far identified 120 basic abilities (only a fraction are measured by standard IQ tests) involved in intellectual functioning. These abilities apparently are learned but not, as might be supposed, by

differentiation of a general intellectual ability. The idea of a sentence in language development, for example, appears to start out as a gross one-word utterance. As development proceeds, the sentence idea is differentiated into its elaborate mature form. This is apparently not true with intelligence. The Garrett hypothesis—that the infant begins life with an innate core of intellectual ability that, with development, subdivides into the various mature abilities of the intellect—is a hypothesis opposed by the balance of evidence.

How, then, is intellect acquired, if not by a process of differentiation from a single gross ability to a multitude of specific abilities? The best available answer is that each ability is learned separately. From birth the person learns how to bring together and utilize the various abilities of intellect. How well any particular combination develops will depend on how effectively it has been exercised, which is to say, how well it has been learned.

Table 9-1. Levels of adaptive behavior*

	Preschool age, 0-5; maturation and development	School age, 6-21; training and education	Adult, 21; social and vocational adequacy
Level I (mild)	Can develop social and communication skills; minimal retardation in sensorimotor areas; rarely distinguished from normal until later age	Can learn academic skills to approximately 6th grade by late teens; cannot learn general high school subjects; needs special education, particularly at secondary school age levels ("educable")	Capable of social and vocational adequacy with proper education and training; frequently needs supervision and guidance under serious social or economic stress
Level II (moderate)	Can talk or learn to communicate; poor social awareness; fair motor development; may profit from self-help; can be managed with moderate supervision	Can learn functional academic skills to approximately 4th grade level by late teens if given special education ("educable")	Capable of self-maintenance in unskilled or semiskilled occupations; needs supervision and guidance when under mild social or economic stress
Level III (severe)	Poor motor development; speech is minimal; generally unable to profit from training in self-help; little or no communication skills	Can talk or learn to communicate; can be trained in elemental health habits; cannot learn functional academic skills; profits from systematic habit training ("trainable")	Can contribute partially to self-support under complete supervision; can develop self-protection skills to a minimal useful level in controlled environment
Level IV (profound)	Gross retardation; minimal capacity for functioning in sensorimotor areas; needs nursing care	Some motor development present; cannot profit from training in self-help; needs total care	Some motor and speech development; totally incapable of self-maintenance; needs complete care and supervision

*Modified from Sloan and Birch (1955); from Chinn, P., Drew, E., and Logan, D., *Mental Retardation: a Life Cycle Approach*. St. Louis: The C. V. Mosby Co. (1975).

The prospect of acquiring a specific ability on one hand depends on being exposed in the environment to information in the various forms in which it can be discriminated. On the other hand, it depends on hereditary limits of the individual's sensory and motor equipment for exposing himself to the environment. Probably it depends more on the characteristically human discrimination, recognition, storage, retrieval, and processing operations for which man's brain was apparently designed. Rarely, however, does one reach his hereditary limits; room for improving intellectual abilities is almost always available (Guilford, 1967).

Although developed from quite different origins, the popular views of Piaget (1964) on how intellectual abilities are acquired are not especially at odds with Guilford's. Piaget describes a structure of cognitive abilities, whereas Guilford describes a structure of factors of intellect; both structures are assembled by learning. What makes Piaget's conception especially appealing to clinicians and teachers is the idea of sequential development of these abilities. He conceives of cognition as evolving through stages. The hopeful implication for retarded children is that an intellectual deficit can be seen as failure to master an earlier cognitive function that is a prerequisite for higher-level tasks. Failure is avoided by beginning training with essential low-level skills that lay the foundation for success with higher cognitive levels.

Piaget's prodigious work and that of his legion of followers describes these stages (Beard, 1969; Bruner, Olver, and Greenfield, 1967). Beginning with sensorimotor skills in infancy, development progresses through a period of concrete operations during childhood. Concepts of classes, relations, and numbers are established at this time as a foundation for the level of abstract thinking that is entered at adolescence. Most retarded children do not progress beyond the concrete operations of foundation laying, and the more severely retarded may hardly get started, if they begin at all. During this period, of course, normal children master all aspects of language. We will consider the relationship of cognitive development and language development later in this chapter.

Conditions for mental retardation

From what conditions does mental retardation, with its speech disturbances, stem? Basically, it arises from conditions that affect the chemistry or structural integrity of the nervous system or from those which affect the learning of cognitive abilities. The AAMD *Manual on Terminology and Classification* (Grossman, 1973) includes ten etiologic categories:

1. Infection and intoxication (e.g., congenital rubella or syphilis)
2. Trauma or physical agents (e.g., head wounds or birth injury)
3. Metabolism or nutrition (e.g., phenylketonuria or galactosemia)
4. Gross postnatal brain disease (e.g., neurofibromatosis or intracranial neoplasm)
5. Diseases or conditions of unknown prenatal influence (e.g., hydrocephaly or microcephaly)
6. Chromosomal abnormality (e.g., Down's syndrome or cat's cry syndrome)
7. Gestational disorder (e.g., prematurity or postmaturity)
8. Psychiatric disorder (e.g., autism or schizophrenia)
9. Environmental influences (e.g., sensory deprivation or institutional environment)
10. Other conditions (i.e., biologic conditions of unknown etiology)

Category 9, environmental influences, accounts for the vast majority of mental retardation, 80% to 85% of which is mild to moderate. Fortunately, this is the group most amenable to training. Only 15% to 25% of retardation is known to be caused by the discernible biologic conditions in the first eight categories. In this relatively small portion, however, are found those with greatest de-

ficiency (Gearheart, 1975; Chinn, Drew, and Logan, 1975).

The effects of these conditions are usually not discrete; they can interact in all sorts of combinations. Unfortunately, the persons least able to cope are often hit hardest. For instance, a culturally deprived mother existing on a subsistence diet is especially vulnerable to disease. If she conceives a child who, because of prenatal metabolic disturbance or infection, is born deaf and blind, then her child enters the world deprived of major sources of sensory information for constructing intellectual abilities. Perhaps she must work, leaving her child to the probable fate of being environmentally unstimulated, a condition that may affect brain chemistry and that certainly affects the opportunity to learn how to learn. Fig. 9-1 summarizes some of the main ways in which disease, social, and nutritional factors can interact to disable learning and intelligence.

Environmental deprivation. Neither rats, dogs, monkeys, nor children profit from deprivation. At best, a pallid environment in early life is only slightly injurious, but it can also leave disabling effects. The need for social stimulation of different types and amounts probably changes with age and from one species to another. With monkeys, for example, deprivation of experience with peers seems to be more damaging than deprivation of experience with mothers, especially during the third to sixth month (Harlow and Harlow, 1962). With slowly developing, long-dependent human infants, mothers are probably more important at least during the first few years, and effects of deprivation vary from one age to another.

Moreover, different types of deprivation probably have different effects: early sensory deprivation disturbs perception, whereas social and emotional deprivation affects social functioning. Intellectual impairment is not appreciable if deprivation occurs during the first 3 months, but it is considerable if it occurs between 3 and 12 months, the period during which Hebb (1949) hypothesizes that early perceptual learning is being established with neurophysiologic development of cell

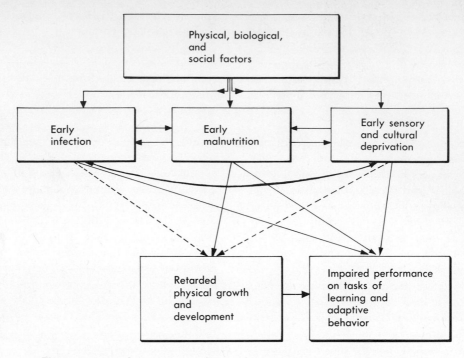

Fig. 9-1. Interrelations among factors that contribute to mental retardation.

assemblies and phase sequences (Yarrow, 1961; Guilford, 1967; Schiefelbusch, 1967). Clearly, as Lyle (1959, 1960) has shown, an institutional environment is hazardous to normal development of language.

Chemical impairment. When chemical processes (enzyme chemistry in synaptic conduction for short-term memory; protein synthesis for long-term memory) are impaired, learning ability can be disabled (Guilford, 1967; Nirenberg, 1967). These impairments can result from drugs and, more often, from nutritional or metabolic disorders (Eichenwald and Fry, 1969; Heber, 1959; Brozek and Grande, 1960; Hicks, 1960; Sokoloff, 1960). Although many chemical effects on specific intellectual abilities remain a mystery, a deficiency of oxygen and of thyroid secretion in infants, if not corrected, has been found to result in severe mental retardation.

Brain damage. Disease, infection, growths, poisoning, and injury can damage neural tissue with consequent impairment of intellect. The effects of damage depend on the extent and the location. Although intellectual and speech abilities cannot be localized in the brain with the specificity that phrenologists once acclaimed, still, different regions are vital to different functions (Piercy, 1964). The cerebrum (particularly the frontal cortex, once thought to be supreme in intellectual functioning) is now seen as an apparatus that provides refined discriminations to lower centers in the thalamus, limbic system, and reticular formation. It is these lower centers that integrate information for purposive behavior. Damage to them is considered much more devastating than to the cortex—when they are impaired, attention and even consciousness are also impaired (Guilford, 1967).

SPEECH EFFECTS OF LEARNING AND INTELLECTUAL DISABILITIES

During the last decade, a surge of interest in language problems of cognitively disabled children has occurred. The idea that intellect is an immutably static capacity fixed by ge-

---

Comprehensive reviews of forerunners of this work have been published by Jordan (1967), McCarthy (1964), Schiefelbusch (1969), and Spradlin (1967).

netic endowment has given way to the more optimistic views of Piaget (1964). Most workers have adopted his idea that intelligence increases as the child masters progressively higher stages of cognitive development. In this sense, the level of retardation reflects where in the hierarchy of cognitive abilities the child must begin if he is to show progress. As noted earlier, the retarded child usually does not progress beyond the concrete thinking that normal children use as a stepping-stone to abstract thinking. Whether language development retards cognitive development or vice versa is problematic. Wide agreement exists that they are intimately intertwined (Schiefelbusch, 1972).

Considering how abstract the structure of language is, the level of intellect required for mastering at least the mechanics of an elementary grammar is surprisingly low. Perhaps this fact is additional evidence of man's being uniquely endowed with a special auditory mechanism that allows him to understand and acquire speech (Studdert-Kennedy, 1975). Although the retarded can learn a vocabulary of words and sentences with which they can make responses, their difficulty is with using language meaningfully to understand and express ideas (Hass and Hass, 1972).

Piaget, Vygotsky, and Bruner propose slightly different versions of how language functions in development of a child's ability to think. Piaget's (1964) position is that the infant evokes sensorimotor imagery of his experience, with which words are associated. During early childhood, words are tied to concrete objects and events and are used to help master imagery of the world. The child's speech is used privately to help him organize his images. This, then, is what Piaget calls the *egocentric* use of language. Only later, when forced by social demands, does the child begin to consider the listener's point of view. It is then that he begins to adapt his speech to social concerns of communicating ideas.

Vygotsky (1962) regarded egocentric speech as being essentially social in its beginnings. Gradually it is transformed into private language. As *inner speech*, it is no longer tied to concrete situations or social contexts. Wordless perception of the world shifts to verbally guided perception of that concrete world. Eventually with development of inner speech, the world that is perceived becomes largely an abstract representation expressed in words. Thus the cognitive abilities of abstract thinking, which are especially lacking in the retarded, have their basis in meaningful language. As far as Vygotsky was concerned, impairment of language is tantamount to impairment of intelligence. By the same token, he saw habilitation of language as a prime approach to improvement of intelligence.

Bruner, Olver, and Greenfield (1966) have taken a position not very much different from Vygotsky's. From their research, they have concluded that for a child to use language for thinking, the organization of his perception of the world must parallel and be congruent with the organization of his language. In other words, for the child to make sensible statements about the real world, he must perceive relationships in it in essentially the same way as the grammar of his language permits him to express those relationships.

One of Bruner's reasons for suspecting that cognition and language are organized normally under control of the same principles is the ease with which the normal child swiftly masters syntax. By contrast, he spends all of childhood, much of adolescence, and sometimes much of adulthood grasping semantic implications and nuances of the words and sentences he uses. It is as though he must first firmly grasp the grammatical rules that permit him to express in words the relationships he has observed in life. Then, apparently, he is prepared to proceed with refining his use of language to express the shades of meaning he intends.

Bruner contends that the child's intellect grows as he constructs and tests a model of reality with three techniques: action, imagery, and symbolism. He must act in accordance with the physical reality of the world if he is to live in it successfully. Were he to leap from a bridge and expect to fly, his model of reality would be sharply altered if he survived and extinguished if he did not survive. His imagery of the world also develops predictably within the constraints of what he can hear, see, feel, smell, and taste. Similarly, his symbolic representation of his experience must conform to the relationships he has observed in the world as it exists if what he says is to have any meaning. It is the inability to use language symbolically to represent reality that is a prime mark of the retarded child's intellectual deficit.

Language development of mentally retarded children

Fig. 9-2 shows several important considerations in language development. First, it shows that below a mental age of 5 years, speech acquisition correlates roughly with amount of retardation, until at a mental age of 1 year no language is found. Second, it shows that the IQ in mentally retarded children (shown with heavy black lines) decays with age until it reaches a plateau at puberty. The same is true with language skills. Whereas the normal child has language fully established by age 4 years, a retarded child with an IQ of approximately 45 will not reach the threshold of grammatical language until adolescence. Third, the graph shows that below this threshold, full language will never be acquired. Moreover, the farther the child is below the threshold, the more primitive will be whatever language does develop. These results are essentially congruent with older studies reviewed by Matthews (1971).

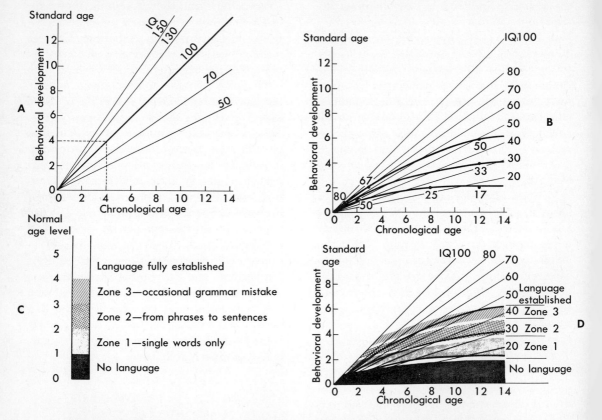

Fig. 9-2. Relationship between development of IQ and language. **A,** Nonverbal IQ (behavioral development plotted against chronological age). **B,** Changes in nonverbal IQ of retarded children who will reach IQ levels of 17, 33, and 50 at age 12. **C,** Normal age levels of language development. **D,** Language development expectations for retarded children shown in relation to nonverbal IQ and chronological age. (From Lenneberg, E., *Biological Foundations of Language.* New York: John Wiley & Sons, Inc. [1967].)

Confirmations and puzzlements. The speech of mentally retarded children provides puzzlements and confirmations. These children offer confirmation that mastery of articulation and mastery of language are largely unrelated. Some who can barely understand language, who have a vocabulary of less than fifty words, and who mostly babble can articulate their nonsense comprehensibly. More typically, those with reasonably good linguistic skills, when they speak, are virtually unintelligible. Mongoloid children, especially, confirm the conclusion in Chapter 4 that extensive babbling, dependence on adults, and imitation are not sufficient factors (even though they may be necessary) for language acquisition. If these factors were sufficient, the affectionate, imitative, babbling mongoloid child would be linguistically supreme.

Another confirmation, again following Lenneberg's (1967) argument, is that language emerges according to a schedule of evolvement; one set of events sets the stage for subsequent events. The developmental pattern is not bizarre; it follows the normal course, but at a retarded rate. As with the normal child, once across the language threshold, they stop babbling, they attempt to speak in words and phrases, they have a vocabulary of fifty words or more, and they understand spoken commands.

The puzzlement is why these children tend to have such poor articulation. Were the whole answer to articulation development Mowrer's autism theory (1952)—that children learn intelligible speech through identification much as do talking birds—then

---

Does Siegel (1969) agree with Mowrer's autism theory of speech acquisition?

---

mongoloids should have superb articulation, even if they had nothing to say. They fit perfectly the conditions generally considered essential for perfection of intelligible speech: they babble profusely, are affectionate, and most likely receive affectionate care—yet more often than not their speech is incomprehensible (Lenneberg, 1967).

Types of speech problems of mentally retarded children

Depending on the severity of the mentally retarded group studied, up to 95% have been found with defective speech (Schiefelbusch, 1963; Matthews, 1971; Schiefelbusch, Copeland, and Smith, 1967). The types of problems found can be largely inferred from the preceding discussion. Delayed language development is a predominant characteristic. Below the threshold of language acquisition, primitive forms of grammar such as single words and phrases predominate; they may be articulated comprehensibly but usually are not. Those who finally reach this threshold will pass through normal stages of speech acquisition but, depending on intelligence, at a slower rate. The fact that they can construct a fully grammatical sentence does not imply that they can speak or understand sentences of any length or complexity. To the contrary, this ability is very much a function of intelligence (Lenneberg, 1967).

Mentally retarded children who acquire full language are still subject to the types of speech problems of the normal population, only more so. Disorders of articulation abound. They seem to take the same form as those in the normal population, but they occur in greater abundance. Numerous voice problems have been found in a few studies. An incidence of stuttering as high as 45% has been reported for mongoloids, but why a problem of fluency would be a function of intelligence is puzzling. A more recent study of 216 patients in a state hospital revealed only one stutterer and one clutterer, an incidence close to normal (Sheehan, Martyn, and Kilburn, 1968; Matthews, 1971; Bangs, 1942; Schiefelbusch, 1963; Schiefelbusch, Copeland, and Smith, 1967).

SPEECH PATHOLOGIST'S RESPONSIBILITY IN TREATMENT OF LEARNING AND INTELLECTUAL DISABILITIES

A decade ago many speech pathologists still viewed the problem of mental retardation as a wasteland to be avoided. They saw communicative disorders of this group as discouragingly difficult to rehabilitate. In the last several years, however, this attitude has changed. The possibility is being explored that much "retarded" behavior can be modified under carefully designed conditions of learning. Schlanger (1967), for example, points to nine characteristics of the mentally retarded that presumably affect language, such as short attention span, poor auditory memory, poor grammar, minimal speech content, and the like. He suggests that many of these characteristics are learned in defective form. Hence, by implication, they should be subject to improvement by learning.

Responsibility for referral

Because a primary symptom of mental deficiency is delayed speech development, the speech pathologist often has the first professional encounter with these children. Concerned parents, hoping against hope, frequently want not to see the full scope of their child's problem. They may focus on speech and press for its correction. Obviously, in such cases the speech pathologist must deal with a multiple problem. He must initiate a series of referrals to specialists who can provide the child with maximal opportunities; these referrals will probably begin with a physician and may include psychologists, educators, social workers, and so on. He must counsel sympathetically with the parents to help them accept the reality of the child's condition, which entails more than a speech problem. Finally, he must provide whatever corrective help is possible for the communicative disorder.

Responsibility for treatment and research

Still, within the framework of what can be done for the learning and intellectual disabilities, a program of behavioral modification has much efficacy. Although the causes of mental retardation may justify the physiologic emphasis usually built into diagnostic procedures, the fact that even the biochemistry of learning can be altered by exercise and stimulation is becoming clearer. Not only can defective communication *result* from mental retardation, it can also *contribute* to a retarded condition. Moreover, we have not yet entered the era of pharmaceutical aids to learning and intelligence (although that day may be close). Until it arrives, rehabilitation will undoubtedly remain with efforts to modify behavior and improve the environment.

Speech pathologists and psychologists alike are currently pursuing programs of behavioral modification to determine how far the abilities of the mentally retarded can be expanded. Agreement prevails that approaches to the improvement of speech can be developed for retarded persons of all ages and all levels of development, that strategies for care and training can be improved, that early development of speech skills may facilitate acquisition of adaptive behavior, and that these gains are proportional to professional imagination and dedication (Schiefelbusch, 1963, 1969; Schiefelbusch, Copeland, and Smith, 1967).

The answers—résumé

1. What is the nature of learning and intellectual disabilities that affect speech?

As learning and intellectual functions are impaired sufficiently to produce mental retardation, meaningful use of language is progressively affected. These functions can be disabled by early environmental deprivation; by drugs, nutritional deficits, and metabolic disorders that affect the chemistry of memory and recall; and by brain damage, especially in the speech areas of the dominant hemisphere.

2. What are the speech effects of learning and intellectual disabilities?

The more severely mentally retarded a child is, the slower will be his rate of speech acquisition. If his mental age at puberty is much below 5 years, he will not have sufficient intelligence to cross the threshold of grammatical language. The farther below the threshold, the more primitive will be his phrases and words. Above the threshold, which is remarkably low considering the level of abstraction of linguistic structure, the child will be able to master grammatically accurate sentences. The farther above the threshold, the more complex will be the sentence that can be understood and spoken, and the larger will be the vocabulary.

Intelligibility of articulation especially is a prevalent problem among mentally retarded individuals, but mastery of language and mastery of articulation are largely unrelated. One can speak grammatically and unintelligibly, or vice versa. The other types of speech disorders found in a normal population also appear among mentally retarded persons.

3. What is the speech pathologist's responsibility in the treatment of learning and intellectual disabilities?

Because retarded speech development is an early sign of mental retardation, the speech pathologist is often sought first for professional help. He must initiate a series of referrals to specialists who can provide the full range of needed services for the retarded child. He must counsel sympathetically with concerned if not distraught parents to help them face the reality of their child's condition. He must also provide appropriate rehabilitative services for defective speech. Perhaps his greatest service in the long view will be to demonstrate the extent to which modification of communicative behavior can improve the conditions of retardation. A major responsibility of the speech pathologist is to identify sharply those responses that must be acquired if normal speech is to develop.

REFERENCES

Bangs, J., A clinical analysis of the articulatory defects of the feeble-minded. *J. Speech Dis.*, **7**, 343-356 (1942).

Beard, R., *An Outline of Piaget's Developmental Psychology for Students and Teachers*. New York: Basic Books, Inc. (1969).

Brozek, J., and Grande, F., Abnormalities of neural function in the presence of inadequate nutrition. In Field, J., Magoun, H., and Hall, V. (Eds.), *Handbook of Physiology*. (Sec. I) *Neurophysiology*. (Vol. II) Washington, D.C.: American Physiological Society (1960).

Bruner, J., Olver, R., and Greenfield, P., *Studies in Cognitive Growth*. New York: John Wiley & Sons, Inc. (1966).

Chinn, P., Drew, C., and Logan, D., *Mental Retardation: a Life Cycle Approach*. St. Louis: The C. V. Mosby Co. (1975).

Eichenwald, H., and Fry, P., Nutrition and learning. *Science*, **163**, 644-648 (1969).

Gearheart, B., and Litton, F., *The Trainable Retarded: a Foundations Approach*. St. Louis: The C. V. Mosby Co. (1975).

Grossman, H., *Manual on Terminology and Classification in Mental Retardation*. Washington: American Association on Mental Deficiency (1973).

Guilford, J., *The Nature of Human Intelligence*. New York: McGraw-Hill Book Co. (1967).

Harlow, H., and Harlow, M., Social deprivation in monkeys. *Scient. Am.*, **207**, 136-146 (1962).

Hass, W., and Hass, S., Syntactic structure and language development in retardates. In Schiefelbusch, R. (Ed.), *Language of the Mentally Retarded*. Baltimore: University Park Press (1972).

Hebb, D., *The Organization of Behavior*. New York: John Wiley & Sons, Inc. (1949).

Heber, R., A manual on terminology and classification in mental retardation. (Monogr. Suppl. No. 2) American Journal of Mental Deficiency, **64**, (1959).

Hicks, S., Disturbances of neural function in the presence of congenital disorders. In Field, J., Magoun, H., and Hall, V. (Eds.), *Handbook of Physiology*. (Sec. I) *Neurophysiology*. (Vol. II) Washington, D.C.: American Physiological Society (1960).

Jordan, T., Language and mental retardation: a review of the literature. In Schiefelbusch, R., Copeland, R., and Smith, J. (Eds.), *Language and Mental Retardation*. New York: Holt, Rinehart & Winston, Inc. (1967).

Lenneberg, E., *Biological Foundations of Language*. New York: John Wiley & Sons, Inc. (1967).

Lyle, J., The effect of an institutional environment upon the verbal development of imbecile children. I. Verbal intelligence. *J. ment. defic. Res.*, **3**, 122-128 (1959).

Lyle, J., The effect of an institutional environment upon

the verbal development of imbecile children. II. Speech and language. *J. ment. defic. Res.*, **4**, 1-13 (1960).

Matthews, J., Speech problems of the mentally retarded. In Travis, L. (Ed.), *Handbook of Speech Pathology and Audiology* (2nd ed.) New York: Appleton-Century-Crofts (1971).

McCarthy, J., Research on the linguistic problems of the mentally retarded. *Ment. Retard. Absts.*, **2**, 90-96 (1964).

Mowrer, O., Speech development in the young child. I. The autism theory of speech development and some clinical applications. *J. Speech Hearing Dis.*, **17**, 263-268 (1952).

Nirenberg, M., The genetic code. In Quarton, G., Melnechuk, T., and Schmitt, F. (Eds.), *The Neurosciences.* New York: Rockefeller University Press (1967).

Piaget, J., *Origins of Intelligence.* New York: International Universities Press (1964).

Piercy, M., The effects of cerebral lesions on intellectual functions: a review of current research trends. *Br. J. Psychiat.*, **110**, 310-352 (1964).

Schiefelbusch, R., Introduction: language studies of mentally retarded children. *J. Speech Hearing Dis.*, Monogr. Suppl. No. 10, pp. 3-7 (1963).

Schiefelbusch, R., The development of communication skills. In Schiefelbusch, R., Copeland, R., and Smith, J. (Eds.), *Language and Mental Retardation.* New York: Holt, Rinehart & Winston, Inc. (1967).

Schiefelbusch, R., Language functions of retarded children. *Folia Phoniatrica*, **21**, 129-144 (1969).

Schiefelbusch, R., *Language of the Mentally Retarded.* Baltimore: University Park Press (1972).

Schiefelbusch, R., Copeland, R., and Smith, J., *Language and Mental Retardation.* New York: Holt, Rinehart & Winston, Inc. (1967).

Schlanger, B., Issues for speech and language training of the mentally retarded. In Schiefelbusch, R., Copeland, R., and Smith, J. (Eds.), *Language and Mental Retardation.* New York: Holt, Rinehart & Winston, Inc. (1967).

Sheehan, J., Martyn, M., and Kilburn, K., Speech disorders in retardation. *Am. J. ment. Defic.*, **73**, 251-256 (1968).

Siegel, G., Vocal conditioning in infants. *J. Speech Hearing Dis.*, **34**, 3-19 (1969).

Sokoloff, L., Metabolism of the central nervous system in vivo. In Field, J., Magoun, H., and Hall, V. (Eds.), *Handbook of Physiology.* (Sec. I) *Neurophysiology.* (Vol. II) Washington, D.C.: American Physiological Society (1960).

Spradlin, J., Procedures for evaluating processes associated with expressive and receptive language. In Schiefelbusch, R., Copeland, R., and Smith, J. (Eds.), *Language and Mental Retardation.* New York: Holt, Rinehart, & Winston, Inc. (1967).

Studdert-Kennedy, M., From continuous signal to discrete message: syllable to phoneme. In Kavanagh, J., and Cutting, J. (Eds), *The Role of Speech in Language.* Cambridge, Mass.: The M.I.T. Press (1975).

Vygotsky, L., *Thought and Language.* Cambridge, Mass.: The M.I.T. Press (1962).

Yarrow, L., Maternal deprivation: toward an empirical and conceptual re-evaluation. *Psychol. Bull.*, **58**, 459-490 (1961).

Chapter 10

Personality and emotional disturbances

Questions

NATURE OF PERSONALITY AND EMOTIONAL DISTURBANCES THAT AFFECT SPEECH

Personality and emotional disturbances are classified in four major groups: *neurosis, psychosis, character disorders,* and *psychosomatic disorders.* The essence of the differences between the first two categories is captured in the facetious distinction made by some: neurotics build castles in the air; psychotics live in them. In neurosis, personality illness does not involve impairment of the ego function of reality-testing. By contrast, psychosis is distinguished by grossly distorted perception of and response to reality.

Whereas the personality disorders of neurotics and psychotics are marked by characteristic symptoms, in a character disorder the personality disturbance is *acted out* in characteristic overt behavior. Thus neurotic or psychotic symptoms of a personality disorder may involve inner difficulties not directly observable, whereas the conflicts of an individual with a character disorder are on public display in ways more troublesome to others than to himself.

Psychosomatic disorders are organic diseases to which emotional conflicts contribute. Sometimes called *organ neuroses* and by official American Psychiatric Association terminology *psychophysiologic autonomic and visceral responses*, they differ from psychoneurotic reactions by involving physiologically based symptoms in autonomically controlled organs not subject to volitional control (Coleman, 1956).

Although we cannot attribute specific speech disorders to specific types of psychopathology with much confidence, still, persons with character disorders as well as with psychosis, psychosomatic disorders, and neurosis have speech problems. It behooves us to be familiar with at least the major features of these personality disturbances.

Neurotic adjustments

Neurosis is a term sired by Freud, nurtured by his disciples, and abused by almost everyone else. It designates an illness diagnosed by the presence of covert or overt neurotic symptoms. *Neurotic conflict*, on the other hand, is indicative of the use of neurotic defense mechanisms as the ego attempts to reestablish equilibrium. This condition is often described as *emotional disturbance* (Kessler, 1966). While everyone can be said to be neurotic in the sense that all of us probably resort at times to unhealthy defense mechanisms, we cannot say that everyone has a neurosis. Not all neurotic conflicts lead to neurotic symptoms. All forms of neurosis, however, do reflect the inability of the ego to cope with environmental stress. When a relatively healthy personality succumbs to extreme stress, as in battle, the condition is called *traumatic neurosis*. With an unhealthy personality, mild stress can produce a *psychoneurosis* (Hofling and Leininger, 1960). Most of the personality problems with which speech pathologists are concerned involve psychoneuroses.

Types of psychoneuroses. The major types of psychoneuroses classified by the American Psychiatric Association are anxiety reaction, conversion reaction, dissociative reaction, phobic reaction, obsessive-compulsive reaction, and depressive reaction. The last is so similar to psychotic depression that it will be discussed in that section.

Anxiety reaction. The simplest form of psychoneurosis is an anxiety reaction. It is a straightforward consequence of ego failure to cope. The symptoms are either direct expressions of anxiety (fear, sweating, and the like) or of ego fatigue from the conflict (tension, poor concentration, irritability, and so on).

Conversion reaction. Conversion reaction is of particular interest to us because it is thought to be involved in functional aphonia and stuttering. It is a major type of *hysteria*—hence the term *conversion hysteria*. The distinguishing symptom is slight to total failure of a sensory or voluntary muscle mechanism when no organic disability exists. Conversion symptoms have meaning. They are translations of psychologic conflicts into body language. The ego, unable to resolve the conflict adaptively, resorts to the fundamental defense mechanism of repression (Table 10-1), which removes the conflict from consciousness and allays anxiety. Then to buttress this defensive solution, the ego effects a compromise between id strivings for gratification, superego demands for punishment, and realistic restrictions of society: a body function is converted to an ego-defensive purpose. For example, loss of voice can gratify dependency needs, punish for hostile feelings, and successfully curtail verbal aggression.

Dissociative reaction. The other type of hysteria is a dissociative reaction that compartmentalizes experience. The symptom is amnesia, and the major ego-defensive mechanism, as in conversion hysteria, is repression. Unacceptable memories are dissociated by selective repressive barriers, sometimes sufficiently to yield such multiple personalities as Dr. Jekyll and Mr. Hyde or "the three faces of Eve."

Phobic reaction. Sometimes called "anxiety hysteria," a phobia is dread of something not realistically dangerous. This symptom represents a relatively simple neurosis in which the ego, unable to tolerate "free-floating" anxiety, uses defense mechanisms, first of repression and then of projection and displacement (Table 10-1), to find a scapegoat. One can develop phobic symptoms from *acrophobia* to *zenophobia* and then assiduously avoid (at the risk of irrational fear) anything from heights to strangers.

Obsessive-compulsive reaction. Obsessions and compulsions are attempts by the ego to resolve unacceptable id impulses of hostility and aggression. The principal defensive mechanisms used are regression, isolation, reaction-formation, and undoing (Table 10-1). The result is a compromise solution among id, superego, and reality. In an obsession, irrational and unwanted thoughts persistently recur. The symptom of compulsion is an irrational act performed to avoid anxiety or to dispel an obsession. The child who avoids walking on cracks and the adult who feels better after straightening a picture exhibit mild normal compulsions. The conscientious housewife on a rare vacation who worries whether she turned off the stove experiences a mild obsession.

Psychotic adjustments

The etiology of psychosis may be organic, functional, or some mixture of the two. *Organic* psychoses result from disease or injury of the central nervous system from malnutrition, glandular deficiency, traumatic head injury, certain infections, and certain chemical conditions (to which LSD may be related). Most organic psychoses tend to be permanent.

Psychoses for which organic etiology cannot be demonstrated are classified as *functional*. They may be divided into two major groups: disorders of *affect* and disorders of *thought*. The latter, comprising schizophrenic reactions, are strongly suspected of hereditary predisposition. Although psychotic and neurotic symptoms overlap. neurotic individuals seldom become psychotic even with increased stress and frustration. Psychotic reactions often develop suddenly, without much warning except for social iso-

lation. It is as though neurosis and psychosis are independent adjustments for coping with excessive stress, with psychosis being a much more immature and maladaptive adjustment.

Types of functional psychosis. Because of the complexity of psychotic problems and their relative infrequency for the speech pathologist's concern, we will sketch them only in broadest outline while looking a bit closer at *autism*, in which speech problems loom larger more frequently. The major forms of psychosis are *manic-depression, schizophrenia*, and *paranoia*.

Manic-depression. The manic-depressive person may show either euphoria or melancholy of psychotic intensity. Both reactions involve disturbances of mood and self-esteem, and both are recurrent and of limited duration. The depressed phase of this psychosis is the most serious of several other forms of depression ranging from "blue" spells, grief and mourning, and neurotic depressions, through psychotic depressions. Although thought and behavior are affected when these moods are of psychotic proportions, they are not distorted severely by delusions and hallucinations.

Schizophrenia. Schizophrenic reactions are primarily thought disorders that, among the psychoses, are marked by greatest deterioration of personality and widest range of characteristics. The most universal features include *apathy, associative looseness* (disjointed thoughts), *autistic thinking* (dreamlike thinking), and *ambivalence* (particularly an admixture of hate, fear, and love).

The four traditionally recognized types of schizophrenic reactions are *catatonic, paranoid, simple*, and *hebephrenic*. Catatonia,

---

What other psychotic and neurotic reactions and mental disorders are described in the American Psychiatric Association's official publication, *Diagnostic and Statistical Manual: Mental Disorders* (1962)?

---

with acute onset and best prognosis, presents two main clinical pictures: *catatonic stupor* and *catatonic excitement*. They may alternate in quick succession. The paranoid type is one of the largest groups of schizophrenia. The major feature is extreme suspicion, typically a manifestation of delusions of persecution, sometimes with matching auditory hallucinations. The simple type of schizophrenia is least conspicuous, revealed more by eccentricities and ineffectual adjustments than by delusions and hallucinations. It develops slowly and may remain arrested for long periods. The hebephrenic type develops gradually, is least accessible to treatment, and has the poorest prognosis. Reflecting almost total disintegration of personality, with bizarre delusions and hallucinations, the hebephrenic patient utterly disregards social conventions: he eats with his fingers and masturbates, urinates, and defecates in public.

Paranoia. Paranoid reactions are quite similar to the paranoid type of schizophrenia. The major differences are that, in paranoia, age of onset is generally later, hallucinations are absent, and delusions are organized into an internally consistent system. The paranoid individual may give a superficial impression of near normalcy.

Autism. Although autism is only one form of childhood psychosis, it is the most common. In fact, the terms are frequently used interchangeably (Baltaxe and Simmons, 1975). Traditionally, the autistic child has been seen as a product of severe deprivation of parental affection or as having introjected the emptiness that presumably characterizes the parent-child relationship. He appears to be a child who cannot tolerate stimulation, who is anxious and obsessively dedicated to maintaining an undisturbed equilibrium. Because he cannot hold his environment constant, he simply shuts it out and holds himself constant—and he starts doing this from the beginning of life. This is the child about whom, by 4 months of age, parents report: "He lives in a shell," "He is happiest when left alone," "He acts as if people aren't there," and, most startling of all to the mothers, "He never reached out to me to be picked up." He is thought to be able to relate to objects that he can control, but not to people. This traditional explanation is also used to account for his personalized communication system, replete with neologisms and familiar words used with idiosyncratic meanings.

That child-rearing practices alone are sufficient to explain autism is being questioned severely. Bartak and Rutter (1974) have tested this psychogenic theory of autism and concluded that their evidence did not support it. Completely aside from the clinical impression that many autistic children appear to have parents who do all that could be asked, research has shown that autistic behavior is not responsive to environmental conditions (Sorosky and others, 1968).

Infantile autism (along with atypical development, symbiotic psychosis, and certain cases of childhood schizophrenia) may prove to be a manifestation of a syndrome of *perceptual inconstancy.* Children so afflicted are unable to maintain a balanced sensory input; they alternate between being flooded with too much excitation and being deprived of sensation. Evidence of this breakdown in the central nervous system vestibular mechanism, which regulates sensory homeostasis, has been found in rapid eye movements (REM) that accompany dreaming. The mechanism that normally suppresses the neurophysiologic activity of dreaming may permit dream activity to break into waking life of the autistic child (Ornitz and Ritvo, 1968a; Ornitz and others, 1969). Not only is perception disrupted, but, as a consequence, so is ego development, motor behavior, and language (Ornitz and Ritvo, 1968b).

For whatever reason, the fact is becoming increasingly evident that autistic children suffer profound perceptual disturbance of visual as well as auditory and possibly somesthetic processes. Their ability to assemble their experience into sensible form is defective. The result is that they appear unable to understand their world.

Although classified as a psychosis, childhood schizophrenia is different from autism. Evidence is available to support both brain pathology and genetic deficiency as a basis for this disability, although the etiology is far from certain (Rutter and Bartak, 1971; Wing, 1966).

Autism occurs in boys as many as four times as often as in girls, and it is apparently independent of mental retardation. Autistic children can range from high to low in nonverbal intelligence. On the other hand, many of the language deficits found in developmental aphasia are also apparent in autism. The difference between these two problems seems to be in the extent of perceptual involvement. Whereas auditory processing difficulties disable oral language acquisition in developmental aphasia, the autistic child is faced with the more severe problem of visual as well as auditory perceptual disturbance (Churchill, 1972; Wing and Wing, 1971).

Character disorders

Character disorders, also called *personality disorders*, are identified by inadequate behavior, not by specific symptoms such as distinguish among psychoses and neuroses. Some writers describe these problems by level of psychosexual fixation (such as oral personality), others by terms borrowed from neurosis or psychosis (for example, schizoid personality), and others by manner of response (for instance, passive-aggressive personality). The official psychiatric classifications involve five major categories, of which three will be mentioned.

Personality pattern disturbances involve inadequate intellectual, emotional, and social responses that resemble psychotic reactions. Therefore this category is unofficially called *psychotic personality*.

Personality trait disturbances involve excitable and ineffectual responses to minor stress suggestive of neurosis. Because the disturbance is acted out without evidence of symptoms, the term *neurotic personality* is sometimes applied.

Sociopathic personality disturbance, unofficially called *psychopathic personality*, is perhaps the best known of the character disorders. Persons with this disturbance include alcoholics, drug addicts, and sexual deviates, as well as irresponsible, immature, antisocial individuals with little loyalty or judgment.

Psychosomatic disorders

Psychophysiologic autonomic and *visceral disorders* (to use the official terminology of the American Psychiatric Association) are classified according to the organ system affected. No organ system seems to be immune. These disorders range from skin to nervous system reactions and from endocrine to cardiovascular reactions. Two of particular relevance to voice would appear to be *gastrointestinal* and *respiratory reactions*. Although a duodenal ulcer is a typical example of the former and asthma of the latter, laryngeal pathology consequent to vocal abuse would fit well within these categories. Contact ulcers not only involve organic damage to the vocal cords, but they occur mainly in ulcer-prone executive types, suggesting a gastrointestinal as well as a respiratory disorder. Vocal nodules, on the other hand, may be limited to respiratory system damage from hypertensive phonation reflective of emotional disturbance.

SPEECH EFFECTS OF PERSONALITY AND EMOTIONAL DISTURBANCES
Introduction

Clinical evidence leads regularly to the conclusion that speech is affected by personality and emotional disturbances. That strong confirmation of this conclusion is lacking can be attributed more to the complexity of the problem than to the lack of serious study. *Emotion* is a cognitive process, *personality* a hypothetical construct. Both are difficult to define adequately for accurate measurement. Their relations to speech, like shapes in the dark, can be seen better out of the corner of the eye than when observed squarely. Such evidence as exists plus inferences from learning theory, personality theory, and speech development, provide the basis for this chapter.

The effects of personality and emotional disturbances on speech can be explained as the confluence of two major streams of development: personality and speech. The aspect of personality of particular relevance is the development of the *ego* and its *defenses*. The two aspects of speech are the development of the *speaking signal system* and of the *language symbol system.* Emotion is a source of motivation that probably weighs heavily in patterns of personality and communicative behavior reinforced at various stages of development.

Personality development. *Personality* can be viewed usefully as an individual's pattern of *traits.* Traits are relatively static abstractions. They describe only patterns of responses typically utilized. They do not account for the rich variety of exceptions with which each of us defies the pigeonholes that would be so comfortable for others to have us fit. Personality, constructed of traits, is an even higher level of abstraction from which

---

What does Mischel (1969) think of the adequacy of explaining personality in terms of traits?

---

to predict specific responses.

By far the most influential conception of personality has been the psychoanalytic theory. It is at once tantalizing and frustrating. Unlike Venus, born full-blown on her half shell, psychoanalytic insights have been emerging ever since Freud's genius first revealed the unconscious. More like Topsy, the theory has grown every which way. Freud tinkered with it. His disciples tinkered with it. Almost everyone who has used it has tinkered with it. It did not start out as a thing of beauty. It has never been a parsimonious, internally consistent, elegantly simple conception of the human condition. It has been flawed from the beginning by superimposition of an anthropomorphic set of psychic structures on a hydraulic analogy of the economic distribution of psychic energy. It has, now, so many contributors that it resembles the Bible (which, for many, it is) more than a scientific theory. It is a marvelously intricate assemblage of metaphors more than a closely knit unified body of knowledge.

But for all its faults, it has vitality. It has invaded literature, the theater, and religion. It provides the underpinnings for the practice of psychotherapy by many psychiatrists, clinical psychologists, social workers, and some speech pathologists. Wherein lies the

power? It speaks to the depth and breadth of human experience. It comprises a collection of astute observations, most of which are so inexorably mentalistic as to be unmeasurable and untestable, but some of which can be treated as empirical processes subject to scientific analysis. It offers a holistic, if grotesque, interpretation of the rich complexities of human existence. Perhaps most important of all for the clinician with responsibility for problems of mental health, it offers what is thought to be his best basis for predicting and understanding human behavior in all of its inexplicable subtleties and intricacies.

Fortunately, the aspects of psychoanalytic theory of prime interest for us, development of the ego and its defenses, involve relatively testable observations about personality. Let us review ego development briefly before relating it to the development of speech disorders.

Ego development. After birth, the helpless infant does not yet have a sense of identity. His discomforts reflect failures of the environment to meet his pressing needs. To the extent that his psychic apparatus exists, it is all *id*—the anthropomorphic psychic reservoir of primitive instinctual energy that fuels other "agencies" of the mind that will develop. The id operates exclusively at an *unconscious* level and follows the *pleasure-pain principle* avidly. It seeks the pleasure of the immediate discharge of instinctual impulses without regard for consequences, and it seeks immediate relief from pain or discomfort.

The portion of the id that develops self-regulatory functions as it interacts with the external environment becomes the *ego*, the Latin word for "I." It is the sober rational mediator through which we experience our sense of identity. It develops to mediate consciously and unconsciously among irresponsible pressures of the id for immediate gratification and demands of the realistic external world. It meets its responsibilities three ways: by mediating perception of the world, by controlling motor performance, and by controlling impulses. It attempts to mediate the pressure of the id in socially acceptable and sensible fashion.

What determinants of normal personality development in infants does Escalona (1968) describe?

A portion of the ego, the *superego*, is further differentiated to aid in coping with external conflicts with authority figures, especially the child's parents. The superego becomes the judicial voice of conscience that can be heard consciously but that imposes its restrictive effects largely in unconscious, and sometimes unreasoning, ways. It is responsible for such feelings as guilt, shame, and disgust. With its development the ego must now cope with superego restrictions as well as with id pressures and environmental realities. Failure to negotiate successfully among these demands is experienced as *anxiety*, the feeling of threatened loss of ego control. To aid in preserving control and to protect itself from anxiety, the ego utilizes various adaptive and defensive adjustments *(ego defenses)*, which are mainly unconscious.

The use of ego-defensive mechanisms is a necessary part of normal personality development. The infant, faced with the basic problem of differentiating himself from his environment, uses whatever techniques will help him to determine whether the stimuli to which he responds originate from within or without. Too, he must be able to select among stimuli, shutting out those of little importance to whatever response he is making. Otherwise, the ability to focus attention and to ward off anxiety would be imperiled. All ego defenses contribute to these normal ends. Only when overworked do they become *pathogenic* (conducive to psychopathology). As powerful methods for reducing anxiety, they tend to be reinforced strongly when conflict prevails. They can then become pathologic by restricting ego functions, impeding development, distorting one's view of reality, or alienating one from others. Authors vary in how they define and interrelate functions of these various adjustive and defensive mechanisms. Table 10-

1 gives a list of ego defenses and their purposes as offered by Kessler (1966).

The child tends to use these personality adjustment mechanisms selectively at different stages of ego development. The course of this development is thought to follow evolving sources of gratification for primitive id forces. During infancy the most pleasurable region of stimulation is thought to involve the mouth. This is the *oral stage* of *psychosexual development.* The infant's ego is primitive and so must be whatever ego-adjustment mechanisms he uses. Identification and especially sublimation are healthy and normal mechanisms, whereas denial, repression, introjection, projection, displacement, and fixation become pathogenic when used more than occasionally.

Hofling and Leininger (1960) offer a lucid account of ego-adjustment mechanisms used in personality development.

The *anal* stage during the period of muscle training is traversed most successfully when sublimation is the major adjustive technique. By contrast, when this period is traumatic, pathogenic defenses such as reaction formation, undoing, isolation, and regression set the stage especially for obsessive-compulsive neurosis. If the child can progress through the masturbatory self-centered sexual phase (the *phallic* period) to the *genital* stage, he will have reached the highest level of psychosexual development. At this level, he will acquire increasing concern for others as he learns to depend on them for psychosexual gratification. The major ego mechanism with which he will achieve this maturity is identification.

Speech development. Speech and personality presumably interact during their concurrent development. That speech facilitates problem-solving abilities of the ego is readily apparent. How personality affects speech is less obvious. The proposed connection involves a distinction between the language system for symbolizing the *content* of a message and the speaking system for signaling a speaker's *intent.*

Table 10-1. Ego defenses and their purposes*

Mechanism of defense	Purpose
Introjection—psychologic incorporation analogous to the physiologic process of eating *Identification*—involving imitation, incorporation of characteristics of another as one's own	Parts of the environment are taken into the self. Both mechanisms are essential to normal development.
Sublimation—substitution of usually a more acceptable form of gratification for a less acceptable one: thumb sucking for nursing in young children, football for fighting in young males *Hallucination*—a sense of omnipotence presumably typical of contented infants that is experienced by healthy adults in dreams as a type of sensory experience without external stimuli	One form of gratification is substituted for another as a means of allaying tension.
Denial—a primitive form of fantasy thinking in which unwanted realistic conditions are denied *Repression*—a derivative of denial in which unwanted memories are "forgotten"	Unpleasant thoughts are made unconscious. Both mechanisms are often considered basic to other defenses.
Projection—affect (such as anger) acknowledged but attributed to someone other than oneself *Displacement*—one's own affect acknowledged but attributed to some cause other than the real one	Perception of the source of danger is altered to make the situation seem safer.
Fixation—halt in personality development at a stage short of maturity *Regression*—retreat from a painful stage of personality development to an earlier, safer stage	Pervasive ego defenses retard personality development and preserve immaturity.
Reaction formation—adoption of an opposite attitude that counters an original feared impulse (that is, excessive gentleness wards off destructive impulses) *Undoing*—acting out of an opposite attitude to counter a feared impulse (compulsive hand washing to offset feeling of dirtiness) *Isolation*—separation of feeling from thoughts of an event (for example, a steeplejack's thoughts of falling are separated from his fear of it)	These defense mechanisms are sometimes considered to be supplementary to repression for the purpose of preventing the return to awareness of anxiety-provoking feelings.

*Compiled from data taken from Kessler, J., *Psychopathology of Childhood*. Englewood Cliffs, N.J.: Prentice-Hall, Inc. (1966).

The communication of the content of a message must obey rules of language. Semantic rules denote the meaning of symbols. Transformational and phrase structure rules determine word arrangement. Morphophonemic rules determine the arrangement of sounds in words as they are spoken. These rules provide the assurance that information transmitted by the speaker about the relation of one thing to another will be received by the listener, who decodes message content using the same rules. When any linguistic rule is violated, the message risks distortion. Reception of the idea communicated by way of the language system depends on close adherence to the formal arrangement of symbols in the linguistic code (Chapter 3).

But communication goes far beyond the content of what is said. The intent of the speaker is invariably embedded in his message—that is, the speaker desires to have a certain effect on the listener, such as admiration, sympathy, or awe. Intent is closer to connotative than to denotative meaning. It has to do with the essence of one's condition that is signaled, the state of his being as he exists. Words are far removed from existence, however. They identify the classes of objects that exist, never a single object. Because words are abstractions, they can never fully express one's intent.

Compare Maslow's (1949) distinction between coping and expressive behavior with Fearing's (1968) differentiation of intent from content.

The speaking system is probably better adapted to communicate intent than is the language system of symbols for several reasons. First, speaking processes permit a wider variety of individual expression than do symbolic processes. Message content can be preserved whether spoken high or low, loud or soft, strained or relaxed, fluently or disfluently, slowly or rapidly, with articulatory precision or with misarticulations. Garbled grammar or semantic selection of wrong words, on the other hand, can render the message meaningless or at best alter its content. Second, the intent of the communication is generally more urgent than content. The content of speech is comprised of abstract symbols that may require extended periods of digestion before their effects can be seen. Because a speaker's intent is to evoke an effect in his listener, he generally seeks immediate feedback—hence the merit of a signal system uniquely suited to urgent communication (Chapter 3). Third, the form of communication used earliest in development is a vocal signal system of crying, yelling, and screaming, often accompanied by gestures. A prelinguistic system without the capacity for transmitting symbolic message content, it functions exclusively to demand attention to pressing needs of the moment (Chapter 4).

Emotional disturbance and the confluence of speech and personality development. Personality development is marked by the emergence of a sense of identity. Threat to it is experienced as anxiety. As Hayakawa (1962) observed: "The fundamental motive of human behavior is not self-preservation, but preservation of the symbolic self." Thus personality development is an emotional process; the ego must mediate between reality and conflicting *psychodynamic* forces of id and superego. To preserve identity the ego must develop techniques for obtaining satisfying responses from important persons in one's world. The alternative is to develop defensive mechanisms with which the ego can protect itself from having to confront failures in effecting satisfactory impact on the world.

The earliest means available to the in-

fant of making his presence felt is vocal. It is his operant system for signaling intent. Even as an adult, when he can symbolize his emotion in message content, vocal signals will remain a major means of communicating feelings (Davitz and Davitz, 1959). Throughout development—indeed, throughout life—one must be able to signal for a listener the type of response desired irrespective of message content. The speaking system is comprised of vocal components used for this purpose from birth, and their use is integrally associated with ego development. Also, articulatory and speech-flow components of the mature speaking system permit freedom of expression of intent without serious distortion of message content.

Here we arrive at the crux of the proposed relation between speech and personality. With the speaking system one can signal intent as a superscript to the content of a spoken message that affirms or negates it, that demands, petitions, cajoles, persuades, or soothes the listener. If the signal system learned utilizes articulatory, phonatory, or speech-flow processes of the speaking system in ways judged to be abnormal, the result would be defective speech. The more that techniques for signaling intent are utilized in conjunction with ego defenses that reduce anxiety, the more strongly they would be

---

What does Harlow (1954) have to say about the importance of anxiety as a human motivation? What is Pribram's (1967) explanation of the biology of emotion?

---

negatively reinforced, and the more resistant they would be to modification. Thus speaking system defects are generally associated with neurotic adjustments, although rhythm analyses have revealed differences among more serious forms of psychopathology (Dreher and Bachrach, undated). As for the relation of the language system to personality, only when ideational processes are disturbed would symbolization of content be distorted; thus they are typically associated with psychotic adjustments.

Speaking process disorders

Now let us focus on the components of the speaking process to determine more specifically how they are affected by personality and emotional disturbances.

Articulatory-resonatory processes. Rousey (1971), noting the parallel development of primitive drives, ego functions, and speech, has hypothesized the significance of specific vowel and consonant defects. He reasoned that because vowels are predominant during the first 6 months of life, during which primitive effects dominate psychologic existence, vowels are auditory manifestations of drives. Similarly, since consonants appear during the development of perception, awareness, and adaptive and defensive devices, the use of consonants reflects ego development. Thus Rousey sees a general relationship in which the development of consonants describes mastery of instinctual life, whereas difficulty with vowels indicates an immature struggle with primitive drives. Viewing consonantal mastery as an indicator of stages of emotional maturation, he proposes that consonants reflect oral, anal, and phallic periods of psychosexual development according to their time of acquisition.

In an earlier study, Rousey and Moriarty (1965) set up a group of working assumptions, seven of which concerned the significance to personal adjustment of consonantal misarticulations: (1) a frontal lisp is associated with a pregenital level of personality development, (2) a lateral lisp indicates excessive narcissism, (3) a whistle /s/ reflects anxiety, (4) substitutions of /ʒ/ for /ɝ/ and /w/ for /r/ indicate difficulty with impulse control, (5) substitutions of /f/ for /θ/ and /v/ for /ð/ reflect difficulty in the father-child relationship, (6) substitution of /d/ for /ð/ is associated with repressed expression of anger, and (7) distortion of /l/ or substitution of /w/ for it reflects deprivation of early oral needs. Twenty-four children were seen for separate psychiatric and speech examinations. Articulatory performances were evaluated according to working assumptions to arrive at postdictions about personal adjustment that could be compared with psychiat-

ric results. When all working assumptions were lumped together, 83% were accurate. Granted, after-the-fact statements that are supported are weaker than supported predictive statements, in part because for postdiction the possibility cannot be altogether excluded that foreknowledge somehow influenced the results. Even so, systematic postdictions are more convincing by an order of magnitude than uncontrolled clinical observations.

Phonatory processes. Considerably more attention has been given to the relation of personality to voice, which has been discussed extensively in the medical and speech pathology literature, than to articulation. Moses (1954) even titled a book after the problem: *The Voice of Neurosis.* Most discussion of the emotional aspects of voice problems centers more around mute, whispered, and intermittently phonated-whispered speech than around continually phonated speech. The less favored traditional labels for these psychogenic problems are *hysterical aphonia, spastic dysphonia, ventricular dysphonia,* and *functional hoarseness.* The preferred term is *functional dysphonia* or *aphonia* (Aronson, Peterson, and Litin, 1964, 1966; Brodnitz, 1969).

Aronson and his colleagues (1966) did a psychiatric study of twenty-seven functionally aphonic or dysphonic patients and found consistently related situational conflicts that vocal problems resolved at least temporarily. Although none showed serious psychopathology, all gave evidence of a *conversion reaction* (a physical symptom unjustified by physiologic pathology). To a lesser extent the group fitted a *hysterical* type of character (a loosely used term centering around inadequate sexual adjustment), thereby giving some credence to the widely held explanation of functional aphonia as a symptom of *conversion hysteria* (Brodnitz, 1969).

Evidence that voice need not be grossly defective to be affected by personal adjustment can be seen in two studies. In one, three personality types showed three different voice quality profiles (Markel, 1969). In the other, a portion of the Rousey and

Moriarty study (1965), five working assumptions about voice were set up: (1) persistent hoarseness indicates socially distorted sexual identification and functioning, (2) deviation from culturally accepted pitch levels is associated with distorted sexual identity, (3) restricted vocal pitch range indicates constricted expression of sexual drive, (4) breathy voice indicates repressed or denied sexuality, and (5) harshness and nasality express aggression. As with their articulatory evidence, they had insufficient data to test the working assumptions separately. With their postdictions pooled, however, twenty-one out of twenty-three were accurate—again, substantial evidence of the relation of personality to the speaking process.

Speech-flow processes. No other aspect of speech has produced such vigorous and heated controversy about its psychodynamic significance as has the major problem of speech-flow, stuttering. The literature on this topic alone would fill a book. In fact, it has (Murphy and FitzSimons, 1958). A label has even been applied to the ever-expanding collection of theories that posit stuttering as a symptomatic expression of personality disturbance, the *repressed need* theories. Despite persistent interest in the problem, all efforts to demonstrate unique personality characteristics in the stutterer that distinguish him from the nonstutterer have come to naught. True, some studies have shown the relations that experimenters sought, but conflicting results from other studies plus methodologic errors have negated conclusions that could be drawn either way. Dissonance between the clinician and the re-

Compare the conclusions about personality differences between stutterers and nonstutterers reached by Bloodstein and Schreiber (1957), Goodstein (1958), and Sheehan (1958). Do they agree? Do they support psychoanalytic concepts?

searcher is great when it comes to their cognitions about the personalities of stutterers. Clinicians, who work psychotherapeutically, remain convinced that they are observing evidence of personality conflicts; yet re-

searchers have been unable to substantiate it.

Have investigators asked the wrong questions? Perhaps. Comparing stutterers who are supposed to be compulsive with college students who are likely to be compulsive if they are to succeed in school has merely told us that neither group is importantly different one from the other. Have the wrong measures been used? Perhaps. None of the projective and attitude instruments commonly used are noted for reliability or validity. Have the clinicians observed only evidence that confirms their theory? Perhaps. The temptation is always great to see what one wishes to see, and clinical conditions are generally not conducive to observational safeguards. We can conclude only that the issue remains open. The evidence does not require that we accept or reject a connection between stuttering and personality.

Lacking substantive evidence that requires one explanation over another, theories have proliferated. We will only sample them for the essence of how fluency may be functionally related to personality. As might be expected, the most explicit formulation comes from psychoanalysis. Glauber (1958) defined stuttering as a *pregenital conversion neurosis.* "Pregenital" identifies the level of psychosexual development at which personality is

Do psychoanalysts and psychiatrists agree in their explanations of stuttering? Compare Glauber's account with Barbara's (1962), Blanton's (1965), Fenichel's (1945), and Bluemel's (1957).

fixated: a *pregenital* level. Presumably unable to complete a successful identification that would permit progress to a mature genital level, the child *regresses* to an earlier and safer stage of development. "Conversion neurosis" identifies the manner in which the neurotic conflict is converted from an unconscious psychic form to overt physical expression. All conflicting forces—ego, id, and superego—are manifested in the expression. The conflict is between speaking and not speaking.

Because early stages of speech development coincide with the terminal phase of the oral stage of psychosexual development, speech activities are associated with not only oral but also anal, phallic, and, if it is reached, genital levels of development. Thus speech partakes of all of the archaic, instinctual, and sometimes unrealistic symbolism of the primitive levels, as well as of the logical, rational functions of the higher levels. When the ego regresses from a genital to a pregenital fixation, it permits id expression of instinctual impulses and superego prohibitions of them at the more primitive level to which it reverts. Stuttering, then, as a pregenital conversion neurosis is an unconscious symptomatic expression in speech of the conflict between the id (seeking release of erotic and aggressive impulses in a phallic, an anal, or an oral manner) and the ego and superego as they attempt to thwart this release through the act of speech—all of which is superimposed on the stutterer's volitional efforts to carry on a sensible, logical discourse.

The type of clinical evidence from which psychoanalytic theories have been constructed has been presented vividly by Travis (1971). Viewed in this framework, stuttering signals what he described as endless nostal-

---

Consider the explanation by Wyatt and Herzan (1962) of stuttering as the result of a developmental crisis in mother-child relationships. Compare it with Perkins' (1965) proposal that stuttering develops to help the child cope with covert rejection and threatened loss of personal impact. Do these concepts explain stuttering as a conversation reaction?

---

gia for "culturally disavowed, biologically rooted pleasures of sucking, eating, evacuating, and exploring." Such would be the primitive intent expressed if stuttering is indeed a conversion symptom. On the other hand, disfluency may develop as an operant technique for signaling listener attention. Whatever the answer, enough alternate explanations are possible to leave the relation of personality to disfluency veiled in uncertainty.

Language process disorders

Language processes are much more likely to be distorted by psychosis than neurosis.

Although semantic aspects of language may be affected by neurosis, so many talk so much nonsense so much of the time that our culture is exceedingly lenient in the range of linguistic meanings it will accept as normal. One has to be out of the ball park, semantically, before he is excluded from the daily game of interpersonal communication. When his personality is so deteriorated as to disrupt structural aspects of language—especially syntax, about which society is intolerant—he not only is out of the ball park but probably is in the psychiatric ward of a hospital.

In young children especially, our rule of thumb that links speaking process disorders with neurosis, not psychosis, has many exceptions. Psychosis in childhood is generally accompanied by a wide range of communicative disorders, none of which could be called typical. Phonemic, morphemic, syntactic, and semantic disorders can be found. Speaking defects of rate, rhythm, vocal pitch, loudness, and quality may occur. Speech may be severely retarded from the beginning, it may develop normally and then regress to primitive levels with onset of psychosis, or it may cease to be used for communication. The child may have a large vocabulary but fail to combine words into sentences. He may be hypersensitive or totally oblivious to sound (Shervanian, 1967).

In an extensive review, Baltaxe and Simmons (1975) tentatively concluded that language development is more deviant than delayed in childhood psychosis, especially in the autistic type. These children seem able to decode the phonetic surface structure of language well enough to repeat it verbatim. This ability seems to be basic to their abundant *echolalic* responses. What they are not able to do is to detect functional relationships, which is fundamental to recognition of the subject/predicate relationship in a sentence and to the use of language to understand and express meaning. Their inability to make sense of what they hear is probably the reason that the best response they can often manage is echolalic. If a general underlying cognitive deficit is basic to autism, it would tie in with their typical inability to form object relationships, and their insistence on rigidly stereotyped behavior.

In psychotic adults, older children, and adolescents, language difficulties reflect the predominant nature of the symptom as well as the underlying dynamics of the psychotic adjustment. For example, manic symptoms are reflected in an erratically directed stream of ideas that flows out in speech incessantly and rapidly; they come out slurred and telegraphically, with connecting words omitted. A listener is merely an object on whom the manic person dumps his load of verbiage; the listener is not a person with whom to com-

---

Vetter (1969) provides an extensive review of language behavior in psychosis.

---

municate. Depressive symptoms, on the other hand, show up in slow utterance of a retarded flow of ideas, frequently verbalized over and over.

The disordered language of the schizophrenic individual has several typical features. It is as though he turns his abstractions about the world inside out to avoid, as Ruesch (1957) says, sharing "with others his private system of symbolization." He will often use concrete terms for abstract concepts, and general terms for concrete objects. When he says "fork" he may be symbolizing the whole idea of eating and meals, whereas when he says "food" he may be referring to a specific fork. Likewise, he is inclined to use approximate terms for precise ones and to think in almost dreamlike associations: "wagon" may mean train, "boat" may mean water. The following excerpt of a reply to the question, "Why are you in the hospital?" is typical of psychotic speech: "I'm a cut donator, donated by double sacrifice. I get two days for every one. That's known as double sacrifice; in other words, standard cut donator. You know, we considered it. He couldn't have anything for the cut, or for these patients. . . ." (Cameron, 1947).

We cannot be certain whether these language distortions are used purposefully by the schizophrenic patient as red herrings

dragged across the listener's path to prevent understanding and human closeness, or whether, as Eisenson, Auer, and Irwin (1963) suggest, these distortions may be what would happen to the speech of any of us if we operated long enough under high enough stress and anxiety to turn away from social relationships. If the schizophrenic individual is attempting to grapple with anxiety by disconnecting himself from society, then he need not be concerned with logical discourse —his speech is but unmonitored free association unintended for human ears. He is thinking aloud.

SPEECH PATHOLOGIST'S RESPONSIBILITY IN TREATMENT OF PERSONALITY AND EMOTIONAL DISTURBANCES
Responsibility for referral

Traditionally, speech pathologists have limited their responsibility to defective communicative functions. Within this tradition, they have typically referred persons suspected of complicated or complicating emotional and personality problems to psychiatrists and clinical psychologists for diagnosis and treatment. When in doubt, whether because of the complexity of the problem, professional competence, or community restrictions, this course is the most prudent one to follow. Referral, however, does not necessarily terminate ethical responsibility for a patient. The speech pathologist remains responsible for making certain that his referral was properly helpful, for integrating further treatment of any communicative disorder with the program of treatment for which referred, or for retaining primary responsibility for continued therapy, with appropriate consultation for the mental health problem.

Responsibility for consultation

Psychiatric examinations include routine appraisal of speech. Psychiatrists and psychologists are specialists in conditions of the psyche; they may not be equally skilled in observing the fine detail of linguistic and speaking abilities. Yet their judgment may rest, lightly or heavily, on impressions of this behavior. A speech pathologist skilled in such observation can be of inestimable value as a consultant in problems of mental health —especially if some of the connections discussed between speech and personality prove valid. Speaking behavior would then provide explicit clues to psychologic adjustment. The better able the speech pathologist is to appraise oral communication with precision, and the better able he is to understand the conceptual framework within which mental health specialists will fit his information, the greater will be his consultative value.

Responsibility for therapy

A definitive statement of a speech pathologist's responsibility for therapy of emotional and personality disturbances would have as many qualifying clauses as Joseph's coat had colors. Three major considerations are involved: the extent of the disability, the scope of the speech pathologist's preparation and competence, and the established practice within the community. States vary in legal restrictions as to who can do what to whom. Some permit only psychiatrists to utilize psychotherapeutic procedures, whereas other states are more lenient. Some communities in some states with lenient legal limits are, by tradition, jealously restrictive of who is permitted into the inner sanctum of psychotherapeutic practice. As Professor Hill says in *The Music Man:* "You have to know the territory."

Speech pathologists vary widely in their preparation and competence for assuming responsibility for the treatment of mental health problems. A few speech pathologists are also psychiatrists. Some are physicians. Many are clinical psychologists. Some are licensed to practice in their state. Some have the scope of their competence certified by professional organizations; they have the trappings of practitioners to whom people with psychic hurts can turn with confidence for healing. But many speech pathologists hold none of these trappings, and yet by training and experience consider themselves competent. What of them? The answer is that until they obtain the necessary diploma, license, or certificate, their solutions will generally be makeshift. Some may arrange for a formal psychiatric consultant, whereas others may utilize such consultation informally. Still others may try it alone—a rather risky arrangement. Many speech pathologists, however, do not include the responsibility for treating mental health problems within their jurisdiction. They do not deny the existence, importance, or relevance of personality and emotional disturbances to communication—only the propriety of their involvement. They constitute the speech pathologists most likely to refer such problems for treatment.

Probably the ultimate determination of responsibility for the therapy of psychic difficulty is the severity of the problem. Psychosis generally requires confinement; obviously, primary responsibility for treatment is a medical problem. Neurosis involves consistent failure to find effective solutions to certain problems of living. Alteration of the personality sufficiently to resolve neurotic conflict is usually thought to require psychotherapy, often extending for years. The clinician, in effect, assumes responsibility for parenthood (even if the neurotic patient is an adult) and continues the job of raising the patient. Many emotional disturbances, however, are transitory. They do not necessarily reflect the functioning of an immature personality; rather, they can represent temporary failure to find a successful solution to a specific important problem—be it an affair of the heart, the pocketbook, or the business. Most speech pathologists are capable of the counseling that would be helpful in such situations.

The problem that must be faced is how to recognize the nature of the disability before becoming entangled in it. Unfortunately, the less prepared the speech pathologist is to deal with emotional problems, the less prepared he will be to distinguish early evidence of the treacherous from the trivial disorder. Some mental disturbances have deep roots, others shallow, but they can look much the same on the surface. To refer every patient who presents evidence of disturbance for psychologic evaluation would probably mean referring almost every patient. The alternative is adequate preparation of speech pathologists to recognize danger signs for mental health; referrals could then be made when appropriate.

The question with which we will close is the question that has prevailed throughout this chapter: "What is the relationship between disruption in communication and disruption in emotion and personality?" Obviously, if one does not affect the other, then speech pathologists could tend their garden of communicative skills without bothering very much about the brier patch of their mental health neighbors. But what if they do affect each other? How can their treatment be separated and still offer the patient the help to which he is entitled?

Certainly, if speech problems cause emotional problems, remediation of the speech disorder would make sense as good therapy for the consequent emotional distress. If these two types of problems are related by association more than by causation, perhaps an even broader case can be made for separating therapy for them. At present, the ground on which delimitation of a speech pathologist's responsibility for therapy rests is too soft for the erection of a solid conclusion. Were it solid, it would not preclude the ideal speech pathologist's being a therapeutic man for all seasons.

The answers—résumé

1. What is the nature of personality and emotional disturbances that affect speech?

Although specific speech disorders cannot be attributed with confidence to specific types of psychopathology, still, speech problems do appear among all the major groups of personality and emotional disturbances. In neurosis, personality illness does not involve impairment of the ego function of reality-testing so much as impairment of control of the motor apparatus. By contrast, psychosis is distinguished by grossly distorted perception of and response to reality. Personality disturbance in a character disorder, on the other hand, is acted out overtly. Thus the various types of neurotic and psychotic adjustments are characterized by symptoms, whereas character disorders are marked by observable behavioral difficulties. The major groups of psychosomatic disorders are distinguished by symptoms with physiologic bases to which emotional conflicts contribute.

2. How do personality and emotional disturbances affect speech?

Development of personality and development of the speech system (with which the speaker's intent is signaled) and the language system (with which message content is symbolized) proceed concurrently and undoubtedly interact. If the signal system learned utilizes articulatory, phonatory, or speech-flow processes of the speaking system in ways judged as abnormal, the result would be defective speech. The more that speaking techniques for signaling intent are utilized in conjunction with ego defenses that reduce anxiety, the more strongly they are negatively reinforced. Whereas speaking system defects are generally associated with neurotic adjustments, symbolic defects of language are more disrupted by ideational disturbances of psychosis.

3. What is the speech pathologist's responsibility in the treatment of personality and emotional disturbances?

This question may be subdivided into issues of responsibility for referral, consultation, and therapy. The choice to provide therapy or to refer to a competent specialist in mental health problems rests on three considerations: the extent of the disability, the speech pathologist's preparation and competence for treating problems of mental health, and the established legal and professional practices within the community. As for consultation, the issue is unambiguous: many psychodiagnostic decisions involve judgments of speech about which speech pathologists should be prepared to contribute expert appraisals.

REFERENCES

American Psychiatric Association, *Diagnostic and statistical manual: mental disorders* (1962).

Aronson, A., Peterson, H., and Litin, E., Voice symptomatology in functional dysphonia and aphonia. *J. Speech Hearing Dis.*, **29**, 367-380 (1964).

Aronson, A., Peterson, H., and Litin, E., Psychiatric symptomatology in functional dysphonia and aphonia. *J. Speech Hearing Dis.*, **31**, 115-127 (1966).

Baltaxe, C., and Simmons, J., Language in childhood psychosis: a review. *J. Speech Hearing Dis.*, **40**, 439-458 (1975).

Barbara, D., *The Psychotherapy of Stuttering.* Springfield, Ill.: Charles C Thomas, Publisher (1962).

Bartak, L., and Rutter, M., The use of personal pronouns by autistic children. *J. Autism child. Schizo.* **4**, 217-222 (1974).

Blanton, S., Stuttering. In Barbara, D. (Ed.), *New Directions in Stuttering.* Springfield, Ill.: Charles C Thomas, Publisher (1965).

Bloodstein, O., and Schreiber, L., Obsessive-compulsive reactions in stutterers. *J. Speech Hearing Dis.*, **22**, 33-39 (1957).

Bluemel, C., *The Riddle of Stuttering.* Danville, Ill.: The Interstate Printers & Publishers, Inc. (1957).

Brodnitz, F., Functional aphonia. *Ann. Otol. Rhinol. Laryng.*, **78**, 1244-1253 (1969).

Cameron, N., *The Psychology of Behavior Disorders: a Biosocial Interpretation.* Boston: Houghton Mifflin Co. (1947).

Churchill, D., The relation of infantile autism and early childhood schizophrenia to developmental language disorders of childhood. *J. Autism child. Schizo.*, **2**, 182-197 (1972).

Coleman, J., *Abnormal Psychology and Modern Life.* Chicago: Scott, Foresman & Co. (1956).

Davitz, J., and Davitz, L., The communication of feelings by content-free speech. *J. Commun.*, **9**, 6-13 (1959).

Dreher, J., and Bachrach, A., Power spectral density: a methodology for the rhythm analysis of disordered speech. In Sankar, D. (Ed.), *Schizophrenia: Current Concepts and Research.* Hicksville, N.Y.: PJD Publications (undated).

Eisenson, J., Auer, J., and Irwin, J., *The Psychology of Communication.* New York: Appleton-Century-Crofts (1963).

Escalona, S., *The Roots of Individuality.* Chicago: Aldine Publishing Co. (1968).

Fearing, F., Toward a psychological theory of human communication. In Barnlund, D. (Ed.), *Interpersonal Communication: Survey and Studies.* Boston: Houghton Mifflin Co. (1968).

Fenichel, O., *The Psychoanalytic Theory of Neurosis.* New York: W. W. Norton & Co., Inc. (1945).

Glauber, I., The psychoanalysis of stuttering. In Eisenson, J. (Ed.), *Stuttering: a Symposium.* New York: Harper & Row, Publishers (1958).

Goodstein, L., Functional speech disorders and personality: a survey of the research. *J. Speech Hearing Res.*, **1**, 359-376 (1958).

Harlow, H., Motivational forces underlying learning. In *Learning Theory, Personality Theory, and Clinical Research, the Kentucky Symposium.* New York: John Wiley & Sons, Inc. (1954).

Hayakawa, S., Conditions of success in communication. *Bull. Menninger Clinic*, **26**, 225-236 (1962).

Hofling, C., and Leininger, M., *Basic Psychiatric Concepts in Nursing.* Philadelphia: J. B. Lippincott Co. (1960).

Kessler, J., Psychopathology of childhood. Englewood Cliffs, N.J.: Prentice-Hall, Inc. (1966).

Markel, N., Relationship between voice-quality profiles and MMPI profiles in psychiatric patients. *J. abnorm. Psychol.*, **74**, 61-66 (1969).

Maslow, A., The expressive component of behavior. *Psychol. Rev.*, **56**, 261-272 (1949).

Mischel, W., Continuity and change in personality. *Am. Psychol.*, **24**, 1012-1018 (1969).

Moses, P., *The Voice of Neurosis.* New York: Grune & Stratton, Inc. (1954).

Murphy, A., and FitzSimons, R., *Stuttering and Per-*

sonality Dynamics. New York: The Ronald Press Co. (1958).

Ornitz, E., and Ritvo, E., Neurophysiologic mechanisms underlying perceptual inconstancy in autistic and schizophrenic children. *Arch. gen. Psychiat.,* **19,** 22-27 (1968a).

Ornitz, E., and Ritvo, E., Perceptual inconstancy in early infantile autism. *Arch. gen. Psychiat.,* **18,** 76-98 (1968b).

Ornitz, E., and others, The EEG and rapid eye movements during REM sleep in normal and autistic children. *Electroencephalography clin. Neurophysiol.,* **26,** 167-175 (1969).

Perkins, W., Stuttering: some common denominators. In Barbara, D. (Ed.), *New Directions in Stuttering.* Springfield, Ill.: Charles C Thomas, Publisher (1965).

Pribram, K., The new neurology and the biology of emotion: a structural approach. *Am. Psychol.* **22,** 830-838 (1967).

Rousey, C., The psychopathology of articulation and voice deviations. In Travis, L. (Ed.), *Handbook of Speech Pathology and Audiology.* New York: Appleton-Century-Crofts (1971).

Rousey, C., *Psychiatric Assessment by Speech and Hearing Behavior.* Springfield, Ill.: Charles C Thomas, Publisher (1974).

Rousey, C., and Moriarty, A., *Diagnostic Implications of Speech Sounds.* Springfield, Ill.: Charles C Thomas, Publishers (1965).

Ruesch, J., *Disturbed Communication.* New York: W. W. Norton & Co., Inc. (1957).

Rutter, M., and Bartak, L., Causes of infantile autism: some considerations from recent research. *J. Autism child. Schizo.,* **1,** 20-32 (1971).

Sheehan, J., Projective studies of stuttering. *J. Speech Hearing Dis.,* **23,** 18-25 (1958).

Shervanian, C., Speech, thought, and communication disorders in childhood psychoses. *J. Speech Hearing Dis.,* **32,** 303-313 (1967).

Sorosky, A., and others, Systematic observations of autistic behavior. *Arch. gen. Psychiat.,* **18,** 439-449 (1968).

Travis, L., The unspeakable feelings of people with special reference to stuttering. In Travis, L. (Ed.), *Handbook of Speech Pathology and Audiology.* New York: Appleton-Century-Crofts (1971).

Vetter, H., *Language Behavior and Psychopathology.* Chicago: Rand McNally & Co. (1969).

Wing. J., Diagnosis, epidemiology, aetiology. In Wing, J. (Ed.), *Early Childhood Autism: Clinical, Educational and Social Aspects.* Oxford, New York: Pergamon Press (1966).

Wing, L., and Wing, J., Multiple impairments in early childhood autism. *J. Autism child. Schizo.,* **1,** 256-266 (1971).

Wyatt, G., and Herzan, H., Therapy with stuttering children and their mothers. *Am. J. Orthopsychiatry,* **32,** 645-659 (1962).

Applications of
speech pathology

Part III

Disorders of speech

Part III implements another aspect of the central theme of speech pathology as an applied behavioral science: that modification of defective speech requires explicit identification of what is wrong as well as what is right. In Part I, we analyzed the processes and development of language and speaking to determine goals toward which to work for acceptable speech. In Part II, disabilities that can limit the acquisition of normal speech or disrupt it once acquired were explored. Now, in Part III, behavioral characteristics of defective language and speaking will be considered.

Chapter 11

Disorders of language

Questions

1. In what ways can language development be impaired?
2. With what disabilities is delayed language development associated?
3. What are the characteristics of aphasia?
4. With what disabilities are aphasic disorders associated?
5. What is the nature of nonstandard English of disadvantaged children?

Language is more than a useful tool that facilitates communication; more than a collection of individual traits, each independent of the other; more than an appendage tacked onto man by evolution that, if removed, would reduce him to the level of animals. It is a species-specific ability that permeates the crevices of his performance, altering him more profoundly than Shakespeare altered the most routine plot he borrowed for his plays. It is neither an effect nor a cause of cognition; it is at the core of how man apprehends his world. Not a static product of the mind, it is the dynamic manifestation of the functioning of his brain. Every level of language—phonemic, morphemic, syntactic,

and semantic—facilitates the discrimination of relations among classes of objects and among objects as they belong to different classes.

A fundamental function of any language is to represent symbolically the relationships observed in the real world. The other basic function is to provide symbolic referents (e.g., words) to represent objects, situations, ideas, feelings, and so on as they are experienced. This semantic function goes far beyond mere labeling. Words used meaningfully are heavy with connotation. Consider "grief." If you have experienced it, the word may still resonate so strongly for you as to bring tears. So in the broadest sense, a dis-

233

order of language affects either or both of these basic functions. It impairs the ability to discriminate relationships. It limits the ability to think.

Lang Disorder [handwritten margin note]

This chapter will be an exploration of disorders of language. Processes of speech have been divided into those of language and those of speaking. The separation is arbitrary. The production of speech sounds is carried out under the direction of linguistic rules. In order not to disconnect phonemic rules from their phonetic realization, problems of phonology will be analyzed in Chapter 12. Here let us consider those children whose language acquisition has been delayed or distorted, aphasic individuals who have lost some part of the language they once had, and those groups whose nonstandard speech differs from the dominant language of the community.

DELAYED LANGUAGE: IMPAIRMENT OF DEVELOPMENT

What can we say of the child whose language has not developed normally? That he is mentally retarded? Aphasic? Brain-injured? Deaf? Autistic? All these terms have been applied. They are loosely suggestive of etiologic conditions that affect language acquisition. Difficulties arise, however, in the differential diagnosis of these disorders. Fortunately for speech pathologists, such difficulties are not his primary responsibility. Problems of diagnosing somatic disabilities that can contribute to language impairment are mainly in the province of medicine. As Wood (1964) stresses: "Each specialist must stick to his specialty."

The speech pathologist is vitally interested in diagnostic issues, but they are of practical importance to him only insofar as they provide clues for the facilitation of language acquisition. Furthermore, it is in this realm that he makes his unique contribution to diagnosis. His is the responsibility for the accurate description of linguistic performance. The more that is learned of the complexities of language, the more intricate and demanding this responsibility becomes.

Characteristics of delayed language

Describing the characteristics of delayed language is quite a different matter from describing the characteristics of the child with delayed language. These children may be distractible and easily frustrated; have short attention span generally and poor retention for speech specifically; perseverate in what they say; show little creativity, imagination, or self-criticism; show little ability to perceive and organize stimuli; and have problems of learning, behavior, and hearing. These difficulties may be as urgently in need

Do Wood (1964), Myklebust (1957), and Schlanger (1967) present essentially the same descriptions of children with language problems? Do these descriptions differ as the causes of their problems differ?

of attention as the language disorder. Indeed, they may contribute to the language disorder, or the language disorder may contribute to these difficulties; all may stem one way or another from disabling conditions within the child, or within the environment, or both. The language-handicapped child presents a confusing picture.

How can the speech pathologist be of most help? Certainly not by adjusting his professional "blinders" to see only the child's speech and miss how defective communication skills fit with other problems, possibly as consequence, possibly as cause. The speech pathologist must contribute vital information about the condition of language behavior to the diagnosis that will guide medical treatment. At the same time, while holding a clear view of speech acquisition as an interrelated facet of the whole process of biologic and psychologic development, the speech pathologist must have expert knowledge of his trade.

Description of delayed language. What is needed is a description of the child's knowledge of how language works. Put grossly, this knowledge is reflected earliest in his understanding of the speech he hears and, to a lesser extent, in his first attempts to speak. Put specifically, in terms of the mechanics of how a language operates, it is reflected semantically in his ability to find the common

What does Deese (1969) have to say about all that is implied when we "understand" the meaning of a word? Is understanding exclusively a linguistic phenomenon?

features of objects that the meaning of a word denotes, thus enabling him to correctly name things never encountered before. It is reflected *phonemically* in the ability to detect the fact that words with different speech sounds have different meanings. It is reflected *grammatically* in the ability to extract relations among ideas as they are signaled by word classes. (rules)

In this grammatical knowledge the rules of language are the dominant issue. The child's knowledge of how grammar works is reflected *morphologically* in his ability to detect appropriate grammatical categories of words from a vocabulary pool of morphophonemic units. It is reflected *syntactically* in his ability to recognize the organization of phrase-structure units that make grammatical sentences. It is reflected *transformationally* in the operational rules by which these grammatical units can be recognized as one type of sentence or another (Chapter 3).

Description of the ability to comprehend language has been stressed over the ability to produce it because comprehension is basic to production. Normal children understand speech before they can speak. Speech-handicapped children may have no trouble understanding language and yet be unable to produce it adequately. The converse condition, however, is apparently impossible: the child cannot produce language normally if he cannot understand it. The fact that the retarded child can imitate, with echolalia, statements he does not understand is evidence that development of his meaning system has not kept pace with development of the mechanics of his language. Still, the question of how cognitively involved children can learn at least a rudimentary grammar, with all its abstractions and complexities, and yet have far more difficulty learning to use their speech meaningfully is puzzling. Psycholinguists and cognitive theorists are coming more and more to the view that the

speech mechanism for learning the structure of a language, its syntax, is somehow separate from the semantic mechanism (Bruner, Olver, and Greenfield, 1967; Kavanagh and Cutting, 1975). The infant, by virtue of being human, is apparently endowed with the former mechanism, which will facilitate his acquisition of grammar. The latter mechanism, by which symbolic representations of the world are invested with meaning, is intricately involved with cognition. Apparently, this is a more complex operation to master; its functions are most typically affected when language acquisition is delayed (Schiefelbusch, 1972).

As Fig. 11-1 (compiled by Lenneberg [1966] from studies of fairly large samples of Austrian, British, and American children) shows, production of words, phrases, and sentences is so regular for normal children as to provide a fairly clear set of norms for assessing the adequacy of language development. A similar chart could be drawn that would show comprehension regularly preceding production.

The steepness of these curves shows clearly that most normal children pass these language acquisition milestones at about the same time. In other words, they suggest rather sharp divisions between children who develop language normally and those who are delayed. The vast majority of normal children speak words at 12 months, phrases at 18 months, and short syntactic sentences at 36 months. Of course, not all healthy children will meet this schedule; thus delay in speech acquisition does not necessarily mean impairment. Using developmental norms as the criterion, we therefore arrive at this definition: *delayed language is failure to understand or speak the language code of the community at a normal age*. This definition does not say why language is delayed, nor does it indicate whether the reason is pathologic; it merely specifies the condition of delay.

Can language development be accelerated? We come now to a crucial issue. Can a retarded rate of language development be accelerated? The answer apparently depends

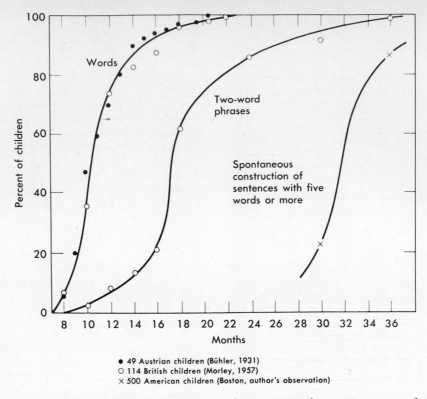

● 49 Austrian children (Bühler, 1931)
○ 114 British children (Morley, 1957)
× 500 American children (Boston, author's observation)

Fig. 11-1. Emergence of language acquisition milestones. Rapid acquisition rates of normal development makes retardation in these skills relatively apparent. (From Lenneberg, E., *Biological Foundations of Language.* New York: John Wiley & Sons, Inc. [1967].)

on the nature and severity of the conditions that impair it. We will examine those conditions next.

Lenneberg (1966, 1969) has assembled impressive evidence that links the stages of language development with physical maturation. Whereas language acquisition need not correlate well with chronologic age (if it did, we would not be concerned with delayed language), the correlation with motor development is remarkably high, even among retarded children (Lenneberg, Nichols, and Rosenberger, 1964). In fact, these courses of development run so parallel that children begin to speak no sooner and no later than when they reach a corresponding stage of physical maturation. Indeed, the parallel is so close that the capacity for language can probably be determined more accurately from motor milestones than from measures of speech de-

velopment. (Lenneberg argues that a child's real capacity for language may be obscured by factors that interfere with speech, such as congenital deafness, childhood schizophrenia, or a deficient environment.)

Following this line of reasoning further, the rate of acquisition of language is apparently impervious to social environment and to unsystematic efforts to hasten its development. It will even survive remarkably haphazard exposures to language—children of deaf parents and those in institutions whose only significant contact with speech is by watching television can manage to acquire language at rates that match their motor milestones. But the connection between motor and language development is apparently not direct; peripheral motor disabilities do not necessarily retard language acquisition. More probably, both reflect physical

— Sph/Motor development paralleled!

maturation of the brain, which apparently must reach about 65% of maturity before language begins (Chapter 4).

If capacity for acquiring language is biologically determined, where can hope be found for the language-handicapped child? Must he await advances in medical science that may eventually offer biochemical modes of treatment? Can nothing be done short of altering his genetic endowment? One thing is clear: such obvious procedures for trying to hasten speech as "motivating" him to talk, as rewarding him for babbling, or as having him imitate words or phrases or even sentences have little value in furthering acquisition of meaningful speech.

What, then, can be done? Innumerable prospects abound, but they have become visible only since the recent advent of psycholinguistics has brought language within the range of behavioral analysis. Extensive work is underway to obtain answers to such questions as the following: What prerequisite abilities (such as brain maturation and cognitive abilities) are essential to language readiness? Can techniques be developed (for instance, the Montessori method for developing motor and sensory skills) that will enhance these readiness abilities? Can the frequency of occurrence of functional units of language be increased by behavioral management procedures? Can the organization of these functional units into syntactic arrangements be facilitated by programming their sequence so that undergirding abilities are mastered prior to undertaking a new level of linguistic complexity? Although final answers are not yet in, those which have been produced hold promise.

Function and structure interact. Perhaps the greatest promise is pointed up when Lenneberg (1969) reminds us that the course of maturation is marked by progression through a sequence of *epigenetic* states. In each state, the child is capable of certain performances that determine to what and how he will respond. From interaction with the environment he develops into a new state that alters the interaction and leads to the development of additional new states.

Man's relation to his world, for instance, would be profoundly different if walking were not a state that developed from crawling.

This principle of epigenesis appears applicable to language, whether it has a biologic foundation or not. Assuming that the maturation of the brain sets the pace for language acquisition, there is evidence that the brain, much like a muscle, develops with exercise. If so, the problem is to determine the types of exercise that will prepare it for language. Viewed behaviorally, the same developmental principle holds. Children are sensitive to successively different aspects of language: they respond earliest to vocal inflections; then to articulatory distinctions that make word recognition possible; and then to extraction of the basic subject-predicate syntactic relation from which are differentiated morphophonemic rules, phrase-structure rules, and transformational rules. Normally, the ability to produce these linguistic distinctions in speech follows closely, but apparently it is not essential to develop each new stage of recognition.

Consider the possible function of semantic development in the delayed language of mentally retarded children. If they are handicapped not so much in ability to learn as in ability to retain what they learn, then the problem of acquiring language could be, at least in part, a problem of memory (Smith, 1959; Carroll, 1967). A moment of introspection while listening will reveal that you must hold all parts of a statement in mind (presumably in short-term memory) until it is finished before deciding whether or not you have heard a complete sentence. Much the same memory requirement holds for speaking. In fact, Carroll (1962) has found that one of the most predictive tests of a normal adult's ability to learn a foreign language is his ability to repeat nonsense syllables after a brief delay in which he does something else. Persons with low language aptitude can echo a pair of nonsense syllables immediately, but if, for example, they perform 10 seconds of mental arithmetic before repeating the nonsense syllables, they cannot remember them. Those of high language aptitude have no trouble.

The foregoing discussion of language aptitude relates to how words facilitate memory. It is also relevant to the work of Vygotsky (1962) and Luria (1961), who assume that children who have an inadequate vocabulary of meaningful words will be handicapped in thinking, remembering, and planning. Luria, for instance, reports an experiment in which children were asked to discriminate candy under covers with two different colors. Until the colors were named, the children had to relearn the discrimination each day. With names, the discrimination was learned two to three times as quickly and was preserved up to a week.

Disabilities associated with delayed language

Development of two fundamental functions of language can be affected. Acquisition of speech, the surface structure of language, can be impaired, so that the child does not use words to label objects and events, or does not assemble what words he does have into grammatical statements. The other functional impairment of cognition is evident when the surface structure is mastered to some extent, but the child has no concept of how to use speech to express ideas. His vocabulary consists of rote words and phrases uttered with little or no meaning.

If these two functions are as autonomous as evidence suggests, then they may reflect processes mediated by separate brain mechanisms (Chapter 5). Were this indeed the case, we would expect to find these two functions affected to the extent that those underlying brain mechanisms were affected. Were both mechanisms defective, both functions would be defective. Possibly, then, it is because these mechanisms are involved to one extent or another that the following conditions impair development of language.

Mental retardation. The speech of the mentally retarded illustrates the autonomy of the two functions of language that can be defective. Minimal mastery of surface structure does not require an IQ much above 50.

With a sophisticated training program, even some of the more severely retarded can acquire the mechanics of language. It is in impairment of the cognitive function of language to express meaning and to think abstractly that we find a correlation with intelligence. Mastery of speech by those who are only subnormal may even be exceptional. Their difficulty lies with the refinement of what they have to say more than with how they say it.

The course of language development for such severely retarded children as those who are afflicted with mongolism or microcephaly, on the other hand, will parallel the progress of their physical maturation, at least until puberty. By early adolescence, the brain has matured, and for unknown reasons, the propensity for learning language falls sharply (Chapter 9).

Puberty sets the ceiling on how far mentally retarded children can progress in speech acquisition. They will move through the regular stages of language development,

---

Does Jordan (1967), in his review of studies of language and mental retardation, include evidence that would alter the picture presented here?

---

but at a slower rate (Newfield and Schlanger, 1968). Whatever mental age they reach by adolescence will determine in large measure how far they will go. As they leave childhood, the acquisition rate will gradually decline until it comes to a complete halt in the early teens. If they progress as far as a mental age of 4 or 5 years, they should have reasonably normal language; if they reach a mental age of 2 years, they should have primitive rudiments of language; if below 2, they are likely to have almost none. Unfortunately, without special help, their linguistic condition will probably remain constant for life (Lenneberg, 1969).

From what has just been said of mentally retarded children, we can see that any disability that prevents normal language development prior to adolescence will effectively and permanently impair language. Thus the capacity to learn language is of practical value only prior to puberty. If it is not tapped during childhood, it will pass, sadly, as an unrealized potential advantage from which no profit was gained. Let us review briefly the disabilities that need not, but may if not corrected early, impair a child's ability to capitalize on his native capacity to learn language.

Deafness. No disability points up the importance of early intervention more than deafness. Children learn to listen and talk naturally without benefit of adult instruction; yet they must be taught to read and write. (Inability to learn to read is a related problem, called *developmental dyslexia*, but it is beyond the scope of this text.) Language capacity seems to be biologically linked to audition. It is little wonder that the congenitally deaf child, regardless of how much language capacity is suggested by his rate of physical maturation, will require special instruction if he is to learn speech. Ironically, he will have to learn it much as an adult would a second language. Even so, his progress will be much faster during childhood than after puberty (Chapter 4).

Moreover, the manner in which language participates in his cognitive maturation will be different from normal, even though the two specialized language mechanisms and their two basic functions, which we postulated, have a good chance of being intact. This is not to say that he will be intellectually impaired. But because he acquires language by instruction rather than by natural processes, and because whatever he does acquire is probably superimposed on, rather than being an integral part of, cognitive development, language will tend to operate differently in his thinking processes (Chapter 9). That his inner language is likely to be different is suggested by the different grammatical constructions he is inclined to use (Chapter 4).

Children with even a brief exposure to language before loss of hearing, though with problems similar to the congenitally deaf, will have less trouble learning it later by instruction. They will profit more if they acquired language prior to deafness, even though their speech subsequently deteriorates so much that they must relearn it in a school for the deaf (Lenneberg, 1969).

Congenital aphasia. Young children who seem normally intelligent, coordinated, and adjusted, with normal homes, yet who fail to develop language, give clearest evidence of being *congenitally* or *developmentally* *aphasic.* These more-or-less alternate terms are used for a form of the condition commonly called *childhood aphasia.* Nothing prohibits such children from being multiply handicapped; they may also be mentally retarded or cerebral palsied or have almost any other combination of afflictions. The aphasic component will then be more difficult to detect (Chase, 1972; Eisenson, 1968; Myklebust, 1971; Wood, 1964).

Wood (1969) discusses childhood aphasia in her monograph on verbal learning. What characteristics of this problem does she describe? Does Hardy (1965) describe the same characteristics?

Found alone, childhood aphasia is characterized by defective functioning of the auditory system. Little wonder that on first inspection, deafness is often suspected in these children. That the defect is due to neural damage is often not detected by neurologic examination but rather is inferred from the nature of the impaired auditory behavior. The fact that the child responds to environmental sounds, but not to speech, rules out the peripheral auditory mechanism as accounting for the problem. The child's difficulty is with auditory perception, memory, integration, and comprehension of speech. This condition is presumably caused by discrete damage to the specialized speech analysis equipment that has evolved largely in connection with the auditory system. The effect on language development is remarkably similar to that of deafness. Because the young child is unable to decode speech, he is unable to understand what he hears, and thus, of course, is also unable to learn to speak (Myklebust, 1971).

Acquired aphasia in children. Strictly speaking, children who have acquired some mastery of language prior to impairment by brain injury are not delayed in language development. Indeed, their problem is different from that of congenitally aphasic children, who have never known language. But even though the damage is in the same cortical areas that produce aphasia in adults, children with acquired aphasia, another form of childhood aphasia, differ from adult aphasics in some ways worth noting here.

One difference is in the effects of injury to the cortical speech areas. In adults, the effects differ according to location of the lesion, but in children the results of localized damage are not so differentiated. The most striking feature is the sharp reduction in the amount of speech used. Unlike all but the most severe adult aphasics, the child often becomes virtually mute. He is reluctant to communicate in any way, whether by speaking, writing, gesturing, or reading. When speech is used, it is usually sparse and telegraphic (Chase, 1972).

Another difference is in the child's remarkable ability to recover. Traumatic insults to speech areas of the brain that would surely render adults severely aphasic can be absorbed better by young children; the younger the child, the better the prognosis. Left hemisphere lesions in prelinguistic children under 2 years of age are possibly no more injurious than right hemisphere lesions. In fact, if injury occurs early enough, the normally dominant left hemisphere can be removed entirely, and the right hemisphere apparently will have the competence to take over language functions. Even children under 4 years of age who have language usually suffer only temporary setbacks by left hemisphere trauma. After a transient period of aphasia, they will often traverse again the stages of language development through which they have already passed. The prospect of recovery remains good until the early teens, at which time the effects of damage tend to remain permanently (Lenneberg, 1966, 1969).

Chase (1972) issues a note of caution, however, about an overly optimistic prognosis. Although children do recover more readily

than adult aphasics, this rapid improvement is usually measured by their increase in speech output. What may not recover so readily is their ability to comprehend such nuances of language as are involved in humor and sarcasm, or to use language as a tool of thought and imagination.

Autism. The psychotic child, a generic label for the *autistic child*, characteristically shows abnormalities of language reminiscent of the aphasic child, but his disorder is generally considered to be more pervasive and profound. Autistic children, whose impairment begins prior to 30 months of age, are aloof, relate more to objects than to people, and avoid physical contact. All of their behavior is depersonalized. These characteristics, understandably, are especially distressing to their mothers. They engage in repetitive, stereotyped, self-stimulatory activity; they may bang their heads so long and so hard as to injure themselves. Their thinking is concrete; they have difficulty with abstractions. Disturbance of language may take the form of mutism, echolalia, or delayed development, and if speech does exist, its usage may be idiosyncratic in word selection, expression, and content. They are generally able to label objects and situations, but not to use language in terms of recognizing or describing functional relationships. The autistic child seems unable to use speech as a vehicle for meaningful communication of ideas (Baltaxe and Simmons, 1975).

Yet these children, if not multiply handicapped with other disabilities such as mental retardation, are generally conceded to be much brighter than they appear. They often have remarkable ability to learn. What accounts for this peculiar pattern of deficits is still an open debate. The parent-infant relationship has long been implicated, and it is certainly not precluded by the growing body of evidence pointing to brain injury. That the damage is not characteristically in the cortical speech areas is suggested by the prevalence of echolalic responses, some of which show evidence of grammatical competence (Chase, 1972).

Research in England is pointing to at least

part of the basis for the effects of autism on language. Hermelin (1971) has shown in a series of experiments that autistic children have no difficulty with immediate auditory memory. They do as well with immediate recall of a series of random words as do normal children. But they do no better when those words are organized into sentences. Their difficulty is in processing temporally structured information. Grammatical organization of words is not helpful to their grasp of what has been said. Moreover, this trouble with patterned information is a generalized cognitive impairment. It affects processing of visual as well as auditory material. It may explain, too, why the echolalic responses Fay (1969) describes are so characteristic of autism. Because children with this problem do not understand what they hear, they echo what is said, whether it be word, syllable, phrase, or sentence.

Perhaps the perceptual inconstancy of early infantile autism is sufficient to hamper language capacity seriously (Ornitz and Ritvo, 1968). Understandably, a child who has monumental difficulty holding perception of his world constant would be expected to have difficulty deciphering the language code (Chapter 10).

Minimal brain dysfunction. Children classified as having *minimal brain dysfunction* (also called *minimal cerebral dysfunction* and *minimal brain damage*) usually show only minor nonspecific neurologic signs, if any. Their brain dysfunction is largely inferred from their behavioral abnormalities, which may or may not include language. Their major problems are hyperactivity, short attention span, impulsiveness, emotional lability, perseveration, clumsiness, and perceptual, cognitive, and memory defects. They may also have reading, writing, spelling, and arithmetic problems. When language problems are found, they usually involve the auditory system in ways similar to those seen in childhood aphasia, suggesting that minimal brain dysfunction can, but need not, lap over and involve the speech areas (Chase, 1972; Wender, 1971).

Learning disabilities. Only three charac-

teristics are common to all children with *learning disabilities:* at least average intelligence, adequate sensory acuity, and a significant discrepancy between the actual level of verbal functioning (especially in reading and arithmetic) and the level that might be expected from intellectual potential and sensory capability. Generally excluded from this category are the visually, auditorially, mentally, and emotionally handicapped as well as the culturally disadvantaged. Children who show the three mandatory characteristics may also exhibit hyper- or hypo-activity, lack of motivation, too much or too little attention, incoordination, perseveration, and perceptual or memory disorders.

In many ways, these children resemble those with minimal brain dysfunction, but the implication of neural deficit is less explicit. Obviously, language is a central problem for them, but usually in its written rather than spoken form. Again, we see evidence of the separateness of the special speech equipment for dealing with auditory manifestations of language from that which deals with it in its other forms (Gearheart, 1973).

APHASIA: IMPAIRMENT OF ACQUIRED LANGUAGE
What aphasia is and is not

Aphasia is one of many possible consequences of brain injury. In some ways it is the most dramatic and devastating. Unlike delayed language, it strikes those nearing or past their prime of life who have already acquired speech: presidents, kings, and paupers alike are leveled. Aphasic language is not entirely bizarre. Though the disorder may range from mild to severe, the difference between aphasic and nonaphasic disruptions is largely one of degree. All of us lose words, garble syntax, and misunderstand what we read and hear—aphasic persons just experience more disruptions (Schuell, 1965).

As Tikofsky (1966) reminds us, aphasia is only one manifestation of the effects of brain injury on communication. *Aphasia* is impairment of the ability to use language. As such, it cuts across all language modalities; it impairs the ability to read and write as well as to speak and listen; it is not specific to audition or to vision. Furthermore, it affects learning and personality. Aphasics require more time to respond and to shift responses. The more severely affected they are, the more primitive are their learning strategies. They can learn, but they are less flexible and require optimal conditions free of distractions. As for personality, rarely does aphasia make its victim more lovable. New traits are not acquired, but old ones, particularly undesirable ones, are intensified. Fortunately, recovery includes improvement of personality (Eisenson, 1973).

What aphasia is not. Neurologic disabilities that impair the perception of sensory input produce *agnosia* that involves specific sensory channels. Hence, persons with *auditory agnosia* have trouble making sense of what they hear. With *visual agnosia, what they see is meaningless*, whereas with *tactile agnosia*, they do not recognize objects that they touch (Eisenson, 1973). On the motor output side *apraxia*, too, is specific to the mode of verbal expression. The apraxic person knows what he wants to say, but with *oral verbal apraxia*, he will have trouble making his articulators speak the right sounds; with *motor agraphia*, his fingers will not write what he intends (Chapter 5).

Not only can brain damage produce input and output communication problems related to, but different from, aphasia; so, too, can it produce integrative disorders of cognition that Darley (1964) calls *confused language* and *generalized intellectual impairment*. In these disorders, the person can put together grammatical, intelligible sentences but may have difficulty keeping the point he is trying to make in focus. These high-level problems are closely related to aphasia. In the broadest sense they are *semantic defects*; the ability to formulate an idea and keep the intended meaning in mind long enough to express it is impaired. Here, we confront the nebulous relations among language, thought, and intelligence (Deese, 1969; Vygotsky, 1962). Thinking and intelligence involve symbolic processes, but not all symbolism is verbal; it comes in many nonverbal forms, such as art and music.

What aphasia is. Because thought and language are intimately, though fuzzily, connected, we will consider their interrelations in aphasia within this definition: *aphasia is impairment by localized cerebral pathology of the acquired ability to understand and use the language code of the community*. This definition excludes delayed language in which acquisition of linguistic rules is impaired. Once these rules are learned, children as well as adults can have their knowledge of them disabled by aphasia. Also excluded as the central concern in aphasia are input and output disorders of agnosia and apraxia, along with nonverbal ideational disorders. It is not that these other impairments are unimportant, and not that they cannot accompany aphasia. Because the brain functions as an integrated organ, damage in one area tends to affect overall neural function. Not surprisingly, damage that produces aphasia is also likely to produce nonlinguistic communication consequences (Tikofsky, 1966).

Aphasia described

Neurologic descriptions. The prevailing theme of this chapter, indeed of this book, still prevails: we seek a behavioral description of aphasia. From almost the beginning of recorded history, however, aphasia has been known to follow head injury. Small wonder that neurologic descriptions have predominated. Neurologists such as Broca, Wernicke, Jackson, Head, Weisenberg, and McBride have looked at the aphasic person's performance with a diagnostic eye for clinical signs of neural disability. Despite wide variations in terminology, their observations of aphasic behavior have been remarkably perceptive. Still, neurologic premises were

---

Tikofsky (1966) and Schuell and Jenkins (1961) have reviewed some currently important approaches to aphasia and differences in terminology. Do they agree in the approach that should be emphasized? Do Wepman and Jones (1966) and Spreen (1968) agree with them?

Weisenberg
McBride: receptive/expressive
aphasia

apparent in early descriptions. Weisenberg and McBride's (1935) substitution of "receptive" and "expressive," for instance, altered the terminology more than the underlying neurologic concept.

After World War II, when head-injury cases filled Veteran's Administration hospitals, speech pathologists became extensively involved in attempts to rehabilitate persons with aphasia. The extensive statistical analyses of Schuell and her colleagues (1961, 1964), who studied a large number of aphasic persons, led them to the conclusion that aphasia is a unidimensional language deficit, so much so that they rejected the need for traditional motor-sensory, expressive-receptive subcategories. Whether viewed as a neurologic deficit, a visual-verbal response, or an auditory-verbal response, their evidence showed a "pure" language loss in aphasia. Basing their argument on patient responses to a multitude of tasks in eighteen tests of linguistic performance, they recognized that these tasks probably involve various levels in the hierarchy of linguistic abilities. Thus, though demonstrating that language is a single dimension, they do not claim this single dimension to be a single linguistic skill; each of their testing tasks may well tap several levels of ability in the linguistic hierarchy.

Localization theories. The idea that specific speech and language behavior is mediated by specific brain mechanisms in specific locations has had a long and rocky history. This strict localization view began with Broca and Wernicke in the middle of the nineteenth century. It was opposed by Jackson and Head, who argued that the brain operates as a functional unit. Neither extreme position now seems tenable, but from both of them have come various sophisticated versions of a localization concept. Goldstein led the way with the idea that a given cortical area is important according to the influence it has on the brain as a whole. Thus he could accept Weisenberg and McBride's (1935) position that expressive (motor) aphasia involves a lesion in Broca's area, whereas receptive (sensory) aphasia is caused by damage in the

left temporal lobe (Eisenson, 1973; Tikofsky, 1966).

Various versions of localization are proposed by such modern theorists as Luria (1970), Geschwind (1970), Pribram (1971), Penfield and Roberts (1959), and Goodglass and Kaplan (1972). Luria's position resembles Goldstein's: the brain is a differentiated system in which its parts are responsible for different aspects of the unified whole. Since Geschwind has narrowed cortical location of lesions that produce different effects on such discrete functions as naming, he differentiates localization of damage that produces two types of *anomia*. Pribram, on the other hand, sees language and aphasic impairments as involving interaction of cortical and subcortical systems rather than of discrete cortical locations. Penfield and Roberts' position is somewhere between Geschwind's and Pribram's. They have localized discrete speech functions in various areas of the cortex, but they have also conceived what they call the "centrencephalic system," involving integrating mechanisms in the upper brain stem, as being heavily involved in the formulation of ideational language (Chapter 5).

From Goodglass and his investigators have come extensive correlations of brain injury and language behavior. These correlations are known as the *Boston Classification System*. The feature of the system of particular interest here is that it was constructed to give a reliable basis for neurologic diagnosis and localization of the site of lesion. The main differentiation is between *fluent* and *nonfluent aphasia*. The most typical nonfluent aphasia involves damage in Broca's area. This type is roughly equivalent to what is identified by such other terms as motor aphasia, expressive aphasia, and, of course, Broca's aphasia. The patient's speech is halting, garbled, telegraphic, and generally deficient in the planning and execution of coordinated speech sequences. Darley and his Mayo Clinic colleagues (1975) hold that this disorder should be called *apraxia of speech*. (BROCA 5)

Of the fluent aphasias, lesions in Wernicke's area are most commonly found.

Hence another name for this type is Wernicke's aphasia, or, sometimes, receptive aphasia or sensory aphasia. The mechanics of speech are essentially normal: speech is fluent, rhythmic, intelligible, and grammatical—but it is empty. It lacks content and meaning (Brookshire, 1973).

The foregoing is only a sampling of the major types of aphasia and the correlated lesions described in the Boston Classification System. Other subtypes, such as *conduction aphasia* and *transcortical motor aphasia,* are too numerous to be discussed in detail here.

Much less is known about neural functions required for recovery from aphasia than about those which are damaged to produce it. Is the function transferred from the normally dominant left hemisphere to the right? This transfer seems to be a strong possibility in preadolescent children who suffer from aphasia. Whatever the mechanism, the prognosis for recovery is far better prior to puberty than after the establishment of laterality in the early teens (Lenneberg, 1966).

It is not certain what functions are performed by portions of the dominant hemisphere that equip it so uniquely to mediate speech. A strong case is being built that one if not *the* crucial function performed by the dominant temporal lobe is the timing of incoming stimuli. Because discriminations of temporal sequences of sounds, syllables, words, and phrases are fundamental to speech perception, Efron (1963) has suggested that a central problem in aphasia may be a manifestation of disruption of the timing mechanism. He and Edwards and his associates (1965, 1966) have presented impressive evidence that aphasic persons are far less able to determine the temporal order of speech stimuli than are normal persons or than are brain-injured persons who are not aphasic.

On the other hand, the degree of impairment of the ability to determine auditory sequence correlates inversely with the severity of aphasia and is greater in expressive than receptive aphasia. What this peculiar correlation possibly signifies is that the timing mechanism serves the mechanical function of decoding and encoding the grammatical structure of language. The mechanism for connecting meaning with language, which, when defective, would produce the most profound losses of aphasia, is apparently separate from the timing equipment.

We again confront the limits of inferring what a person can do from an inadequate understanding of his mechanisms for doing it. The brain and language are both far too complex and our knowledge of them still too meager to say with much certainty what a neurologically damaged person will and will not be able to do. Clinically, the safest and most humane approach is to determine empirically the behavioral performance of which an aphasic person is capable and to build a remedial program on this foundation.

Psycholinguistic descriptions. Perhaps the most germinal linguistic analysis of aphasia has been Jakobson's (1961, 1966) theoretical formulation. Though his study is not based on personal observations of many aphasic persons, though his theory is related to a neurologic motor-sensory dichotomy as presented by Luria (1964), and though some of his ideas and hypotheses have been challenged, Jakobson has nonetheless been instrumental in promoting a linguistic analysis. Of his three linguistic dichotomies within which aphasic persons can vary, the basic dichotomy between *selection* and *combination* will illustrate his approach.

Selection has to do with the semantic process of choosing the word that best expresses the concept, whereas combination has to do with the syntactic process of combining words according to rules of the grammatical code and of arranging sentences in whatever order one chooses to express an idea. Jakobson sees combination as the primary problem when encoding (motor) ability is impaired. Since the speaker knows the ideas he is attempting to relate, his chief difficulty is not in finding the desired word but in combining the words in the proper arrangement. Conversely, selection is the primary difficulty when decoding (sensory) ability is defective. The reason is that the listener does not know what the speaker is attempting to say until the entire statement is complete; he must grasp the whole utterance to determine the meaning of key individual words. Of decoding and encoding processes, decoding ability is more widespread and basic than is the ability to encode; the ability to understand speech is fundamental to the ability to use it.

A psycholinguistic approach to aphasia has become popular in recent years. In addition to Jakobson, Osgood and Miron (1963) have followed it, as have Goodglass and his colleagues (1958, 1960, 1968a, b) and Tikofsky (1968). Wepman and Jones (1966) have carried it farthest. They noted that linguistic ability, as revealed by formal tests requiring structured responses to a limited number of tasks, is often different from the picture aphasic persons present when speaking in an unstructured conversational situation. By utilizing both formal tests and free speech samples, they have performed an analysis of different aspects of language ability that are impaired in aphasia.

Behavioral characteristics of aphasia. The results of analyses of Wepman and Jones (1966) are shown in the following comparison in Table 11-1 of stages of aphasia and stages of normal speech development. Wepman and Jones hypothesize that aphasia involves language regression; the more severe the impairment, the greater is the regression. An implication of this challenging idea, as yet untested, is that recovery would follow sequentially through these stages. Observe, though, that the developmental stages Wepman and Jones list describe the typical sequence of speech-acquisition events for normal children but do not describe causal relationships. For example, children babble before they talk, but whether a child babbles a little or a lot will not make much difference in his acquisition of language. Regardless of the fate of this regression hypothesis, the description of different types of language impairment still stands as the most comprehensive analysis of aphasic speech available so far (Spreen, 1968).

The basic types of aphasia that Wepman and Jones first described were *syntactic, semantic, and pragmatic.* Syntactic impairment affects morphology and syntax: forming proper morphemes for tense or gender and using words grammatically suffer most. Semantic impairment is seen in aphasic persons whose speech flows on in grammatical form but is limited to frequently used but imprecise words. It is considered more severe than syntactic aphasia for the same reason that Jakobson considers decoding more basic than encoding: understanding is basic to performance. An even greater impairment of understanding is seen in pragmatic disorders. This type of aphasia is revealed in the failure to comprehend a stimulus or situation. Pragmatic aphasic persons retain good phonologic control of speech-flow but do not understand what is being said to them, nor do they seem to understand what they are saying. The result is *neology*—they manufacture new words because they do not keep the rules of morphology and syntax straight.

That the two most recently developed categories, *jargon* aphasia and *global* aphasia, represent more severe impairments seems sensible. Wepman and Jones (1966) see jargon as resembling pragmatic aphasia, the difference being that with jargon the aphasic person not only fails to understand what he is saying but says it unintelligibly. With global aphasia no speech is available; loss of language is complete. Though Wepman and Jones have evidence that recovery from prag-

Table 11-1. Parallel sequences of recovery from aphasia and development of speech*

Development of speech	Recovery from aphasia
No speech	Global aphasia
Babbling	Jargon aphasia
Fortuitous speech	Pragmatic aphasia
Substantive symbols	Semantic aphasia
Grammar	Syntactic aphasia

*Based on data from Wepman, P., and Jones, L., Studies in aphasia: a psycholinguistic method and case study. In Carterette, E. (Ed.), *Brain function*. (III) *Speech, Language, and Communication*. UCLA Forum in Medical Sciences No. 4. Los Angeles: University of California Press (1966).

matic aphasia progresses through semantic and syntactic levels, they are much less certain that people with global aphasia would have to progress through jargon en route to whatever recovery they can achieve.

Howes and Geschwind (1964) found from analysis of free speech that aphasic persons can be divided into a fluent type and a nonfluent type. Which is more severe? How do these types compare with the ones discussed here?

On one side, we see aphasia as a single dimension in the sense that language involves a unified set of rules that operate irrespective of input or output modality. Of course, linguistic impairment can be selectively accompanied by visual or auditory input disorders or by oral or written output disorders (Schuell and Jenkins, 1961; Jones and Wepman, 1965). On the other side, we see what has been evident throughout discussions of language: aphasia has component parts that can be described linguistically. When these parts are analyzed in generative grammar as functional units, the impaired language processes that are involved can be described behaviorally and biologically.

Psycholinguistic analysis of aphasia, though popular now, is still in its infancy. The types of aphasia described here are gross; they are roughly equivalent to describing language in terms of semantics, grammar, and phonology. These descriptions only begin to reveal the language processes involved in language learning. They probably also fall short of what we need to know about language impairment in aphasia. The need to define a functional unit of language behavior would seem to be as great for therapy of aphasia as for acceleration of delayed language.

Although the value of a generative grammar approach would appear relevant, Wepman and Jones (1966) have commented in a dialogue with Lenneberg that phrase-structure and transformational analyses have not been perfected sufficiently to permit useful application to aphasic language structure; at least attempts made so far have not been successful. As Lenneberg in this dialogue observed, the only classifications of aphasia

that have proved valuable are very gross systems useful in localizing lesions. Part of the problem is in finding which linguistic dimensions have behavioral relevance for people with aphasia. For instance, the analysis of words by part of speech, by syllable length, or by concrete versus abstract reference has little differentiating value (Jones and Wepman, 1965). The impression that aphasic persons have more trouble with nouns than with other parts of speech may merely reflect the fact that they, like normal speakers, have trouble with nouns because nouns have a relatively low frequency of occurrence and therefore are probably not as well learned (Spreen, 1968).

Brown (1968) proposed what may prove to be a germinal model for central and peripheral behavior in aphasia. Similar to a model of generative grammar, the basic idea shown in Fig. 11-2 is that a central language process transforms meaning into language and language into meaning. Four behavioral components, shown in the diagram, are required: the ability to symbolize meaning with words, the ability to combine words syntactically, the ability to hold language and meaning of ongoing events in memory, and the ability to select quickly and appropriately from various input and output channels and a vocabulary pool. Damage to any component of the central language process degrades the concordance between meaning and language. Discordance between word and meaning can range from mild groping for a missing word to gross distortions of unrecognizable neologisms; discordance between syntactic rules and inner meaning can range from telegraphic speech to the fluent agrammatical, nonsensical flow of jargon. Impaired retention disrupts the understanding of what is being said and the expression of a complete idea, whereas impaired ability to select, focus, and shift input channels produces perseveration and distraction.

Regardless of the difficulty, the need remains for a system of analysis of aphasic language that will permit identification of linguistic behavioral steps that must be taken to restore impaired language. Some encour-

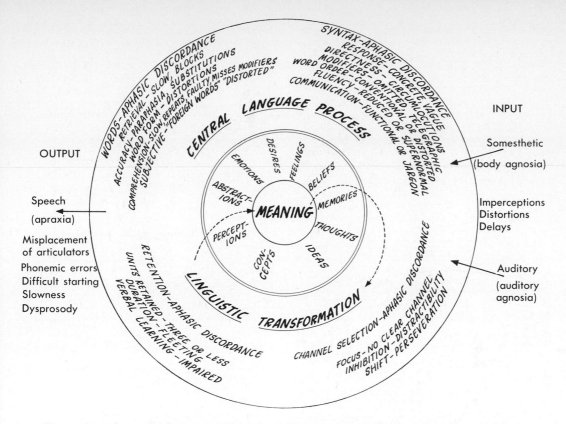

Fig. 11-2. Aphasia in relation to central language processes, agnosia, and apraxia. (Modified from Brown, J. R., A model for central and peripheral behavior in aphasia, a paper presented at the Academy of Aphasia meeting [1968].)

aging efforts in this direction are already under way (Holland, 1969; Porch, 1971). The challenge has vistas that boggle the imagination. Aphasia is characterized by more than gross impairments that can be detected by formal testing. Speech may be altered in ways difficult to quantify with traditional methods: it may be impoverished, simplified, or distorted; the speaker's "style" may be subtly impaired. Since twenty to 600 different dimensions are used in statistical analyses of literature to define an author's style, we may need an equally elaborate scheme to capture the many dimensions of aphasic speech (Spreen, 1968). What Luria (1966) calls the "language sense"—the ability to hold one idea in mind long enough to relate it meaningfully to another—may also be impaired. If Efron (1963) is right, though, at least an aspect of aphasia may prove to be an impairment not so much of linguistic pro-

cesses as of timing processes that are basic to language function.

NONSTANDARD ENGLISH OF DISADVANTAGED CHILDREN
Substandard language?

Ghetto children have been viewed as verbally destitute. They have often been included among those with delayed language. Research has shown that children of economically disadvantaged families acquire impoverished speech; their comprehension of language is poor, and they lack the vocabulary to express themselves. Their pronunciation and articulation are inaccurate. Their grammar is immature and incorrect. Worse yet, because of linguistic impoverishment, they are thought to be handicapped in thinking: in generalizing, categorizing, and problem-solving (Bernstein, 1960; Bereiter, 1965; Deutsch, 1965; Engelmann, 1964;

Gerber and Hertel, 1969; John and Gold-stein, 1964; Raph, 1965). That lower-class, unlike middle-class, mothers are vague and authoritarian in their use of language, that they are too exhausted from just managing to survive to talk to their children, and that they do not know how to stimulate or reinforce speech learning are all considered to be parts of the explanation of this presumed linguistic deprivation (Hess, Shipman, and Jackson, 1965; Raph, 1967; Schiefelbusch, 1967a,b).

An alternate view

These findings are apparently reliable. They all point in the same direction: the speech of ghetto children is different from the English that most children learn. Several insuperable problems arise, however, if we view this difference as evidence of delayed language. To begin, since the majority of children in a ghetto show the same speech characteristics, we would have to say that this majority all have delayed language. We have seen that anyone who reaches a mental age of 4 years will have to be deaf, severely psychotic, or totally isolated from speech not to acquire the language of his environment. The logical conclusion, then, would be that most ghetto children are grossly mentally retarded—and also that most adults in the ghetto have not reached a mental age of 4 years. It is their speech that the children learn.

This leaves the view that ghetto speech is a *subcultural language* (Labov, 1966; Shuy, Wolfram, and Riley, 1968). If "subcultural" is equated with "substandard," as educators and psychologists have shown some inclination to do, a dilemma remains. Linguists

---

Cazden (1966) has reviewed the evidence on subcultural language learning. Does he conclude that these children are linguistically deficient? If so, under what conditions?

---

have disproved the notion of a "primitive" language. Each language has its own system for signaling relations grammatically. Differences in these systems make for differences in relations that languages can signal

best. One can, for example, signal relations of time and plurality or singularity with much greater facility in English than in Chinese. Yet, who is to argue that Chinese is primitive or substandard?

The alternate view proposed here, that subcultural languages are not substandard, does not say that subcultural speech will not pose problems. Indeed, it may be a grossly inadequate tool of communication outside of the subculture. It is fitted to the special needs of its own group. But if those needs are different or require fewer discriminations than in the larger community, the child who knows only his own lingo can be severely handicapped when he moves beyond his culture, first in school and later as an adult. He will need an enlarged and different vocabulary. He will need different morphologic and phrase-structure rules, and he will need different articulation and pronunciations.

Black English. America is a linguistic conglomerate of dialects in which nonstandard English is spoken. The one that has dominated the scene in recent years is that of disadvantaged black children, particularly in Northern urban areas. Equivalently disadvantaged white children have probably suffered in school because a reason for their nonstandard English is not announced by physical evidence of their race. Their dialects are likely to be attributed to ignorance, whereas teachers are apt to use race as an explanation of black dialects (Shuy, 1972).

Baratz (1968, 1969) has done a forceful job of demonstrating that the differences in speech of disadvantaged black children are characteristic of speech of their culture. Nothing is wrong with their ability to learn language, since what they do learn is, indeed, the language of their community. It is as expressive, logical, complex, and rule-governed as any other dialect. True, it differs from standard English in phonology, vocabulary, and grammar. The words "toe" and "told" or "bowl" and "bold" are not likely to be discriminated as having different sounds. "Cat" may mean anything from carrot to a four-legged feline to a "big black dude." "She sick" and "She be sick" are grammatical constructions that signal when she is sick: in the first instance she is sick right now, whereas in the second she is habitually sick. To say, "She be here tomorrow," would reflect incompetence with this aspect of black English (Abrahams and Troike, 1972; Burling, 1973).

Jarring as this speech may be to the cultured white ear, the question of whether nonstandard English is substandard is waning as an issue. Black English is substandard only if one assumes that it should sound like some other dialect, such as that of middle-class, white America. Actually, the important questions about nonstandard English have not been answered. An especially relevant one is this: "Does the dialect spoken in the home affect language acquisition?" Being raised in a disadvantaged environment affects language, but whether the cause is the dialect or the condition of being disadvantaged is undetermined (Shuy, 1972).

The answers—résumé

1. In what ways can language development be impaired?

Delayed language is the failure to understand or speak the language code of the community at a normal age. What is delayed is the knowledge of how language works. Semantically, the ability to classify objects with words that carry appropriate meanings can be impaired. Phonologically, the ability to determine that words with different speech sounds have different meanings can be impaired. Grammatically, the ability to use morphemic, phrase-structure, and transformational rules to signal meaningful relations among ideas can be impaired. Delayed language does not specify a pathologic condition, nor does it denote why language is delayed; it only specifies that acquisition has not proceeded according to developmental norms.

2. With what disabilities is delayed language development associated?

Either or both of two basic functions of the brain mechanisms of language can be disabled. One appears to be the mechanical function of decoding and encoding units of language into grammatical speech. The other is the more fundamental function of transforming language into meaning, and meaning into language. Disabling conditions in which these functions are typically involved include mental retardation, deafness, childhood aphasia, autism, minimal brain dysfunction, and sometimes learning disabilities.

3. What are the characteristics of aphasia?

Aphasia is the impairment by localized cerebral pathology of the acquired ability to understand and use the language code of the community. Because it affects all language modalities, it is different from, though closely related to and complicated by, transmission difficulties: input disabilities (visual, auditory, or tactile agnosia) and output disabilities (oral verbal apraxia or motor agraphia). As a defect in the use of a unified set of linguistic rules, it can selectively involve components of the process by which meaning is transformed into language, and language into meaning. With advances in psycholinguistic analyses of aphasia, clearer delineation of functional units of aphasic language should become available.

4. With what disabilities are aphasic disorders associated?

Aphasia is language impairment subsequent to injury of the dominant cerebral hemisphere. Especially indicated is the centrencephalic system, involving areas of the dominant temporal and frontal lobes and integrating mechanisms in the upper brain stem. A crucial function of the temporal area appears to be the timing of stimuli, which, if disrupted, would make perception and integration of speech difficult if not impossible. Short-term memory ability, necessary for holding sounds, words, and phrases and for decoding or encoding speech, also seems to be affected.

5. What is the nature of nonstandard English of disadvantaged children?

Nonstandard English can be viewed as the "native" language of a subculture; it functions as the effective means of communication within that group. It is "substandard" only if viewed as a deviant form of standard speech. Those who use it outside of the subculture, however, can be seriously handicapped by differences in vocabulary, grammar, articulation, and pronunciation.

REFERENCES

Abrahams, R., and Troike, R., *Language and Cultural Diversity in American Education.* Englewood Cliffs, N.J.: Prentice-Hall, Inc. (1972).

Baltaxe, C., and Simmons, J., Language in childhood psychosis: a review. *J. Speech Hearing Dis.,* **40,** 439-458 (1975).

Baratz, J., Language in the economically disadvantaged child: a perspective. *Asha,* **10,** 143-145 (1968).

Baratz, J., Language and cognitive assessment of Negro children: assumptions and research needs. *Asha,* **11,** 87-91 (1969).

Bereiter, C., Academic instruction and preschool children. In Corbin, R., and Crosby, M. (Eds.), *Language Programs for the Disadvantaged.* Champaign, Ill.: National Council of Teachers of English (1965).

Bernstein, B., Language and social class. *Br. J. Sociol.,* **11,** 271-276 (1960).

Brookshire, R., *An Introduction to Aphasia.* Minneapolis: BRK Publishers (1973).

Brown, J., A model for central and peripheral behavior in aphasia. Paper read at the Academy of Aphasia, Rochester, Minn. (1968).

Bruner, J., Olver, R., and Greenfield, P., *Studies in Cognitive Growth.* New York: John Wiley & Sons, Inc. (1966).

Burling, R., *English in Black and White.* New York: Holt, Rinehart, & Winston, Inc. (1973).

Carroll, J., The prediction of success in intensive foreign language training. In Glaser, E. (Ed.), *Training Research and Education.* Pittsburgh: University of Pittsburgh Press (1962).

Carroll, J., Psycholinguistics in the study of mental retardation. In Schiefelbusch, R., Copeland, R., and Smith, J. (Eds.), *Language and Mental Retardation.* New York: Holt, Rinehart & Winston, Inc. (1967).

Cazden, C., Subcultural differences in child language: an interdisciplinary review. *Merrill-Palmer Quart. Behav. Developm.,* **12,** 185-219 (1966).

Chase, R., Neurological aspects of language disorders in children. In Irwin, J., and Marge, M. (Eds.),

Principles of Childhood Language Disabilities. New York: Appleton-Century-Crofts (1972).

Darley, F., *Diagnosis and Appraisal of Communication Disorders.* Englewood Cliffs, N.J.: Prentice-Hall, Inc. (1964).

Darley, F., Aronson, A., and Brown, J., *Motor Speech Disorders.* Philadelphia: W. B. Saunders Co. (1975).

Deese, J., Behavior and fact. *Am. Psychol.,* **24,** 515-522 (1969).

Deutsch, M., The role of social class in language development and cognition. *Am. J. Orthopsychiatry,* **35,** 24-25 (1965).

Edwards, A., and Auger, R., The effect of aphasia on the perception of precedence. In *Proceedings of the 73rd Annual Convention of the American Psychological Association.* Washington, D.C.: American Psychological Association, pp. 207-208 (1965).

Edwards, A., and Ebbin, J., Speech sound discrimination of aphasics when intersound interval is varied. In *Proceedings of the 74th Annual Convention of the American Psychological Association.* Washington, D.C.: American Psychological Association, pp. 201-202 (1966).

Efron, R., Temporal perception, aphasia and déjà vu. *Brain,* **86,** 403-424 (1963).

Eisenson, J., Developmental aphasia (dyslogia): a postulation of a unitary concept of the disorder. *Cortex,* **4,** 184-200 (1968).

Eisenson, J., *Adult Aphasia: Assessment and Treatment.* New York: Appleton-Century-Crofts. (1973).

Engelmann, S., *Cultural Deprivation and Remedy.* Champaign: University of Illinois, Institute for Research on Exceptional Children (1964).

Fay, W., On the basis of autistic echolalia. *J. Commun. Dis.,* **2,** 38-47 (1969).

Fay, W., and Butler, B., Echolalia, IQ, and the developmental dichotomy of speech and language systems. *J. Speech Hearing Res.,* **11,** 365-371 (1968).

Gearheart, B., *Learning Disabilities: Educational Strategies.* St. Louis: The C. V. Mosby Co. (1973).

Gerber, S., and Hertel, C., Language deficiency of disadvantaged children. *J. Speech Hearing Res.*, **12**, 270-280 (1969).

Geschwind, N., The varieties of naming errors. *Cortex*, **3**, 97-112 (1967).

Geschwind, N., The organization of language and the brain. *Science*, **170**, 940-944 (1970).

Goodglass, H., A psycholinguistic study of aggrammatism. In Zale, E. (Ed.), *Language and Language Behavior*. New York: Appleton-Century-Crofts (1968a).

Goodglass, H., Studies on the grammar of aphasia. In Rosenberg, S., and Koplin, J. (Eds.), *Developments in Applied Psycholinguistics Research*. New York: The Macmillan Co. (1968b).

Goodglass, H., and Berko, J., Aggrammatism and inflectional morphology in English. *J. Speech Hearing Res.*, **3**, 257-267 (1960).

Goodglass, H., and Kaplan, E.: *Boston Diagnostic Aphasia Examination*. Philadelphia: Lea & Febiger (1972).

Goodglass, H., and Mayer, J., Aggrammatism in aphasia. *J. Speech Hearing Dis.*, **23**, 99-111 (1958).

Hardy, W., On language disorders in young children: a reorganization of thinking. *J. Speech Hearing Dis.*, **30**, 3-16 (1965).

Hass, W., and Hass, S., Syntactic structure and language development in retardates. In Schiefelbusch, R. (Ed.), *Language of the mentally retarded. Baltimore: University Park Press (1972)*.

Hermelin, B., Rules and language. In Rutter, M. (Ed.), *Infantile Autism: Concepts, Characteristics, and Treatment*. Edinburgh: Churchill, Livingstone, Ltd. (1971).

Hess, R., Shipman, V., and Jackson, D., Some new dimensions in providing equal educational opportunity. *J. Negro Ed.*, **34**, 220-231 (1965).

Holland, A., Some current trends in aphasia rehabilitation. *Asha*, **11**, 3-7 (1969).

Howes, D., and Geschwind, N., Quantitative studies of aphasic language. In Riach, D., and Weinstein, E. (Eds.), *Disorders of Communication*. Baltimore: The Williams & Wilkins Co. (1964).

Jakobson, R., Aphasia as a linguistic problem. In Saporta, S. (Ed.), *Psycholinguistics*. New York: Holt, Rinehart & Winston, Inc. (1961).

Jakobson, R., Linguistic types of aphasia. In Carterette, E. (Ed.), *Brain function. (III) Speech, Language and Communication*. UCLA Forum in Medical Sciences No. 4. Los Angeles: University of California Press (1966).

John, V., and Goldstein, L., The social context of language acquisition. *Merrill-Palmer Quart. Behav. Developm.*, **10**, 265-275 (1964).

Jones, L., and Wepman, J., Language: a perspective from the study of aphasia. In Rosenberg, S. (Ed.), *Directions in Psycholinguistics*. New York: The Macmillan Co. (1965).

Jordan, T., Language and mental retardation: a review of the literature. In Schiefelbusch, R., Copeland, R., and Smith, J. (Eds.), *Language and Mental Retardation*. New York: Holt, Rinehart & Winston, Inc. (1967).

Kavanagh, J., and Cutting, J., *The Role of Speech in Language*. Cambridge, Mass.: The M.I.T. Press (1975).

Labov, W., *The Social Stratification of English in New York City*. Washington, D.C.: Center for Applied Linguistics (1966).

Lenneberg, E., Speech development: its anatomical and physiological concomitants. In Carterette, E. (Ed.), *Brain function, (III) Speech, Language, and Communication*. UCLA Forum in Medical Sciences No. 4 Los Angeles: University of California Press (1966).

Lenneberg, E., On explaining language. *Science*, **164**, 635-643 (1969).

Lenneberg, E., Nichols, I., and Rosenberger, E., Primitive stages of language development in mongolism. *Res. Publ. Ass. Res. nerv ment Dis.*, **42**, 119-137 (1964).

Luria, A., *The Role of Speech in the Regulation of Normal and Abnormal Behavior*. New York: Liveright Publishing Corp. (1961).

Luria, A., Factors and forms of aphasia. In de Reuck, A., and O'Connor, M. (Eds.), *Disorders of Language*. Boston: Little, Brown & Co. (1964).

Luria, A., *Human Brain and Psychological Processes*. New York: Harper & Row, Publishers (1966).

Luria, A., *Traumatic Aphasia*. The Hague: Mouton (1970).

Myklebust, H., Aphasia in children—language development and language pathology. In Travis, L. (Ed.), *Handbook of Speech Pathology*. New York: Appleton-Century-Crofts (1957).

Myklebust, H., Childhood aphasia: an evolving concept. In Travis, L. (Ed.), *Handbook of Speech Pathology and Audiology*. New York: Appleton-Century-Crofts (1971).

Newfield, M., and Schlanger, B., The acquisition of English morphology by normal and educable mentally retarded children. *J. Speech Hearing Res.*, **11**, 693-706 (1968).

Ornitz, E., and Ritvo, E., Perceptual inconstancy in early infantile autism. *Arch. gen. Psychiatry*, **18**, 76-98 (1968).

Osgood, C., and Miron, M., *Approaches to the Study of Aphasia*. Urbana: University of Illinois Press (1963).

Penfield, W., and Roberts, L., *Speech and Brain Mechanisms*. Princeton, N.J.: Princeton University Press (1959).

Porch, B., Multidimensional scoring in aphasia testing. *J. Speech Hearing Res.*, **14**, 776-792 (1971).

Pribram, K., *Languages of the Brain*. Englewood Cliffs, N.J.: Prentice-Hall, Inc. (1971).

Raph, J., Language development in socially disadvantaged children. *Rev. educ. Res.*, **35**, 389-400 (1965).

Raph, J., Language and speech deficits in culturally-disadvantaged children. *J. Speech Hearing Dis.*, **32**, 203-215 (1967).

Schiefelbusch, R., The development of communication skills. In Schiefelbusch, R., Copeland, R., and Smith, J. (Eds.), *Language and Mental Retardation*. New York: Holt, Rinehart & Winston, Inc. (1967a).

Schiefelbusch, R., Language development and language modification. In Haring, N., and Schiefelbusch, R. (Eds.), *Methods in Special Education*. New York: McGraw-Hill Book Co. (1967b).

Schiefelbusch, R., *Language of the Mentally Retarded*. Baltimore: University Park Press (1972).

Schlanger, B., Issues for speech and language training of the mentally retarded. In Schiefelbusch, R., Copeland, R., and Smith, J. (Eds.), *Language and Mental Retardation*. New York: Holt, Rinehart & Winston, Inc. (1967).

Schuell, H., *Differential Diagnosis of Aphasia with the Minnesota Test*. Minneapolis: University of Minnesota Press (1965).

Schuell, H., and Jenkins, J., The nature of language deficit in aphasia. In Saporta, S. (Ed.), *Psycholinguistics*. New York: Holt, Rinehart & Winston, Inc. (1961).

Schuell, H., Jenkins, J., and Jiminez-Pabon, E., *Aphasia in Adults*. New York: Harper & Row, Publishers (1964).

Shuy, R., Language problems of disadvantaged children. In Irwin, J., and Marge, M. (Eds.), *Principles of Childhood Language Disabilities*. New York: Appleton-Century-Crofts (1972).

Shuy, R., Wolfram, W., and Riley, W., *Field Techniques in an Urban Language Study*. Washington, D.C.: Center for Applied Linguistics (1968).

Smith, D., Speculations: characteristics of successful programs and programmers. In Galanter, E. (Ed.), *Automatic Teaching: the State of the Art*. New York: John Wiley & Sons, Inc. (1959).

Spreen, O., Psycholinguistic aspects of aphasia. *J. Speech Hearing Res.*, **11**, 467-480 (1968).

Tikofsky, R., Language problems in adults. In Reiber, R., and Brubaker, R. (Eds.), *Speech Pathology*. Amsterdam: North-Holland Publishing Co. (1966).

Tikofsky, R., Contemporary issues in aphasia. In Zale, E. (Ed.), *Language and Language Behavior*. New York: Appleton-Century-Crofts (1968).

Vygotsky, L., *Thought and Language*. Cambridge, Mass.: The M.I.T. Press (1962).

Weisenberg, T., and McBride, K., *Aphasia*. New York: Commonwealth Fund (1935).

Wender, P., *Minimal Brain Dysfunction in Children*. New York: Wiley Interscience (1971).

Wepman, J., and Jones, L., Studies in aphasia: a psycholinguistic method and case study. In Carterette, E. (Ed.), *Brain Function*. (III) *Speech, Language and Communication*. UCLA Forum in Medical Sciences No. 4. Los Angeles: University of California Press (1966).

Wood, N., *Delayed Speech and Language Development*. Englewood Cliffs, N.J.: Prentice-Hall, Inc. (1964).

Wood, N., *Verbal Learning*. Dimensions in Early Learning Series. San Rafael, Calif.: Dimensions Publishing Co. (1969).

Chapter 12

Disorders of articulation-resonance

Questions

1. What are the characteristics of disorders of articulation-resonance?
2. With what disabilities are articulatory-resonatory disorders associated?

CHARACTERISTICS OF ARTICULATORY-RESONATORY DISORDERS

Articulatory disorders, a convenient synonym for disorders of articulation-resonance (Chapter 3), reflect some degree of imprecision in speech sound production. The extent of articulatory *defectiveness* is determined by the judgment of either speaker or listener; the determination of an articulatory *problem* is the private concern of the speaker. The extent of the disorder can be judged by the following criteria:

1. Intelligibility. This criterion is the crucial linguistic test—how well can one recognize what was said?
2. Cultural speech standards. Acceptability of accents within a language vary.

One who must function in several cultures will probably need to meet several standards—for example, ghetto children in integrated schools or politicians speaking to constituents in different regions.

3. Vocational goals. Television and radio technicians, for example, will generally need to meet less exacting articulatory standards than will television and radio announcers.
4. Cosmetic acceptability. Occasionally, the appearance of articulatory production is a consideration—a speaker with a prognathic mandible may produce /f/ and /v/ upside down (upper lip against lower teeth), a solution that can

be acoustically acceptable but cosmetically peculiar.

5. Personal satisfaction. This criterion, applicable only to speakers, concerns their preferences for how they want to sound.

What are the characteristics of articulatory disorders? Obviously, since they are judged by ear, they have acoustical characteristics. Because they are produced by mouth, they also have physiologic characteristics. Still, the matter is more complicated. Speech sounds articulated are phonemes in a linguistic system, but as we saw in Chapter 3, phonemes are abstract linguistic classes. They exist only in the listener's ear.

As Denes (1966) and Ladefoged (1966) make clear, no one-to-one relation exists between the articulation of phonemes and any single type of articulatory characteristic. Speech is organized at multiple levels: psycholinguistic, articulatory, physiologic, and acoustical. Although these levels are correlated, none is identical to the other. That they are not identical is pointed up by an experiment of House and his colleagues (1962) on learning to identify acoustical patterns. These investigators synthesized sounds of various complexities and found that learning decreased with complexity. But when they presented the most complex signals of all, natural speech, the ability to learn them increased sharply. This type of evidence suggests that only acoustical patterns that humans can produce with their characteristic vocal tract equipment are readily learned as speech. Such evidence supports the motor theory of speech perception (Liberman and others, 1967). Another example of the lack of correspondence between acoustical characteristics and phonemes we hear is our ability to make voiced/voiceless perceptual distinctions in whispering—for example, between "his" and "hiss" or "eyes" and "ice"—even though the breath stream is entirely voiceless (Chapters 3 and 6).

The lack of correspondence between a physiologic description of a sound and its perception in speech can be illustrated by

assimilative influence (more recently called *coarticulation*) of one sound on almost any other Daniloff (1973). Take /k/ as an example. A standard physiologic description would seem to fit it when it is produced in isolation (and most clinicians begin work on articulatory disorders in isolation). Yet when /k/ is produced in "*k*ey" in contrast with "*c*ool," different adjustments of the tongue are required. In fact, recent studies of coarticulation have shown that nearly all sounds in a syllable influence each other physiologically, the influence coming from such factors as phonetic context, stress, rate, and morphemic boundaries. Ladefoged (1966) sees this influence as evidence that higher linguistic processes control the articulation of phonemes.

Similarly, MacNeilage and DeClerk (1969), looking at their data neurologically, find support for the influence of the syllable on the sounds within it. Still, they do not rule out the possibility that invariant high-level motor commands for each phoneme may be adapted by assimilative influences at lower levels, the neuromuscular level of the "gamma loop" mechanism being one possibility. Although not disagreeing, Daniloff and Moll (1968) find the greatest support in their evidence for Henke's (1966) theory. It explains coarticulation in terms of articulatory features: as a feature of each phoneme produced by a set of distinctive articulatory adjustments is completed, adjustment of that feature begins for the next phoneme in which it will be required. In "boom," for example, when the lip-rounding feature for initial /b/ is completed, adjustment for it in final /m/ begins and carries through the vowel that is thereby inadvertently affected.

Perceptually, speech can be segmented into a linear string of separate phonemes organized into meaningful words. Whether articulatory production of these phonemes can be chopped into matching segments is the question. It is a problem with clinical significance. Should articulatory disorders be treated as defective segments that can be isolated, corrected, and then reinserted into contextual speech? This approach has been typical in speech pathology. Yet coarticulation is so prevalent that a child who has learned how to produce a sound correctly in isolation could, when applying the same phonologic rule in context, produce an articulatory error.

Winitz's (1968) division of articulatory learning into two phases may solve some of the problem. He proposes that the acquisition of phonemic production skills and the association of acquired sounds into integrated linguistic units are not only separate processes but may involve different principles of learning. Carrell (1968) makes a similar distinction by dividing defective articulation into *phonemic errors*, in which speech sound production has not developed correctly, and *contextual errors*, in which the ability to use sounds in normal sequence and with normal prosody is faulty.

On the other hand, Garrett (1968) observes with clinical cogency that regardless of the theoretic considerations, behavioral modification technology is available for efficient remediation of articulation. Whether the basic unit to be corrected is a phonemic segment or a syllable, an auditory discrimination or an oral production, if it can be specified, it can probably be modified. Clearly, disorders of articulation have two faces: a perceptual aspect that permits isolation of discrete phonemic segments, and a phonetic production aspect that involves the continuous flow of articulatory movements. The former involves processes by which we perceive articulatory errors; the latter, processes by which those errors are modified.

Articulatory-resonatory disorders: phonemic perception

Listeners have many names for articulatory disorders, from "baby talk" to "lalling," "oral inaccuracy" to "lisping" (of which more than a dozen varieties can be described). All fit within the following perceptual definition: *Articulation is defective when phonemes are perceived as omitted, substituted, or distorted.* With omissions, phonemes included in normal pronunciations are absent—for example, "Tha wha I eh" being a young

child's truncated effort to say "That's what I said." Omissions make up only about 13% of misarticulations (Templin, 1957). With *substitutions*, incorrect phonemes are substituted for those which would normally be heard—"That'th what I thaid" exemplifying a /θ/ for /s/ substitution. With *distortions*, the correct phoneme is approximated, but not closely enough to be normally acceptable—"That's what I said," for example, being articulated with the /s/ in "said" resembling /z/ but not completely.

These three types of defectiveness can be attributed to the inability to produce all phonemes correctly or to apply phonologic rules properly (the distinction that Winitz makes and that Carrell separates into "phonemic errors" and "contextual errors"). *Additions* are a fourth perceptual type of articulatory defect in which the ability to produce phonemes is not at fault; what is faulty is improper addition of phonemes to words—"That'suh what I saiduh."

Factors related to defective phonemic development. Factors to be considered in this section are generally associated with probability of development of articulatory disorders more than with estimates of severity or predictions of recovery. Too, only factors that conceivably affect phonemic differentiation will be discussed now; those which can disable phonetic production will be considered shortly. Included here will be intelligence, linguistic ability, educational achievement, personal adjustment, socioeconomic status, sibling status, and sex.

Does Powers (1971), in her extensive review of causes of articulatory disorders, find any etiologic factor consistently present?

Intelligence, linguistic ability, and educational achievement. Except for mentally retarded children, who have high probability of developing defective articulation, intelligence has little predictive value of articulatory proficiency in normal children, a conclusion reached by Winitz in 1969 and again by Powers in 1971. Because this relation is essentially the same as that found between language and intelligence, it points to similarities in phonologic and grammatical developmental differentiation (Chapters 9 and 11). The results of the many studies done on the relation of articulation to various grammatical and lexical measures have been inconsistent, however. Still, phonologic and grammatical developments have generally been found to be correlated, especially in young children (Menyuk, 1964; Shriner, Holloway, and Daniloff, 1969; Winitz, 1969). As for the connection between articulatory adequacy and educational achievement, reading and spelling abilities and possibly academic grades appear to suffer with poor articulation (Winitz, 1969). Whether defective articulation impairs these abilities directly or is but a manifestation of underlying linguistic or educational disabilities has not been determined.

Personal adjustment. Terms such as "baby talk" and "infantile speech" identify the impression of both personal adjustment and articulatory adequacy. Dependency and regression are often associated clinically with immature articulation. Aside from the clinical study of Rousey and Moriarty (1965), investigations to demonstrate quantitatively what many clinicians suspect intuitively have been discouraging. Spriestersbach's research review in 1956 and Goodstein's in 1958, along with a subsequent study of maternal adjustment in 1960 (Moll and Darley), have led to the conclusion that neither articulatory defective children nor their mothers are clearly different from those without this problem, although they lean toward more personal difficulties.

As both Spriestersbach and Goodstein observed, many of these studies were undertaken without a specific hypothesis to test. In effect, they were "fishing expeditions" for relationships. Predictably, they returned without much of a catch. By contrast, Rousey and Moriarty had well-defined psychodynamic constructs to test. (See Chapter 10.) Perhaps this accounts for the 83% agreement of independent psychiatric evaluations with their research assumptions about the psychologic significance of various speech sounds: they had seven hypotheses specify-

ing ego-defensive functions of various substitutions and distortions of /s/, /θ/, /ð/, /r/ and /l/.

Socioeconomic and sibling status. After evaluating studies of socioeconomic and sibling status in relation to articulation, Winitz (1969) concluded that both are macrovariables reflecting differences in language stimulation and reinforcement. This theory would explain why more misarticulations are found among children of lower than higher socioeconomic classes. Such class differences in language experience as are found usually work their effects between ages 4 and 7 (Templin, 1957).

Articulatory proficiency favors first-born children and those spaced widely rather than closely in age. Whether this reflects the effects of differences in the frequency or the quality of parental attention or of sibling interaction, the fact remains that sibling status alters language experience. An extreme case in point is *idioglossia*, the idiosyncratic language occasionally developed by twins. With no age difference and with continuous physical and interpersonal closeness, they sometimes develop a unique language, different from their parents, which they alone may understand.

Sex. If girls more than boys are favored in articulatory development, and they may not

Table 12-1. Mean number of articulation errors by grade*

Grade	Mean number of articulation errors
1	13.3
2	10.0
3	8.9
4	7.6
5	7.6
6	8.0
7	3.9
8	4.3
9	4.5
10	4.4
11	3.3
12	3.3

*Based on data from Roe, V., and Milisen, R., The effect of maturation upon defective articulation in elementary grades. *J. Speech Dis.*, **7**, 37-45 (1942).

be, the reasons are opaque. Erection of a bridge of speculations may be unnecessary, however. The results of the many studies done are conflicting, differences reported are small, and they are virtually nonexistent in well-controlled studies (Winitz, 1969). Templin (1963) therefore suspects that sex is of little significance in understanding speech development.

Factors related to severity and recovery. Numerous factors have been used for determining the severity of misarticulations, for selecting sounds with which to begin therapy, and for predicting recovery. Since not all are as valuable as they have seemed, let us look at what is known about them first, and then consider their efficacy.

Maturation and articulatory-resonatory development. Table 12-1 summarizes much of the evidence relating maturation to articulatory disorders. Although probably a macrovariable formed of several other variables,

maturation nonetheless correlates with rapid improvement of articulation through grade 4, tapering off through grade 12.

Table 12-2 shows evidence often used to support the notion of a developmental sequence of speech sounds. Presumably, children improve articulation in an orderly fashion as they mature. The fact that the most frequently misarticulated consonants, shown in Table 12-3, are among those acquired later in the developmental sequence supports the idea that maturational factors are at work. Some speech pathologists hold that this sequence reflects the relative difficulty of these sounds to be discriminated and produced. Seemingly, perfection of those phonemes that are most complex must await maturation of the motor and sensory apparatus. This view, though popular, will probably not withstand careful scrutiny.

Winitz (1969), relying heavily on Irwin's (1947, 1951) studies of infant speech, points out that when developmental evidence gathered from groups is viewed in terms of individual performance, support for sequential development vanishes. He grants the normative picture of orderly development of different sounds at different ages, but he reminds us that sounds at the 7-year level of the developmental scale occur with considerable frequency at 3 years of age. A child of this age, for the most part, has phonetic

Table 12-2. Normal developmental sequence of speech sounds*

Sound	Age correctly produced
m	3.0
n	
ŋ	
p	
f	
h	
w	
j	3.5
k	4.0
b	
d	
g	
r	
s	4.5
ʃ	
ɟ	
t	6.0
θ	
v	
l	
ð	7.0
z	
ʒ	
dʒ	

*Based on data from Templin, M., *Certain Language Skills in Children, Their Development and Interrelationships.* Institute of Child Welfare, Monograph Series No. 26. Minneapolis: University of Minnesota Press (1957).

Table 12-3. Frequently misarticulated consonants*

Con-sonant	Percentage of error	Percentage of children with error	
	Grades 1 to 6	Grade 1	Grade 6
z	45.8	88.1	84.5
hw	40.0	—	44.7
θ	30.3	68.8	45.1
dʒ	30.2	91.2	70.7
d	25.0	70.1	68.8
s	19.9	48.9	32.8
g	18.5	69.1	39.7
ð	16.5	57.3	41.4
v	16.0	53.0	38.4
t	14.0	45.7	55.6

*Based on data from Roe, V., and Milisen, R., The effect of maturation upon defective articulation in elementary grades. *J. Speech Dis.*, **7**, 37-45 (1942).

skills to produce the necessary sounds of speech. Moreover, he demonstrates by his understanding that he discriminates enough phonemes to be able to decipher the morphology and grammar of his language.

Thus the apparent order of sound acquisition probably relates mainly to a child's problems of utilizing long-mastered phonetic skills in differentiating and matching the adult production of words. The developmental sequence does not necessarily reflect motor or sensory maturation, nor does it imply that sounds at one stage must be mastered before those at the next can be acquired. Instead, it points to the sequence by which the child modifies his self-contained (but inaccurate) phonemic system, with its own rules of articulation and pronunciation, to accord with the phonemic and morphologic system of his culture.

We can conclude from studies of maturation that a child has a greater probability of outgrowing an articulatory defect before the fourth grade than after. What age does not reveal are those children who will not improve spontaneously. The clinician who waits until the third or fourth grade to begin treatment risks increased complications and resistance of the problem to correction. Perhaps Van Riper and Erickson's (1969) Predictive Screening Test of Articulation will help clinicians avoid the alternative of a caseload of many children who would improve without help. As for the "normal developmental sequence," contrary to frequent clinical practice, it does not show which error sounds for which child at which age need correction. The order in which sounds are incorporated into speech varies from child to child, and acquisition does not require a specific sequence. No sound appears to be dependent on any other for its development.

Frequency of misarticulation and intelligibility. The phrase "frequency of misarticulation" is ambiguous. It can refer to the number of different sounds misarticulated or to the frequency of occurrence of error sounds in the language. For example, a child could misarticulate four sounds found in the final position of such words as ran*ge*, ju*dge*,

chur*ch*, and pa*th* and still produce a lower absolute number of errors in normal speech than if he misarticulated the single sound /s/. The reason, of course, is that /s/ occurs over three times as often in English as the first four sounds combined (Travis, 1931). In fact, Wood (1949) proposed an "Articulation Index" that weighted each sound to reflect its frequency of occurrence in the language as a means of measuring therapeutic progress. His assumption was that listeners judge the severity of an articulatory problem by number of errors heard. Subsequent research showing the close correspondence between

---

Do Henrikson (1948) and Van Riper and Irwin (1958) think that the Articulation Index is an adequate method of estimating the severity of an articulatory disorder?

---

intelligibility, negative listener judgment, and the number of articulatory errors has supported his assumption (Dietze, 1952; Garwood, 1952; Jordan, 1960; Kleffner, 1952; McWilliams, 1954). Also, as Winitz (1969) concluded after reviewing available evidence, an articulatory error score is one of the few reliable predictors of articulatory improvement, with or without therapy.

We can conclude that frequency of misarticulation not only has predictive value for improvement but is also an index of the extent of impairment of intelligibility and the severity of the disorder. As for the selection of misarticulations for therapy, a clinician would be well advised to choose the error sound that occurs most frequently, provided it is as ready as other misarticulations for correction when tested for stimulability.

Stimulability of misarticulation. The ability to improve an error with auditory stimulation is probably the best test of readiness of a misarticulation for improvement, with or without help. Snow and Milisen (1954) found that misarticulations that improve with imitation of correct production have a good chance of being corrected or of improving spontaneously. Later, Farquhar (1961) found essentially the same result when she compared children's ability to imitate correct production of error sounds with their ability to discriminate their errors; imitative ability was significantly predictive of improvement, whereas auditory discrimination was not.

Type of misarticulation. Whether an error sound is omitted, substituted, or distorted is considered to be indicative of severity, especially by Milisen and his associates (1954), Roe and Milisen (1942), and Wright (1954). Others are in general agreement (Van Riper and Irwin, 1958), and such research as has been done is supportive (Mulder, 1948; Sayler, 1949; Jordan, 1960). The rationale for a relation is as follows: Children perfect articulation by progressively approximating adult speech. The poorer the approximation, the farther they have to go, and thus the more severe the error will be. The hierarchy of severity of the type of misarticulation, then, is (1) omission, in which the sound is not produced and hence is farthest from resembling the correct sound; (2) substitution, in which the child at least recognizes that some sound is needed even though he uses the wrong one; and (3) distortion, in which the correct sound is approximated but not closely enough.

Consistency of misarticulation. For economy, clinicians often test a sound only a few times, usually in *initial, medial,* and *final* (IMF) positions in words. This practice has been severely criticized; it flies in the face of evidence that misarticulations are typically inconsistent (Hahn, 1949; Perkins, 1952; Spriestersbach and Curtis, 1951). This fact carries several clinical implications. First, it means that without detailed testing in a wide range of phonetic contexts, articulatory errors can be easily missed (McDonald, 1964). Second, it means that often among the inconsistencies are some "nuggets of gold," as Van Riper calls them—correct productions of the error sound that can be utilized for therapy. Third, it means that the prognosis for improvement is probably favorable. Van Riper and Irwin (1958) reason that when sounds are stabilized and permanently acquired, they are produced consistently. Theoretically, inconsistency suggests that the process of phonemic learning is still in progress. Yet preliminary research suggests that

children whose error consistency is high or average have similar difficulty learning the correct sound in new words, even though those with the most inconsistency learn it easiest (Baer and Winitz, 1968). Inconsistency of misarticulation as a prognostic index has not lived up to its theoretical potential (Templin, 1966).

Position of misarticulation. In articulation testing, distinctions have long been made among errors occurring in initial, medial, and final positions of words and syllables. Linguistically, IMF distinctions have some merit in that omissions, particularly, are to a large extent a function of position. Templin (1957) found no omissions in initial position in children 7 years of age or older, and regardless of age, omissions were three times as prevalent in final as in medial position and almost six times as prevalent in final as in initial position. Winitz (1969) interprets this phenomenon as indicating that initial sounds carry more information than final sounds, which are the most redundant. They can be dropped without as much loss of intelligibility.

Phonetically, however, McDonald (1964) makes the incontestable point that "the concept of initial, medial, and final consonants has little or no validity" outside of words. But spoken words have no unity linguistically, acoustically, or physiologically. They appear in speech not as entities but as sequences of syllables. Physiologically, consonants release and arrest syllables with various movement sequences that depend on phonetic context, not on IMF positions. Perhaps this explains why Powell and McReynolds (1969) found no generalization from articulatory training in different positions but did find generalization from nonsense syllables to familiar words.

Phonemic difficulty of misarticulation. Speech pathologists have often observed that some sounds are more difficult to teach than others. Powers (1971), reviewing studies of manner and place of articulation, found high agreement that friction sounds requiring the use of the front of the tongue account for the great majority of errors. Although different groups of sounds have been reported as most difficult to acquire, often on the basis of maturation, Scott and Milisen (1954) developed what is probably the most clinically significant list. They ranked sounds in the following order of decreasing difficulty on the basis of correct responses after equal stimulation: /r/, /s/, /z/, /l/, /g/, /v/, /k/, and /f/.

The usual explanation for this relative difficulty of articulation is that some sounds are more complex than others. Although complexity is a possible explanation, Winitz (1969) raises serious doubt that it is adequate. He reminds us that by 18 months of age, an infant has uttered all phonemes but /tʃ/ and /dʒ/, even though he will not incorporate many of them into his phonemic system for several years (Winitz and Irwin, 1958).

Too, typical substitutions closely resemble the correct sound in phonetic features. For example, any lisp utilizes the same fricative process that is required to produce a normal /s/. The feature that differs is the place of articulatory contact of the tongue; yet the place for producing /s/ is practically the same as for /n/ and /t/, sounds that are rarely missed (Winitz, 1969). Further, as Locke (1968) argues, an extremely rare misarticulation, such as /z/ for /k/, is bizarre and probably more severe than a "normal" substitution of /ʃ/ for /s/, precisely because so many features of the former differ (voicing, manner, and place of production), whereas only one (place) differs in the latter. Lewis (1951) makes a similar point when he observes that 81% of substitutions are for sounds the child can already produce; substitutions are replacements of consonants heard by ones relatively more familiar and longer established. Thus whatever differences in articulatory complexity may exist from sound to sound, they apparently do not bear on one's ability to produce most, if not all, phonemes phonetically.

We now come to the crux of Winitz's (1969) thesis that articulatory errors are, for the most part, not so much problems of phonetic production as of mastery of a phonemic system. En route to mastering this system, a child approximates the adult system with one of his own design that is similar but not identical—the greater the dissimilarity, the greater the articulatory defectiveness. Faced with the buzzing confusion of adult speech, the child must separate distinctive phonetic features that make phonemic differences in meaning from nondistinctive features that do not.

Here, the concept of *distinctive features* provides a valuable explanation for the sequence of speech sound acquisition and for the greater phonemic difficulty of differentiating late maturing sounds (Berko and Brown, 1960). Although hypothetical, the idea is that those articulatory adjustments and their acoustical consequences that contrast one phoneme with others are distinctive features for the phoneme. Just as voiceless /s/ differs from voiced /z/ by the vocalic feature, and just as /p/ contrasts with /t/ by the place of articulation, so is /i/ distinct from /e/ by the feature of height of tongue. Such are some commonly used distinctive features of English.

Several universal schemas of distinctive features have been proposed, the one by Jakobson, Fant, and Halle (1952) probably being best known. It is also the one from which Fant (1962) and Jakobson and Halle

---

Crocker (1969) has devised a phonologic model of consonantal development, based on distinctive feature theory and Chomsky's linguistic competence model, that could explain common articulatory substitutions.

(1956) have built modified systems. Others include systems by Miller and Nicely (1955), Chomsky and Halle (1968), and Wickelgren (1965a, b). Differing in the list of features proposed as contrasting, these systems still share the concept that any phoneme in any langauge can be described as a bundle of concurrent distinctive features. As Parker (1976) points out, however, the concept of distinctive features is still fraught with problems that will have to be resolved. Phonemic theories assume a correspondence between abstract linguistic features and the spoken speech signal that does not in fact exist. On the other hand, generative theories do not link linguistic structure to speech production. Despite such unresolved problems, the assumption still seems defensible that the sequence of speech sound acquisition is assumed to be an orderly progression in which the most distinctive phonetic features (such as vowel/consonant and voiced/voiceless contrasts) are learned first, with progressively finer discriminations following (such as the subtle tongue adjustments of /s/, /r/, and /l/).

Auditory discrimination of misarticulation. Van Riper and Irwin (1958) point to auditory acuity as a basic necessity for speech perception, especially in the speech range from 500 to 2,000 Hz, and few would disagree in general. Specifically, however, when the question arises concerning how much acuity is required, agreement wanes. Other considerations prevail. Speech has so many cues by which it can be deciphered and monitored that a clear generalization is nearly impossible. Speech is fraught with redundancy linguistically, physiologically, and acoustically for one who has learned the rules and "feel" of speaking it. His need for auditory acuity is probably less than is that of the child just acquiring speech.

After reviewing evidence linking auditory memory span to articulatory disorders, Van Riper and Irwin (1958) suspect that the two are not commonly related, although as Winitz (1969) points out, the evidence is not conclusive one way or the other. On the other hand, auditory discrimination and articulatory ability are often found to be related, at least in children (Winitz, 1969). Templin (1943) found that children made the most discriminative errors in the same medial and final positions in which they had exhibited the most articulatory errors.

Sherman and Geith (1967) later tested this relation by turning the investigation around. They first selected children with high and low auditory discrimination scores and then checked to see if articulatory skill correlated. It did. The connection is strengthened further by Stitt and Huntington's (1969) finding that speech signal discrimination and identification abilities are related strongly to articulatory proficiency.

More recently, Monnin and Huntington (1974) found that children with defective articulation are specifically deficient in their ability to identify misarticulated sounds. They suspect that production of the sound is a factor in its perception, a possibility that fits with the motor theory of speech perception. Giving impetus to this possibility is the work of Locke and Kutz (1975). They argue from their evidence that misarticulations can be a cognitive as well as a communicative problem. By virtue of producing articulatory errors, misarticulations interfere with accurate rehearsal and consequently with perception and short-term memory for the defective sounds.

On the other hand, Aungst and Frick (1964) found that "traditional" tests (in which one judges the similarity of pairs of nonsense syllables spoken by another) correlate negatively with judgments of the correctness of one's own articulation. Both instantaneous and delayed judgments of one's own speech, however, are related to the consistency of accurate articulation, at least of /r/. Winitz and his associates (1963a,b, 1967) have explored the concept that what is discriminated are distinctive features. Their results generally support the idea that the ease of discrimination is directly related to the number of features by which sounds differ.

Clearly, auditory discrimination and articulation are connected, but available evidence does not yet prove which causes which. Must perceptual proficiency precede improved articulatory production, or is the order reversed? Obviously, the prelinguistic child's perceptual development leads his motor production—he understands speech before he can utter it. But unanswered are the following questions (Winitz, 1969): Do perceptual and motor development proceed at the same rate and in the same order? How do they interact so that understanding can be superior to speaking ability? Does production as well as discrimination proceed by learning phonemic contrasts?

Because the relation between auditory and articulatory abilities is ambiguous, speech pathologists have drawn opposing clinical implications. Van Riper and Irwin (1958), for instance, point to poor auditory awareness as a vital part of the difficulty of articulatory defects in adults, as well as in children, who are often oblivious of their errors. Auditory discrimination, memory span, and phonetic ability—an "ear for speech"—are considered in relation to this lack of awareness. From this point of view, the therapeutic value of ear training is a logical emphasis.

The other side of the issue is stressed by such experts as Milisen (1966). He takes the position that lack of speech awareness is normal, that "the last person to know how he sounds is the speaker himself." He holds that articulatory learning is largely a by-product of a child's interaction with his environment as he learns to talk. The listener judges the adequacy of his speech and is primarily responsible for selectively reinforcing it. With this view, the emphasis is on the production of sounds to which listeners can respond, not on the child's awareness of errors; thus the therapeutic value of ear training is minimized (McDonald, 1964). Fortunately for the clinician, both points of view have proved effective. The applied issue swings mainly on the hinge of which view is the most efficient therapeutically, an issue for which the final word is yet to be written.

Articulatory-resonatory disorders: phonetic production

Whereas articulatory proficiency is judged in terms of the ability to produce phonemic segments of the language, defective articulation is modified by altering the flow of phonetic behavior. New movements of the speech apparatus are learned in the correction of articulatory disorders. Therefore, we will shift the focus from perceptual discrimination problems of phonemic detection to motor learning problems of phonetic production.

Articulatory-resonatory disorders: a problem of motor phonetics? By contrast with the earlier definition of defective articulation as perception of phonemic inaccuracies, the production of correct as well as incorrect speech sounds fits within McDonald's (1964) motor phonetics definition of articulation as "*a process consisting of a series of overlapping, ballistic movements which place varying degrees of obstruction in the way of the outgoing airstream and simultaneously modify the size, shape, and coupling of resonating cavities.*" "Ballistic movements" are the rapid, skilled articulatory movements by which consonants and vowels are produced with resonator adjustments and obstructions. "Overlapping" means that movements for production of forthcoming sounds are in progress while others are being uttered. The linguistic system provides the phonemic targets to guide these speech mechanism movements. Articulatory errors are evidence of misguided movements that miss phonemic targets. Let us review briefly how this process operates.

Stetson (1951), whose work forms the foundation of motor phonetics, observed that all speech utterances involve breath control and respiratory movements. He noted that although the phoneme is the basic linguistic unit of speech perception, the syllable is the basic physiologic unit of speech production. Produced by the smallest *breath pulse*, it consists of a *beat stroke* that releases the *syllable pulse* (vowel), and a *back stroke* that arrests it. Auxiliary consonant movements may accompany the beat and arrest strokes, but not necessarily. What is minimally required is the vowel-like sound of the syllable pulse; it may be a pure vowel, a diphthong, or a semivowel. Consonants, too, may be *simple* (/t/ releases *tea* and arrests *eat*), *compound* (/st/ releases *stop* and arrests *list*), *abutting* (/st/ simultaneously arrests the first and releases the second syllable in *history*), and *double* (/s/ when repeated arrests the first and releases the second syllable in *this sigh* to distinguish it from *this eye*). Each significant movement aspect of a syllable can be the basis of a phoneme; thus the single-syllable word "strength" has seven phonemes.

Although the syllable pulse is the physiologic unit of articulatory significance, it is only the smallest of several expiratory movements found in any statement: a *foot* is the unit built around a stressed syllable that includes whatever unstressed syllables cluster around it; a *breath group* is composed of feet; and a *phrase* is composed of breath groups. All utterances contain all these expiratory movements, ranging from the simplest—a phrase of one breath group con-

---

Stetson's explanation of respiratory physiology is not as well accepted as his theory of the speech effects of expiration. Do Hixon (1973), Netsell (1973), Hoshiko (1960), and Draper, Ladefoged, and Whitteridge (1959) agree with Stetson's description of respiratory muscle action for speech?

---

sisting of a monosyllabic foot ("Yes!")—to phrases of any complexity (see below). As you can see, all these expiratory units, from syllable to phrase, determine patterns of stress —hence they are the backbone of speech prosody. Physiologically, articulatory movements within the syllable cannot be separated from prosodic movements of syllable pulses, feet, breath groups, and phrases. Therefore, as McDonald (1964) stresses, sounds do not exist in isolation; the smallest utterance in which they occur is the syllable.

Because some sounds are presumably more complex and require finer discriminations than others, they should logically require higher levels of motor and sensory development to produce; thus they should develop last. Sensible as this conclusion appears, we have already seen evidence that disproves it, at least in part. The work on infant sounds of Irwin (1947, 1951) and Winitz (1969) shows that by the time the child starts to talk, he has mastered most of the articulatory adjustments he will need, even though he will not incorporate many of them in his speech for several years. The child is apparently in the terminal, not the early, stages of motor and sensory maturation when he says

his first word. The implication is that unless the articulatory process is physiologically disabled, articulatory defects must be attributed generally to problems of phonemic differentiation, not of phonetic production.

Factors that disable phonetic production. Articulation involves the guidance of movements of the speech apparatus to produce auditory and somesthetic feedback that matches the speech sound goal to be achieved. Coordination of movements with feedback effects is practiced during the infant's months of babbling. Having looked at the factors that influence the incorporation of these coordinated movements into a child's phonemic system for speaking his language, we will now examine the factors that can disable the development of phonetic coordinations in the first place.

Disabling conditions are, in the final analysis, physiologic. Although morphologic factors such as a congenital cleft or a prognathic mandible may loom large, still, effects on speech are determined entirely by physiologic movements and positions that can be achieved with existing speech equipment, defective as it may be. Thus three general areas of disabled functioning can impair the development of articulatory coordinations: orofacial, neurologic, and sensory. Speech effects of these disabilities are sometimes identified by their medical terms: *dysglossia* refers to defective articulation associated with orofacial movement defects, *dysarthria* to defective articulation associated with neural control disabilities, and *dysaudia* to defective articulation associated with auditory feedback difficulties (Carrell, 1968). Terms for these conditions are used so loosely that we need not be finicky in our selection. What is important is that we be clear in our concept of how disabilities relate to speech. As West

---

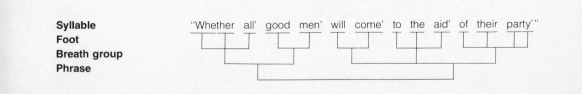

Syllable	
Foot	"Whether all' good men' will come' to the aid' of their party'"
Breath group	
Phrase	

and Ansberry (1968) caution, children vary so much in adjustments and compensatory movements that some are exceedingly facile in surmounting physical handicaps. We must be cautious about seeing simple cause-and-effect relations. When "obvious" disabilities are connected to articulatory defects, the linkage is probably complex (Perkins and Curlee, 1969).

Orofacial disabilities. Diverse orofacial conditions, particularly cleft palate, defective dental structures and tongue and lip status, have been associated with defective articulation (Chapter 8). Spriestersbach (1965) summarized the articulatory problems typically found in studies of cleft palate: (1) development of articulatory skill is retarded; (2) nasal consonants and vowels suffer least, fricatives and affricates most; (3) compensatory adjustments are more likely with simple than with complex speaking tasks; (4) omissions are most prevalent, followed by substitutions of glottal stops for plosives and pharyngeal for oral fricatives; (5) articulatory proficiency varies with the different types of cleft and with differences in ability to impound air orally; and (6) the same person varies in the types of errors he produces. The key to these effects is velopharyngeal incompetence, for which Shelton and his associates (1964, 1965) have found the best clinical index to be articulatory adequacy. In addition, compensatory efforts to achieve velopharyngeal closure, thereby increasing pharyngeal wall movement, are beneficial, whereas those that position tongue against palate and pharyngeal wall are conducive to defective articulation (Brooks, Shelton, and Youngstrom, 1965, 1966).

Probably for many laymen, the most common cause of defective articulation is tongue-tie, technically called *ankyloglossia.* Physicians who once clipped tongues indiscriminately have been reluctant to intervene since McEnery and Gaines (1941) discovered that only four out of 1,000 children with articulatory defects had short frenums. Judging from Fletcher and Meldrum's (1968) evidence, however, the pendulum may have swung too far; lingual mobility may con-

tribute to defective articulation. Ostensibly, the size of tongue should also be a factor; one too large *(macroglossia),* too small *(microglossia),* or nonexistent *(aglossia)* would seemingly affect articulation. Extreme cases undoubtedly produce speech defects, but for those tongue, palate, and lip dimensions that have been compared between superior and inferior speakers, no stable differences have been found (Winitz, 1969). Even in the extremes of such cases of tongue excision as Milisen (1966) and Backus (1940) describe, the ability to compensate adequately is remarkable.

Tongue thrust, a condition in which abnormal lingual pressure is applied to the incisors during swallowing, is an annoyance to speech pathologists, who must cope with whatever articulatory defects relate to it, and a distress to orthodontists, whose dental alignments are displaced. Because so many clouds of clinical smoke have risen about presumed articulatory effects, many speech pathologists have responded to the orthodontist's alarm with programs of "myofunctional therapy" as well as speech therapy. Others have been reluctant to become involved for lack of clear evidence that a relation does exist and, if it does, which causes which (Winitz, 1969; Mason and Profitt, 1974).

In one well-controlled study, the effects on dental alignment of correcting an accompanying lisp were compared with direct correction of the abnormal pattern of swallowing. Using a sigmatism training technique designed to keep the tongue away from the incisors, Stansell (1970) found that sigmatism training reduced dental overjet regardless of tongue-thrust swallow, whereas deglutition training alone was not as effective. Clearly, such evidence points to a functional relationship, but it suggests that speech causes malocclusion more than does tongue-thrust swallow—a rather startling reversal of expectation.

Research results on the effects of dentition on articulation have been at odds from the beginning: Carrell (1936) and Fymbo (1936) reported opposite evidence in the same issue of the same journal. Matters have not improved much with time. Snow's (1961) careful investigation points to at least a weak relationship that Milisen (1966) attributes to such factors as upper more than lower incisor abnormality, frontal more than lateral dental defect, upper and open bite more than overbite, and sudden more than gradual loss of teeth.

Neurologic disabilities. No one seems to doubt that motor control disabilities can affect articulation—the problem is discussed in most texts on speech pathology, usually under the heading of dysarthria. Much of the research and logic by which causal relations have presumably been demonstrated, however, have left much room for uncertainty. For example, as Winitz (1969) has shown after reviewing investigations of motor abilities, motor skills correlate poorly with each other, let alone with articulation. Moreover, specific tests of oral and facial motor control that do correlate with articulatory skill seem unfair. Tests of *diadochokinesia* (rapid repetition of movements), in which defective groups are poorer than normal groups, involve articulatory movements more likely to be practiced in normal than in abnormal articulation.

Even more basic is McDonald's (1964) reservation about the usefulness of diadochokinetic tests. These tests use alternating contractions of opposed muscles, whereas articulatory movements involve simultaneous contraction of different muscles. Differences have been found that may hold up with more careful study; however, as Shelton and his associates (1966) point out, the fact that children with good as well as poor articulation fail tongue motor tasks indicates that such tasks do not identify the disabilities that cause articulatory disorders. Similarly, investigations of physical development have produced divergent results: FitzSimons (1958), for example, found differences, Everhart (1953) did not, but both relied for their information on the vagaries of parental memory of how their children developed.

Lest we become too eager to abandon "organic" in preference to "functional" explanations, the results of Frisch and Handler (1974) should give us pause. They studied twenty children with "functional" misarticulations. Nine of the ten subjects with omissions and seven of the ten with substitutions showed evidence of cerebral damage suggestive of sensory-receptive dysfunction in the left hemisphere. In fact, in a similar study, Yoss and Darley (1974) found a cluster of children with moderate to severe articulatory problems whose difficulty could be described as *developmental apraxia* of speech.

Studies of dysarthria and respiratory physiology particularly are providing a firm foundation for understanding the effects of neurologic disabilities on the speaking process. Darley, Aronson, and Brown, at Mayo Clinic (1969a,b), have demonstrated unequivocally that different types of defective speech mirror different types of abnormal motor functioning—different patterns of dysarthria sound different. Eight clusters of deviant speech dimensions characteristic of seven types of neurologic disease have been identified. Three of those clusters center around articulation and are shown in Table 12-4 in relation to the type of neurologic defect, the disease that caused it, and the consequent neuromuscular movement disabilities that are the core of each cluster of speech dysfunctions. Such work forms the basis for correlating neurophysiologic processes of dysarthria with behavioral characteristics of defective speech.

Hardy (1968), observing that respiratory abnormalities appear to be a basis for defective speech in neuromuscularly handicapped speakers, has been building a body of knowledge that will permit specific therapeutic applications to the "speech/breathing problems" of dysarthric persons. One of his major findings is that respiratory problems can be a consequence of inefficient management of the airstream for speech as well as of weakened respiratory muscles. The result of inefficient control of articulatory mechanisms is excessive expiration when speaking. Such air wastage during speech for those with deficient vital capacity for normal breathing can be severely taxing. Thus dysarthric persons may have a compound problem: paretic respiratory muscles that generate inadequate

Table 12-4. Neuromuscular basis for dysarthric dysfunctions*

Neurologic group	Cluster components	Chief defects of movement and tone	Neurologic defects	Disease system						
				CLR	CHO	DTN	PBP	ALS	BUL	PKN
1 *Articulatory inaccuracy*	Imprecise construction Irregular articulation breakdown Vowels distorted	Inaccurate direction of movement Irregular rhythm of repetitive movements	Ataxia or involuntary movements	++	±	++				
2 *Prosodic excess*	Slow rate Excess/equal stress Phonemes prolonged Intervals prolonged Inappropriate silences	Slow individual movements Slow repetitive movements	Ataxia, involuntary movements, or spasticity	++	++	++	±	++		++
3 *Prosodic insufficiency*	Monopitch Monoloudness Reduced stress Phrases short	Reduced range of individual and repetitive movements	Dystonia, spasticity, or rigidity		+	+	++	++		++
Extension	Variable rate Short rushes Imprecise consonants	Repetitive movements very fast with very limited range	Rigidity		+	++	++	++		
4 *Articulatory-resonatory incompetence*	Imprecise consonants Vowels distorted Hypernasality	Reduced force of movements when associated with reduced range	Spastic paresis							
5 *Phonatory stenosis*	Low pitch Harsh voice Strained-strangled Pitch breaks Voice stoppages Slow rate Phrases short Excess loudness variations	Hypertonus biased toward adductors Sustained or spasmodic in occurrence	Dystonia or spasticity		+	++	++	+		
6 *Phonatory incompetence*	Breathy voice Audible inspiration Phrases short	Weakness of movements	Flaccid weakness					++	++	±
7 *Resonatory incompetence*	Hypernasality Nasal emission Imprecise consonants Phrases short	Weakness of movements	Flaccid weakness					++	++	
8 *Phonatory-prosodic insufficiency*	Monopitch Monoloudness Harsh voice	Hypotonia	Ataxia or flaccidity	+					+	

*From Darley, F., Aronson, A., and Brown, J., Clusters of deviant speech dimensions in the dysarthrias. *J. Speech Hearing Res.*, **12**, 477-478 (1969).

Symbols: ++ = strongly present; + = present; ± = present but fragmentary.

CLR: Cerebellar ataxia   PBP: Pseudobulbar palsy   BUL: Bulbar palsy
CHO: Cho...   ALS: Amyotrophic lateral sclerosis   PKN: Parkinsonism

air supply for speaking and inefficient control of the speech mechanism that wastes such air as is available.

Another neurologic impairment, for which less firm evidence is available than for dysarthria, is *oral verbal apraxia*, by definition a disability of motor formulation of articulated language. Neither aphasia nor dysarthria, it is a disability of the output transmission system that has more to do with motor patterning than linguistic organization or muscular coordination. The oral verbal apraxic individual who once had normal speech seems to have his facility for automatic articulatory control impaired. Understanding of speech and the ability to write may be unaffected, but he will exhibit inconsistent articulatory errors as he gropes for correct positioning of his speech mechanism (Chapter 5).

Sensory disabilities. Two types of sensory feedback, auditory and somesthetic, guide articulatory coordinations. We have already glimpsed the role of audition in the utilization of these coordinations in the development of a mature phonemic system. Now we are concerned with its role in the acquisition of phonetic coordinations, a problem of establishing "ear-vocal reflexes" from which the child learns the acoustical effects of his speech mechanism movements. Unfortunately, we have little more than inference and speculation with which to proceed; we cannot very well tinker with the hearing of very young children in the interests of science. What is known comes mainly from observation of the effects of hearing impairment in infants.

The question here is what a child must be able to hear in order to develop adequate auditory control of speech mechanism movements. Why does the deaf child, for example, who babbles much as does a hearing child, have a characteristic "deaf quality" when he eventually learns to speak (Calvert, 1962)? Is it because he could not hear his own babbling and so has no idea of the sounds he is making? Is it because he cannot hear normal speech and so has no idea of how he should sound? Is it both? What minimal abilities

must he have to detect differences in pitch, loudness, quality, temporal sequence, interval, and duration? What must be his auditory memory span?

We know from studies of older children with normal and defective articulation that differences are often found in auditory discrimination of pitch signals and speech signals; memory span results are too contradictory to point one way or another (Winitz, 1969). What cannot be concluded from these differences, however, is their role in the development of adequate phonetic coordinations. Somewhere between deafness and normal hearing must lie minimal requirements for auditory acuity and for those discriminative abilities essential to the detection of speech. Whether these requirements will be essentially the same for developing ear-vocal reflexes during babbling, for understanding speech prior to learning to speak, and for incorporating articulatory coordinations into a mature phonemic system are questions for which we do not yet have answers.

In one sense the view is even cloudier, but in another sense clearer, for *somesthetic* (body sensation) abilities. It is cloudier in that these abilities are only in preliminary stages of investigation; we have relatively little information on how they are related to any aspect of speech development. It is clearer in that, logically, what is known can be attributed directly to coordination of the speech apparatus for articulation. Because the "feel" of speech is exclusively private, it can only provide guidance for articulatory movements that produce sounds that can be matched by audition to adult phonemic systems. All of this is reminiscent of Van Riper and Irwin's (1958) proposal that we learn speech initially by ear and subsequently guide it automatically by feel.

Practically, our concern with somesthesia goes beyond the component *tactual* and *kinesthetic* senses. It extends to the *haptic system* that includes the neural processes by which these sensory inputs are utilized to perceive one's body in relation to objects and space, the system by which we feel speech. Of the various somesthetic skills, tests of *oral stereognosis* (the identification of object form by exploring it in the mouth) seems most promising. This ability improves through adolescence to adulthood; it seems related to articulation and particularly to oral motor control, being decidedly inferior for aphasic and cerebral-palsied dysarthric persons (Chapter 6).

In fact, Bloomer (1967) has suggested that when somesthetic disabilities are found, they resemble oral motor apraxias; they are congenital, not acquired; and they are likely to involve impairment of the neural transmission system rather than of sensory receptors. True as this description may be, a very few rare cases of somesthetic disability have apparently been located. The two persons who have been studied for several years at the National Institutes of Health have seemed normal in all respects, even neurologically and in the ability to understand speech, but neither has acquired intelligible articulation. They both failed oral stereognosis tests completely, have difficulty moving the speech mechanism, and yet can swallow and breathe normally (Bosma, Grossman, and Kavanagh, 1967). Whatever the basis of somesthetic difficulty, the fact seems clear that these disabilities, infrequent as they may be, can loom large in the development and maintenance of articulatory coordinations.

Modification of phonetic production. Regardless of the reason that speech sounds are in error, their correction requires modification of phonetic production, a point stressed by McDonald (1964). Shelton and his research group (1967; Elbert, Shelton, and Arndt, 1967) see articulatory improvement as a problem of motor learning that follows the sequence from acquisition to generalization to automatization. As Cratty (1967) concludes from experimental evidence, the motor learning process clearly divides into several component phases of skill development. First is the learner's ability to remember directions for the task. A second phase involves organizing discrete portions of the task into larger components that permit increased rate, accuracy, and smoothness. The final phase is not as clearly defined by evidence but seems to involve automatization such as Paillard (1960) proposed. All phases, however, fit within the definition of motor learning as "a stable change in a skill with practice" (Cratty, 1967). By "practice" is meant more than mere repetition; practice is repetition with a purpose. The motor task is solved and resolved with techniques perfected with each trial (Cross, 1967; Bernstein, 1967).

Motor learning vis-à-vis articulatory-resonatory skills. The first step in applying motor learning principles to improvement of articulation requires the acquisition of the desired phonetic skill. The "feel" and sound of producing a phoneme properly must replace erroneous motor adjustments. Here, two approaches are particularly helpful. If careful testing of articulation has revealed phonetic contexts within which the correct sound occurs with some consistency, they can be utilized as a starting point for the acquisition of the desired phoneme. For instance, /s/ is likely to be produced accurately in the consonantal blend /kstr/ of "extra," whereas the probability of its being defective is great in the medial position of "useless" (Perkins, 1952). On the other hand, factors other than phonetic context appear to be related to consistency and may hold clinical significance (Shelton, Wright, and Arndt, undated).

The other approach, though similar, involves shaping the sound to the desired form. Studies of phonemic generalization have shown that improvement of one sound generalizes to phonetically similar but not to highly dissimilar sounds, the transferred improvement being greatest when the two sounds differ by no more than two distinctive features (Winitz and Bellerose, 1963b; Elbert, Shelton, and Arndt, 1967). As an example, correction of /z/ would probably generalize to /s/, which differs only by the distinctive feature of voicing. Thus, if instances of accurate production of /s/ could not be obtained but of /z/ were available, therapy could begin by shaping /z/ to its voiceless cognate /s/. By capitalizing on such similarities, phonemes already produced normally can be shaped to replace defective phonemes.

With an articulatory skill acquired, it must then be generalized to a variety of phonetic and linguistic contexts. Changes in phonetic environment and speech prosody tend to pull newly found skills out of line. The long-utilized technique of strengthening sounds in phonetically varied nonsense syllables is now sanctioned by research results as well as clinical experience (Powell and McReynolds, 1969). Shames (1957) has even suggested carrying the use of nonsense syllables one step farther by incorporating them into structured jargon to facilitate phonetic carryover. As for generalizing new skills into varied linguistic contexts, Van Riper (1963) has long advocated (complete with a wealth of examples) a progression from nonsense syllables to unfamiliar words, to familiar words, to phrases, and then to sentences.

Automatization in daily speech is the ultimate and most difficult test of articulation. Until motor skills become automatic they tend to deteriorate back to error patterns established earlier. Shames (1957) investigated why sounds learned in the clinic were not used in connected speech. Typical reasons were that stopping to correct "old" with "new" sounds is irritating, and that "deliberate" articulation distorts phrasing, rate, and inflection, making speech artificial. Basically, the problem of automatization is one of establishing stimulus control of the articulatory response, a crucial and vexing problem of therapy, and one that we will look at more closely in Chapter 16.

The answers—résumé

1. What are the characteristics of disorders of articulation-resonance?

Disorders of articulation have a perceptual aspect that permits linguistic isolation of discrete phonemic segments and a phonetic production aspect that involves the continuous flow of articulatory movements. Perceptually, articulation is defective when phonemes are perceived as omitted, substituted, or distorted. Factors related to severity and prognosis for the acquisition of a normal phonemic system are age and the frequency, type, consistency, position, phonemic difficulty, phonemic discrimination, and stimulability of misarticulations. Phonetically, articulatory production is defective when speech mechanism movements do not automatically produce the sounds of the adult phonemic system.

2. With what disabilities are articulatory-resonatory disorders associated?

Defective phonemic development is associated with auditory disabilities (particularly that affect discrimination of speech), mental retardation and commensurate linguistic and educational abilities, socioeconomic and sibling status (presumably reflecting differences in language stimulation and reinforcement), and possibly personal adjustment. Phonetic production can be impaired by orofacial disabilities (especially cleft palate), apraxic and dysarthric neurologic disabilities, and sensory disabilities of audition and somesthesia. These disabilities impair structures that move for speech, their neural control, and feedback of the "feel" and sound effects of those movements.

REFERENCES

Aungst, L., and Frick, J., Auditory discrimination ability and consistency of articulation of /r/. *J. Speech Hearing Dis.*, **29**, 76-85 (1964).

Backus, O., Speech rehabilitation following excision of the tip of the tongue. *Am. J. Dis. Child.*, **60**, 368-370 (1940).

Baer, W., and Winitz, H., Acquisition of /v/ in "words" as a function of the consistency of /v/ errors. *J. Speech Hearing Res.*, **11**, 316-333 (1968).

Berko, J., and Brown, R., Psycholinguistic research methods. In Mussen, P. (Ed.), *Handbook of Research Methods in Child Development*. New York: John Wiley & Sons, Inc. (1960).

Bernstein, N., *The Coordination and Regulation of Movements*. Long Island City, N.Y.: Pergamon Press, Inc. (1967).

Bloomer, H., Oral manifestations of dysdiadokokinesis with oral astereognosia. In Bosma, J. (Ed.), Symposium on Oral Sensation and Perception. Springfield, Ill.: Charles C Thomas, Publisher (1967).

Bosma, J., Grossman, R., and Kavanagh, J., A syndrome of impairment of oral perception. In Bosma, J. (Ed.), *Symposium on Oral Sensation and Perception*. Springfield, Ill.: Charles C Thomas, Publisher (1967).

Brooks, A., Shelton, R., and Youngstrom, K., Compensatory tongue–palate–posterior pharyngeal wall relationships in cleft palate. *J. Speech Hearing Dis.*, **30**, 166-173 (1965).

Brooks, A., Shelton, R., and Youngstrom, K., Tongue-palate contact in persons with palate defects. *J. Speech Hearing Dis.*, **31**, 14-25 (1966).

Calvert, D., Deaf voice quality: a preliminary investigation. *Volta Rev.*, **64**, 402-403 (1962).

Carrell, J., A comparative study of speech-defective children. *Arch. Speech*, **1**, 179-203 (1936).

Carrell, J., *Disorders of Articulation*. Englewood Cliffs, N.J.: Prentice-Hall, Inc. (1968).

Chomsky, N., and Halle, M., *The Sound Pattern of English*. New York: Harper & Row, Publishers (1968).

Cratty, B., *Movement Behavior and Motor Learning*. Philadelphia: Lea & Febiger (1967).

Crocker, J., A phonological model of children's articulation competence. *J. Speech Hearing Dis.*, **34**, 203-213 (1969).

Cross, K., Role of practice in perceptual-motor learning. *Am. J. phys. Med.*, **46**, 487-510 (1967).

Daniloff, R., Normal articulation processes. In Minifie, F., Hixon, T., and Williams, F. (Eds.), *Normal Aspects of Speech, Hearing, and Language*. Englewood Cliffs, N.J.: Prentice-Hall, Inc. (1973).

Daniloff, R., and Moll, K., Coarticulation of lip rounding. *J. Speech Hearing Res.*, **11**, 707-721 (1968).

Darley, F., Aronson, A., and Brown, J., Clusters of deviant speech dimensions in the dysarthrias. *J. Speech Hearing Res.*, **12**, 462-496 (1969a).

Darley, F., Aronson, A., and Brown, J., Differential diagnostic patterns of dysarthria. *J. Speech Hearing Res.*, **12**, 246-269 (1969b).

Denes, P., Discussion. In Carterette, E. (Ed.), *Brain function*. (III) *Speech, Language, and Communication*. UCLA Forum in Medical Sciences, No. 4. Los Angeles: University of California Press, pp. 221-225 (1966).

Dietze, H., A study of the understandability of defective speech in relation to errors of articulation. Master's thesis. University of Pittsburgh (1952).

Draper, M., Ladefoged, P., and Whitteridge, D., Respiratory muscles in speech. *J. Speech Hearing Res.*, **2**, 16-27 (1959).

Elbert, M., Shelton, R., and Arndt, W., A task for evaluation of articulation change. I. Development of methodology. *J. Speech Hearing Res.*, **10**, 281-288 (1967).

Everhart, R., The relationship between articulation and other developmental factors in children. *J. Speech Hearing Dis.*, **18**, 332-338 (1953).

Fant, G., Descriptive analysis of the acoustic aspects of speech. *Logos*, **5**, 3-17 (1962).

Farquhar, M., Prognostic value of imitative and auditory discrimination tests. *J. Speech Hearing Dis.*, **26**, 342-347 (1961).

FitzSimons, R., Developmental, psychosocial, and educational factors in children with nonorganic articulation problems. *Child Developm.*, **29**, 481-489 (1958).

Fletcher, S., and Meldrum, J., Lingual function and relative length of the lingual frenulum. *J. Speech Hearing Res.*, **11**, 382-390 (1968).

Frisch, G., and Handler, L., A neuropsychological investigation of "functional disorders of speech articulation." *J. Speech Hearing Res.*, **17**, 432-445 (1974).

Fymbo, L., The relation of malocclusion of the teeth to defects of speech. *Arch. Speech*, **1**, 204-216 (1936).

Garrett, E., Speech pathology: some principles underlying therapeutic practices, discussion. *Asha*, **10**, 203-204 (1968).

Garwood, V., An experimental study of certain relationships between intelligibility scores and clinical data of persons with defective articulation. Doctoral dissertation. Ann Arbor: University of Michigan (1952).

Goodstein, L., Functional speech disorders and personality: a survey of the research. *J. Speech Hearing Res.*, **1**, 359-376 (1958a).

Goodstein, L., Functional speech disorders and personality: methodological and theoretical considerations. *J. Speech Hearing Res.*, **1**, 377-381 (1958b).

Hahn, E., An analysis of the delivery of the speech of first grade children. *Quart. J. Speech*, **35**, 338-343 (1949).

Hardy, J., Respiratory physiology: implications of current research. *Asha*, **10**, 204-205 (1968).

Henke, W., Dynamic articulatory model of speech production using computer. Doctoral dissertation. Cambridge, Mass.: The Massachusetts Institute of Technology (1966).

Henrikson, E., An analysis of Wood's Articulation Index. *J. Speech Hearing Dis.*, **13**, 233-235 (1948).

Hixon, T., Respiratory function in speech. In Minifie, F., Hixon, T., and Williams, F. (Eds.), *Normal Aspects of Speech, Hearing, and Language*. Englewood Cliffs, N.J.: Prentice-Hall, Inc. (1973).

Hoshiko, M., Sequence of action of breathing muscles during speech. *J. Speech Hearing Res.*, **3**, 291-297 (1960).

House, A., and others, On the learning of speechlike vocabularies. *J. verb. Learning verb. Behav.*, **1**, 133-143 (1962).

Irwin, O., Development of speech during infancy: curve of phonemic frequencies. *J. exper. Psychol.*, **37**, 187-193 (1947).

Irwin, O., Infant speech: consonantal position. *J. Speech Hearing Dis.*, **16**, 159-161 (1951).

Jakobson, R., Fant, G., and Halle, M., *Preliminaries to Speech Analysis*. Acoustics Laboratory, Technical

Report 13. Cambridge, Mass.: The Massachusetts Institute of Technology (1952).

Jakobson, R., and Halle, M., *Fundamentals of Language.* The Hague: Mouton Publishers (1956).

Jordan, E., Articulation test measures and listener ratings of articulation defectiveness. *J. Speech Hearing Res.*, **3**, 303-319 (1960).

Kleffner, F., A comparison of the reactions of a group of fourth grade children to recorded examples of defective and nondefective articulation. Doctoral dissertation. Madison: University of Wisconsin (1952).

Ladefoged, P., Discussion. In Carterette, E. (Ed.), Brain function. (III) *Speech, Language, and Communication.* UCLA Forum in Medical Sciences, No. 4. Los Angeles: University of California Press, pp. 197-198 (1966).

Lewis, M., *Infant Speech, a Study of the Beginnings of Language.* New York: Humanities Press, Inc. (1951).

Liberman, A., and others, Perception of the speech code. *Psychol. Rev.*, **74**, 431-461 (1967).

Locke, J., Questionable assumptions underlying articulation research. *J. Speech Hearing Dis.*, **33**, 112-116 (1968).

Locke, J., and Kutz, K., Memory for speech and speech for memory. *J. Speech Hearing Res.*, **18**, 176-191 (1975).

MacNeilage, P., and DeClerk, J., On the motor control of coarticulation in CVC monosyllables. *J. acoust. Soc. Am.*, **45**, 1217-1233 (1969).

Mason, R., and Profitt, W., The tongue thrust controversy: background and recommendations. *J. Speech Hearing Dis.*, **39**, 115-132 (1974).

McDonald, E., *Articulation Testing and Treatment: A Sensory-Motor Approach.* Pittsburgh: Stanwix House, Inc. (1964).

McEnery, E., and Gaines, F., Tongue-tie in infants and children. *J. Pediatr.*, **18**, 252-255 (1941).

McWilliams, B., Some factors in the intelligibility of cleft-palate speech. *J. Speech Hearing Dis.*, **19**, 524-527 (1954).

Menyuk, P., Comparison of grammar of children with functionally deviant and normal speech. *J. Speech Hearing Res.*, **7**, 109-121 (1964).

Milisen, R., Articulatory problems. In Rieber, R., and Brubaker, R. (Eds.), *Speech Pathology.* Amsterdam, North-Holland Publishing Co. (1966).

Milisen, R., and others, The disorders of articulation: a systematic clinical and experimental approach. *J. Speech Hearing Dis.*, *Monog. Suppl.* 4 (1954).

Miller, G., and Nicely, P., An analysis of perceptual confusions among some English consonants. *J. acoust. Soc. Am.*, **27**, 338-352 (1955).

Moll, K., and Darley, F., Attitudes of mothers of articulatory-impaired and speech-retarded children. *J. Speech Hearing Dis.*, **25**, 377-384 (1960).

Monnin, L., and Huntington, D., Relationship of articulatory defects to speech-sound identification. *J. Speech Hearing Res.*, **17**, 352-366 (1974).

Mulder, R., A case study of the growth of verbal responses in preschool children, Master's thesis. Columbus: Ohio State University (1948).

Netsell, R., Speech physiology. In Minifie, F., Hixon, T., and Williams, F. (Eds.), *Normal Aspects of Speech, Hearing, and Language.* Englewood Cliffs, N.J.: Prentice-Hall, Inc. (1973).

Paillard, J., The patterning of skilled movements. In Field, J., Magoun, H., and Hall, V. (Eds.), *Handbook of Physiology.* (Sect. I) *Neurophysiology.* (Vol. III) Washington, D.C.: American Physiological Society (1960).

Parker, F., Distinctive features in speech pathology: phonology or phonemics? *J. Speech Hearing Dis.*, **41**, 23-39 (1976).

Perkins, W., Methods and materials for testing articulation of [s] and [z]. *Quart. J. Speech*, **38**, 57-62 (1952).

Perkins, W., and Curlee, R., Causality in speech pathology. *J. Speech Hearing Dis.*, **34**, 231-238 (1969).

Powell, J., and McReynolds, L., A procedure for testing position generalization from articulation training. *J. Speech Hearing Res.*, **12**, 629-645 (1969).

Powers, M., Functional disorders of articulation—symptomatology and etiology. In Travis, L. (Ed.), *Handbook of Speech Pathology and Audiology.* New York: Appleton-Century-Crofts (1971).

Roe, V., and Milisen, R., The effect of maturation upon defective articulation in elementary grades, *J. Speech Dis.*, **7**, 37-45 (1942).

Rousey, C., and Moriarty, A., *Diagnostic Implications of Speech Sounds.* Springfield, Ill.: Charles C Thomas, Publisher (1965).

Sayler, H., The effect of maturation upon defective articulation in grades seven through twelve. *J. Speech Hearing Dis.*, **14**, 202-207 (1949).

Scott, D., and Milisen, R., The effect of visual, auditory and combined visual-auditory stimulation upon the speech responses of defective speaking children. *J. Speech Hearing Dis.*, *Monogr. Suppl.* 4, pp. 37-43 (1954).

Shames, G., Use of the nonsense-syllable in articulation therapy. *J. Speech Hearing Dis.*, **22**, 261-263 (1957).

Shelton, R., Brooks, A., and Youngstrom, K., Articulation and patterns of palatopharyngeal closure. *J. Speech Hearing Dis.*, **29**, 390-408 (1964).

Shelton, R., Brooks, A., and Youngstrom, K., Clinical assessment of palatopharyngeal closure. *J. Speech Hearing Dis.*, **30**, 37-43 (1965).

Shelton, R., Elbert, M., and Arndt, W., A task for evaluation of articulation change. II. Comparison of task scores during baseline and lesson series testing. *J. Speech Hearing Res.*, **10**, 578-585 (1967).

Shelton, R., Wright, V., and Arndt, W., Context, consistency, and remediation of /r/ and /s/. Unpublished manuscript (undated).

Shelton, R., and others, Identification of persons with articulation errors from observation of nonspeech movements. *Am. J. Phys. Med.*, **45**, 143-150 (1966).

Sherman, D., and Geith, A., Speech sound discrimination and articulation skill. *J. Speech Hearing Res.*, **10**, 277-280 (1967).

Shriner, T., Holloway, M., and Daniloff, R., The relationship between articulatory deficits and syntax in speech defective children. *J. Speech Hearing Dis.*, **12**, 319-325 (1969).

Snow, K., Articulation proficiency in relation to certain dental abnormalities. *J. Speech Hearing Dis.*, **26**, 209-212 (1961).

Snow, K., and Milisen, R., The influence of oral versus pictorial representation upon articulation testing results. *J. Speech Hearing Dis.*, *Monogr. Suppl.* 4, pp. 29-36 (1954).

Spriestersbach, D., Research in articulation disorders and personality. *J. Speech Hearing Dis.*, **21**, 329-335 (1956).

Spriestersbach, D., The effect of orofacial anomalies on the speech process. Proceedings of the Conference: Communicative Problems in Cleft Palate. *Asha Rep.*, **1**, 111-128 (1965).

Spriestersbach, D., and Curtis, J., Misarticulation and discrimination of speech sounds. *Quart. J. Speech*, **37**, 483-491 (1951).

Stansell, B., Effects of deglutition training and speech training on dental overjet. *J. South. Calif. dent. Assoc.*, **38**, 423-437 (1970).

Stetson, R., *Motor Phonetics: a Study of Speech Movements in Action.* Amsterdam: North-Holland Publishing Co. (1951).

Stitt, C., and Huntington, D., Some relationships among articulation, auditory abilities, and certain other variables. *J. Speech Hearing Res.*, **12**, 576-593 (1969).

Templin, M., A study of sound discrimination ability of elementary school pupils. *J. Speech Dis.*, **8**, 127-132 (1943).

Templin, M., *Certain Language Skills in Children: Their Development and Interrelationships.* Institute of Child Welfare, Monograph Series No. 26. Minneapolis: University of Minnesota Press (1957).

Templin, M., Development of speech. *J. Pediatr.* **62**, 11-14 (1963).

Templin, M., The study of articulation and language development during the early school years. In Miller, G., and Smith, F. (Eds.), *The Genesis of Language.* Cambridge, Mass.: The M.I.T. Press (1966).

Travis, L., *Speech Pathology.* New York: Appleton-Century-Crofts (1931).

Van Riper, C., *Speech Correction: Principles and Methods.* Englewood Cliffs, N.J.: Prentice-Hall, Inc. (1963).

Van Riper, C., and Erikson, R., A predictive screening test of articulation. *J. Speech Hearing Dis.*, **34**, 214-219 (1969).

Van Riper, C., and Irwin, J., *Voice and Articulation.* Englewood Cliffs, N.J.: Prentice-Hall, Inc. (1958).

West, R., and Ansberry, M., *The rehabilitation of Speech.* New York: Harper & Row, Publishers (1968).

Wickelgren, W., Distinctive features and errors in short-term memory for English vowels. *J. acoust. Soc. Am.*, **38**, 583-588 (1965a).

Wickelgren, W., Distinctive features in short-term memory for English consonants. *J. acoust. Soc. Am.*, **39**, 388-398 (1965b).

Winitz, H., Speech pathology: some principles underlying therapeutic practices. *Asha*, **10**, 202-203 (1968).

Winitz, H., *Articulatory Acquisition and Behavior.* New York: Appleton-Century-Crofts (1969).

Winitz, H., and Bellerose, B., Effects of pretraining on sound discrimination training. *J. Speech Hearing Res.*, **6**, 171-180 (1963a).

Winitz, H., and Bellerose, B., Phoneme-sound generalization as a function of phoneme similarity and verbal unit of test and training stimuli. *J. Speech Hearing Res.*, **6**, 379-392 (1963b).

Winitz, H., and Irwin, O., Syllabic and phonetic structure of infants' early words. *J. Speech Hearing Res.*, **1**, 250-256 (1958).

Winitz, H., and Preisler, L., Effect of distinctive feature pretraining in phoneme discrimination learning. *J. Speech Hearing Res.*, **10**, 515-530 (1967).

Wood, K., Measurement of progress in the correction of articulatory speech defects. *J. Speech Hearing Dis.*, **14**, 171-174 (1949).

Wright, H., Reliability of evaluations during basic articulation and stimulation testing. *J. Speech Hearing Dis.*, Monogr. Suppl. 4, pp. 20-27 (1954).

Yoss, K., and Darley, F., Developmental apraxia of speech in children with defective articulation. *J. Speech Hearing Res.*, **17**, 339-416 (1974).

Chapter 13

Disorders of phonation

Questions

1. What are the characteristics of disorders of phonation?
2. With what disabilities are phonatory disorders associated?

PHONATORY DISORDERS: A BEHAVIORAL PROBLEM

Phonatory disorders involve defective vocal behavior. By contrast, laryngeal disabilities involve anatomic defects and physiologic dysfunction of the vocal mechanism. Vocal production can affect the vocal mechanism and vice versa; persistent vocal abuse, for example, is a common cause of such laryngeal lesions as nodules. In this sense, the term *functional disorders of voice* is meaningful: vocal function can lead to laryngeal pathology. Conversely, abnormal laryngeal conditions typically interfere with normal phonation, so much so that when the larynx must be surgically removed, a complete substitute for normal phonation is needed. The laryngologist's specialty is the laryngeal condition, whereas the speech pathologist's specialty is behavior of vocal production. This chapter is about the latter: disorders of phonation with and without a larynx.

Phonatory disorders with a larynx

Behavioral characteristics of voice. Whether defective phonation reflects abnormal functions of a normal larynx (functional voice disorders") or of a defective larynx ("organic disorders"), the problem that the speech pathologist must manage is the vocal behavior involved. Since considerably more research has been done on the physiology of phonation and respiration than on the behavioral aspects of vocal production, this chapter rests heavily on clinical evidence.

Although voice is usually described in terms of pitch, loudness, and quality, only the first two are independent dimensions of vocal production. Quality is multidimensional, reflecting interaction of at least six parameters. These parameters are the independent behavioral elements by which vocal production is controlled: *pitch*, *loudness*, *voicing*, *vocal constriction*, *vocal mode*, and *vocal focus*. Each can be regulated separately of the others, although typically they interact. The independent factors are controlled by the speaker to generate the breath stream of speech (Perkins, 1971a). Two dependent dimensions, *vocal effort* and *vocal smoothness*, can also be described. Since they interact necessarily with independent dimensions, they cannot be controlled separately (Chapter 3).

Optimal vocal behavior. The objective of this behavioral analysis is to account for all normal and abnormal vocal conditions with a minimum of vocal elements, six independent and two dependent dimensions being proposed as sufficient. To determine whether a dimension is produced defectively, we must have a clear idea of how it would be produced optimally. Criteria for assessing optimal vocal production are therefore necessary.

Although *esthetic standards* of the culture and *acoustical standards* of comprehension must be considered in evaluating optimal phonation, the dominant criterion for the speech pathologist is *vocal hygiene*. Any form of vocalization abusive to the larynx would, by any conceivable standard, be undesirable. Fortunately, esthetic, acoustical, and hygienic criteria are not incompatible provided vocal hygiene is accorded prime importance. An efficient voice achieves maximum acoustical output, flexibility, and esthetic gratification with minimal effort. To strive for pitch or loudness levels by pushing the voice will impede acoustical output and flexibility. Similarly, to strain for quality will yield unpleasant tone. Maximum realization of acoustical and esthetic goals is achieved when voice is produced efficiently, therefore effortlessly, therefore hygienically (Perkins, 1957, 1971b).

These six independent and two dependent dimensions proposed would be present in any vocal sound. All must be considered: at any instant voice is produced at a specific pitch, with some level of loudness, voicing, focus, and vocal constriction, all of which are regulated within a specific vocal mode, require a specific amount of vocal effort, and are controlled with some amount of smoothness. Because these dimensions interact, they must be evaluated as an integral set of elements that functions holistically, an injunction that accords with Brodnitz' (1965) view. For instance, when the average speaker raises pitch, loudness and constriction follow. Similarly, when loudness is increased, pitch and constriction follow. In fact, a mark of vocal skill is the ability to control each independent dimension independently. The poorer the vocal production, the more the dimensions interact, the greater the probability of vocal abuse, and the more the speech pathologist must evaluate all vocal elements in a holistic context.

The specification of optimal function is quite different from the specification of normal. Optimum is best, whereas normal is average. Persons with vocal problems vary widely in their needs for optimal production. Some use voice infrequently and in quiet settings. They may get by with production so poor that it does not even qualify as normal, let alone optimal. Others will require higher standards. The clinician should be prepared to offer as much help as a vocally handicapped person needs. By aiming for optimal function that yields optimal vocal balance and efficiency, therapy can be terminated at whatever distance from this objective is deemed adequate.

Deviant vocal behavior. Deviations from optimum have characteristic features that we will examine briefly before analyzing vocal disorders for their behavioral components.

Pitch is generally an accomplice, not the culprit, in vocal abuse, a position supported by one of the few investigations of voice therapy (Laguaite and Waldrop, 1964). Pitch works traumatic effects only by interaction with constriction. If all pitches were produced free of constriction—the goal of vocal

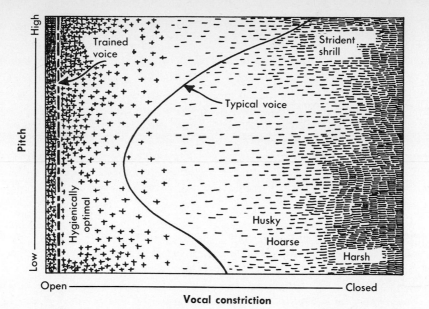

Fig. 13-1. Interaction of pitch with constriction. The tendency to interact increases above and below the lower midpitch range. Pluses indicate hygienic production, minuses vocally abusive production. (From Perkins, W., Vocal function: assessment and therapy. In Travis, L. [Ed.], *The Handbook of Speech Pathology and Audiology.* New York: Appleton-Century-Crofts [1971].)

training—the entire range would be optimal. As Fig. 13-1 shows, though, constriction interacts with high and low pitches for most speakers. The more the interaction, the more vocal effort is required to maintain loudness. Pitches above optimum are typically associated with strident, shrill, tense voices. They tend to abuse the vocal folds at the point of maximum displacement, the middle of the vibrating glottis. Pitches below optimum are more apt to be associated with voices described as harsh, hoarse, husky, and rough.

Loudness tends to interact in a straight-line function with constriction, as you can see in Fig. 13-2; the greater the loudness, the greater the constriction. With constriction, vocal efficiency drops, so that increased vocal effort is required to achieve loudness. This interaction tends to amplify whatever form of vocal abuse is in the making. Whereas the pitch-constriction interaction tends to select different locations for vocal trauma (vocal nodules at high pitches, contact ulcers at

low ones), loudness and constriction combine to supply the power to make the selected form of vocal abuse traumatic. Were voice produced softly, regardless of pitch-constriction interaction, no pathology would be likely to develop. A three-way interaction among loudness, pitch, and constriction is probably necessary to account for functional abuse of the vocal cords.

Voicing (the dimension concerned with the extent to which the breath stream is converted to tone by glottal vibrations) interacts with constriction as shown in Fig. 13-3. The reason for this interaction involves loudness and vocal effort. The level of voicing is normally a function of the loudness level required: one does not whisper (voiceless) when a shout (voiced) is needed. Furthermore, vocal effort generally increases directly as the need for loudness increases. Thus a speaker's inclination is to increase voicing along with effort to meet loudness requirements. With a healthy larynx, a breathy voice tends to have little constriction be-

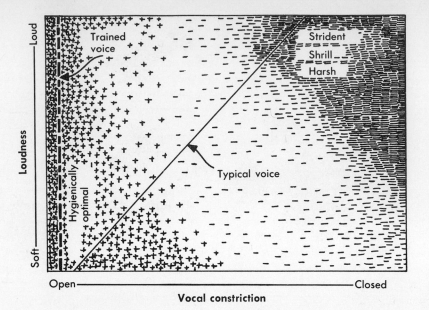

Fig. 13-2. Interaction of loudness with constriction. The tendency to interact increases progressively with increased loudness. Interaction is minimal at all loudness levels in an optimally produced voice. (From Perkins, W., Vocal function: assessment and therapy. In Travis, L. [Ed.], *The Handbook of Speech Pathology and Audiology.* New York: Appleton-Century-Crofts [1971].)

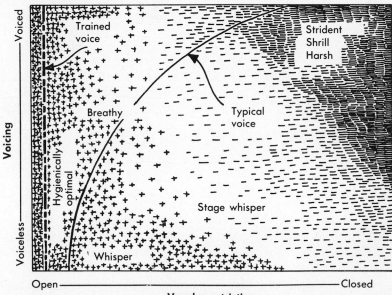

Fig. 13-3. Interaction of voicing with constriction. When loudness is minimal, the tendency to interact decreases as breathiness increases. If loudness is achieved with a whisper, however, constriction generally increases. (From Perkins, W., Vocal function: assessment and therapy. In Travis, L. [Ed.], *The Handbook of Speech Pathology and Audiology.* New York: Appleton-Century-Crofts [1971].)

cause breathiness is rarely used when loudness is needed (an exception is a stage whisper, which is usually produced with strain). With laryngeal disability that precludes full voicing, constriction is typically found because of the increased effort required to achieve loudness with excessive airflow. Frequently in such cases, a louder, less constricted voice can be achieved by reducing effort. Physiologically, reduction of effort involves reducing subglottal pressure to the optimal level that a particular larynx can utilize for generation of its most powerful glottal pulses. Beyond this optimal level, the vocal folds will either leak air with loss of vocal power, or, to resist excessive pressure, the individual may squeeze the false vocal folds and laryngeal inlet closed, which is the ultimate in vocal constriction. Either way, despite inefficiency, the potential for tissue damage is reduced because the cords do not close with the force they achieve in full voicing.

That vocal constriction (the feeling of openness or closedness of the throat) is a key to vocal hygiene has been often reiterated. Like weeds in a garden, constriction has no useful place in the cultivated (or uncultivated) voice. It serves to limit all independent dimensions. Like weeds, it tends to spread, thriving on one of its accomplices, vocal effort, with which it is apparently reflexively related. In fact, the only way subglottal pressure can be achieved is with laryngeal resistance to exhalation. Because the natural tendency is to increase loudness by increasing vocal effort (subglottal pressure), this increase, in the inefficient voice, is typically countered by vocal constriction, which increases laryngeal resistance, reduces loudness, and hence requires more effort, which is resisted with more constriction, and so the spiral goes. By contrast, the optimal condition to be emulated for efficient phonation occurs with each inhalation in a healthy vocal tract: the throat expands to offer minimal

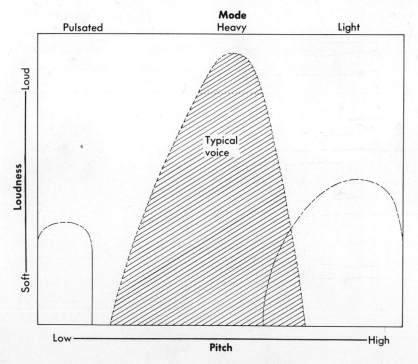

Fig. 13-4. Interactions among mode, pitch, and loudness. Heavy vocal mode permits the widest pitch and loudness ranges, pulsated vocal mode the narrowest. (From Perkins, W., Vocal function: assessment and therapy. In Travis, L. [Ed.], *The Handbook of Speech Pathology and Audiology.* New York: Appleton-Century-Crofts [1971].)

resistance to incoming air. Only in the pathologic condition of inspiratory dyspnea would the vocal tract be as constricted on inhalation as it is for inefficient vocal production on exhalation.

Deviant vocal mode (register) is more often a problem of inadequate loudness (acoustical criterion) or deviation from cultural standards (esthetic criterion) than of vocal abuse (hygienic criterion). You can see in Fig. 13-4 the approximate relative ranges of pitch and loudness for each mode. Obviously, heavy voice holds considerable advantage in flexibility over pulsated and, to a lesser extent, light voice. Probably the most frequently troublesome mode problem in our culture is *mutational voice* in adolescent boys and occasionally adult males. Usually for psychologic reasons, adolescent males shift to light voice at puberty to resist the vocal change a growing larynx would force on them if they retained heavy voice. In *virilization,* the female voice becomes heavy and masculine, generally because of hormonal imbalance (Damsté, 1967). All modes can be produced hygienically or abusively. Pulsated voice, however, seems to impose the narrowest limits on constriction and effort, it offers the least potential for abuse. Although light and pulsated voices are of restricted value for social communication, they have hygienic value that can be utilized as therapeutic means to an end—a normal voice.

Vocal focus (the feeling of location of the tone, from floating high in the head to being squeezed from low in the throat) is pivotal to efficient vocal production. Although pitch, like focus, can be altered along a continuum from high to low, the two dimensions are entirely separate. For instance, a tone with low focus pushed from a tight throat can be produced with a range of pitches from low to high. With low focus, constriction is virtually impossible to avoid, as shown in Fig. 13-5. As you might surmise, vocal abuse is invariably associated with low focus. Conversely, high focus is a powerful antidote for constriction. A voice focused high in the head feels as though it "floats," as though it were disconnected from the throat. It feels effortless to produce, and yet the tone, being relatively free of noise, carries clearly. The actor relies on high focus to "project" his voice in a large auditorium without seeming to shout. Similarly, the production of the professional singer's extraordinary pitch and loudness ranges requires a high focus (Chapter 3).

Most of what needs to be said about deviant vocal effort has been said. Any pattern of breath control that elicits vocal constric-

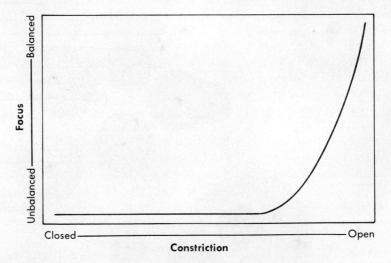

Fig. 13-5. Interaction of focus with constriction. Only with high focus can minimal constriction be maintained at high loudness levels. With soft, breathy tones, abusive effects of constriction associated with middle and low focal levels can be minimized.

tion, is unsteady, or limits vital capacity deviates from optimum. *Clavicular breathing* (upper chest breathing) tends to be ruled out on all three counts. Since vocal effort is required in some amount for all vocal dimensions, it is necessarily ubiquitous. Constriction is not. Constricted vocal production cannot exist without effort, but effort can, and should, be exerted without constriction.

Irregularity in the smoothness of control of any vocal dimension, with the possible exception of constriction, deviates from optimum. Acoustical studies of frequency, intensity, and harmonic components of voice have consistently shown irregularity associated with pitch, laryngeal pathology, harshness, or constriction (Coleman, 1969; Lieberman, 1963; Wendahl, 1963, 1966; Bowler, 1964; Koike, 1967, 1969; Yanagihara, 1967; Beckett, 1969). These results involve irregularities of pitch, loudness, and voicing particularly and are heard as roughness. Irregular control of vocal mode involves "breaks" in pitch sometimes heard in adolescent male voices. Irregular control of vocal effort is likely to be heard as tremor in pitch and loudness effects, a diagnostic sign of certain neuromotor disabilities (Darley, 1964). On the other hand, irregular control of constriction could be considered advantageous; even intermittent lessening of constriction points to some ability, albeit variable, to improve vocal production.

Behavioral analysis of disorders of the voice. Traditional medical distinctions between functional and organic disorders of the voice can be confusing for the speech pathologist whose responsibility is to correct deviant vocal behavior. Certainly we should know the behavioral effects of laryngeal pathologies described by such authorities as Brodnitz (1967), Moore (1971), Luchsinger and Arnold (1965), Van Riper and Irwin (1958), Cooper (1973), and Greene (1957). From the standpoint of vocal behavior, however, a speaker with a normal larynx can exhibit a performance similar to that of a

Would West and Ansberry (1968) agree with this statement of the speech pathologist's responsibility?

speaker with laryngeal paralysis, endocrine disturbance, muscular or mucosal disorders, neoplasms, or dysarthric dysphonia. Regardless of laryngeal condition, our task is to know what a speaker does vocally that is defective.

Unfortunately, vocal disorders have persistently resisted exact definition. As Murphy (1964) says, they are described by a language of metaphor, ranging from "pear shaped" to "metallic." Aside from ambiguities of metaphoric terms, Brodnitz (1967) cautions that the "as if" is quickly forgotten; we can easily come to believe in our metaphors. Murphy has collected over sixty terms used for normal and abnormal voice. Nine current texts use twenty-seven terms for defective voice. Of these, only twelve are in more than one text, and of these twelve, only two, "nasality" and "hoarseness," are used by all. The next six contenders, on which at least four texts agree, are, in order of preference, "breathy," "harsh," "strident," "denasal," "husky," and "metallic." Unfortunately, "husky" is synonymous with "breathy" in two texts and with "hoarse" in another; "harsh" means "metallic" or "strident" in one, "strident" and "intense" in another, and "throaty" in still another; and "strident" is equivalent to "guttural," "strained," "shrill," "harsh," or "metallic." Obviously, this gordian knot of intertwined terminology hardly provides a lucid description of defective vocal behavior.

Fig. 13-6 displays an attempt to give order to this problem. The thesis is that most of the confusion arises from lack of agreement on terms descriptive of perception of normal as well as defective vocal quality. Because of the infinite phonatory-respiratory physiologic adjustments possible with either a healthy or disabled larynx, and because each adjustment produces a different vocal quality, the problem is to agree on categories (and terms to label categories) for the sounds produced by all these adjustments.

The speech pathologist's difficulties extend farther, however. Being responsible for modifying as well as describing defective voice, he must be able to specify the vocal behavior to be controlled. The proposal

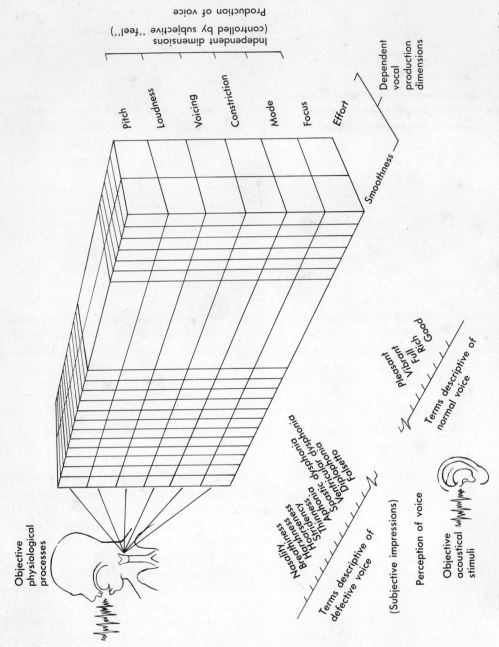

Fig. 13-6. Model of vocal production dimensions as determinants of perception of voice. Perception of normal and abnormal voice quality is conceived as a product of the combination of six independent and two dependent vocal elements.

offered is that six independent and two dependent dimensions of vocal production are necessary, and possibly sufficient, to account for the endless variety of normal and defective vocal sounds produced.

This concept, though verified in clinical practice, is exceedingly difficult to test thoroughly in the research laboratory, mainly because of poor correspondence between vocal physiology and "feel" as well as sound of voice, the two sensory feedback modalities by which phonation is guided. Low-frequency harmonic components of voice are particularly distorted for self-perception by bone conduction feedback. The result: no one ever sounds to himself as he sounds on a tape recording heard only by air conduction. Clinical impression suggests that greater stability exists between the "feel" of voice and vocal physiology, at least for those aware of such sensations. This is not to contend at all that these somesthetic impressions describe vocal physiology accurately. To say that a tone feels focused in the head is not intended to be descriptive of where it is actually produced physiologically or acoustically. The point is that these sensations provide stable guidance for vocal production. Furthermore, they can be raised to awareness with practice.

The need is to supplement, not replace, perceptual with production terminology. Both are required. Production terms, however, must describe behavioral elements by which phonation is regulated. Therefore, the eight parameters proposed have been developed to be unidimensional. Although they typically interact, each independent element can be measured and controlled separately along a single scale. By contrast, perceptual terms descriptive of normal as well as disordered voice reflect interaction of all aspects of vocal production. If reliably established, they would provide convenient economical descriptions of these patterns of complex interactions, but they would be of little value in providing explicit information by which vocal production could be controlled and modified.

Perception vis-à-vis production of vocal disorders. The difficulty with the description of perception of voice is not so much with the terms per se as with lack of agreement as to meanings. Those terms listed in Fig. 13-6 are far from exhaustive (which is why the figure shows room for expansion of terms for both defective and normal voice). Even though judges in one study (Thurman, 1953) agreed reasonably well on the first six of these terms for voice disorders, in another (Bradford, Brooks, and Shelton, 1964) a frequently used term, "hypernasality," was found unreliable. Failure to agree on the sounds to describe as nasal should not be surprising in view of several possibilities for confusion. First, nasality is mainly a transmission problem of resonance more than a tone generation problem of phonation (Fairbanks, 1960). As such, it can be a disorder of *hypernasality* with excessive nasal resonance, of *hyponasality* with the nose occluded (often called *denasality*), of "hooty" nasality with excessive air escape as in cleft palate speech, or of "twangy" nasality with vocal tract tensions (Brodnitz, 1965; Luchsinger and Arnold, 1965; Vennard, 1964). Yet, *nasality* is one of the most universally used terms in voice literature.

Hoarseness is descriptive of the early warning sound of laryngitis, vocal abuse, and serious pathology (Moore, 1971; Williamson, 1945; Yanagihara, 1967; Zinn, 1945). Even though used as universally as "nasality," it is usually described with an even wider variety of subtypes and synonyms. Like harshness, nasality is one of the more frequently investigated disorders of voice (Bowler, 1964; Wendahl, 1963; Rees, 1958; Michel and Hollien, 1968).

Perhaps *falsetto* is the easiest condition to recognize (the sound of light vocal mode); as a result it is probably the least ambiguous of most voice terms. *Aphonia,* too, identifies an unambiguous condition—no voice. Whether to speak of *hysterical aphonia* and confirm the opinion of neurotic symptom, or to call the condition *functional aphonia* and avoid unpleasant implications while leaving the door ajar for various other causes, indicates possible disagreement only about the etiology of the condition (Aronson, Peterson, and Litin, 1964; Brodnitz, 1965, 1969a). The same is true of *diplophonia,* a term that denotes double pitch, one pitch usually normal and the other low. Two structures in the vocal tract vibrating at different rates produce this distinctive sound, but opinions vary as to which two structures (Luchsinger and Arnold, 1965; Moore, 1971; Murphy, 1964; Van Riper and Irwin, 1958).

With *ventricular dysphonia,* the point of agreement is that the ventricular folds (false vocal folds) vibrate, but the ability to detect this fact by the sound of the voice is dubious. Brodnitz (1969b) indicates that it is easily confused with excessive constriction and cannot be properly diagnosed without stroboscopic examination. Perhaps as much disagreement surrounds the condition called *spastic dysphonia* as any. Some think it sounds like ventricular dysphonia (Murphy, 1964). Some call it "laryngeal stuttering" (Brodnitz, 1965). Most believe it is a psychogenic problem (Bloch, 1965; Kiml, 1965). Some point to evidence that it can be of neurologic origin (Robe, Brumlik, and Moore, 1960; Aronson and others, 1968a, b).

But all seem agreed that it is a problem resistant to effective treatment.

The foregoing has been a sampling of terms descriptive of different types of defective voice. Some are associated with misuse of a normal larynx, others of an impaired larynx. Regardless, the proposal here is that all are produced by adjustments of our eight vocal dimensions. Obviously, these vocal dimensions could be combined in a multitude of other patterns of defective voice. In effect, this type of analysis extends the distinctive feature concept of phonology from articulation to phonation. Just as phonemes are produced by combining different distinctive articulatory features, so are optimum and defective types of phonation produced by distinctive combinations of vocal elements. Summed up in Table 13-1 for each type of perceived phonatory defect are those production elements which necessarily seem to deviate from optimum.

Basic to Table 13-1 is the idea that each instant of phonation involves an adjustment of each vocal dimension. Were a specific sound to be produced, all eight production elements would have to be specified, just as a musical score specifies the note each instrument in an orchestra will play at a given

Table 13-1. Defective vocal production dimensions of typical disorders of voice

Perceived phonatory defect	Vocal dimensions that necessarily deviate from optimum							
	Pitch	Loud-ness	Voicing	Constric-tion	Mode	Focus	Effort	Smooth-ness
Nasal escape			Breathy					
Nasal twang				High		Low		
Breathiness			Breathy					
Harshness	Low			High		Low	High	Rough
Hoarseness	Low		Breathy			Low		Rough
Stridency	High	High		High		Low	High	
Thinness		Low		High		Low	Low	
Aphonia		Low	Whisper					
Spastic dysphonia	Low	Low	Breathy	High		Low	High	Rough
Ventricular dysphonia	High or low			High		Low	High	Rough
Diplophonia	Double pitch		Breathy					Rough
Falsetto	High				Light voice			

instant. Were one interested only in the melody, he would not need a fully orchestrated musical score. Similarly, our interest at the moment is only in the basis of phonatory disorders. Thus, to avoid the confusion of unnecessary details, we have specified deviations from optimum production for only those dimensions essential to a particular disorder. The fact that the remaining elements are unspecified implies that they involve any adjustment that is either optimal or a deviation secondary to the basic problem (for example, excessive airflow is the primary problem of "breathiness"—the result is often inadequate loudness, for which effort and constriction typically increase in compensatory effort, but none of these possible secondary reactions is indicated in the table).

Speech without a larynx

One century ago speech without a larynx was no problem; laryngeal cancer terminated in death, not laryngectomy. Today, the American Cancer Society (1955) estimates that 3,000 persons annually survive surgical removal of the larynx to join the more than 25,000 now alive in the United States. For these individuals, the breath stream of speech can no longer be produced by laryngeal phonation; a substitute method of sound generation is required.

Two basic alternatives are available: *alaryngeal speech* or an *artificial larynx*. Alaryngeal speech utilizes a *neoglottis*, also called a *pseudoglottis*, and an air pocket to activate it at some level of the esophageal-vocal tract. Historically, four types of alaryn-

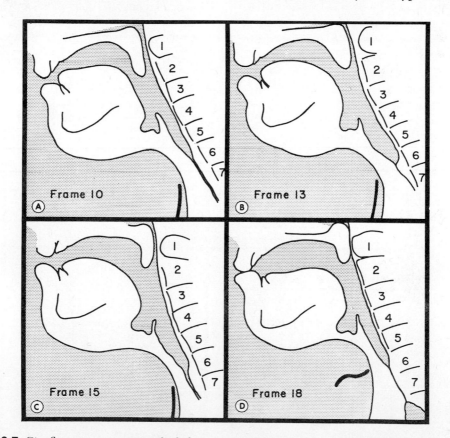

Fig. 13-7. Cinefluorogram tracings of inhalation method of air intake. The four frames shown are in preparation for /pa/. The esophageal air reservoir appears in Frame 18, six frames prior to beginning of phonation. (From Diedrich, W., and Youngstrom, K., *Alaryngeal Speech.* Springfield, Ill.: Charles C Thomas, Publisher [1966].)

geal speech have been described: *buccal*, *pharyngeal*, *esophageal*, and *gastric*. Each is named for location of the air bubble, whether in the mouth, throat, esophagus, or stomach. Of these, only one is used extensively: *esophageal speech* (Diedrich, 1968). Recently, however, a new surgical procedure, the *Asai technique*, has added a new form of alaryngeal speech in selected cases. An artificial larynx is what the name implies, a device for generating sound that, when applied to the vocal tract, activates air in the resonators for speech modulation.

Esophageal speech. Esophageal speech involves a method of inflating an air reservoir in the gullet used to activate vibration of a neoglottis near the top of the esophagus. Let us examine the behavioral mechanisms of air intake and expulsion.

Air intake. Two basic methods are used to inflate the esophageal reservoir: *inhalation* and *injection.* The inhalation method, also called *suction* or *breathing*, is much preferred by Hodson and Oswald (1958) in England and by Seeman (1958) in Prague. Air is apparently "sucked" into the esophagus by rapid downward movement of the diaphragm. With skilled speakers, air is not swallowed, nor does it enter the stomach. The cinefluorogram tracings in Fig. 13-7 show mouth and throat actions of the inhalation method.

The injection method has been described as involving two techniques: *tongue-pumping* and *glossopharyngeal-press*, or *plosive-injection*. From available evidence, however, Snidecor (1969) and Diedrich and Youngstrom (1966) have concluded that these tech-

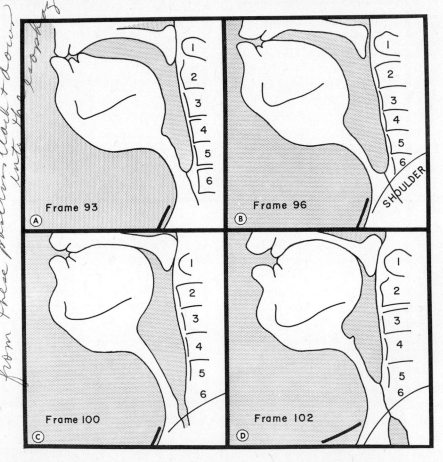

Fig. 13-8. Cinefluorogram tracings of glottal press method of air injection. Tongue action, as shown in preparation for /u/, is essential for this method. (From Diedrich, W., and Youngstrom, K., *Alaryngeal Speech.* Springfield, Ill.: Charles C Thomas, Publisher [1966].)

niques are interrelated components of a basic pattern of air injection. Electromyographic and x-ray evidence shows, however, that they are separable (Shipp, 1970; Diedrich and Youngstrom, 1966). In one the tongue pumps air into the esophagus in rapid, swallowlike motions. In the other, endorsed by Damsté (1959) and Moolenaar-Bijl (1953), the throat is relaxed, and air in the oropharyngeal cavity is compressed from consonant positions /p/, /t/, or /k/ back and down into the esophagus, as shown in Fig. 13-8.

These methods are not exclusive; they can be used in whatever combination works best for the individual. The inhalation method can yield excellent results but it requires considerable energy that may exclude it as feasible for enfeebled persons. Because respiratory inhalation must accompany it, considerable noise in the tracheostoma tends to accompany vigorous effort. Too, whichever method permits fastest intake of the most air (usually the inhalation method) is a consideration (Isshiki, 1969). Also important is the method, or combination of methods, that dilates the entire esophagus. Superior speakers tend to have a larger available air supply (Diedrich and Youngstrom, 1966) and to hold what air they do take in higher in the esophagus than poorer speakers (Snidecor, 1969).

Air expulsion. Agreement prevails about mechanisms of sound generation by expulsion of esophageal air. Normally, intake and expulsion operate in synchrony with respiratory inhalation and exhalation, but the relation is complex (Isshiki and Snidecor, 1965). Synchrony on inhalation is necessary with the inhalation method but not always needed with the injection method; expulsion of esophageal air seems to be coordinated with pulmonary exhalation regardless of method (Isshiki, 1969).

The vibratory segment that functions as the neoglottis is considered to be the *pharyngoesophageal junction*. This junction is thought to be comprised usually of the cricopharyngeus muscle, but x-ray evidence indicates that fibers from the inferior constrictor and superior esophageal sphincter are also probably involved. Curiously, little relation

has been found between the length of the surgically reconstructed pharyngoesophageal junction and the quality of speech (Robe and others, 1956; Finkbeiner, 1969; Diedrich and Youngstrom, 1966). According to Brodnitz (1969b), however, radiation treatment tends to impair softness and vibratory capacity of the pseudoglottis. The ability to relax the throat is essential for expulsion as well as intake. Speech often becomes impossible when tension mounts. On the other hand, control of tension and airflow in the neoglottis would seem necessary to explain the ability to vary pitch (Snidecor, 1969).

Pitch, loudness, quality, and time. Several investigators have studied the fundamental frequency of alaryngeal speech. Much of this work has been done on superior speakers in order to determine the limits that can be achieved. In general, as Fig. 13-9 shows, esophageal speech is an octave lower than laryngeal speech, a condition that poses several problems (Snidecor and Curry, 1960; Rollin, 1962; Curry, 1969). Shipp (1967) has shown clearly that alaryngeal speech is more acceptable at high than low fundamental frequencies. No doubt the distorting effect of low frequencies on pitch perception contributes to lack of acceptance. When superior alaryngeal speakers were compared with superior normal speakers for pitch variability, the alaryngeal group was judged to have "restricted pitch range"—even though their frequency range was 13.2 tones in comparison with only 10.5 for normal speakers (Snidecor and Curry, 1960). Too, low fundamental frequency reduces vowel intelligibility by producing acoustical overlap of formants one and two of adjacent vowels (Rollin, 1962).

Loudness, like pitch, is lower in esophageal than in normal speech. Hyman (1955) found a 79 dB intensity level for normal speakers, and a 73 dB level for esophageal speakers. More recently, 95 dB peaks for normal speakers have been reported, in contrast with 85 dB in esophageal speech. The intensity range even in superior alaryngeal speech is more limited: 20 dB in comparison with 45 dB in normal speech (Snidecor and Isshiki, 1965).

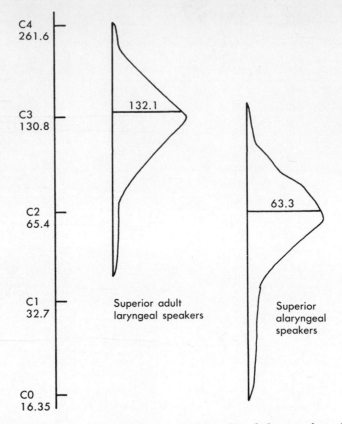

C4 261.6

C3 130.8

132.1

63.3

C2 65.4

C1 32.7

Superior adult laryngeal speakers

Superior alaryngeal speakers

C0 16.35

Fig. 13-9. Pitch frequencies of superior laryngeal (normal) and alaryngeal speakers. Although average pitch levels for the two groups differ by about an octave, individual speakers vary widely. (From Snidecor, J., *Speech Rehabilitation of the Laryngectomized.* [2nd ed.] Springfield, Ill.: Charles C Thomas, Publisher [1969].)

The single most descriptive term for the quality of esophageal speech is "hoarse." Considering the relative crudeness of the neoglottis in comparison with the intricately refined structure of a normal larynx, we can marvel that esophageal quality is as good as it is. Apparently, it can gradually improve for 5 or more years (Palmer, 1970). Additionally, the characteristically irregular vibratory patterns and indistinct harmonic structure of esophageal quality also reduce vowel intelligibility. Coupled with these problems, frequently, is an annoying respiratory noise (Nichols, 1969).

A prime criterion for the development of esophageal speech is the ability to take in air and produce an easy, natural flow of sound without apparent attention or effort (Wepman and others, 1953). By studying superior speakers who had achieved this criterion, Snidecor (1969) determined that they averaged somewhat fewer than 5 words per air charge at an average rate of 120 words per minute. Such a fast rate is not necessary, however, for a person to be a superior speaker, nor are long phrases essential (normal phrase length is 12.5 words). More important is the ability to take a fast air charge (in about 0.5 second) for use in clear, easy speech at a reasonable rate.

Asai speech. Because the Asai surgical technique (Chapter 7) was developed and has been used longer in Japan than in the United States, most of the following discussion is based on the study by Snidecor and Isshiki of five Japanese Asai speakers (Snidecor, 1969). In general, they are superior to esophageal but inferior to normal speakers.

The neoglottis, which connects the pharynx and the trachea, is activated by normal exhalation. Hence speech can be available without training after completion of therapy.

With the same air supply as for normal speech, the ability of Asai speakers to approach normal in the management of air is understandable. They use about the same volume as normal speakers, which is greater than that used in esophageal speech. They tend to waste air in breathy production more than esophageal speakers, but even so they are still better able to sustain phonation of a vowel or to count on one breath. They approach normal pitch and loudness levels, and their speaking rate can be normal, far beyond esophageal speakers, who at best approach low normal. This difference in rate points up the complexity of the role of phonation and respiration in articulatory coordinations. Once learned for normal speech, these coordinations are difficult to master in altered form for esophageal speech.

The Asai technique with its speech advantages has serious drawbacks, nonetheless. Miller (1969), who has done much of the early surgical work with it in the United States, says that he would not encourage it for a laryngectomee with excellent esophageal voice. Furthermore, patients must be selected carefully if the operation is to have much chance of success. Three operations and a convalescent period are required. Too, food and drink tend to leak through the dermal tube into the trachea. Perhaps the most serious drawback for those who must use their hands while talking (for example, waitresses) is that for speech, the tracheal stoma must be closed by finger pressure.

Artificial larynx. The relative value of esophageal speech versus that of an artificial larynx is a traditional issue in rehabilitation of the laryngectomized person. A prevailing attitude has been that esophageal speech is preferable as a more natural, convenient, and economical—though no more intelligible and not as loud—substitute for normal voice (Diedrich and Youngstrom, 1966). This attitude has apparently been effective: the American Cancer Society estimates that 69% of laryngectomized persons use esophageal speech.

Snidecor (1969) points out circumstances, however, in which an artificial larynx might be preferred. First, the aged, lacking the motivation and strength to learn alaryngeal speech, may find an artificial larynx adequate for their limited communicative needs. Younger persons may also fit this category. Second, physical limitations such as stenosis of the esophagus or recurrence of disease may preclude the development of an adequate neoglottis. Diedrich and Youngstrom (1966) take a sensible position: the issue is not esophageal speech versus artificial larynx. Rather, it is the selection of the combination that will best meet the patient's need. In early postoperative months, for example, when the laryngectomee would otherwise be reduced to communication by writing, an artificial larynx offers several merits. It helps meet immediate needs for speech. It provides a known alternative that helps offset frustration and despair for those who later fail in attempts to learn alaryngeal speech. It also aids in the development of articulatory skill that will be needed for esophageal speech. Still, arguments for and against an artificial larynx are numerous, and the controversy remains alive (Lauder, 1968).

Use of an artificial larynx. Successful speech with an artificial larynx depends on generating sound either pneumatically or electronically, transmitting it to the resonating cavities, and modulating it with articulatory-resonatory processes. Speech aids vary in how they generate and transmit sound. Early models were reed instruments driven by breath pressure that fed sound into the mouth by an intraoral tube. Modern descendants of the pneumatic larynx are still in use, primarily in Japan. They require considerable respiratory exertion, and the tongue and tube tend to interfere with each other. An electronic version of the pneumatic larynx is available, and intraoral models that eliminate the tube are being developed. The neck type of vibrators also eliminates oral tube problems but require careful placement on the skin to work well. Perhaps the most universal difficulty with electronic vibrators is in learning to turn them on and off in synchrony with speech.

An artificial larynx does not automatically provide intelligible speech. Clear articulation of vowels requires considerable exaggeration of tongue and lip movements. Coordinations for consonantal articulation are quite different from normal speech. Whether the device is pneumatic or electronic, it only sets molecules into vibration; it does not produce the airflow required for plosives and fricatives. Their production depends on learning to impound buccal air and coordinate its release. With skill, reasonably normal speaking rates (probably under 150 words per minute) can be achieved (Diedrich and Youngstrom, 1966; Snidecor, 1969).

DISABLING CONDITIONS ASSOCIATED WITH PHONATORY DISORDERS

The phonatory process can be affected by laryngeal, bronchopulmonary, neurologic, orofacial, sensory, emotional, and personality disturbances and by environmental conditions. Let us review how these problems can interfere with the generation of the breath stream of speech.

Bronchopulmonary disabilities

Bronchopulmonary disabilities can loom as large for laryngectomized persons as for speakers with a larynx. Such diseases as emphysema and bronchial asthma can reduce the vital capacity close to the limits needed to sustain life without additional respiratory exertion. For laryngectomees with sharply reduced vital capacity, an artificial pneumatic larynx or the inhalation method of esophageal speech, both of which require vigorous respiratory effort, would probably be precluded. For speakers with a larynx, limited vital capacity will shorten the length of phrases that can be sustained, especially with inefficient phonation. This limitation can be serious for those who use voice professionally. For most, the bigger problem is maintenance of steady subglottal pressure,

a problem more related to the respiratory musculature, which is not as prone to disease or injury (Chapter 7).

Laryngeal disabilities

Normal voice requires that the cords close firmly in each vibratory cycle to permit buildup of sufficient subglottal pressure to produce a glottal pulse. The cords must vibrate in synchrony, and the glottal edges must be smooth. Moore (1957) lists five laryngeal conditions that can interfere with this requirement:

1. Those which limit adduction of the cords (adductor paralysis, ankylosis of the cricoarytenoid joints, interarytenoid growths)
2. Those which disrupt synchrony of vibration of smooth approximation of the cords (growths, edema, scars, asymmetric arytenoid approximation, excessive mucus)
3. Those which alter the contractile ability of the cords (tensor paralysis, myasthenia laryngis)
4. Those which alter the mucosal surface of the cords, thereby producing phonatory noise (excessive sticky mucus, loose mucous membrane, dry mucosa, scars)
5. Those in which essential tissue is destroyed (total or subtotal laryngectomy, injury, destructive disease)

To this list could be added endocrine conditions that alter the size of the larynx (mutational changes in males, virilization of the female voice).

Orofacial disabilities

Certainly resonance effects of cleft palate and other forms of velopharyngeal incompetence and resonance effects of obstructions in the nasal cavity are major factors in the perception of nasality and denasality. Probably, too, resonator adjustments affect phonatory efficiency, but this relation has not been demonstrated conclusively (Brooks and Shelton, 1963). The prevalent "hooty" quality of cleft palate suggests a functional relation of some sort among velopharyngeal incompetence, excessive airflow, and vocal inefficiency (Chapter 8).

Neurologic disabilities

Vocal consequences can follow damage to upper as well as lower motor neurons. The most common lower motor neuron paralyses are usually attributed to injury of the recurrent laryngeal nerve, often in connection with thyroid surgery. Depending on whether one or both nerves are damaged, and on whether superior as well as recurrent branches are involved, the pattern of paralysis will be unilateral or bilateral, incomplete or complete. If incomplete and unilateral, the disabled cord will usually be fixed in an adducted paramedian position that will permit reasonably normal vibration (and voice) of the healthy cord. If complete neural supply to a cord is impaired, an intermediate position that will make normal vibration and voice difficult is more likely.

Dysphonic effects of upper motor neuron lesions have been studied by Aronson and

Table 13-2. Summary of voice symptoms and associated factors in psychogenic and neurologic dysphonias*

	Spastic dys-phonia†	Mixed psycho-genic dys-phonia-aphonia	Essential tremor	Pseudo-bulbar palsy	Amyo-trophic lateral sclerosis	Bulbar palsy	Cere-bellar ataxia	Parkin-sonism	Total
Low pitch level	+	+	+	+	+	+	+	+	8
Pitch breaks	+	+	+	+	+	+	+	−	7
Monopitch	+	+	+	+	+	+	+	+	8
Tremor (con-textual)	+	+	+	+	+	−	+	−	6
Harshness	+	+	+	+	+	+	+	+	8
Strain-strangle	+	−	+	+	+	−	+	−	5
Irregular voice stoppages	+	−	+	+	−	−	−	−	3
Regular voice stoppages	+	−	+	−	−	−	−	−	2
Lingual paresis; asymmetry; dysarthria	−	−	−	+	+	+	+	+	5
Velopharyngeal paresis; asymmetry; hypernasality	−	−	−	+	+	+	−	−	3
Marked improve-ment with therapy	−	+	−	−	−	−	−	−	1
Course									
Gradually worse	+	−	+	+	+	+	+	+	7
Always present	+	−	+	+	+	+	+	+	7
Worse under emotional stress or fatigue	+	+	+	+	+	+	+	+	8
Voice spon-taneously returns to normal	−	+	−	−	−	−	−	−	1

*From Aronson, A., and others: Spastic dysphonia. II. Comparison with essential (voice) tremor and other neurologic and psychogenic dysphonias. *J. Speech Hearing Dis.*, **33**, 219-231 (1968).
†+ = Often present; − = often absent.

his associates at Mayo Clinic (1968b). Table 13-2 summarizes their clinical findings of the relative presence or absence of voice disorders in a comparison of "psychogenic" and "neurologic" dysphonias. The most striking point in this table is that spastic dysphonia, generally considered to be a psychogenic problem, more closely resembles the neurologic dysphonias (Chapter 5).

Sensory disabilities

Control of phonation is dependent on the "feel" as well as on the sound of voice. Little evidence is available, however, about the relation between somesthetic disabilities and voice disorders. Even the effects of auditory disabilities on phonation can be kept minimal unless severe loss precedes the acquisition of speech. Perhaps because the child learns vocal patterns of intonation as his first imitation of adult speech, or perhaps for less obvious reasons, voice seems particularly resistant to deterioration with hearing loss. For laryngectomized individuals, by contrast, hearing is crucial. Without experience in alaryngeal speech, they must hear themselves to develop adequate intelligibility, loudness, or quality. Too, they must be able to hear respiratory and air-injection noises if they are to eliminate these distractions (Chapter 6).

Emotional and personality disturbances

Voice is often considered to be the mirror of emotions and personality. Moses (1954) wrote a book on the subject—*The Voice of Neurosis*. Rousey and Moriarty (1965) have presented evidence from clinical research that indicates the psychodynamic significance of such voice disorders as hoarseness, pitch deviations, breathiness, harshness, and nasality. Murphy (1964) has discussed the effects of emotional states on breathing as well as personality and parent-child conditions for learning abnormal and neurotic vocal patterns (Chapter 10).

Brodnitz (1965), though, has shown how such psychologic factors affect voice through laryngeal hyperfunctions and hypofunctions. At the hypofunctional extreme is "functional" or "hysterical" aphonia in which the speaker, by whispering, appears to have given up the will to speak (Brodnitz, 1969a). At the hyperfunctional extreme are spastic dysphonia and ventricular dysphonia. Whether such excessive effort is more symptomatic of psychologic than of neurologic disorder, the fact remains that they are a gross form of hyperfunctional phonation. Between these extremes are the more frequent abusive forms of hyperfunctional phonation that typically involve excessive pitch, loudness, constriction, effort, and faulty respiratory control. From these hyperfunctional patterns come such consequences as laryngitis, nodules, polyps, and, more often with low-pitched, "throaty" voices of men, contact ulcers. Neither hyperfunctional nor hypofunctional, mutational voice problems in males are fraught with psychologic difficulties, especially with problems of dependency.

Successful rehabilitation of laryngectomized persons depends more on emotional and personality factors than on any others. Stoll (1958) lists often-held fears that, though sometimes exaggerated, are realistic: fear of death, cancer, operations, permanent loss of voice, loss of job, loss of friends or security, impaired appearance, old age, and uselessness. As if these fears were not enough, there is also fear of failure to learn a new method of speaking. Not surprisingly, the aggressively extroverted individual much involved in professional and social activities is the one who is most likely to learn to speak effectively.

Environmental conditions

Disorders of voice can arise directly or indirectly from environmental conditions. A dependent adolescent boy who resists "voice change" may be supported in his maladjustment by a dominant, overprotective mother. A child may be a member of a vocally competitive family in which he must shout to gain attention. An adult may have to talk constantly over noise, speak loudly and often to large groups, or use his voice in any of innumerable other conditions that invite vocal strain. Adjustment of loudness is virtually reflexive to such social conditions as the distance between speaker and listener, the background noise level, the size of the room, the size of the audience, the loudness of feedback of one's own voice, and so on. These or similar circumstances can have such powerful effects as to override all therapeutic measures. Persistent recurrence of vocal nodules and polyps after surgical removal is not uncommon in patients who continue old social patterns of voice usage.

The 69% of laryngectomees who have learned a new voice face special problems when they return home and to work (American Cancer Society, 1955). Careful attention is usually necessary to understand what is said, a requirement that can be taxing for family and friends, let alone fellow workers and strangers. In fact, a number of laryngectomees are employed because they can use small but efficient amplifiers. To improve, laryngectomees must speak as much as possible. Yet women especially are often embarrassed by their rough, low-pitched speech and must be encouraged. Many listeners, not understanding the laryngectomee's needs, react in unproductive ways. Greene (1957) tells of a transport driver who was as depressed by tender sympathy of a waitress as by being teased about his belching voice. Gardner (1966) found that of the 46% of wives whose husbands avoided, pitied, or babied them on their return home, only 65% succeeded in learning esophageal speech. By contrast, of the 54% whose husbands were supportive, 82% succeeded.

The answers—résumé

1. What are the characteristics of disorders of phonation?

Phonation is the behavior of vocal production. Phonatory disorders are, therefore, behavioral aberrations judged abnormal by deviation mainly from a criterion of vocal hygiene as well as from acoustical and cultural standards. Potentially unlimited in variety, disorders (such as hoarseness, harshness, aphonia) are inefficient interactions among six independent (pitch, loudness, voicing, constriction, mode, and focus) and two dependent (effort and smoothness) behavioral dimensions of vocal production.

The laryngectomized person must use a substitute for phonation with a larynx: alaryngeal speech or an artificial larynx. Several varieties of both are available, esophageal speech being used most frequently. It requires learning to inflate an air reservoir in the esophagus by inhalation or injection techniques and, by controlling air expulsion, setting a neoglottis at the neck of the esophagus into vibration. The sound generated is lower in pitch and slower in rate than normal. It also tends to be less intelligible and hoarse. Surgical procedures such as the Asai technique make speech that is closer to normal more easily available for selected cases. An artificial larynx, either electronic or pneumatic, is easier to learn to use than esophageal speech but has many of the same difficulties and limitations in addition to those uniquely its own.

2. With what disabilities are phonatory disorders associated?

Various conditions can disable normal phonation. Laryngeal disabilities have primary effects if they limit adduction of the cords; disrupt synchrony of vibration; alter contractile ability, mucosal surface, or size; or destroy essential tissue. Neurologic effects range from the laryngeal paralyses of damaged lower motor neurons to the neurologic dysphonias of disabled upper motor neurons. Emotional and personality conditions provide the basis for vocally inefficient hyperfunctional and hypofunctional patterns of phonation, either as a result of emotional tension or as symptomatic expression of personality conflict. Environmental conditions conducive to strained loud speech are especially damaging.

Disabling conditions for laryngectomized speakers are considerably different than for speakers with a larynx. Bronchopulmonary disabilities that reduce vital capacity close to the limits needed to sustain life preclude the use of the inhalation method of air intake or a pneumatic type of artificial larynx, both of which have high effort requirements. Auditory disabilities can reduce feedback and hence interfere with successful learning of a new method of speech. Emotional, personality, and social conditions are of overriding importance for laryngectomized persons. With their special fears, realistically centered around death, they need continuous support plus strong needs to communicate if they are to learn to speak well again.

REFERENCES

American Cancer Society and International Association of Laryngectomies, Report, October 13, 1955.

Aronson, A., Peterson, H., and Litin, E., Voice symptomatology in functional dysphonia and aphonia. *J. Speech Hearing Dis.*, **29**, 367-380 (1964).

Aronson, A., and others, Spastic dysphonia. I. Voice, neurologic, and psychiatric aspects. *J. Speech Hearing Dis.*, **33**, 203-218 (1968a).

Aronson, A., and others, Spastic dysphonia. II. Comparison with essential (voice) tremor and other neurologic and psychogenic dysphonias. *J. Speech Hearing Dis.*, **33**, 219-231 (1968b).

Beckett, R., Pitch perturbation as a function of subjective vocal constriction. *Folia Phoniatrica*, **21**, 416-425 (1969).

Bloch, P., Neuro-psychiatric aspects of spastic dysphonia. *Folia Phoniatrica*, **17**, 301-364 (1965).

Boone, D., *The Voice and Voice Therapy.* Englewood Cliffs, N.J.: Prentice-Hall, Inc. (1971).

Bowler, N., A fundamental frequency analysis of harsh vocal quality. *Speech Monogr.*, **31**, 128-134 (1964).

Bradford, L., Brooks, A., and Shelton, R., Clinical judgment of hypernasality in cleft palate children. *Cleft Palate J.*, **1**, 329-335 (1964).

Brodnitz, F., *Vocal Rehabilitation.* Rochester, Minn.: American Academy of Ophthalmology and Otolaryngology (1965).

Brodnitz, F., Semantics of the voice. *J. Speech Hearing Dis.*, **32**, 325-330 (1967).

Brodnitz, F., Functional aphonia. *Ann. Otol. Rhinol. Laryng.*, **78**, 1243-1255 (1969a).

Brodnitz, F., Personal communication (1969b).

Brooks, A., and Shelton, R., Incidence of voice disorders other than nasality in cleft palate children. *Cleft Palate Bull.*, **13**, 63-64 (1963).

Coleman, R., Effect of median frequency levels upon the roughness of jittered stimuli. *J. Speech Hearing Res.*, **12**, 330-336 (1969).

Cooper, M., *Modern Techniques of Vocal Rehabilitation.* Springfield, Ill.: Charles C Thomas, Publishers (1973).

Curry, E., Acoustical measurement and pitch perception in alaryngeal speech. In Snidecor, J. (ed.), *Speech Rehabilitation of the Laryngectomized.* Springfield, Ill., Charles C Thomas, Publisher (1969).

Damsté, P., The glosso-pharyngeal press. *Speech Pathol. Ther.*, **2**, 70-76 (1959).

Damsté, P., Voice change in adult women caused by virilizing agents. *J. Speech Hearing Dis.*, **32**, 126-132 (1967).

Darley, F., *Diagnosis and Appraisal of Communication Disorders.* Englewood Cliffs, N.J.: Prentice-Hall, Inc. (1964).

Diedrich, W., The mechanism of esophageal speech. *Ann. N.Y. Acad. Sci.*, **155**, 303-317 (1968).

Diedrich, W., and Youngstrom, K., *Alaryngeal Speech.* Springfield, Ill.: Charles C Thomas, Publisher (1966).

Fairbanks, G., *Voice and Articulation Drillbook.* New York: Harper & Row, Publishers (1960).

Finkbeiner, E., Surgery and speech, the pseudoglottis, and respiration in total standard laryngectomy. In Snidecor, J. (Ed.), *Speech Rehabilitation of the Laryngectomized.* Springfield, Ill.: Charles C Thomas, Publisher (1969).

Gardner, W., Adjustment problems of laryngectomized women. *Arch. Otolaryng.*, **83**, 31-42 (1966).

Greene, M., *The Voice and Its Disorders.* London: Sir Isaac Pitman & Sons, Ltd. (1957).

Hodson, C., and Oswald, M., *Speech Recovery After Total Laryngectomy.* Baltimore: The Williams & Wilkins Co. (1958).

Hyman, M., An experimental study of artificial-larynx and esophageal speech. *J. Speech Hearing Dis.*, **20**, 291-299 (1955).

Isshiki, N., Airflow in esophageal speech. In Snidecor, J. (Ed.), *Speech Rehabilitation of the Laryngectomized.* Springfield, Ill.: Charles C Thomas, Publisher (1969).

Isshiki, N., and Snidecor, J., Air intake and usage in

esophageal speech. *Acta Otolaryng.*, **59**, 559-574 (1965).

Kiml, J., Recherches expérimentales de la dysphonie spastique. *Folia Phoniatrica*, **17**, 241-300 (1965).

Koike, Y., Application of some acoustic measures for the evaluation of laryngeal dysfunction (abstract). *J. acoust. Soc. Am.*, **42**, 1209 (1967).

Koike, Y., Vowel amplitude modulations in patients with laryngeal diseases. *J. acoust. Soc. Am.*, **45**, 839-844 (1969).

Laguaite, J., and Waldrop, W., Acoustic analysis of fundamental frequency of voice before and after therapy. *Folia Phoniatrica*, **16**, 183-192 (1964).

Lauder, E., The laryngectomee and the artificial larynx. *J. Speech Hearing Dis.*, **33**, 147-157 (1968).

Lieberman, P., Some acoustic measures of the fundamental periodicity of normal and pathologic larynges. *J. acoust. Soc. Am.*, **35**, 344-353 (1963).

Luchsinger, R., and Arnold, G., *Voice-Speech-Language*. Belmont, Calif.: Wadsworth Publishing Co., Inc. (1965).

Michel, J., and Hollien, H., Perceptual differentiation of vocal fry and harshness. *J. Speech Hearing Res.*, **11**, 439-443 (1968).

Miller, A., First experiences with the Asai technique for vocal rehabilitation after total laryngectomy. In Snidecor, J. (Eds.), *Speech Rehabilitation of the Laryngectomized*. Springfield, Ill.: Charles C Thomas, Publisher (1969).

Moolenaar-Bijl, A., Connection between consonant articulation and the intake of air in oesophageal speech. *Folia Phoniatrica*, **15**, 212-215 (1953).

Moore, P., Voice disorders organically based. In Travis, L. (Ed.), *Handbook of Speech Pathology and Audiology*. New York: Appleton-Century-Crofts (1971).

Moses, P., *The Voice of Neurosis*. New York: Grune & Stratton, Inc. (1954).

Murphy, A., *Functional Voice Disorders*, Englewood Cliffs, N.J.: Prentice-Hall, Inc. (1964).

Nichols, A., Loudness and quality in esophageal speech and the artificial larynx. In Snidecor, J. (Ed.), *Speech Rehabilitation of the Laryngectomized*. Springfield, Ill.: Charles C Thomas, Publisher (1969).

Palmer, J., Clinical expectations in esophageal speech. *J. Speech Hearing Dis.*, **35**, 160-169 (1970).

Perkins, W., The challenge of functional disorders of voice. In Travis, L. (Ed.), *Handbook of Speech Pathology*. New York: Appleton-Century-Crofts (1957).

Perkins, W., Vocal function: a behavioral analysis. In Travis, L. (Ed.), *Handbook of Speech Pathology and Audiology*. New York: Appleton-Century-Crofts (1971a).

Perkins, W., Vocal function: assessment and therapy. In Travis, L. (Ed.), *Handbook of Speech Pathology and Audiology*. New York: Appleton-Century-Crofts (1971b).

Rees, M., Harshness and glottal attack. *J. Speech Hearing Res.*, **1**, 344-349 (1958).

Robe, E., Brumlik, J., and Moore, P., A study of spastic dysphonia: neurologic and electroencephalographic abnormalities. *Laryngoscope*, **70**, 219-245 (1960).

Robe, E., and others, A study of the role of certain factors in the development of speech after laryngectomy: 1. Type of operation; 2. Site of pseudoglottis; 3. Coordination of speech with respiration. *Laryngoscope*, **66**, 173-186, 382-401, 481-499 (1956).

Rollin, W., A comparative study of vowel formants of esophageal- and normal-speaking adults. Doctoral dissertation. Detroit: Wayne State University (1962).

Rousey, C., and Moriarty, A., *Diagnostic Implications of Speech Sounds*. Springfield, Ill.: Charles C Thomas, Publishers (1965).

Seeman, M., Pathology of the esophageal voice. *Folia Phoniatrica*, **10**, 44-50 (1958).

Shipp, T., Frequency, duration, and perceptual measures in relation to judgments of alaryngeal speech acceptability. *J. Speech Hearing Res.*, **10**, 417-427 (1967).

Shipp, T., EMG of pharyngoesophageal musculature during alaryngeal voice production. *J. Speech Hearing Dis.*, **13**, 184-192 (1970).

Snidecor, J., *Speech Rehabilitation of the Laryngectomized*. Springfield, Ill.: Charles C Thomas, Publisher (1969).

Snidecor, J., and Curry, E., How effectively can the laryngectomee expect to speak? *Laryngoscope*, **70**, 62-67 (1960).

Snidecor, J., and Isshiki, N., Vocal and air use characteristics of a superior male esophageal speaker. *Folia Phoniatrica*, **17**, 217-232 (1965).

Stoll, B., Psychological factors determining the success or failure of the rehabilitation program of laryngectomized patients. *Ann. Otol. Rhinol. Laryng.*, **67**, 550-557 (1958).

Thurman, W., The construction and acoustic analyses of recorded scales of severity for six voice quality disorders. Doctoral dissertation. Lafayette, Ind.: Purdue University (1953).

Van Riper, C., and Irwin, J., *Voice and Articulation*. Englewood Cliffs, N.J.: Prentice-Hall, Inc. (1958).

Vennard, W., An experiment to evaluate the importance of nasal resonance. *Folia Phoniatrica*, **16**, 146-153 (1964).

Wendahl, R., Laryngeal analog synthesis of harsh voice quality. *Folia Phoniatrica*, **15**, 241-250 (1963).

Wendahl, R., Laryngeal analog synthesis of jitter and shimmer auditory parameters of harshness. *Folia Phoniatrica*, **18**, 98-108 (1966).

Wepman, J., and others, The objective measurement of progressive esophageal speech development. *J. Speech Hearing Dis.*, **18**, 247-251 (1953).

West, R., and Ansberry, M., *Rehabilitation of Speech*. New York: Harper & Row, Publishers (1968).

Williamson, A., Diagnosis and treatment of seventy-two cases of hoarse voice. *Quart. J. Speech*, **31**, 189-202 (1945).

Yanagihara, N., Significance of harmonic changes and noise components in hoarseness. *J. Speech Hearing Res.*, **10**, 531-541 (1967).

Zinn, W., The significance of hoarseness. Transactions of the American Laryngological, Rhinological, and Otological Society, pp. 133-134 (1945).

Chapter 14

Disorders of speech-flow

Questions

1. What are the characteristics of stuttering?
2. With what disabilities is stuttering associated?
3. What are the characteristics of cluttering?
4. With what disabilities is cluttering associated?

DEFINING SPEECH-FLOW DISORDERS

Stuttering is the enigma of speech pathology. Not long ago more had been written about it than most other communicative disorders combined. What has been learned, for the most part, is what adult stutterers do as a group; we are relatively uncertain about how or why individual stutterers behave as they do. Although people think that they can detect a stutterer when they hear one, we still lack agreement on a satisfactory definition of an act of stuttering, let alone of a person who stutters. What is this elusive problem? Why does it persistently escape the nets of scientific inquiry?

Characteristics of speech-flow

Stuttering, although the most notorious, is only one type of breakdown in the flow of speech. Let us review the five temporal dimensions of speech sound flow and their disorders so that we may put stuttering into perspective (Chapter 3).

The first dimension is *sequence:* the order in which sounds must occur if they are to have linguistic significance. Turn the sequence of sounds around in "top", and you will have "pot"; reverse the "v" and "l" in "relevant", and you have the nonsense word "revelant." Failure to arrange sounds in proper order is generally considered to be a pronunciation more than a speech problem. Such failure may place one's level of education and social sophistication in question, but alone it is not likely to require a speech pathologist for correction.

The second dimension is *duration:* the length of time during which any phonetic element occurs. When phonetic duration is defective, the problem is articulatory, since phonemic perception is affected by phonetic duration. More typically, the problem is prosodic, involving syllable and word stress that is dependent on duration, as well as pitch and loudness cues, for detection. Defective duration, then, may distort intelligibility, contribute to mispronunciations, or affect a speaker's expression of intent.

The third dimension is *rate:* the speed with which phonetic elements of whatever dura-

tion are articulated with each other. Because phonetic elements can be combined into various linguistic units, rate is often measured in several forms: rate of articulation of speech sounds, rate of utterance of syllables, and rate of speaking words. Although any of these forms can be unusually fast or slow, deviations when considered alone are rarely judged as defective. The staccato delivery of a Walter Winchell is tolerated so long as articulation and fluency are unaffected. When intelligibility is impaired, as it is in cluttering, rate can be a serious problem.

The fourth dimension is *rhythm:* the timing pattern of phonetic elements. Not only do sounds pour forth at a rate and in a sequence that can be specified, but they also flow out with varying segmental and language rhythms. These are the rhythms by which the elements of speech are coordinated into intelligible utterances. With faulty segmental rhythm, fluency is imperiled. With faulty language rhythm, comprehension is jeopardized.

The fifth dimension is *fluency* of flow: the vital characteristic of how smoothly sounds are articulated with each other. Society is tolerant of some forms of disrupted fluency—hence the term *normal disfluency* (in the jargon of speech pathology)—and intolerant of others, such as stuttering.

Disorders of speech-flow

Disorders of fluency, rhythm, and rate have several major names: *stuttering, stammering,* and *cluttering.* American speech pathologists do not generally distinguish between stuttering and stammering. To the extent that a distinction is made, stuttering usually refers more to involuntary repetitions, stammering to involuntary speech stoppages. Because a speaker may do both in the same breath, use of the two terms is more confusing than helpful. Thus we will follow the precedent in the United States and avoid the term "stammering." "Stuttering" will be used to include the meaning of "stammering."

Cluttering is a term widespread in the European medical literature that has re-

Temporal Aspects of Speech —
sequence, duration, rate, rhythm, fluency

ceived attention recently in this country. It is ambiguous because it connotes so many neurologic and behavioral features; yet what it denotes when peeled to its bare essentials is behavior that, in some ways, is difficult to distinguish from stuttering. Still, cluttering is an umbrella under which can be gathered a wide array of neurologic conditions that affect fluency, rhythm, and rate.

Read Weiss' (1964) definition of the obligatory characteristics for a diagnosis of cluttering. Are these symptoms that would not occur in stuttering? Are secondary facilitative symptoms needed to separate cluttering from stuttering?

The names used to describe these conditions are abundant; the medically uninitiated mind boggles at the prospect of understanding differences among tachyphemia, leipophemia, barylalia, and tumultus sermonis. Even this tongue-twisting collection does not exhaust the supply of words that we can, gratefully, summarize under *cluttering*.

STUTTERING
Psychologic characteristics

What a person does who stutters can be described in terms of his observable performance (overt behavior) and his thoughts and feelings (cognition or covert behavior). Neither a behavioral nor a cognitive account alone is sufficient to describe any person psychologically, a truism especially true of persons who stutter. From the outside looking in, for instance, stuttering can be quite different from what it is from the inside looking out. Some who complain most bitterly about their stuttering are rarely heard to do anything that anyone else would call by that name. Are they stutterers? A listener would say "no." The answer from the inside of persons with the problem is a resounding "yes."

Behavioral description. We will start our investigation of stuttering by looking at the evidence open to public inspection: what a person does when he stutters. Simple as this task may seem, it has, in fact, proved troublesome, not because stuttering cannot be identified, but because the dividing line between stuttering and normal disfluency is ambiguous. Whether fluency or disfluency is normal or abnormal is a matter of judgment. As Johnson (1961a) and his students have demonstrated, the evaluation of "stuttering" is in large part in the ear of the listener as well as in the mouth of the speaker. No absolute difference separates fluency from disfluency or "normal disfluency" from stuttering. The booby traps around this problem are plentiful. We must be careful, for example, not to confuse the definition of stuttering with the definition of a stutterer. Were we to define a stutterer as one who does what stutterers do, the world's entire population would probably have to be said to stutter: normal speakers do what many stutterers do —but apparently not as often.

Still, stuttering is surely woven of some common threads. The problem is to isolate and define them. An accurate definition is essential as a basis for reaching agreement as to what it is that we are trying to understand. This is no small problem, and it probably accounts for more confusion about stuttering than any other factor. The trap can be the method of testing the reliability of judgments. Whereas observers typically show high agreement in judgments of the total number of words stuttered, they disagree grossly in the identification of specific words stuttered (Young, 1969). The reliability index based on the agreement of frequency judgments has been used widely (Sander, 1961). It is appropriate for group studies of conditions under which the total amount of stuttering varies, but it offers a false sense of judgmental accuracy for inquiries into the exact nature of this problem. If we are to investigate or modify what a stutterer does when he stutters, we must be able to identify an instance of stuttering (Young, 1969). Yet neither experts nor stutterers agree with many more than half of their own judgments of specific moments of stuttering (Curlee, 1970; Perkins, 1969). A step toward solution of the reliability issue is to identify more precisely the disfluency behavior judged as abnormal.

Forms of disfluency judged as stuttering.

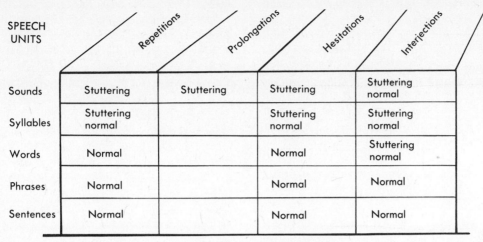

SPEECH UNITS	Repetitions	Prolongations	Hesitations	Interjections
Sounds	Stuttering	Stuttering	Stuttering	Stuttering normal
Syllables	Stuttering normal		Stuttering normal	Stuttering normal
Words	Normal		Normal	Stuttering normal
Phrases	Normal		Normal	Normal
Sentences	Normal		Normal	Normal

JUDGMENTS OF DISFLUENCY

Fig. 14-1. Types of disfluency and size of speech units as determinants of judgments of stuttering. Only with sounds can all types of disfluency occur. The larger the speech unit, the more apt a disfluency to be judged as normal.

What forms of disfluency are listeners inclined to judge as stuttering? Two types of evidence are available for the judgment: auditory and visual. You can demonstrate reasonably well for yourself what research has shown about auditory judgments. Set up an

---

Wendell Johnson (1961b) stimulated considerable inquiry about the kinds of disfluency considered as stuttering. What did he and his associates conclude in their monograph? Did their work extend, corroborate, or contradict that of Boehmler (1958) and of Williams and Kent (1958)?

---

arrangement, such as in Fig. 14-1, in which you try out different types* of disfluency with different units of speech: sounds, syllables,

---

*The fluent flow of speech can be disrupted by *repetition* of a unit of speech of any size, from sounds to sentences, by *prolongation* of sounds, by *hesitation* before utterance of any unit of speech, and by *interjection* of any unit—such as the all-American "uh"—between words (phrase and sentence interjections are possible but not typical). Because many hesitations are easily perceived as prolongations, some experts, such as Wingate (1964b), identify them both as prolongations. Without "hesitations," however, stoppage of air on plosives cannot be described, because plosives cannot be prolonged.

words, phrases, and sentences. Observe which combinations are heard as normal disfluency and which as abnormal (stuttering).

If your judgments resemble the bulk of those studied, they will be approximately as shown in Fig. 14-1 (Johnson, 1961b; Boehmler, 1958; Williams and Kent, 1958; Luper and Mulder, 1964; Wingate, 1964b). Speech sound and syllable disfluencies tend to be judged as stuttering, whereas disfluencies on larger units of speech (phrases and sentences) tend to be judged as normal. Although unitary sound repetitions, prolongations, and hesitations are regularly judged as stuttering and the person who speaks them as a stutterer (Huffman and Perkins, 1974), interjections depend on whether or not the speaker has been judged to be a stutterer. If he has, any interjection—whether of phrase, word, syllable, or sound—is likely to be heard as a postponement tactic to avoid stuttering, and hence it may be deemed a feature of stuttering. If he is considered to be a normal speaker, his interjections even of unitary sounds will probably be heard as normal.

Only on phones do all types of disfluency occur. They are among speech units that are repeated and interjected. Although hesitations may appear between sentences, phrases, words, and syllables, in the final analysis they always occur, of necessity, before sounds, an observation that has led Wingate (1969b) to define stuttering as a "phonetic transition defect." Similarly, the only speech unit that can be prolonged is a phone. Although speech sound disfluencies typify stuttering, they are found in the speech of normal speakers as well (Johnson, 1961a). As you can see, then, a stutterer can hardly be defined as a person who does what stutterers do without including ourselves as stutterers.

If "primary" characteristics of stuttering do not define a stutterer, what about the so-called "secondary" characteristics? They presumably develop as struggle reactions to the "primary" stuttering. Of the few studies of such characteristics of stuttered speech, that of Prins and Lohr (1968) is the most comprehensive. These authors found, among other things, that as a group both visible and audible characteristics of moments of stuttering occurred inconsistently. Only two visible phenomena were typical: suspension of jaw and lip activity and eyelid movement. Contrary to prevailing clinical opinion, although visible evidence of the struggle to speak was seen occasionally (tension in the speech mechanism and face, oscillatory movements of eyes and lips, and head jerks), it was not common. Another popular opinion was also not supported, namely that a consistent sequence of responses is used to terminate stuttering once it occurs (for example, eye blinks followed by head jerks followed by tongue protrusions, and so on). By and large, the stuttering that Prins and Lohr observed was not consistent in sequence or pattern.

Severity judgments of stuttering. The basis for a definition of stuttering has, so far, been limited to features by which the occurrence of acts of stuttering could be identified. The identification of the severity of stuttering is an additional matter. Again, we confront the problem of separating description from evaluation. The severity cannot be described any more objectively than can the act of stuttering. Judgments of severity involve evaluations mainly of frequency, tension, and duration of sound and syllable disfluencies (Young, 1961).

To what does an observer respond for his judgments of severity? The frequency of disfluency is the easiest cue to measure (hence most is known about it). One study showed that if a speaker uses a double rather than a single pattern of repetition of a syllable (if he says "Sa-Sa-Saturday" instead of "Sa-Saturday"), he more than doubles the probability that his speech will be judged as defective and that he, as a person, will be judged as a stutterer. But if he uses a single repetition pattern, he can get away with up to eight syllable repetitions per hundred words before people will decide that the disfluencies heard are not those of nervousness but of stuttering (Sander, 1963).

Other related factors may influence judgments of severity, but no one has paid much attention to them yet. For example, are people more likely to hear stuttering if disfluencies occur more at the beginning than at the middle or end of a word? Will they hear stuttering if disfluencies are closely spaced rather than far apart? Is it stuttering if disfluencies involve speech revisions on sounds, syllables, or words that were intended to be spoken?

A more nebulous determinant of severity is the effort, tension, or strain exerted to produce disfluency, the factor that presumably differentiates "primary" from "secondary" stuttering (McDearmon, 1968). Although strain does increase the likelihood of judgments of stuttering and stutterer, it apparently does not contribute as much to severity as clinical impression would suggest. Huffman and Perkins (1974) found that it did not affect these judgments as much as did the type of speech sound disfluency.

Too, prolongations, hesitations, and repetitions disrupt articulatory and syllabic rhythms of speech (*dysrhythmia*). The greater the struggle with disfluencies, the greater the dysrhythmia. Although this notion has not been put to direct experimental test, it is supported indirectly by Prins and Lohr (1968), who report prolongations as being most consistently associated with stuttering severity. That they did not find struggle occurring frequently does not preclude the fact that greater struggle is possible with prolongations than with other types of disfluency. Still, it is virtually inconceivable that opinions of severity would not match closely the amount of struggle during a disfluency. Were a speaker in prolonged conversation to have only one disruption of fluency and rhythm, in which he spent 30 seconds pushing and straining to articulate a single sound, few would doubt that he stutters.

Subtle aspects of disfluency and dysrhythmia also affect judgments of stuttering. These effects are seen in the detection of stuttering from tape recordings that have had the obvious speech stoppages removed (Wendahl and Cole, 1961). In other words, something happens to fluency, rate, and rhythm in the vicinity of a moment of stuttering that signals its occurrence to an observer, even when the disruption per se has been deleted. Some clinicians think that the flow of speech begins to become "sticky" with tension as the moment of stuttering approaches. This may actually occur, and among the cues may be a greater number of 150 to 250 msec pauses in the fluent speech of stutterers than of nonstutterers (Love and Jeffress, 1971).

Whether one listens to stuttering, or both looks and listens, appears to make little difference in most judgments of severity or, for that matter, of frequency of stuttering. Severity seems to be evaluated by how much the speaker distorts the normal flow of speech. We usually detect these distortions by listening, but facial contortions or other visual evidence of struggle will lead us to conclude that stuttering is severe even when the speech heard is not grossly deviant (Williams, Wark, and Minifie, 1963).

Stuttering defined. Although stuttering is basically a judgment about how a person is disfluent, factors other than manner of disfluency and dysrhythmia affect that judgment: Is the listener a stutterer? Does he regard the speaker as a stutterer? Is he a speech clinician, layman, or the child's parent (Johnson and others, 1959)? Thus a definition of

the act of stuttering must include the listener's contribution to the judgment.

The basic contribution, though, is the speaker's disfluency. All judgments of stuttering need not involve phrase, word, or syllable disfluencies, but they do involve disfluent articulation of sounds. They reflect difficulty in starting the first sound in words and syllables (Johnson and Brown, 1935). Conceivably, they could also involve difficulty in initiating subsequent sounds within a syllable. Thus whether these articulatory disfluencies occur in initiation of an utterance or in transitions between syllables or sounds, they necessarily involve abnormal timing of speech movements for starting sounds. This is the behavior most likely to be judged as stuttering. The following statement therefore defines what the stutterer does that the listener can observe as abnormal: *Stuttering is the abnormal timing of speech sound initiation.*

Five ideas are implied in this definition. First, any type of disfluency that could be judged as abnormal would qualify: repetition, prolongation, and hesitation would be major candidates. Second, any location of sound initiation that could be judged as abnormal would qualify: the first sound in an utterance (where most stuttering occurs) is inevitable; in articulatory transitions between sounds is also inevitable; between syllables is probable; between words, phrases, or sentences is possible. In brief, groping for a word is generally judged as normal; struggling to produce a sound is abnormal. Third, any basis for judging severity of disfluency is implied: intensity of struggle, duration of prolongation, number of repetitions, frequency of disfluency, and extent of dysrhythmia are usually involved. Fourth, any listener bias independent of the speech being judged would be reflected. Fifth, although this is a relatively objective listener's definition of stuttering, it can include the speaker as his own listener.

Stutterer defined. Apparently the basis on which the label "stutterer" is assigned is similar to that for judging acts of stuttering (Huffman and Perkins (1974). Conceivably, one could argue that a *stutterer* be defined as a person who stutters. Sheehan's (1958a) definition,* however, is broader:

A stutterer may be defined as a person who shows, to a degree that sets him off from the rest of the population, any one or more of the following groups of symptoms: (1) blockings, stickings, grimaces, forcings, repetitions, prolongations, or other rhythm breaks or interruptions in the forward flow of speech; (2) fear or anticipation of blockings, fear of inability to speak, or related symptoms prior to words or speaking situations; (3) a self-concept which includes a picture of himself as a stutterer, a stammerer, speech blocker, or a person lacking normal speech fluency.

The merit of defining a stutterer is strictly that of assigning a convenient label, a convenience fraught with substantial objections. Almost everyone from time to time does what is defined as stuttering. Aside from the uselessness of a definition that includes the bulk of the populace, the person who does stutter can be fluent as much as is the person not considered to stutter. Presumably, by identifying stutterers we can compare them with nonstutterers to find why they are different. Were a difference to be found, though, that could account for the stuttering, we would then face the peculiar problem of having to explain for many of these people how they can be fluent more often than they are disfluent.

A more profitable and defensible comparison is between stuttered and fluent (or even normally disfluent) speech; the act, not the person, must therefore be defined. Finally, the most important objection to the label is that it carries a stigma. Since a person is not necessarily more lovable by virtue of being known as a stutterer, let us attempt to remember that this label does not identify anything about a person other than the manner in which he judges himself or is judged by others to be disfluent.

Observable conditions related to stuttering. Let us turn now to conditions under which stuttering has been observed to vary.

---

*From Sheehan, J., Projective studies of stuttering. *J. Speech Hearing Dis.*, **23**, 18-25 (1958).

Only in recent years have we glimpsed beneath the shrouds of uncertainty that have veiled the exact nature of stuttering. You will probably be less than surprised, then, to learn that speech pathologists still do not exude great confidence in their knowledge of the conditions related to it.

The two main lines of inquiry have departed from opposite observations. Those impressed with differences between stutterers and nonstutterers have compared these groups. The prevailing hypothesis in early work was that stutterers are different; more recently it has been that they are not. This approach has been prevalent. By contrast, those who have seen the major differences as being between what the stutterer does when speaking normally and when stuttering have compared his performance under these two conditions. Adherents of this view, now being utilized more frequently, hold that a comparison of stutterers and nonstutterers will be more profitable after we know the nature of what the stutterer does differently when he stutters from when he speaks normally. Both approaches have been used to provide evidence about the following conditions.

Everyday conditions that reduce or increase stuttering. The conditions most revealing of the nature of stuttering would be those which invariably reduce or increase it. They may not exist in everyday life, but a few come close. Stuttering rarely seems to occur during singing, speaking in unison, speaking in synchrony with a rhythmic beat, speaking alone or to animals, or swearing. Wingate (1969a) suggested that "artificial" fluency often involves doing something different with the voice from what is done when stuttering is present. Many other conditions reduce stuttering partially for some; none eliminates it completely for all.

What did Bloodstein (1950) find when he asked 204 stutterers about 115 conditions that might reduce their stuttering?

On the other side of the problem are those everyday conditions that increase stuttering.

Whereas singing, for instance, virtually ensures its elimination, nothing seems to ensure its occurrence. The closest approximations include speaking during recovery from an operation or when a person is exhausted, is called on to speak in class, or is in a prolonged state of fear. As with the reduction of stuttering, an abundance of daily conditions will increase it for some; none increases it for all.

Adaptation effect. Distinct from everyday situations are laboratory conditions that have been used to study stuttering. The one that has received the most attention during the last two decades is called *adaptation:* the decrease of stuttering with successive reading of the same passage. This effect is so stable for stutterers collectively that group adaptation curves are quite predictable. But as Williams, Silverman, and Kools (1968) have shown, the adaptation effect does not appear to differentiate stutterers from nonstutterers as was thought; rather, it is characteristic of normal disfluency of normal speakers as well.

Gray (1965) has worked out a table with which he can predict how much stuttering will decrease from reading to reading if its frequency during the first reading is known. Will this prediction be accurate for individuals who stutter or just for groups?

The adaptation effect, probably because of its stability and resemblance to a learning extinction curve, has figured in considerable theorizing and research about stuttering as learned behavior. In fact, it has been suggested as a predictive measure of therapeutic success because it presumably reveals the extent to which stuttering is learned. The best controlled test of this possibility, however, has shown that adaptation measures and therapeutic progress are neither consistently nor highly related (Prins, 1968). Some are unconvinced, too, that decrements seen in repeated readings have anything to do with the extinction of stuttering as a learned response, especially if it is a feature of such apparently unextinguishable, universally present behavior as normal disfluency. Moreover, the annoying fact persists that not all persons who stutter follow the crowd under

---

What is Wingate's (1966a,b) conclusion about the similarities between adaptation and experimental extinction?

---

adaptation conditions—a few nonconformists increase stuttering on repeated readings. In other words, the adaptation effect is typical of groups of stutterers but not necessarily of each individual who stutters (Cullinan, 1963).

Consistency effect. Another laboratory phenomenon that has enjoyed some attention has been the *consistency effect.* It is the tendency for stuttering to occur on the same words during successive readings of a passage. The point of interest about consistency is that it implies the ability to anticipate an act of stuttering. Otherwise, so the argument goes, how could a person consistently stutter on the same words (Bloodstein, 1961)? Again, this is an effect that appears to be characteristic of disfluency in general. It is not unique to stuttering per se, except as stuttering involves disfluency (Williams, Silverman, and Kools, 1969b; Neelley and Timmons, 1967).

Punishment. More recently, with the advent of operant conditioning in the analysis of stuttering behavior, additional situations have been found that have predictable effects on stuttering. Several investigators have shown that by controlling the consequences of stuttering, as well as of normal disfluency, stuttering can consistently be made to de-

---

Martin and Siegel (1966a,b) shocked stuttering and rewarded fluency, and Quist and Martin (1967) verbally punished stuttering. Similarly, Siegel and Martin (1965a,b) and Brookshire and Martin (1967) punished normal disfluency. Did they find the same results? Do Shames, Egolf, and Rhodes (1969, 1976) find clinical value in an operant conditioning approach?

---

crease. When punishment of various sorts, ranging from shock to saying "wrong" is made directly contingent, the frequency of stuttering invariably declines. Earlier work had shown that stuttering increases with shock, but in these early studies shock was administered during *periods* of stuttering, not immediately after *acts* of stuttering. The ability of stutterers to control their speech when faced with the prospect of punishment is not surprising; they can often refrain from stuttering at least temporarily when consequences are sufficiently threatening.

Unfortunately, even if threat reduces stuttering to zero, when it is removed, stuttering bounces back in full force, suggesting that it can be suppressed but not eliminated by punishment. Perhaps Brutten's (1975) explanation accounts for this phenomenon. He makes a convincing case that those aspects of stuttering that are instrumentally (operantly) conditioned are the aspects that predictably decrease in frequency when punished. He argues that the involuntary core of stuttering is not subject to manipulation by contingent consequences, which would explain why stuttering is not extinguished when treated as an operant response.

Linguistic factors. Emerging interest in language has extended to normal disfluency and stuttering. From this direction of inquiry is coming strong evidence that linguistic decision-making factors weigh heavily in all types of disfluency. A forerunner was Brown's (1945) description of four word attributes (initial phoneme, grammatical function, sentence position, and word length) that appeared to control the loci of stuttering in adults. Similar linguistic attributes were reconfirmed by I. Taylor (1966), who found that adults stuttered mainly on the initial consonants of relatively long words that are nouns, verbs, adverbs, or adjectives and that occur early in a sentence. Silverman and Williams (1967a,b) noted, however, that not only stuttering but normal disfluency as well is influenced by these factors. By contrast, Bloodstein and Gantwerk (1967) reported evidence that children's stutterings were distributed more or less randomly, with some tendency toward pronouns and conjunctions, a finding opposed by the research of Williams, Silverman, and Kools (1969a), who found loci of both stuttering and normal disfluency to be the same as for adults. This disagreement remains to be resolved.

Recent attempts to explain disfluency have related it to the linguistic encoding processes. Goldman-Eisler (1958) led the way by showing that hesitation pauses in normal speech tend to reflect verbal planning. They occur at points of greatest uncertainty, which, by implication from communication theory, means that they are also points of highest information (Chapter 3). Subsequently, several investigators have demonstrated that stuttering, too, is associated with high points of information (Quarrington, 1965; Schlesinger and others, 1965; Soderberg, 1967; I. Taylor, 1966).

Although Lanyon (1968, 1969) presented evidence that he thought attributed increased stuttering to the greater difficulty of speaking long words than to their greater information value, Soderberg (1971) showed that these discrepant findings could well have resulted from an interaction effect occurring between long words and information on disfluency types. He demonstrated that repetitions were associated with long low-information words and prolongations with long high-information words. These results suggest that more difficult decision making is involved in prolongations than in repetitions. When long words were eliminated, however, and sampling of one-syllable words was sufficiently large, stuttering in general related to high-information words.

Too, MacKay and Bowman (1969) have demonstrated linguistic factors that facilitate the rate of speech production: rehearsal at semantic, syntactic, and phonologic levels all increased maximum rate. According to Soderberg (1971), information is not related to consistency of stuttering and only partially accounts for the adaptation effect. Still, it is clearly a major determinant of disfluency in general and stuttering in particular.

This discussion is not an exhaustive catalog of observable conditions related to stuttering. Many stutterers are mute on a telephone, whereas some are more fluent. Many are paralyzed by authority, but some wax eloquent. Many find that the tongue wags fluently when they are intoxicated, whereas some cannot make it wag at all. Many have "Jonah" sounds and words that they devote their lives to avoiding, but the sounds or words that are whales of difficulty for one are but minnows in another's stream of speech-flow. We have looked only at those conditions for which at least a modicum of research evidence is available. Too, we will reserve such conditions as masking, delayed auditory feedback, and rhythm for discussion in connection with their possible biologic explanations.

Cognitive description of stuttering. A safari through the cognitive experiences of people who stutter is fraught with the perils of trekking through a jungle. Nothing is clearly visible; the shapes of what we think we see are ill-defined; everything seems to be intertwined with everything else. To achieve a semblance of organization, let us separate as best we can that part of cognition concerned with the act of stuttering from that part mainly concerned with the person who does the stuttering.

Expectancy to stutter. The subjective clues by which stutterers detect their own stuttering are not entirely clear. Still, Lanyon (1967) has been able to construct a paper-and-pencil scale of attitudes and behavior that discriminates among three levels of severity as well as between stutterers and nonstutterers. This scale generally reflects Johnson's identification of cognitive components of stuttering in his definition: "Stuttering is an anticipatory, apprehensive, hypertonic avoidance reaction" (Johnson and others, 1948). Every major word in the definition describes a subjective condition. In other words, stuttering is what Johnson said a speaker does when he expects it, dreads it, and becomes tense in anticipation of it and in his attempt to avoid it.

From this germinal idea of what the stutterer experiences has sprung more inquiry than from any other single theory. Investigators have reasoned that if stuttering is what

What parallel did Johnson and others (1948) draw between stuttering and tight-rope walking?

the stutterer does when he hesitates to hesitate, then he must be able to anticipate where and when he will have trouble maintaining fluency. This reasoning has led to research on expectancy and on the sounds, words, grammatical elements, and situations that persons who stutter presumably learn to fear. Research has not shown, however, that stutterers do attach fear to stuttered words, nor do these words have special meaning or affect (Spahr, 1968; Peterson, 1969).

The ability of stutterers to anticipate their acts of stuttering has been demonstrated many times—for groups. For a group, stuttering occurs more frequently when it is expected than when it is not. Even the length of blocks can be predicted with some accuracy. Moreover, when expectancy is reduced, so is stuttering (Milisen, 1938). In fact, when expectancy is punished, not only is it reduced, but so is stuttering (Curlee and Perkins, 1968). The consistency effect, mentioned earlier, is also used as an argument for expectancy: to stutter consistently on the same words time after time implies the ability to foresee difficulty on them. The only blemish on this monolithic picture of expectancy is that practically no one who stutters predicts all of his blocks accurately. Martin and Haroldson (1967) reported that only half of the words on which difficulty was anticipated were actually stuttered. Some persons have practically no expectancy of stuttering even though they may stutter severely.

Concealment devices. Much of the stutterer's distress is with his covert attempts to conceal his overt abnormalities of stuttering. *Avoidance* strategies of circumlocution or word substitution are used to evade feared words altogether. An interesting side benefit of this strategy is often the development of a large vocabulary. *Postponement* tactics serve the purpose of delaying initiation of a feared word until the possibility of saying it normally improves. This tactic involves pauses, repetitions of words or phrases, or interjections of stereotyped expressions, such as "you know" or "like well uh," over and over until the feared word is finally attempted. *Starting* maneuvers, of which "uh" prefixed to the feared word is typical, are used to help initiate the difficult first sound. *Escape* techniques, ranging from stomping a foot to blinking the eyes, are used to "break" the block. Then, to ward off future anticipation of difficulty, *antiexpectancy* measures may be used. This can involve speaking in a monotone, using different pitch or loudness levels, or using any other change in speech that the stutterer may be trying in his effort to reduce his dread of becoming stuck (Van Riper, 1971).

Distraction. After reviewing hypothetic conditions under which stuttering is reduced, Bloodstein (1950) concluded that *distraction* from the expectancy of stuttering was one of two conditions primarily responsible. Although this explanation has prevailed for years, Biggs and Sheehan (1969) alone of recent advocates have put it to the test as an alternate explanation of the effects of contingent punishment. Using a "mildly aversive" tone, they found that whether contingent or not, stuttering was reduced. The difficulty with interpreting this result as support for a distraction hypothesis is that it could just as well have produced its effects as a masking tone, the effects of which must probably be attributed to factors other than distraction.

By contrast, several studies have virtually discredited distraction as a viable explanation of reduced stuttering. For one thing, the construct is cognitive, and hence difficult to prove or disprove. Still, if stuttering is reduced when attention is distracted from the expectation of difficulty, then with continued exposure to a particular distraction, its uniqueness would wear off and its value should be reduced. Such has not been the case where rhythm or masking noise has been used (Cherry and Sayers, 1956; Trotter and Lesch, 1967; Perkins and Curlee, 1969; Brady, 1968, 1969). Too, conditions contrived to be maximally distracting have not reduced stuttering when they have not involved such guaranteed stutter-reducers as rhythm, masking noise, retarded rate, and the like (Beech, 1967; Beech and Fransella, 1969; Perkins, 1969). Finally, the technique of "shadowing" that Cherry and Sayers used required greater concentration on speech, not distraction from it; yet it was notably effective in reducing stuttering.

Level of aspiration. Compared with nor-mal speakers, stutterers set lower levels of aspiration and predict more modest performance within range of probable success (Sheehan and Zelen, 1955). This difference is attributed to stutterers' greater defensiveness and desire to avoid risk of failure. The extent to which this modest goal-setting behavior is learned directly or indirectly from parents is clouded by conflicting research. Goldman and Shames (1964a,b) found parents of older children with long-standing stuttering making excessively high performance demands. Partial replication of their study, however, revealed that mothers of young beginning stutterers set significantly lower goals, whereas fathers did not differ in goal setting from the fathers of nonstutterers (Quarrington, Seligman, and Kosower, 1969). As Adams (1969) observed after reviewing studies of psychologic differences between stutterers and nonstutterers, "children who stutter may be youngsters whose speech, fluency and associated behaviors are, for some reason, disrupted far out of proportion to the intensity of the emotional stimuli that precipitate the disturbance." In any event, "stutterers aspire to significantly less than do normal speakers."

Reduced awareness. Another cognitive feature pursued from time to time is reduced awareness during stuttering. Hill (1944b) interpreted physiologic data as indicating that stuttering was nearly identical with reflexive startle accompanied by reduced awareness. Clinical studies have pointed to reduced awareness during stuttering (Johnson and Solomon, 1937; Froeschels and Rieber, 1963). Herren (1931) found in an experimental study that rhythmic bulb-pressing during speaking was disrupted by stuttering. Recent experimentation has shown, though, that if awareness is reduced, it does not affect discriminations of tactual, auditory, or visual stimuli, nor is reduction in these senses a necessary condition for stuttering (Perkins, 1969).

Time pressure. What may be an important cognitive aspect of stuttering has received relatively little attention: time pressure, in which a person feels pressured to hurry and say what is to be said. Probably everyone *time pressure* expect a stutterer to become anxious in anticipation of speaking. Because listeners are expected to endure this performance, a feeling of guilt is not surprising either. These feelings he reports; who can know them bet-

feels this pressure on occasion, but stutterers may be especially susceptible to it (Sheehan, 1958a; Stunden, 1965; Cooper, 1970). They seem compelled to speak rapidly; some dislike speaking slowly more than they dislike stuttering. Severe stutterers even judge the duration of a speaking experience as considerably longer than do those who stutter little

---

Ringel and Minifie (1966) used the concept of *protensity* to measure judgments of duration of speaking time. How did they apply this idea to stuttering?

Wischner (1952) and later Sheehan, Cortese, and Hadley (1962) had stutterers draw pictures of how they feel before, during, and after an act of stuttering. Did they obtain the same results? Do the pictures agree with the verbal account here?

---

or not at all. The evidence is not yet clear enough to tell us whether these speculations about time pressure apply to all acts of stuttering, to all stutterers regardless of their stuttering, or only to some stutterers some of the time.

Moreover, if time pressure is a key ingredient, we have little more than speculation as to its source. It may be a feeling of urgency to speak quickly before the listener stops listening. It may be a disguised feeling of aggressively attacking the listener with words—stuttering increases with covert expression of aggression but decreases when the expression is overt (Hager, 1975). It may be a feeling of urgency to speak quickly before the fluent flow of speech is gummed up by the unnecessary movements of stuttering.

Cognitive description of stutterers. So much for a subjective view of stuttering; now let us look inside the stutterer. The person who does the stuttering is often characterized as anxious, guilty, frustrated, hostile, and dependent. One school of thought maintains that he has these feelings because he stutters, another, that he stutters because of the feelings. Admittedly, sorting out a stutterer's cognitions about his stuttering from those about himself is an artificial distinction—here we can become easily lost in the cognitive jungle. With this warning posted, we will tiptoe into the wilderness.

Stuttering: a phobia? Seemingly, stuttering is unpleasant—it exacts a price. That it occurs involuntarily makes frustration, anxiety, and guilt understandable. One would

ter than he? Still, the suspicion lingers that the picture he paints may not be complete. A consistent feature of his painting is tension. If one is anxious, frustrated, or guilty, he cannot simultaneously be relaxed. Yet workers who have looked for physiologic evidence of anxiety and emotional arousal have, so far, found it only in the speech musculature (Sheehan and Voas, 1954)—stutterers do not seem to be viscerally distressed by stuttering (M. Taylor, 1966), nor is it systematically reduced by deconditioning of anxiety (Gray and England, 1972).

Stuttering: an addiction? The persistence of stuttering raises the possibility that it may not be a speech phobia, but that it may be comprised more of relief than of fear and pain. It behaves more like an addiction than a phobia. Those who treat emotionally handicapped persons have long observed that the prognosis for recovery from a phobia is much better than from an addiction. In fact, phobias tend to cure themselves. The reason is readily apparent. To be irrationally fearful of something is to be phobic about it. Disprove the needless basis for fear and the phobia disappears. An addiction, however, is acquired and maintained by its reinforcing consequences (temporary and ultimately devastating as they may be). Addictions may be suppressed, but when punishment ceases, they have an annoying tendency to recur.

So it is with stuttering. Its frequency can be reduced by many of the conditions already discussed, but when they are removed, stuttering returns undiminished. Its persistence points either to fluency failure induced by realistic fear that no amount of rational thinking will explain away or to contingent reinforcing consequences. As Siegel (1969) points out, the possibility that fear of stuttering increases stuttering is almost excluded by growing evidence that contingent punishment of disfluency invariably reduces it. Its persistence must be a consequence of reinforcement. Several sources of reinforcement are available, at least in theory:

1. The most defensible source derives from the simple truism that what one does is what one learns (Deese and Hulse, 1967). Whatever manner of disfluency stutterers utilize in order to speak will become an integral part of their patterns of speech. All that need be demonstrated for this source of reinforcement is that speaking is reinforcing. The fact that stutterers speak despite stuttering provides that demonstration.

2. Tension reduction at the completion of stuttering is held to be reinforcing (Sheehan and Voas, 1954). Essentially, this explanation is masochistic, since it says stuttering persists because it is such a relief to stop. This relief may be a source of reinforcement, but Luper's (1956) test of the hypothesis tended to oppose this possibility.

3. A more demonstrable source is in listener effects of stuttering. If we assume that attention is reinforcing, stuttering could easily be acquired and maintained by this source alone (Goldiamond, 1969). Stuttering dramatically and effectively demands attention, negative as it often may be. Too, listener attention is held longer during stuttered than fluent speech. The more insecure and hungry for attention the stutterer, the more reinforcement for his stuttering. Perhaps it is for this reason that stutterers are so typically resentful of being stopped or helped during stuttering.

4. A possible source of reinforcement may be the obvious secondary gains. Some persons use stuttering wittingly. They have found that it can pay off. For instance, young men who stutter discover occasionally that some girls find stuttering attractive, whereas others dislike it. Not surprisingly, they often become selective in situations in which they stutter.

5. Another possible source of reinforcement is the relief of unresolved needs by stuttering. Strong feelings of aggression and dependency often attributed to stutterers are thought to be relieved neurotically by stuttering. Viewed in this light, stuttering is a masked plea for nurturance and an equally obscured protest of aggressive independence.

Glauber (1958) elaborates this view theoretically, Travis (1971) elaborates it by interpretation of stutterer's dreams and metaphors, and Perkins (1965) elaborates it by relating stuttering to a fantasy system that preserves a strong self-image.

Psychotherapists arrive regularly at the conclusion that stuttering relieves more stress than it generates. Social consequences are not denied but are merely viewed as the price the stutterer is willing to pay for symptomatic relief. But when these repressed feelings are compared with those of the nonstutterer, no one has yet been able to find much difference, at least with personality tests.

Goodstein (1958) and Sheehan (1958b) have reviewed the evidence from personality tests of stutterers and nonstutterers. Do they conclude that people who stutter have different personalities from people who do not?

Cognitive uncertainties. Here among uncertainties of cognitive phenomena, without hard facts to build on, theories have proliferated. Too frequently has the question been: "In whose theory do you believe?" or "With whose point of view are you identified?" Too seldom have crucial questions been asked and definitive answers produced that exclude further work in unproductive directions (Chapter 2). Much of the research appears to have been undertaken and interpreted more to prove than to test a point. The literature is a graveyard of hopeful leads encased in the concrete of devotion to theories and buried in an avalanche of jargon, ex post facto studies, ad hoc reporting of casual observations, and one-shot-thesis research. The acidity of these ad hominem debates, once sufficient to cause ulcers, now hardly produces indigestion. Devotion to theories and theorists is waning. Perhaps we will soon have some reasonably certain answers about how stuttering functions in the life of a stutterer.

Biologic characteristics

A small mountain of data from biologic studies of stuttering has accumulated during the last half century. Almost every organic condition that can be conceived has been investigated in the search for a cause. There have been explorations seeking genetic disabilities: witness studies of sex differences, of stuttering in families of twins, of stuttering in families of stutterers, of differences in developmental history, and even of differences in intelligence. There have been explorations seeking sensory disabilities: studies of deafness and hearing loss; of artificially masked sound of speech; of oral, tactile, and kinesthetic sensitivity and discrimination; of oral and tactile anesthesia; of delays in auditory feedback of one's own speech; and of differences in auditory phase angle. There have been explorations seeking metabolic disabilities: studies of diabetes, epilepsy, allergy; of disease among stutterers; and of various pharmaceutic effects. There have been explorations seeking neurologic disabilities: studies of laterality, of cerebral dominance, of change in handedness, of various brain-wave rhythms, of perseveration, of general and oral motor coordination, of coordination at different speaking rates, and of speaking in time with rhythm. And there have been explorations seeking organic bases for emotional disabilities: studies of biochemistry; of the effects of various tranquilizers; and of physiologic responses during startle, during stuttering, and during anxiety (the measures have ranged from respiration rate, heart rate, and blood pressure through skin conductance and resistance, palmar sweat, electromyography, and electroencephalography, to eye movement and pupillary reflex).

Are stutterers biologically different? From all this work we should know much about the organic bases of stuttering. What has been learned, though, is that stutterers cannot be differentiated biologically as a group from normal speakers. Certainly, individual stutterers who deviate radically from the norm

---

Perkins (1970) reviewed the physiologic research. Did he find evidence of a biologic basis for stuttering?

---

can be found; the same is true with nonstutterers. Common characteristics can be found among stutterers, but similar characteristics are common to nonstutterers. Research born of various theories, hypotheses, hunches, intuitions, and trial-and-error speculations has been contradictory. Uncertainty, especially in the older studies, stems from the failure to control important variables, from lack of information about experimental conditions, and from inadequate treatment of data. Consequently, those who assume the burden of proving a biologic difference cannot muster convincing evidence. Conversely, if those who would make the opposite case were to assume a similar burden of proof, their position would also be tenuous—the fact that no biologic difference has yet been found does not prove that none exists.

The sum of the matter is that we are almost, but not quite, as uncertain now about whether stutterers are biologically different as we were 30 years ago. The greater prevalence of stuttering among males still begs for explanation (Schuell, 1947). The cerebral dominance imbalance remains an open issue, especially with the recent finding that the normal "right ear effect" (a reflection of cerebral dominance) is smaller in stutterers than nonstutterers (Curry and Gregory). Phonetic skill, with its motor coordinations for prosody, is significantly poorer in stutterers than nonstutterers (Wingate, 1967). A substantial lead comes from Stromsta's (1956, 1959, 1962) extensive work, which demonstrates relative auditory phase angle differences, between stutterers and nonstutterers, of bone-conducted sound, differences that diminish with higher pitches of female voices. The most persuasive lead, however, has been apparent for years in such everyday conditions as singing and whispering. Recent research on laryngeal involvement has turned up a rare phenomenon in stuttering: an invariant relationship, possibly the only one in captivity. Without exception, stuttering diminishes and all but vanishes as the complexity of the coordinations of phonation with articulation and respiration are simplified (Perkins and others, 1976).

Is stuttering biologically different? When the spotlight of investigation was on the *person* who stutters, constitutional predisposition theories were rampant. Searchers were sniffing for evidence of dysphemia, spasmophemia, strephosymbolia, cerebral dominance—in fact, for any somatic variant that could distinguish stutterers from nonstutterers. Sizable differences would be reported by one investigator only to be contradicted by the next. Interestingly, the sizes of differences have been inversely proportional to the rigor of observations and inferences. Successful replication has not distinguished attempts to delineate stutterers from nonstutterers.

As the focus of research has shifted from the person who stutters to the act of stuttering, stricter definitions of what he actually does that is defective have evolved. When stuttering behavior is made explicit, observations become relatively stable. By organizing biologic evidence around five questions about *stuttering*, we can encompass the scope of it and also obtain a clearer picture of what is known.

What biologic conditions surround the onset of stuttering? Although no biologic predisposition to develop stuttering has been incontestably demonstrated, the facts that the problem predominates among males in all cultures, tends to run in families, and develops among those prone to speech sound disfluency attest to some predisposing influence. Of course, Sheehan and Martyn (1967) may be right about why stuttering appears to prevail in families—parents of stutterers, being sensitive to the problem, become "bird watchers," scanning each other's family tree for signs of stutterers roosting there. More stutterers are found because more looking is done.

If stuttering is a familial problem, however, the fact that it could be culturally trans-

mitted through a conducive psychologic climate does not preclude its relation to constitutional factors. The syllable disfluencies of stuttering occur when phonatory, articulatory, and respiratory synergies are mistimed (Adams, 1974). They happen considerably more frequently in the speech of preschool stutterers, as well as older, confirmed stutterers, than in the speech of normal speakers (Floyd and Perkins, 1974). Stuttering, then, appears to have its origin in children whose speech coordination skills are marginal. Obviously, the implication is that children who develop stuttering may be born with a deficient biologic mechanism for coordinating speech. That such a mechanism could be inherited is not surprising. Research interest in a genetic difference has been rekindled (Andrews and Harris, 1964). Whether conclusive evidence will be found that such a difference exists remains to be seen.

Should a genetic difference be discovered, we still need not invoke the stigma of pathology. People vary in any skill. Some are naturally coordinated, some are not. Certainly one of the most complex skills of all is coordinating, at extraordinarily rapid rates, the 100 or more muscles used for speech. People undoubtedly vary in this ability, some being able to time all the movements of speech easily, and some having difficulty. The possibility that young children, who are not adept at this ability, are the ones who have the greatest chance of developing stuttering seems entirely credible. The intricacies of speech being what they are, the wonder is that only one in a hundred persons stutter.

What biologic conditions precede acts of stuttering? The preparation to stutter is similar to the physiologic reactions in a startle

---

Hill (1944b, 1954) has compared stuttering and startle responses and has even produced "stuttering" in nonstutterers. What conditions did he find produced the most "stuttering"?

---

response. Similarity, however, does not demonstrate identity. Were identity assumed, we could just as well conclude that all startle responses are acts of stuttering, a conclusion that might be startling to startled nonstutterers.

What biologic conditions occur during acts of stuttering? Since the biochemical changes associated with stuttering characteristically occur in anyone who increases muscular activity or becomes emotional, they are probably consequences of stuttering (Hill, 1944a). Several studies have shown that a person tends to "freeze" when he stutters (Herren, 1931; Johnson and Solomon, 1937; Froeschels and Rieber, 1963). Although his movements may freeze, his thinking need not; he can make discriminative judgments as well during even severe blocks as during fluent speech (Perkins, 1969). In one of the few attempts to obtain accurate measures of autonomic processes during the brief event of stuttering, autonomic nervous system responses of fear or anxiety were not observed to rise before or fall after an act of stuttering (M. Taylor, 1966).

As for central nervous system responses during and after acts of stuttering, the point of greatest tension in the speech musculature has been found just prior to termination of a block (Sheehan and Voas, 1954). What this evidence means is another matter. It could indicate fear of continuing speech, mounting pressure to terminate stuttering the longer it continues, or that stuttering helps maintain homeostasis. (Shivering, for example, is a reflexive device for raising body temperature; it continues, and sometimes increases, in intensity until an adequate internal temperature is achieved. Muscular exertion of stuttering could conceivably serve an analogous purpose.)

Robert West, a pioneer of speech pathology, theorized about the biologic purpose of stuttering (1958). What function did he think it served?

What biologic conditions are associated with the perpetuation of stuttering? Lacking a clear biologic explanation, the popular notion in recent years has been that stuttering is learned by reinforcement through anxiety reduction, a troublesome reason. "Anxiety" has so many meanings and measures that it

is almost meaningless—and unmeasurable. Another frustration with this explanation comes from violation of common sense. To say that stuttering persists because it reduces anxiety is similar to the apocryphal explanation of why the man beat himself on his head with a hammer: it felt so good when he stopped.

Two recent investigations move doubt closer to certainty that moments of stuttering are not a function of anxiety. Gray and England (1972), using electroskin conductance (ESC) and evaporative water loss (EWL) as operational measures of anxiety, concluded after extensive longitudinal study of the effects of reciprocal inhibition that "anxiety and stuttering apparently do not exist in a one-to-one, or necessarily positive, relationship." This conclusion is buttressed by Ingham and Andrews (1971).

Dabul and Perkins (1973), on the other hand, in a test of an observation of Sheehan, Cortese, and Hadley (1962) that stuttering appears to be a contradiction to the principle of homeostasis, devised an experiment in which they measured systolic blood pressure (SBP). Hypothesizing that stuttering is, indeed, a mechanism for maintaining homeostasis, they used shock to increase SBP (seen in Fig. 14-2 as the increment in Post I over preexperimental measures) and then compared the relative effects of stuttering with fluency, chewing, finger tapping, and silence —conditions selected to control for linguistic, motor exertion, and time factors equivalent to stuttering. Their results are readily apparent in the graph. The dramatic SBP reduction effected by stuttering applied not only for the group but for each of sixteen adult subjects without exception, clear evidence that stuttering is a more powerful mechanism for reducing SBP than shock is for increasing it. We must resist the temptation, however, of viewing SBP as an established measure of anxiety or any other feeling. It is a complex physiologic response (as are ESC and EWL) that participates in a variety of psychologic conditions, of which anxiety (whatever it may be) is only one. That SBP when elevated by stress may be affected

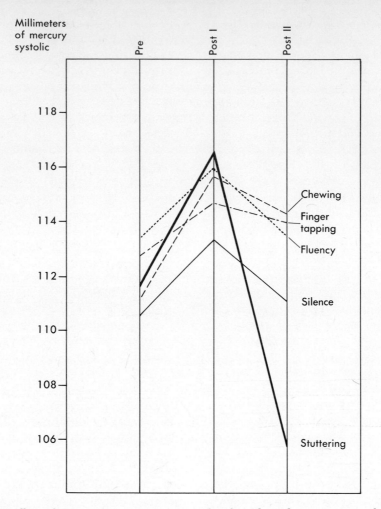

Fig. 14-2. Effect of stuttering in comparison with selected conditions on stress-heightened systolic blood pressure. The effect of shock on SBP is seen in the rise from Prestress to Post I stress. Stuttering reduced SBP substantially more than any other equated condition.

consistently by stuttering is clear; the psychologic significance of this functional relation is not.

What biologic conditions are associated with the reduction of stuttering? Among the few things known reasonably well about stuttering are the conditions that will reduce it. Phonetic skill is proving to be a key factor. A growing body of evidence points to motor coordination for speech as being important, perhaps fundamental. That stuttering involves disruption of phonetic coordinations is seen most directly in studies of rhythm, prosody, and motor rehearsal. Complete reduction of stuttering during singing or with imposition of fixed rhythm has long been known clinically. The *rhythm effect* has been investigated systematically (Beech, 1967; Beech and Fransella, 1969; Brady, 1968, 1969; Meyer and Comley, 1969). Invariably, stuttering is reduced and sometimes eliminated when the person is being paced, for example, by a metronome.

On a different tack, Wingate (1966a,b, 1967) has looked at the relations of stuttering to prosody and to "sound-mindedness" required to translate "slurvian" speech ("scence owe weevil") into normal speech ("see no evil"). He found that altering prosody from one adaptation trial to the next significantly

paced speech → < S

reduced the usual decrease in stuttering, indicating that although words in the passage remained the same, altering the rhythm of speaking them increased the likelihood of stuttering. As for effects of slurvian speech that depend heavily on prosodic deciphering for translation, here is one of very few factors on which nonstutterers are significantly different from and more adept than stutterers.

Approaching stuttering from the standpoint of types of rehearsal, Brenner, Perkins and Soderberg, compared no rehearsal, silent rehearsal with and without lip movement, whispered rehearsal, and aloud rehearsal for effects on stuttering. They found that aloud rehearsal reduced subsequent stuttering significantly more than any of the other conditions. Because rehearsal conditions varied presumably in the phonetic coordinations involved, their results suggest that incorporation of vocal adjustments involve more complex coordinations for fluent speech than articulatory movements without voice.

Closely related to rhythm is rate. Goldiamond (1965) demonstrated that by establishing very slow reading rates (about 30 words per minute), stuttering could be eliminated, with rarely an exception, in a large number of adult stutterers. Curlee and Perkins (1969), in replicating and confirming his work, extended it to social speech by developing a system of conversational rate control. They have demonstrated that under laboratory conditions, fluency established at slow rates can be maintained by gradually approximating normal rates.

Effective as rate control can be when used systematically, it is clearly not solely responsible for reduced stuttering. In Brenner's rehearsal experiment, not only did rate correlate poorly with frequency of stuttering, but rate was generally faster after aloud rehearsals when stuttering was reduced most. Too, in comparative studies of rate and rhythm, rhythm has operated independently of rate as the distinctly more effective condition for reduction of stuttering (Beech, 1967; Beech and Fransella, 1969; Ingham, 1975; Perkins

and others, 1974). The results of these studies suggest strongly that rate works its effect by facilitating rhythmic coordinations for normal speech prosody.

Masking, usually with white noise, has also been shown to reduce stuttering. Cherry and Sayers (1956) were the first to show the reduction of stuttering when it is masked with high-intensity filtered white noise, the effect being much greater with noise below 500 Hz than above. Subsequently, Maraist and Hutton (1957) reported a decrease in the severity of stuttering with 50 dB masking and close to normal speech at 90 dB. Similarly, Sutton and Chase (1961) found that white noise clearly improved speech, but so did the wearing of earphones without noise, and so did noise during silence preparatory to speaking.

Relatively prolonged reductions of stuttering have also been reported with the use of portable clinical masking units (Trotter and Lesch, 1967; Perkins and Curlee, 1969). On the other hand, Murray (1969) found that the majority of his subjects still stuttered without much reduction under white noise. Whether his discrepant result can be attributed to use of unfiltered (20 to 20,000 Hz) rather than filtered (below 500 Hz) noise awaits investigation. Masking effects may be part of a larger effect produced by reduced hearing; stuttering is apparently a rarity among deaf and severely hard-of-hearing persons (Backus, 1938; Harms and Malone, 1939).

Delayed auditory feedback (DAF) effects have received considerable attention lately, originally because they seemed to produce stuttering artificially, and more recently because they have been instrumental in procedures to reduce it. The numerous studies of DAF effects, first described by Lee (1951) as "artificial stutter," have been reviewed by Yates (1963). More recently, Soderberg (1969) compared and evaluated studies of short- and long-term DAF effects and DAF with masking effects. He concluded that (1) DAF reduces the stutterer's rate of speech and frequency of stuttering; (2) with reduced rate, DAF can be eliminated and fluency still be maintained; and (3) DAF with retarded

Table 14-1. Number and rate of physiologic adjustments involved in speaking aloud (voiced), whispering, and articulating silently (lipped)*

Condition	Speech adjustment	Adjustment rate	Respiratory alveolar pressure	Phonatory: transglottal pressure					Vocal tract modulation: supraglottal pressure
				Effective mass	Elasticity	Viscosity	Abduction	Adduction	
Voiced	Pitch	Phrase	▨						
		Syllable							
		Phone		■	■	■		■	
	Loudness	Phrase	▨						
		Syllable							
		Phone		■	■	■		■	
	Voiced/voiceless	Phrase	▨						
		Syllable							
		Phone		■				■	
	Articulatory	Phrase	▨						
		Syllable							
		Phone							■
Whispered	Pitch	Phrase							
		Syllable	XXXXXX					XXXXX	
		Phone							
	Loudness	Phrase							
		Syllable	XXXXXXX					XXXXX	
		Phone							

Lipped		Phrase								
	Voiced/voiceless	Syllable							XXXXX	
		Phone								
		Phrase								
	Articulatory	Syllable			XXXXXXX					
		Phone								
		Phrase								
	Pitch	Syllable								
		Phone								
		Phrase								
	Loudness	Syllable								
		Phone								
		Phrase								
	Voiced/voiceless	Syllable								
		Phone								
		Phrase								
	Articulatory	Syllable								
		Phone								

*The slowest adjustments are from phrase to phrase, the most rapid are from phone to phone (about 14 ± 2 per second), and in between are syllable-to-syllable adjustments (about 6 ± 2 per second).

rate reduces stuttering more effectively than masking without rate retardation. Subsequent research by Curlee and Perkins (1969) supports his first two conclusions; they used DAF to establish a slow rate and then phased it out. They have observed, too, that with attempts to maintain normal rate under DAF, the effect is to disrupt rather than to instate fluency.

Two other DAF studies must be noted. One by MacKay (1968) traced the development of the delay interval maximally disruptive of normal speech. For young children, a feedback delay of 0.5 second is maximally disruptive, for older children it shortens to 0.4 second, and for adults it is about 0.2 second. Children's speech, however, is more disrupted at all intervals than is adult speech. Too, the slower a person's maximum speaking rate, the longer the maximally disruptive interval. Because the maximum speaking rate increases with age, MacKay sees some common factor as relating speech disruption, maximum speaking rate, and maximally disruptive delay intervals. The other study to be noted, in a somewhat similar vein, revealed the puzzling evidence that the speech of adult females is maximally disrupted by somewhat longer delay intervals—0.27 second—than is that of males—0.18 second (Mahaffey and Stromsta, 1965).

Drug effects of all sorts, too, have been investigated, especially the use of the tranquilizer meprobamate. The fact that those drugs used to reduce anxiety have not reduced stuttering significantly is another indication that stuttering is not a function of anxiety, as it has been thought to be (Perkins, 1970). Such differences as have been observed typically have been under less-than-rigorous conditions of observation.

A common thread running through most of the conditions that reduce stuttering, and especially the more powerful ones that virtually eliminate it, is laryngeal activity of one form or another. As Wingate (1969a) observed, conditions that produce "artificial" fluency seem to involve the stutterer's doing something different with his voice. One of his difficulties is with initiating phonation during speech (Adams and Reis, 1971, 1974). He is also slower than the normal speaker in non-speech tasks of initiating and terminating phonation (Adams and Hayden, in press). Disruption of reciprocity of vocal cord adduction and abduction for voiced and voiceless sounds has even been photographed and studied electromyographically during stuttering (Freeman and Ushijima, 1975).

All these implications of voice in stuttering led to our *discoordination hypothesis* that syllable disfluencies are largely a function of the complexity of phonatory coordinations with articulation and respiration. We reasoned that this complexity could be progressively simplified by changing from normal voicing to whispering to articulating silently. Table 14-1 shows that not only are the number of physiologic adjustments sharply reduced with these simplifications, but so, too, are the speeds with which they occur (Perkins and others, 1976).

Considering how unpredictable stuttering has been in the intensive search for clues, the most remarkable feature of this experiment was the consistency of results. When complexity of phonatory coordinations was reduced with whispering, stuttering decreased radically in almost all subjects. When complexity was further simplified with silent articulation, any remaining stuttering was virtually eliminated. These results have been the same without exception in over a hundred stutterers.

Developmental characteristics

Development of stuttering in the speaker. Research has documented what any parent can attest: children are generally disfluent; they back and fill their way through speech from their earliest pronouncements. Many, of course, remain disfluent all the way to the grave. How some become stutterers is not so obvious, however. Since repetitions of sentences, phrases, and words are likely to seem normal—most of us, children especially, do much repeating—we need not be greatly concerned about disfluencies on these larger units of speech. Disruptions of the smooth flow of initiations of speech sounds are the culprits; they are apt to sound abnormal, and hence to become stuttering.

Parents generally report that their child started to stutter soon after starting to talk, with 3 and 4 being peak years. No one ever seems to hear stuttering before a child learns to speak. This observation hardly seems notable until we realize that infants during their first 2 years normally produce more than one fourth of their vocal-play sounds with repetitions (Winitz, 1961). In other words, the very disfluencies (on sounds and syllables) that are judged as stuttering in speech are rarely if ever heard as stuttering in prelinguistic utterances. Judgments of stuttering are usually made only about sound and syllable disfluencies in the context of language.

A sensible question would be: "Do children who stutter show more disfluencies on sounds and syllables than do nonstuttering children?" Addressed both tangentially and directly, the answer clearly seems to be

The evidence for this answer comes from numerous studies. This evidence is utilized by Johnson (1955, 1959) and by Wingate (1962a) in reaching divergent conclusions.

"yes." The only differences in disfluency that consistently appear between stuttering and nonstuttering children are syllable and sound repetitions, and especially sound prolongations. Moreover, to the extent that differences in disfluency can be detected between boys and girls (for whom stuttering is less prevalent), greater syllable and sound disfluencies are found in boys. These differences are not absolute; children vary widely in disfluencies, regardless of whether or not they are judged as stutterers (Wingate, 1962a). What does appear to be absolute is the difference in frequency of syllable disfluencies of preschool children who stutter and those who do not. Those who do stutter have been found to have a frequency of syllable disfluencies ranging from 7% to 14%. Those who do not stutter did not exceed 3%. Frequency of syllable disfluencies of those two groups did not even come close to overlapping, as would be expected if stuttering does indeed

develop from normal disfluency (Floyd and Perkins, 1974).

Children who develop stuttering show various forms of disruption. Some repeat, whereas others prolong (repetitions are sometimes called "clonic blocks"; prolongations and hesitations are called "tonic blocks"). Pressure applied to force speech out can range from negligible in any easy repetition to considerable effort, struggle, and strain even in a child as young as 2 years of age (Bloodstein, 1960). Along this line, Stromsta (1965) found, in a 10-year follow-up of childhood disfluencies labeled by parents as stuttering, that spectrographic analyses of the original disfluency patterns had good prognostic value. Of twenty-seven children showing lack of formant transition and phonatory stoppage (characteristic of articulatory prolongations and hesitations), twenty-four were stuttering 10 years later. Of eleven who did not show this pattern, ten claimed not to stutter. The four not accurately described by the analyses were among eight whose spectrograms were difficult to classify. Thus the presence of pressure symptoms in early stages of disfluency appears to be predictive of probable development of stuttering.

In any event, general agreement can be found on four features that characterize the acquisition of stuttering:

1. It begins for the majority between the ages of 2 and 7 years.
2. Onset is marked by fragmentation of syllables and words, sometimes with accompanying tension.
3. It fluctuates in severity, so that the course of development is not steady. Periods of weeks or months may go by with no difficulty, only to be followed by a sharp increase in severity that oscillates from one level to another.
4. It changes with time; beginning forms differ from advanced forms. A young child beginning to show signs of stuttering will become either better or worse. If he struggles with his fragmented syllables and words, his stuttering is likely to become more complicated and change from episodic to chronic.

Spontaneous recovery. About half the chil-

½ children spontaneously recover by puberty

dren who stutter will recover without therapy by puberty (Milisen and Johnson, 1936; Glasner and Rosenthal, 1957). Apparently, as many as four out of five who have ever stuttered will recover from it, most without help, by the time they reach college (Sheehan and Martyn, 1966, 1967). Of these, the majority will recover during early adolescence (Wingate, 1964a; Shearer and Williams, 1965), a rather surprising finding in view of the turbulence and stress usually associated with these teenage years. As Young (1975) notes, however, the prevalence of stuttering often reported for adults is the same as for children, *prevalence* 1%, which raises questions either about the accuracy of prevalence estimates or about the number who actually recover.

Equally as perplexing as the occurrence of stuttering is the remission of it. How and why so many recover is a mystery. Most have had no professional help, and the majority of those who have had help do not attribute their improvement to therapy. The most typical reason for recovery is likely to be, "I just seemed to outgrow it." The fact that recovery seems to be gradual gives credence to this maturational explanation. The most likely admonition that a recovered stutterer will offer is, "Slow down, take your time," followed by "Calm down, develop a better attitude." Although possible reasons for recovery are varied, and although recovery can occur apparently at any age, four signs are likely to indicate a poor prognosis for complete recovery: (1) severe stuttering, (2) complete blockings rather than syllable repetitions at onset, (3) a *poor prognosis* self-concept as a stutterer, and (4) late onset of recovery from stuttering (Sheehan and Martyn, 1966; Martyn and Sheehan, 1968; Stromsta, 1965).

Environment for the development of stuttering. The "nature versus nurture" debate has raged around stuttering for years. It still persists. Three decades ago and earlier, the prevailing notion was that stuttering was basically a product of nature; it was thought to be rooted in the constitution of the stutterer. The tide then changed. The prevailing idea has been that stuttering is produced by nurture as a learned reaction to environmen-tal stress—the source of stress depends on the theory of stuttering. Let us look briefly at what is known about the environment within which stuttering develops.

Two approaches have been pursued. The most popular in speech pathology has been to study environmental conditions to which the child could react by "monstrifying" his "primary" speech disruptions into full-blown "secondary" stuttering. The more popular approach in fields where psychoanalytic concepts prevail—clinical psychology and psychiatry—has been to look for environmental conditions conducive to neuroses, from which stuttering emerges as a symptomatic expression of personal maladjustment and conflict. Both approaches are concerned with subjective attitudes notoriously difficult to determine accurately. The essence of results

---

Johnson and others (1959) interpreted the evidence in terms of how environmental stress contributes to the development of stuttering. Does Wingate (1962b) agree with him? What does Goodstein (1958) think of the evidence about the effects of stress on personal adjustment?

---

from studies of parental attitudes and personalities and of environmental conditions in other cultures (ranging from polar Eskimo to African Bantu) is that whatever the conditions for stutterers may be, they are not discernibly different from those for nonstutterers.

Granted the possibility that parents of stutterers are overprotective, subtly critical, and perfectionistic, especially of speech; nonetheless, these parents are not severely maladjusted, nor do they have unusual personalities, nor is any such tendency clearly apparent in other cultures. In fact, such negative attitudes, maladjustments, or sensitivities for speech as do exist could be attributed easily to the fact that having a child who stutters is in itself cause for concern. If anything, the mothers, at least, are less overtly rejecting of their children than are those of nonstutterers. Maternal rejection seems to be essentially covert—as though the mother is trying to do the best she can and does not want to see the possibility that she may feel rejecting

environment

Covert rejection

(Kinstler, 1961). Were we to gamble on the best lead for a source of environmental stress, this factor of covert rejection would be one of choice. Yet, too much importance should not be assigned here because many children grow up surrounded by as much, if not more, covert rejection than do stutterers—and never stutter.

If environmental stress does operate to produce either neurosis or avoidance of stuttering, presumably such stress could be seen in the effects it produces. Aside from the argument that stuttering is such an effect, no other unusual consequences are visible, although Broida (1962) found some evidence that boys who stutter seem unusually ambivalent in sex-role identification despite strong preference for the male role. All in all, stutterers may be a bit tense, defensive, withdrawn, and, in general, oversocialized, but as a group they are not severely maladjusted or neurotic. They can, however, as individuals be just as neurotic or psychotic as nonstutterers. The only consistent difference between the two groups is that stutterers stutter.

Theories of stuttering

We will now turn to theories of stuttering. Possibly the most discernible feature of this problem is the abundance of explanations generated for it. Most fit within the three categories that Johnson (1958) described as the *anticipatory-struggle* point of view, the *repressed-need* point of view, and the *breakdown* point of view. These different views have guided most theorizing, research, and clinical thinking along separate paths. The one most heavily traveled in speech pathology has been built around the idea that stuttering is essentially a problem of hesitating to hesitate. These are the anticipatory-struggle theories, of which many of the learning theory and operant analyses are modern versions. The path traveled by those with a preference for psychoanalytic conceptions has been one on which stuttering is seen as a symptom of psychoneurosis: the repressed-need theories. The oldest path, dating back to antiquity and still traveled by those with a

biologic persuasion, has been that stuttering is a reflection of some sort of organic condition. From this line of thought have come the breakdown theories. All these points of view are often called theories, but many have been offered, mainly by astute observers of the clinical scene, as opinions. Let us look at some of these observers and their ideas to sample a few of the explanations that have been advanced for stuttering.

Anticipatory-struggle theories. Wendell Johnson was the fountainhead for the view that stuttering is what a person learns to do when he struggles to be fluent. His idea is that stuttering develops from normal disfluency. Not a symptom or reflection of a constitutional defect, stuttering is an avoidance reaction that an otherwise normal speaker learns to use when he anticipates struggling to speak. The vigor of this concept as developed by Johnson and his students turned the thrust of inquiry from a search for constitutional differences between stutterers and nonstutterers to a search for the conditions that lead to the stutterer's development of struggle reactions.

Johnson (1942, 1944, 1946, 1967) continued to work on this concept until his death. Originally it was called the *diagnosogenic theory*, also the *semantogenic theory*: "diagnosogenic" because the genesis of stuttering was considered to be in the misdiagnosis of normal disfluency as stuttering; "semantogenic" because the misdiagnosis was purported to be based on semantic confusion about the pejorative label "stuttering." The genesis of stuttering in this view is presumed to be in the child's efforts to avoid normal disfluencies because they are mislabeled as stuttering. A child stutters when he attempts to avoid doing what he thinks will be called stuttering.

As Johnson's thinking evolved, he put more and more emphasis on the role of the listener until this formulation came to be called the *interactional theory*, and sometimes the *evaluational theory*. The theory in this form says that the probability of developing stuttering increases, first, as the adults in a child's world set high standards of fluency

① anticipatory struggle — S → problem of hesitating to hesitate
② repressed need — symptom of neurosis
③ break-down — organic in nature

and react negatively to disfluency, and second, as the child's speech is marked by considerable disfluency.

Although serious doubts exist about how normal all disfluencies are in the speech of a child who is identified as a stutterer and about how different are the standards of fluency among parents of stuttering children (Wingate, 1962a,b,c), still Johnson demonstrated once and for all that stuttering exists in the ear of the listener. Stuttering is a judgment rendered about disfluencies from the mouth of a speaker. This truth is one of the most solid rocks on which a valid concept of stuttering can be built.

Several unifying assumptions tie together the opinions of those whose work has been classified under the *anticipatory-struggle* banner. They are that stutterers are essentially normal, that stuttering is learned behavior, and that what is learned are expectations of difficulty and the struggle responses to cope with them. The selection of a specific word on which to stutter is determined by the stutterer's expectation of failure in speaking it. Anticipating difficulty, he becomes so cautious as he approaches the word and attacks it with so much force, that, like the Sunday golfer who swings wildly and misses, any possibility of saying it fluently dwindles. Of course, the more he fails, the more he confirms his conviction that he will fail, and thus, the more he does fail.

These unifying assumptions prevail in many theories and therapies of stuttering. Van Riper (1972), who disavows a theory of stuttering but has nonetheless exerted long-standing pervasive influence on therapy, has done much to develop the idea that the preparation to stutter is a major part of the problem of stuttering. Williams (1957, 1971) stresses an analysis of what the person who stutters does to deviate from normal. He holds that by approaching speech as an easy endeavor (as do normal speakers) rather than as a difficult task (as do stutterers), the "stuttering" behavior tends to evaporate.

Sheehan (1953, 1968, 1969, 1970, 1975), working from a learning theory framework, has embroidered anticipatory-struggle into his *conflict theory* that has evolved into a *role-conflict theory* in which stutterers are seen as struggling with false roles in dealing with feelings of shame, guilt, and concealment. He has proposed that stuttering is an approach-avoidance conflict that results from competitive urges to speak and not to speak.

Bloodstein (1974, 1975a,b) has presented the most explicit argument that stuttering develops from the anticipation of difficulty in speaking. He maintains that stuttering begins with a child's fragmentation of larger linguistic units, such as sentences and phrases. With continued uncertainty about how to organize syntactic structures, motor planning difficulties become more apparent in fragmentations of smaller units of speech: words, syllables, and sounds. These fragmentations are characteristic of the repetitions of older stutterers. With them go tensions that result in the prolongations of stuttering. Fragmentations and tensions arise when, for any reason, a stutterer expects trouble in speaking. This idea extends the source of anticipated trouble from disfluency to delayed speech, articulatory difficulty, or any other difficulty that leads a child to view speech as something with which he must struggle.

Using Bloodstein's and Johnson's analyses of stuttering as an outgrowth of normal disfluency, Shames and Sherrick (1963) assumed stuttering to be operant behavior and showed how it could develop and be maintained by complex schedules of reinforcement and punishment. This idea has subsequently provided the basis for a system of therapy (Shames and Egolf, 1976). With primary interest in children, Luper (1968) has appraised learning-theory concepts in the understanding and therapy of stuttering.

The most complex analysis of stuttering as learned behavior is the *two-process theory* offered by Brutten and Shoemaker (1967, 1969) and elaborated by Brutten (1975). Viewing stuttering as conditioned disintegration of speech behavior, they theorized that it has two component elements: classically conditioned emotional responses disruptive of normal speech, and instrumentally condi-

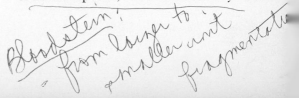

tioned stuttering responses. As they see it, modification of stuttering requires extinction of both classes of response.

Repressed-need theories. Proponents of repressed-need theories vary as to the exact nature of the needs served by the symptom of stuttering, but all assume that stuttering is a disguised manifestation of unspeakable feelings. All see stuttering as a psychoneurotic disorder involving psychodynamic conflicts of the ego as it attempts to mediate compromise solutions among the competing demands of social reality, the id, and the superego. Stutterers, for these theorists and clinicians, are to some extent maladjusted and to some extent neurotic (Chapter 10).

Many researchers have made important contributions to an understanding of the psychodynamics of stutterers. Among them are Murphy and FitzSimons (1960), speech pathologists; Wyatt (1958), a psychologist; Blanton (1965), a psychiatrist; and Barbara (1962) and Glauber (1958), psychoanalysts. Probably the person whose impact has been greatest among speech pathologists is Lee Travis. Trained as a psychologist, he was one of the influential founders of speech pathology. In his early professional years, working as a research scientist (and counting among his students such distinguished men of stuttering as Wendell Johnson and Charles Van Riper), he was interested in the neurophysiology of stuttering. Later, when he directed his attention to therapy of the disorder, he turned to a psychoanalytic conception. After thousands of hours of psychotherapy with thirty stutterers, Travis (1957) summarized his impressions as follows*:

> With almost monotonous repetition our stutterers advertised their unconscious preoccupation with the salvaging of some remnants of their early physical enjoyment. They revealed endlessly a nostalgia for their culturally disavowed, biologically rooted pleasures of sucking, eating, evacuating, and exploring. So frequently their revelations told of their lonely longing for the most primitive, raw, and earthy sensory and motor enjoyments and delights. When early training began its attack upon these pleasures of the flesh, our stutterers must have had three purportful reactions: anger, which met with triumphant counteranger and which ended in being repressed by fear; a loss of oneness with themselves; and finally, a crippling of interpersonal relationships, significantly with the parents.

Breakdown theories. Stuttering has perplexed men from antiquity. It has been treated with everything from putting pebbles into the mouth to cutting the tongue out of the mouth. Only relatively recently has the focus shifted from soma to psyche. Two of the men most responsible for founding speech pathology and giving it a vigorous start, Robert West and Lee Travis, devoted much of their professional lives to a search for a constitutional basis for stuttering. Eisenson (1975), too, has long pursued an organic lead: the possibility that the majority of stutterers are constitutionally inclined to perseverate, that is, to persist in a mental or motor act longer than normal.

Although Travis turned from his neurophysiologic investigations of cerebral dominance (1931) to psychologic studies, some still suspect that laterality and dominance play a role in stuttering. West, on the other hand, pondered the organic bases of stuttering throughout his distinguished career. He forged intriguing speculations about the physiologic mechanism that determines the onset and the termination of an act of stuttering (West, 1958). His idea that seems most prophetic, however, concerns the evolution of articulatory automaticity.*

> When . . . automaticity fails to develop, speech is interlaced with hesitation and repetition. Apparently, this faculty is slower to evolve than the other two, symbolization and abstraction. We may, therefore, think of stuttering as a residuum of delayed evolution. . . . Articulatory dysautomaticity may thus be viewed as the survival of a rather general status of primitive human beings. In the long view, as milleniums pass, stuttering should lessen in frequency.

---

*From Travis, L. (Ed.), *Handbook of Speech Pathology.* New York: Appleton-Century-Crofts (1957), p. 944.

*From West, R., and Ansberry, M., *The Rehabilitation of Speech.* New York: Harper & Row, Publishers (1968), p. 116.

Recent theorizing about the biologic bases of stuttering has focused mainly on laryngeal involvement. After reviewing the vast literature of stuttering, Van Riper (1971) concluded that the core of the disorder is a disruption of timing of the motor sequences of speech, which, of course, are comprised of phonation as well as respiration and articulation. Adams (1974) has proposed that control and coordination of subglottal and supraglottal pressures along with glottal resistance are the major determinants of both fluency and stuttering.

Summary of theories. The three major theoretical approaches are conflicting in some aspects and complementary in others. They represent attempts to integrate information about different aspects of the problem: some are addressed to the nature of stuttering, others to how it develops, and others to the nature of the person who stutters. In a sense, these are not theories; certainly they are not formal theories such as are found in physics. Although each has had its staunch advocates, none has satisfied all; yet each seems to hold a segment of the answer to the riddle of stuttering. Let us conclude, then, by assembling current knowledge into an integrated framework that could lead us to a better understanding of stuttering.

Leads to understanding of stuttering

Were we to follow the leads that appear best, four major factors could be hypothesized as interacting to yield stuttering, much as is shown schematically in Fig. 14-3. These factors are not mutually exclusive (as they can seem to be when discussed as "anticipatory-struggle theories," "repressed-need theories," or "breakdown theories"). Without doubt, stuttering develops through the interaction of multiple factors. Different patterns of interaction probably account for individual differences in stuttering. Two general factors, linguistic-motor coordinations and psychodynamic conflicts, are shown on the left of Fig. 14-3 as determinants of fluency. Whether a child is disfluent because of linguistic-motor incoordinations of psychodynamic conflicts, the more abnormal his

speech sound initiations, the more likely his speech is to be judged as stuttering and he as a stutterer. The two factors on the right, listener response and speaker attitude, reflect judgments of disfluency as stuttering or normal. From these judgments would stem the speaker's response to disfluency and his identity as "normal speaker" or "stutterer."

Linguistic-motor coordinations. If the continuous high-speed performance required for normal speech is contemplated, the linguistic-motor processes of Fig. 14-3 would weigh heavily in determining fluency on theoretical grounds alone. Consider the task. First is the problem of translating semantic-syntactic-morphemic decisions on what is to be said into phonetic sequence. Here, linguistic decision-making is involved. Once arranged, the sound sequence flows normally at a rate too fast to be controlled other than automatically. Articulatory movements of over a hundred muscles must be coordinated with extraordinary precision to arrive at the right position at precisely the right time. The slightest error in timing of any of these movements would, logically, disrupt the fluent flow of sound initiations and articulatory transitions, the very disfluencies typically judged as stuttering. The opportunities for mistiming motor signals are plentiful; they could be in various aspects of cortical motor patterning or transmission, in somesthetic or auditory feedback, in cerebellar coordination of movement, or in any combination thereof. Just as neural timing must surely be coordinated by rhythm, so much speech.

No evidence contradicts linguistic-motor processes as basic to fluency; much supports it strongly. Uncertainty in linguistic decision making is regularly found to be related to normal disfluency and stuttering. As for motor coordination, auditory feedback conditions are consistently associated with fluency effects: delayed auditory feedback disrupts fluency unless speaking rate is retarded; masking of low-frequency, voiced components of speech reduces stuttering; and adjustment of the air-bone conducted phase angles can block phonation. Rhythm effects are paramount: stuttering is reduced more consistently and completely with the imposition of rhythm than with any other condition, and stutterers are relatively poor in prosodic skills, which sets the rhythm of normal speech.

The suspicion that phonatory coordinations seem especially related to fluency has been confirmed. This lead arose from several sources. We knew that neither silent rehearsal with lip movements nor whispered rehearsal reduces stuttering as much as aloud rehearsal, perhaps because control of laryngeal-respiratory movements is more complex and rapid than is control of any other part of the speech apparatus. (Prosody requires

pitch and loudness adjustments for each syllable, and articulation requires voiced/voiceless adjustments for each phoneme.) We knew that rate affects fluency, but probably by facilitating rhythmic coordination of speech. Retarded rate reduces stuttering but not as effectively as rhythm, and maximum speaking rate is related to some common factor affecting disfluency. Thus the stage was set for finding that simplification of the complexity of phonatory coordinations with articulation and respiration greatly reduced stuttering during whispering. During silent articulation stuttering was virtually eliminated. Other factors undoubtedly contrib-

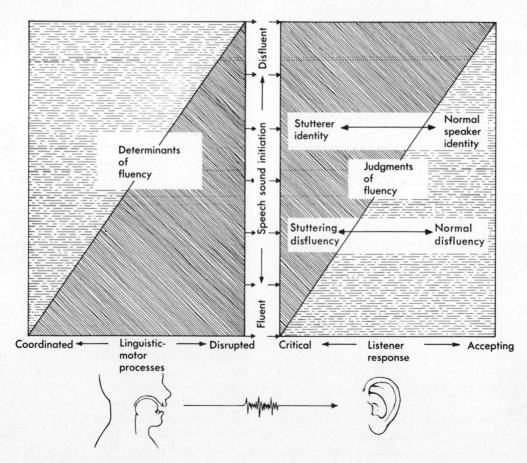

Fig. 14-3. Hypothetical factors of stuttering. Linguistic-motor processes and psychodynamic adjustment determine the fluency of speech sound initiation. Listener response and speaker attitude determine judgments of disfluency as stuttering and of the speaker as a stutterer.

ute to stuttering, but whatever their contributions, they must somehow be exerted through the motor coordination mechanisms of speech.

Perhaps Newman's point in *The Pianist's Problems* will prove instructive*:

Every teacher knows the student who makes so many mistakes in his playing that he figuratively stutters at the piano, and he knows that the habit can be just about as hard to cure as stuttering. I remember a young lady in a conservatory who practiced doggedly, day in and day out, for several months, at Bach's Two-Part Invention in F minor. I began to listen to her when I noticed how every measure was peppered with trials and errors before the right notes appeared. Presently, I realized that this was extremely successful practice, if not from the young lady's or Bach's standpoint, at least from the standpoint of muscular coordination; for every mistake that had once been an accident was now a well-learned, thoroughly mastered, integral part of the piece, a part that could be counted on with certainty to appear each time the piece was repeated.

Not only do the motor skills of the pianist approach those of the speaker in speed and complexity, so may the pianist's solution for avoiding errors hold a parallel for the acquisition of fluent speech: learn desired movements correctly from the beginning. Whereas the pianist slows down to ensure accuracy, the young child typically launches his speech at close to full speed. To the extent that fluency cannot be maintained, disfluency prevails; it is practiced and learned as the motor pattern of speech. Perhaps the old parental admonition to "slow down" has merit, especially since slowing down is one of the tactics to which recovered stutterers ascribe their spontaneously acquired fluency.

Psychodynamic conflict. The other major basis for disfluency shown in Fig. 14-3 is psychoneurotic conflict. Disfluency would wax and wane as conflict and need for the symptom rise and fall. Defensively, disfluent

---

*From Newman, W. S., *The Pianist's Problems*. (2nd ed.) New York: Harper & Row, Publishers (1956), pp. 104-105.

speech can be conceived as an unconscious attempt to block open expression of unacceptable thoughts and feelings. Expressively, the biting, spitting, chewing, and sucking components of stuttering can be viewed as unconscious efforts to gratify early unresolved needs through the act of speaking. These defensive and expressive functions have been elaborated in various forms by various theorists.

That psychodynamic conflict is a determinant of fluency has not been put to a crucial test. Perhaps the strongest support is that some stutterers, with no direct attention to speech, have been "cured" with psychotherapy. On the other hand, such treatment is far from universally effective. Even if it were, uncertainty would persist: no solid evidence points unambiguously to connections between mental health and speech fluency. The reason is that so many factors intervene between psychotherapeutic ministrations and measurable effects of treatment. Lack of evidence in no way demonstrates that psychodynamic conflict does not affect fluency. But if it does, the link is probably not semantic; research shows that even though words may have special meanings for stutterers, stuttering is not a function of those meanings. Too, since stuttering involves sound more than word disfluencies, stuttering would have to be related to the symbolic significance of stuttered sounds, a difficult case to make for sounds spoken fluently more often than stuttered.

Listener response. As Fig. 14-3 shows, listener reactions to disfluency can conceivably contribute to the speaker's evaluation of himself as a stutterer. That listener judgments vary is undoubtedly true. That parents of stutterers make similar judgments or that they are consistently more hypercritical of disfluency than parents of nonstutterers is far from demonstrated fact; some parents appear to exhibit positive responses.

Paradoxically, negative listener attention would be uniquely suited to reinforce disfluency, an identity of stutterer, and struggle behavior to speak. On the premise that even negative attention can be reinforcing (it could be better than none at all), disfluency heard as stuttering demands attention to *how* an idea is spoken, whereas attention in normal speech is commanded mainly by *what* is said. Speech judged as stuttering is almost assured of more attention, and therefore more reinforcement, than normal speech. Ironically, by virtue of negative rather than positive attention, the child would identify the very disfluencies being reinforced as the crux of his problem. The chain of events would spiral. The more he would struggle to speak, the more concern would be heaped on his disfluent speech, the more resistant to extinction it would become, the less success he would have in preventing its occurrence— and thus the more convinced he would become that he is a stutterer.

Speaker attitude. Fig. 14-3 also shows two types of consequences that can be hypothesized as stemming from speaker insecurity. With one, the more insecure a person is, the more vulnerable he is to criticism and to the conviction that disfluency is abnormal, that it is to be avoided, and that speaking is generally a difficult task requiring struggle. With the other, the more insecure a person is, the more he needs a "crutch" to help manage life and a cause on which to hang vague fears and anxieties. Thus he has less need for evidence of negative listener reaction or of abnormal disfluency to be convinced that his basic flaw is stuttering.

Evidence that stutterers become sensitive about their speech difficulty is seen in various forms: in increased struggle and avoidance tactics of advanced stages of stuttering, in apparent susceptibility to time pressure, in the probability that with the expectancy of stuttering will come stuttering, and in poor prognosis for spontaneous recovery of those who struggle severely to speak and who have assumed a stutterer's identity. With evidence that disfluency is typically reduced with contingent punishment, however, the possibility that stuttering is the stutterer's struggle to avoid negative listener response to disfluency seems improbable. Were that response

punishing, stuttering would decrease, not increase. Too, however stutterers may feel about themselves and their speech, the popular view that fear of stuttering produces stuttering is contradicted by available evidence: autonomic nervous system measures of anxiety do not rise before nor fall after a moment of stuttering, and deconditioning of anxiety does not reduce stuttering with much consistency.

From clinical, physiologic, and behavioral studies comes support for the concept that speaker insecurity offers fertile soil for the growth of stuttering as an ego-protective problem to which one's failures could be assigned. Psychotherapists have long observed that stuttering in children can be eliminated by resolving conflicts and insecurities in the child and his parents that do not directly involve speech. Too, stutterers tend to set relatively low levels of aspiration for themselves. Physiologically, stuttering may function as a powerful homeostatic mechanism to reduce stress-heightened systolic blood pressure, suggesting that it functions somehow to relieve tension. From demonstrations that stuttering is operant behavior stems a necessary conclusion: when its contingent consequences are aversive it decreases, when reinforcing it increases. Stuttering is probably acquired and maintained by its reinforcing consequences—the more secure a person is, the more he needs attention and ego protection—and hence the more strongly are disfluency and a self-image of stutterer reinforced.

CLUTTERING

Cluttering is an established diagnostic category among European phoniatrists, who, being physicians, have discussed it in medical terms. The concept has gained recognition in recent years among American speech pathologists, but it is difficult to discuss and evaluate within the frame of reference of a behavioral science because the ideas and terminology are rooted in a "disease model" as distinct from a "behavioral model." Whereas a behavioral account describes observations of what a person does irrespective of the underlying physiologic condition, an etiologic account distinguishes among what are inferred as various pathologic bases of a disorder. Viewed from the standpoint of a disease model, cluttering seems to be different from stuttering. Viewed from a behavioral standpoint, to capture a difference between stuttering and cluttering is like trying to bottle fog: it evaporates when enclosed within the confines of explicit definitions.

Does cluttering differ from stuttering?

The study of cluttering seems to be suffering many of the definitional growing pains that have harassed the study of stuttering. The vaguer the question, the vaguer is the definition of the phenomenon to be studied and the higher the tower of nosologic Babel is likely to grow. Across the centuries, stutterers have been so patently different that the obvious question has been: "What makes stutterers different from nonstutterers?" The same question has been applied to clutterers. Definition of the phenomenon to be studied has tended to slop over from what the stutterer *does* when he stutters to what the stutterer *is* whether he is stuttering or not. The same has happened to cluttering. The implication is that persons who stutter or clutter are more characterized by their stuttering or cluttering than by their human condition. The next step has been to catalog those impressions that seem to distinguish stutterers and clutterers. The raw materials are then at hand for the erection of an impressive nomenclatural edifice. For stuttering we have seen spasmophemia stacked on dysphemia, cerebral dominance built on strephosymbolia; now for cluttering we find such staggering terminologic blocks being fitted together as tachyphemia, tachylalia, leipophemia, barylalia, battarismus, and paraphrasia praeceps!

Cluttering defined. As with stutterers, for whom we have searched in every nook and cranny of their psyches and somas for clues as to why they are different (with little success), so with clutterers, trails fan out through their lives, with most traffic stretching across the linguistic landscape. Weiss defines cluttering as follows*:

Cluttering is a speech disorder characterized by the clutterer's unawareness of his disorder, by a short attention span, by disturbances in perception, articulation and formulation of speech and often by excessive speed of delivery. It is a disorder of the thought processes preparatory to speech and based on a hereditary disposition. Cluttering is the verbal manifestation of Central Language Imbalance, which affects all channels of communication (e.g., reading, writing, rhythm and musicality) and behavior in general.

Behavioral similarities. Luchsinger and Arnold (1965) list twenty-eight points for comparison of stutterers and clutterers that range from graphologic findings to musical talent. Still, only two are concerned with what the person *does* when he speaks: stutterers block tonically or clonically, whereas clutterers stumble and jerk rapidly. Thus we are brought back to the main point. When we define the *behavior* that separates clutterers from stutterers, the difference vanishes. Weiss (1964) points out that the majority of symptoms of cluttering are facultative—that is, they are often, but not necessarily, present. Only a few are obligatory: lack of awareness of the disorder (presumably comprised largely of facultative symptoms), short attention span, and excessive repetitions in speech. Even if we include "lack of awareness" as a behavioral characteristic, a dubious inclusion, the only obligatory behavior of clutterers that an American speech pathologist might not expect to find among his stutterers is short attention span. Because this "symptom" is only a clinical impression that the clutterer's attention must be short because of the short-lived improvement in other "symptoms" when he concentrates on them, this distinction, too, is doubtful, especially when we remember that stutterers notoriously sift through the mesh of college speech-screening examinations by concentrating on not stuttering for the brief duration of these speaking chores.

---

*From Weiss, D., *Cluttering*. Englewood Cliffs, N.J.; Prentice-Hall, Inc. (1964).

If, having played the devil's advocate, this analysis were correct, then we would have two overlapping general terms for a phenomenon that could be specified by some as stuttering and others as cluttering, or more exactly, by organicists as dysphemia and behaviorists as disfluency.

Rate and rhythm disorders of cluttering

Despite the uncertainty as to whether or not cluttering can be distinguished from stuttering, the fact remains that cluttering does direct attention to problems of rate and rhythm not emphasized in consideration of stuttering. Shepherd's (undated) description of cluttered speech, for example, stresses excessive rate *(tachylalia)* and erratic rhythm *(dysrhythmia)* as typical symptoms that lead to garbled speech that can be unintelligible. Involving articulatory distortions, slurring of sounds, syllables, and words, and sound transpositions reminiscent of "slurvian speech" and "spoonerisms," this speed-tumbled speech can be interspersed briefly with a lagging, drawling, abnormally slow rate *(bradylalia)*, but with little improvement in intelligibility (Bradford, undated).

Behaviorally, then, cluttering *(tachyphemia)* is a useful term for identifying problems of rate and rhythm; to the extent that it includes problems of fluency, it overlaps stuttering. Clutterers can do what stutterers do—struggle with disfluency—but additionally clutterers tumble erratically through speech, blurring intelligibility as they go.

Etiology of cluttering. Etiologically, cluttering is considered to be one of many symptoms of a general language disability: grammatical deficiency, impaired reading ability, bizarre handwriting, poor musical ability, and bodily incoordinations. Whether or not the constitutional bases ascribed to cluttering are, in fact, valid causal explanations cannot be determined from existing evidence.

Two lines of research have been pursued. Genetic investigations have been prompted by the basic tenet of cluttering theory, that central language imbalance is hereditary.

Thus heredity is considered to be the etiology of true cluttering as distinguished from symptomatic cluttering, which is thought to be caused by neurologic involvement, the other line of research. Considerably more work has been done on the neurology of cluttering than on its genetic transmission, which remains for the most part a clinical impression that it runs in families (Weiss, 1964).

European electroencephalographic studies have shown, with one exception, more irregularity in the records of clutterers than of stutterers, who in turn produce more irregularities than are found in normal EEG records produced by presumably normal speakers (Luchsinger and Landolt, 1951, 1955; Morávek and Langová, 1962; Streifler and Gumpertz, 1955). Weiss (1964) cautions that these results are questionable: that EEG recordings do not show the neural activity of deep-lying brain structures presumably involved in cluttering, that interpretation of abnormality from recordings is highly individual except for gross conditions such as epilepsy, and that the subject's state of relaxation and emotional condition have considerable effect on records produced. We could add that more careful consideration of the rules of scientific design and inference would make their results more credible. When performances of subjects are presented as percentages, when these performances are not compared with performances of control subjects, when behavior under observation could just as well have produced the physiologic results as vice versa, and when great inferential leaps are made from limited observations to sweeping physiologic explanations, then confidence in sizable differences, even on sizable samples, dwindles.

Not only can cluttered speech be defective in more ways than stuttered speech, but it can also be accompanied by other language disabilities. All in all, cluttering would appear to reflect a more profound disability than stuttering. Viewed in this light, the European research that consistently shows more neurologic disability among clutterers than stutterers gains in credibility.

The answers—résumé

1. What are the characteristics of stuttering?

Stuttering is a judgment rendered mainly of speech sound disfluencies; it can be characterized by factors that determine disfluency and that determine judgments of what stuttering is and who stutterers are. Disfluency judged both as normal and stuttered shows adaptation and consistency effects for reasons not entirely apparent. Disfluency is known to vary, though, with linguistic uncertainty, rhythm, rate, delayed auditory feedback, masking, prosodic and phonetic skill, contingent punishment and reinforcement, and especially with simplification of coordinations of phonatory with articulatory and respiratory adjustments. It probably does not vary systematically with anxiety. The possibility that disfluency varies with psychodynamic conflict is more clinical conjecture than demonstrated fact. Too, up to 80% of children thought to stutter will "outgrow it" by adulthood.

Both listener response and speaker attitude probably contribute to the development and maintenance of stuttering. Although listener reactions to disfluency vary in severity, parents of stutterers do not seem to be much different from parents of nonstutterers. Speakers who become stutterers, however, are more severely disfluent and develop the self-concept of stutterer. That they may be insecure and vulnerable to hypercritical listeners is seen in increased struggle and avoidance tactics of advanced stages of stuttering, in relatively low levels of aspiration, in apparent susceptibility to time pressure, and in susceptibility to reinforcement of stuttering by its consequences—a necessary conclusion if stuttering is the operant behavior it appears to be.

2. With what disabilities is stuttering associated?

Despite years of mostly fruitless search for biologic causes of stuttering, a few leads have survived contradictory evidence or have appeared from relatively sophisticated modern research. The greater prevalence of stuttering among males than females, poorer prosodic skills and a smaller "right ear effect" in stutterers than nonstutterers, relative phase angle differences between stutterers and nonstutterers of bone-conducted sound, and the virtual elimination of stuttering with simplification of phonatory coordinations with articulation and respiration are suggestive of physiologic bases of disfluency that could develop into stuttering. To consider these differences as disabilities, however, would require a thin line between normal and abnormal.

3. What are the characteristics of cluttering?

More frequently described by medically oriented European phoniatrists than by behaviorally oriented speech pathologists, cluttering is generally considered to be a verbal manifestation of central language imbalance involving all forms of communication. Out of its many "symptoms" only a few are characteristic: lack of awareness of the disorder, short attention span, and excessive repetitions. Also consistently emphasized are excessive rate, erratic rhythm, and garbled speech.

4. With what disabilities is cluttering associated?

Phoniatrists distinguish between true cluttering, thought to be genetically transmitted, and symptomatic cluttering, caused by neurologic disability. That it runs in families is largely clinical impression; that it is associated with neurologic disability is fairly well supported by electroencephalographic research.

REFERENCES

Adams, M., Psychological differences between stutterers and nonstutterers: a review of the experimental literature. *J. Communication Dis.*, **2**, 163-170 (1969).

Adams, M., A physiologic and aerodynamic interpretation of fluent and stuttered speech. *J. Fluency Dis.*, **1**, 35-47 (1974).

Adams, M., and Hayden, P., The ability of stutterers and nonstutterers to initiate and terminate phonation during production of an isolated vowel. *J. Speech Hearing Res.*, **19**, 290-296 (1976).

Adams, M., and Reis, R., The influence of the onset of phonation on the frequency of stuttering. *J. Speech Hearing Res.*, **14**, 639-644 (1971).

Adams, M., and Reis, R., The influence of the onset of phonation on the frequency of stuttering: a replication and reevaluation. *J. Speech Hearing Res.*, **17**, 752-754 (1974).

Andrews, G., and Harris, M., *The Syndrome of Stuttering*. London: Heinemann Medical Books, Ltd. (1964).

Backus, O., Incidence of stuttering among the deaf. *Ann. Otol. Rhinol. Laryng.*, **47**, 632-635 (1938).

Barbara, D., *The Psychotherapy of Stuttering*. Springfield, Ill.: Charles C Thomas, Publisher (1962).

Beech, R., Stuttering and stammering. *Psychology Today*, **1**, 49-51, 61 (July, 1967).

Beech, R., and Fransella, F., Explanations of the "rhythm effect" in stuttering. In Gray, B., and England, G. (Eds.), *Stuttering and the Conditioning Therapies*. Monterey, Calif.: Monterey Institute for Speech and Hearing (1969).

Biggs, B., and Sheehan, J., Punishment or distraction? Operant stuttering revisited. *J. abnorm. Psychol.*, **74**, 256-262 (1969).

Blanton, S., Stuttering. In Barbara, D. (Ed.), *New Directions in Stuttering*. Springfield, Ill.: Charles C Thomas, Publisher (1965).

Bloodstein, O., A rating scale study of conditions under which stuttering is reduced or absent. *J. Speech Hearing Dis.* **15**, 29-36 (1950).

Bloodstein, O., The development of stuttering. I. Changes in nine basic features. *J. Speech Hearing Dis.*, **25**, 219-237 (1960).

Bloodstein, O., The development of stuttering. III. Theoretical and clinical implications. *J. Speech Hearing Dis.*, **26**, 67-82 (1961).

Bloodstein, O., The rules of early stuttering. *J. Speech Hearing Dis.*, **39**, 379-394 (1974).

Bloodstein, O., *A Handbook on Stuttering*. Chicago: National Easter Seal Society for Crippled Children and Adults (1975a).

Bloodstein, O., Stuttering as tension and fragmentation. In Eisenson, J. (Ed.), *Stuttering: a Second Symposium*. New York: Harper & Row, Publishers (1975b).

Bloodstein, O., and Gantwerk, B., Grammatical function in relation to stuttering in young children. *J. Speech Hearing Res.*, **10**, 786-789 (1967).

Boehmler, R., Listener responses to nonfluencies. *J. Speech Hearing Res.*, **1**, 132-141 (1958).

Bradford, D., A framework of therapeusis for articulation therapy. In *Studies in Tachyphemia*. New York: Speech Rehabilitation Institute (undated).

Brady, J., A behavioral approach to the treatment of stuttering. *Am. J. Psychiatry*, **125**, 843-848 (1968).

Brady, J., Studies on the metronome effect on stuttering. *Behav. Res. Ther.*, **7**, 197-204 (1969).

Brenner, N., Perkins, W., and Soderberg, G., The effect of rehearsal on frequency of stuttering. *J. Speech Hearing Res.*, **15**, 483-486 (1972).

Broida, H., An empirical study of sex-role identification and sex-role preference in a selected group of stuttering male children. Doctoral dissertation. Los Angeles: University of Southern California (1962).

Brookshire, R., and Martin, R., The differential effects of three verbal punishers on the disfluencies of normal speakers. *J. Speech Hearing Res.*, **10**, 496-505 (1967).

Brown, S., The loci of stutterings in the speech sequence. *J. Speech Dis.*, **10**, 181-192 (1945).

Brutten, E., Stuttering: topography, assessment, and behavior change strategies. In Eisenson, J. (Ed.), *Stuttering: a Second Symposium*. Harper & Row, Publishers (1975).

Brutten, E., and Shoemaker, D., *The Modification of Stuttering*. Englewood Cliffs, N.J.: Prentice-Hall, Inc. (1967).

Brutten, E., and Shoemaker, D., Stuttering: the disintegration of speech due to conditioned negative emotion. In Gray, B., and England, G. (Eds.), *Stuttering and the Conditioning Therapies*. Monterey, Calif.: Monterey Institute for Speech and Hearing (1969).

Cherry, C., and Sayers, B., Experiments upon the total inhibition of stammering by external control, and some clinical results. *J. psychosom. Res.*, **1**, 233-246 (1956).

Cooper, D., The effects of unknown time on the frequency of stuttering. Unpublished research. Los Angeles: University of Southern California (1970).

Cullinan, W., Stability of adaptation in the oral performance of stutterers. *J. Speech Hearing Res.*, **6**, 70-83 (1963).

Curlee, R., Reliability of estimates of instances of stuttering. Unpublished manuscript. Los Angeles: University of Southern California (1970).

Curlee, R., and Perkins, W., The effect of punishment of expectancy to stutter on the frequencies of subsequent expectancies and stuttering. *J. Speech Hearing Res.*, **11**, 787-795 (1968).

Curlee, R., and Perkins, W., Conversational rate control therapy for stuttering. *J. Speech Hearing Dis.*, **34**, 245-250 (1969).

Curry, F., and Gregory, H., A comparison of stutterers and nonstutterers on three dichotic tasks. Unpublished manuscript. Chicago: Northwestern University (undated).

Dabul, B., and Perkins, W., The effects of stuttering on systolic blood pressure. *J. Speech Hearing Res.*, **16**, 586-591 (1973).

Deese, J., and Hulse, S., *The Psychology of Learning.* New York: McGraw-Hill Book Co. (1967).

Eisenson, J., Stuttering as perseverative behavior. In Eisenson, J. (Ed.), *Stuttering: a Second Symposium.* New York: Harper & Row, Publishers (1975).

Floyd, S., and Perkins, W., Early syllable dysfluency in stutterers and nonstutterers: a preliminary report. *J. Commun. Dis.*, **7**, 279-282 (1974).

Freeman, F., and Ushijima, T., Laryngeal activity accompanying the moment of stuttering: a preliminary report of EMG investigations. *J. Fluency Dis.*, **1**, 36-45 (1975).

Froeschels, E., and Rieber, R., The problem of auditory and visual imperceptivity in stutterers. *Folia Phoniatrica*, **15**, 13-20 (1963).

Glasner, P., and Rosenthal, D., Parental diagnosis of stuttering in young children. *J. Speech Hearing Dis.*, **22**, 288-295 (1957).

Glauber, I., The psychoanalysis of stuttering. In Eisenson, J. (Ed.), *Stuttering: a Symposium.* New York: Harper & Row, Publishers (1958).

Goldiamond, I., Stuttering and fluency as manipulable operant response classes. In Krasner, L., and Ullman, L. (Eds.), *Research in Behavior Modification.* New York: Holt, Rinehart & Winston, Inc. (1965).

Goldiamond, I., Personal communication (1969).

Goldman, R., and Shames, G., Comparisons of the goals that parents of stutterers and parents of nonstutterers set for their children. *J. Speech Hearing Dis.*, **29**, 381-389 (1964a).

Goldman, R., and Shames, G., A study of goal-setting behavior of parents of stutterers and parents of nonstutterers. *J. Speech Hearing Dis.*, **29**, 192-194 (1964b).

Goldman-Eisler, F., Speech analysis and mental processes. *Language & Speech*, **1**, 59-75 (1958).

Goodstein, L., Functional speech disorders and personality: a survey of the research. *J. Speech Hearing Res.*, **1**, 359-376 (1958).

Gray, B., Theoretical approximations of stuttering adaptation: statement of predictive accuracy. *Behav. Res. Ther.*, **3**, 221-227 (1965).

Gray, B., and England, G., Some effects of anxiety deconditioning upon stuttering frequency. *J. Speech Hearing Res.*, **15**, 114-122 (1972).

Hagen, A., An experimental investigation of the relationship between frequency of stuttering and open expression of aggression. Doctoral dissertation. Los Angeles: University of Southern California (1965).

Harms, M., and Malone, J., Hearing and stammering. *Ann. Otol. Rhinol. Laryng.*, **48**, 658-662 (1939).

Herren, R., The effect of stuttering on voluntary movement. *J. Exper. Psychol.*, **14**, 289-298 (1931).

Hill, H., Stuttering. I. A critical review and evaluation of biochemical investigations. *J. Speech Dis.*, **9**, 245-261 (1944a).

Hill, H., Stuttering. II. A review and integration of physiological data. *J. Speech Dis.*, **9**, 289-324 (1946b).

Hill, H., An experimental study of disorganization of speech and manual responses in normal subjects. *J. Speech Hearing Dis.*, **19**, 295-305 (1954).

Huffman, E., and Perkins, W., Dysfluency characteristics identified by listeners as "stuttering" and "stutterer." *J. Commun. Dis.*, **7**, 89-96 (1974).

Ingham, R., Operant methodology in stuttering therapy. In Eisenson, J. (Ed.), *Stuttering: a Second Symposium.* New York: Harper & Row, Publishers (1975).

Ingham, R., and Andrews, G., The relation between anxiety reduction and treatment. *J. Commun. Dis.*, **4**, 289-301 (1971).

Johnson, W., A study of the onset and development of stuttering. *J. Speech Dis.*, **7**, 251-257 (1942).

Johnson, W., The Indians have no word for it. I. Stuttering in children. *Quart. J. Speech*, **30**, 330-337 (1944).

Johnson, W., *People in Quandaries: the Semantics of Personal Adjustment.* New York: Harper & Row, Publishers (1946).

Johnson, W. (Ed.), *Stuttering in Children and Adults.* Minneapolis: University of Minnesota Press (1955).

Johnson, W., Introduction: the six men and the stuttering. In Eisenson, J. (Ed.), *Stuttering: a Symposium.* New York: Harper & Row, Publishers (1958).

Johnson, W., Measurements of oral reading and speaking rate and disfluency of adult male and female stutterers and nonstutterers. *J. Speech Hearing Dis., Monogr. Suppl.* 7, pp. 1-20 (1961a).

Johnson, W. (Ed.), Studies of speech disfluency and rate of stutterers and nonstutterers. *J. Speech Hearing Dis., Monogr. Suppl.* 7 (1961b).

Johnson, W., and Brown, S., Stuttering in relation to various speech sounds. *Quart. J. Speech*, **21**, 481-496 (1935).

Johnson, W., and Solomon, A., Studies in the psychology of stuttering. IV. A quantitative study of expectation of stuttering as a process involving a low degree of consciousness. *J. Speech Dis.*, **2**, 95-97 (1937).

Johnson, W., and others, *Speech Handicapped School Children.* New York: Harper & Row, Publishers (1948).

Johnson, W., and others, *The Onset of Stuttering.* Minneapolis: University of Minnesota Press (1959).

Johnson, W., and others, *Speech Handicapped School Children.* New York: Harper & Row, Publishers (1967).

Kinstler, D., Covert and overt maternal rejection in stuttering. *J. Speech Hearing Dis.*, **26**, 145-155 (1961).

Lanyon, R., The measurement of stuttering severity. *J. Speech Hearing Res.*, **10**, 836-843 (1967).

Lanyon, R., Some characteristics of nonfluency in normal speakers and stutterers. *J. abnorm. Psychol.*, **73**, 550-555 (1968).

Lanyon, R., Speech: relation of nonfluency to information value. *Science*, **164**, 451-452 (1969).

Lee, B., Artificial stutter. *J. Speech Hearing Dis*, **16**, 53-55 (1951).

Love, L., and Jeffress, L., Identification of brief pauses in the fluent speech of stutterers and nonstutterers, *J. Speech Hearing Res.*, **14**, 229-240 (1971).

Luchsinger, R., and Arnold, G., *Voice-Speech-Language.* Belmont, Calif.: Wadsworth Publishing Co., Inc. (1965).

Luchsinger, R., and Landolt, H., Elektroencephalographische Untersuchungen bei Stotterern mit und ohne Poltererkomponente. *Folia Phoniatrica*, **3**, 135-150 (1951).

Luchsinger, R., and Landolt, H., Über das poltern, das sogenannte "Stottern mit Polterkomponente und deren Beziehung zu den Aphasien." *Folia Phoniatrica*, **7**, 12-43 (1955).

Luper, H., Consistency of stuttering in relation to the

goal gradient hypothesis. *J. Speech Hearing Dis.*, **31**, 336-342 (1956).

Luper, H., An appraisal of learning theory concepts in understanding and treating stuttering in children. In Gregory, H. (Ed.), *Learning Theory and Stuttering Therapy.* Evanston, Ill.: Northwestern University Press (1968).

Luper, H., and Mulder, R., *Stuttering Therapy for Children.* Englewood Cliffs, N.J.: Prentice-Hall, Inc. (1964).

MacKay, D., Metamorphosis of a critical interval: age-linked changes in the delay in auditory feedback that produces maximal disruption of speech. *J. acoust. Soc. Am.*, **43**, 811-821 (1968).

MacKay, D., and Bowman, R., On producing the meaning in sentences. *Am. J. Psychol.*, **82**, 23-39 (1969).

Mahaffey, R., and Stromsta, C., The effects of auditory feedback as a function of frequency, intensity, time, and sex. De Therapia Vocis et Loquelae. (Vol. II). Societatis Internationalis Logopaediae et Phoniatriae, XIII Congressus Vindobonae Anno MCMLXV, *Acta* (Aug., 1965).

Maraist, J., and Hutton, C., Effects of auditory masking upon the speech of stutterers. *J. Speech Hearing Dis.*, **22**, 385-389 (1957).

Martin, R., and Haroldson, S., The relationship between anticipation and consistency of stuttered words. *J. Speech Hearing Res.*, **10**, 323-327 (1967).

Martin, R., and Siegel, G., The effects of response contingent shock on stuttering. *J. Speech Hearing Res.*, **9**, 340-352 (1966a).

Martin, R., and Siegel, G., The effects of simultaneously punishing stuttering and rewarding fluency. *J. Speech Hearing Res.*, **9**, 466-475 (1966b).

Martyn, M., and Sheehan, J., Onset of stuttering and recovery. *Behav. Res. Ther.*, **6**, 295-307 (1968).

McDearmon, J., Primary stuttering at the onset of stuttering: a reexamination of data. *J. Speech Hearing Res.*, **11**, 631-637 (1968).

Meyer, V., and Comley, J., A preliminary report on the treatment of stammer by the use of rhythmic stimulation. In Gray, B., and England, G. (Eds.), *Stuttering and the Conditioning Therapies.* Monterey, Calif.: Monterey Institute for Speech and Hearing (1969).

Milisen, R., Frequency of stuttering with anticipation of stuttering controlled. *J. Speech Dis.*, **3**, 207-214 (1938).

Milisen, R., and Johnson, W., A comparative study of stutterers, former stutterers and normal speakers whose handedness has been changed. *Arch. Speech*, **2**, 61-86 (1936).

Morávek, M., and Langová, J., Some electrophysiological findings among stutterers and clutterers. *Folia Phoniatrica*, **14**, 305-316 (1962).

Murphy, A., and FitzSimons, R., *Stuttering and Personality Dynamics.* New York: The Ronald Press Co. (1960).

Murray, F., An investigation of variably induced white noise upon moments of stuttering. *J. Commun. Dis.*, **2**, 109-114 (1969).

Neelley, J., and Timmons, R., Adaptation and consistency in the disfluent speech behavior of young stutterers and nonstutterers. *J. Speech Hearing Res.*, **10**, 250-256 (1967).

Newman, W., *The Pianist's Problems.* (2nd ed.) New York: Harper & Row, Publishers (1956).

Perkins, W., Stuttering: some common denominators. In Barbara, D. (Ed.), *New Directions in Stuttering.* Springfield, Ill.: Charles C Thomas, Publisher (1965).

Perkins, W., Stuttering and discriminative awareness. Final Report, Social Rehabilitation Services Research Grant No. RD-2275-S. University of Southern California (1969).

Perkins, W., Physiological studies. In Sheehan, J. (Ed.), *Stuttering: Research and Therapy.* New York: Harper & Row, Publishers (1970).

Perkins, W., and Curlee, R., Clinical impressions of portable masking unit effects in stuttering. *J. Speech Hearing Dis.*, **34**, 360-362 (1969).

Perkins, W., and others, Replacement of stuttering with normal speech. III. Clinical effectiveness. *J. Speech Hearing Dis.*, **39**, 416-428 (1974).

Perkins, W., and others, Discoordination of articulation with phonation and respiration. *J. Speech and Hearing Res.*, **19**, 509-522 (1976).

Peterson, H., Affective meaning of words as rated by stuttering and nonstuttering readers. *J. Speech Hearing Res.*, **12**, 337-343 (1969).

Prins, D., Pre-therapy adaptation of stuttering and its relation to speech measures of therapy progress. *J. Speech Hearing Res.*, **11**, 740-746 (1968).

Prins, D., and Lohr, F., Behavioral dimensions of stuttered speech. *J. Speech Hearing Res.*, **15**, 61-71 (1972).

Quarrington, B., Stuttering as a function of the information value and sentence position of words. *J. abnorm. Psychol.*, **70**, 221-224 (1965).

Quarrington, B., Seligman, J., and Kosower, E., Goal setting behavior of parents of beginning stutterers and parents of nonstuttering children. *J. Speech Hearing Res.*, **12**, 435-442 (1969).

Quist, R., and Martin, R., The effect of response-contingent verbal punishment on stuttering. *J. Speech Hearing Res.*, **10**, 795-800 (1967).

Ringel, R., and Minifie, F., Protensity estimates of stutterers and nonstutterers. *J. Speech Hearing Res.*, **9**, 289-296 (1966).

Sander, E., Reliability of the Iowa Speech Disfluency Test. *J. Speech Hearing Dis.*, *Monogr. Suppl.* **7**, pp. 21-30 (1961).

Sander, E., Frequency of syllable repetition and stutterer judgments. *J. Speech Hearing Res.*, **28**, 19-30 (1963).

Schlesinger, I., and others, Stuttering, information load, and response strength. *J. Speech Hearing Dis.*, **30**, 32-36 (1965).

Schuell, H., Sex differences in relation to stuttering. Parts I and II. *J. Speech Dis.*, **11**, 277-298; **12**, 23-38 (1947).

Shames, G., and Egolf, D., *Operant Conditioning and the Management of Stuttering.* Englewood Cliffs, N.J.: Prentice-Hall, Inc. (1976).

Shames, G., Egolf, D., and Rhodes, R., Experimental programs in stuttering therapy. *J. Speech Hearing Dis.*, **34**, 30-47 (1969).

Shames, G., and Sherrick, C., A discussion of nonfluency and stuttering as operant behavior. *J. Speech Hearing Dis.*, **28**, 3-18 (1963).

Shearer, W., and Williams, J., Self-recovery from stuttering. *J. Speech Hearing Dis.*, **30**, 288-290 (1965).

Sheehan, J., Theory and treatment of stuttering as an approach-avoidance conflict. *J. Psychol.*, **36**, 27-49 (1953).

Sheehan, J., Conflict theory of stuttering. In Eisenson,

J. (Ed.), *Stuttering: a Symposium.* New York: Harper & Row, Publishers (1958a).

Sheehan, J., Projective studies of stuttering. *J. Speech Hearing Dis.*, **23**, 18-25 (1958b).

Sheehan, J., Stuttering as self-role conflict. In Gregory, H. (Ed.), *Learning Theory and Stuttering Therapy.* Evanston, Ill.: Northwestern University Press (1968).

Sheehan, J., The role of role in stuttering. In Gray, B., and England, G. (Eds.), *Stuttering and the Conditioning Therapies.* Monterey, Calif.: Monterey Institute for Speech and Hearing (1969).

Sheehan, J., *Stuttering: Research and Therapy.* New York, Harper & Row, Publishers (1970).

Sheehan, J., Conflict theory and avoidance-reduction therapy. In Eisenson, J. (Ed.), *Stuttering: a Second Symposium.* New York: Harper & Row, Publishers (1975).

Sheehan, J., Cortese, D., and Hadley, R., Guilt, shame, and tension in graphic projections of stuttering. *J. Speech Hearing Dis.*, **27**, 129-139 (1962).

Sheehan, J., and Martyn, M., Spontaneous recovery from stuttering. *J. Speech Hearing Res.*, **2**, 121-135 (1966).

Sheehan, J., and Martyn, M., Methodology in studies of recovery from stuttering. *J. Speech Hearing Res.*, **10**, 396-400 (1967).

Sheehan, J., and Voas, R., Tension patterns during stuttering in relation to conflict, anxiety-binding, and reinforcement. *Speech Monogr.*, **21**, 272-279 (1954).

Sheehan, J., and Zelen, S., Level of aspiration in stutterers and nonstutterers. *J. abnorm. soc. Psychol.*, **51**, 83-86 (1955).

Shepherd, G., Phonetic description of cluttered speech. II. In *Studies in Tachyphemia.* New York: Speech Rehabilitation Institute (undated).

Siegel, G., Review of stuttering and learning theory. *J. Commun. Dis.*, **2**, 174-189 (1969).

Siegel, G., and Martin, R., Experimental modification of disfluency in normal speakers. *J. Speech Hearing Res.*, **8**, 235-244 (1965a).

Siegel, G., and Martin, R., Verbal punishment of disfluencies in normal speakers. *J. Speech Hearing Res.*, **8**, 245-251 (1965b).

Silverman, F., and Williams, D., Loci of disfluencies in the speech of nonstutterers during oral reading. *J. Speech Hearing Res.*, **10**, 790-794 (1967a).

Silverman, F., and Williams, D., Loci of disfluencies in the speech of stutterers. *Percept. Mot. Skills*, **24**, 1085-1086 (1967b).

Soderberg, G., Linguistic factors in stuttering. *J. Speech Hearing Res.*, **10**, 801-810 (1967).

Soderberg, G., Delayed auditory feedback and the speech of stutterers: a review of studies. *J. Speech Hearing Dis.*, **34**, 20-29 (1969).

Soderberg, G., Relations of word information and word length to stuttering disfluencies. *J. Commun. Dis.*, **4**, 9-14 (1971).

Spahr, F., Frequency of stuttering as a function of connotative word meaning. Doctoral dissertation. Los Angeles: University of Southern California (1968).

Streifler, M., and Gumpertz, F., Cerebral potentials in stuttering and cluttering. *Confin. Neurol.*, **15**, 344-359 (1955).

Stromsta, C., A methodology related to the determination of the phase angle of bone-conducted speech sound energy of stutterers and nonstutterers. Doctoral dissertation. Columbus: Ohio State University (1956).

Stromsta, C., Experimental blockage of phonation by distorted sidetone. *J. Speech Hearing Res.*, **2**, 286-301 (1959).

Stromsta, C., Delays associated with certain sidetone pathways. *J. acoust. Soc. Am.*, **34**, 392-396 (1962).

Stromsta, C., A spectrographic study of dysfluencies labeled as stuttering by parents. De Therapia Vocis et Loquelae. (Vol. I). Societatis Internationalis Logopaediae et Phoniatriae, XIII Congressus Vindobonae Anno MCMLXV, *Acta* (August, 1965).

Stunden, A., The effects of time pressure as a variable in the verbal behavior of stutterers. Doctoral dissertation. Los Angeles: University of California at Los Angeles (1965).

Sutten, S., and Chase, R., White noise and stuttering. *J. Speech Hearing Res.*, **4**, 72 (1961).

Taylor, I., What words are stuttered? *Psychol. Bull*, **65**, 233-242 (1966).

Taylor, M., An investigation of physiological measures in relation to the moment of stuttering in a group of adult males. Doctoral dissertation. Los Angeles: University of Southern California (1966).

Travis, L., *Speech Pathology.* New York: Appleton-Century-Crofts (1931).

Travis, L., The unspeakable feelings of people with special reference to stuttering. In Travis, L. (Ed.), *Handbook of Speech Pathology and Audiology.* New York: Appleton-Century-Crofts (1971).

Trotter, W., and Lesch, M., Personal experiences with a stutter-aid. *J. Speech Hearing Dis.*, **32**, 270-272 (1967).

Van Riper, C., *The Nature of Stuttering.* Englewood Cliffs, N.J.: Prentice-Hall, Inc. (1971).

Van Riper, C., *Speech Correction: Principles and Methods.* Englewood Cliffs, N.J.: Prentice-Hall, Inc. (1972).

Weiss, D., *Cluttering.* Englewood Cliffs, N.J.: Prentice-Hall, Inc. (1964).

Wendahl, R., and Cole, J., Identification of stuttering during relatively fluent speech. *J. Speech Hearing Res.*, **4**, 281-286 (1961).

West, R., An agnostic's speculations about stuttering. In Eisenson, J. (Ed.), *Stuttering: a Symposium.* New York: Harper & Row, Publishers (1958).

West, R., and Ansberry, M., *The Rehabilitation of Speech.* New York: Harper & Row, Publishers (1968).

Williams, D., A point of view about "stuttering." *J. Speech Hearing Dis.*, **22**, 390-397 (1957).

Williams, D., Stuttering therapy for children. In Travis, L. (Ed.), *Handbook of Speech Pathology and Audiology.* New York: Appleton-Century-Crofts (1971).

Williams, D., and Kent, L., Listener evaluations of speech interruptions. *J. Speech Hearing Res.*, **1**, 124-131 (1958).

Williams, D., Silverman, F., and Kools, J., Disfluency behavior of elementary-school stutterers and nonstutterers: the adaptation effect. *J. Speech Hearing Res.*, **11**, 622-630 (1968).

Williams, D., Silverman, F., and Kools, J., Disfluency behavior of elementary-school stutterers and nonstutterers: loci of instances of disfluency. *J. Speech Hearing Res.*, **12**, 308-318 (1969a).

Williams, D., Silverman, F., and Kools, J., Disfluency behavior of elementary-school stutterers and nonstutterers: the consistency effect. *J. Speech Hearing Res.*, **12**, 301-307 (1969b).

Williams, D., Wark, M., and Minifie, F., Ratings of stuttering by audio, visual, and audiovisual cues. *J. Speech Hearing Res.*, **6**, 91-100 (1963).

Wingate, M., Evaluation and stuttering. I. Speech characteristics of young children. *J. Speech Hearing Dis.*, **27**, 106-115 (1962a).

Wingate, M., Evaluation and stuttering. II. Environmental stress and critical appraisal of speech. *J. Speech Hearing Dis.*, **27**, 244-257 (1962b).

Wingate, M., Evaluation and stuttering. III. Identification of stuttering and the use of a label. *J. Speech Hearing Dis.*, **27**, 368-377 (1962c).

Wingate, M., Recovery from stuttering. *J. Speech Hearing Dis.*, **29**, 312-321 (1964a).

Wingate, M., A standard definition of stuttering. *J. Speech Hearing Dis.*, **29**, 484-489 (1964b).

Wingate, M., Prosody in stuttering adaptation. *J. Speech Hearing Res.*, **9**, 550-556 (1966a).

Wingate, M., Stuttering adaptation and learning. I. The relevance of adaptation studies to stuttering as "learned behavior." *J. Speech Hearing Dis.*, **31**, 148-156 (1966b).

Wingate, M., Slurvian skill of stutterers. *J. Speech Hearing Res.*, **10**, 844-848 (1967).

Wingate, M., Sound and pattern in "artificial" fluency. *J. Speech Hearing Res.*, **12**, 677-686, (1969a).

Wingate, M., Stuttering as phonetic transition defect. *J. Speech Hearing Dis.*, **34**, 107-108 (1969b).

Winitz, H., Repetition in the vocalizations and speech of children in the first two years of life. *J. Speech Hearing Dis.*, *Monogr. Suppl.* **7**, pp. 55-62 (1961).

Wischner, G., Anxiety-reduction as reinforcement in maladaptive behavior: evidence in stutterers' representations of the moment of difficulty. *J. abnorm. soc. Psychol.*, **47**, 566-571 (1952).

Wyatt, G., A developmental crisis theory of stuttering. *Language & Speech*, **1**, 250-264 (1958).

Yates, A., Delayed auditory feedback. *Psychol. Bull.*, **60**, 213-232 (1963).

Young, M., Predicting ratings of severity of stuttering. *J. Speech Hearing Dis.*, *Monogr. Suppl.* **7**, pp. 31-54 (1961).

Young, M., Response-by-response agreement for marking moments of stuttering. Paper presented at the American Speech and Hearing Association Convention (1969).

Young, M., Onset, prevalence, and recovery from stuttering. *J. Speech Hearing Dis.*, **40**, 49-58 (1975).

Part IV

Clinical practice of speech pathology

Part IV is a presentation of methods of assessing and remediating defective speech. Here we turn from what the speech pathologist needs to know about the nature of speech processes to what he needs to know about measuring, evaluating, and modifying these processes.

Chapter 15

Assessment of disorders of speech

Questions

1. What is the purpose of examining language and speaking behavior?
2. What principles guide the assessment of disorders of speech?
3. How can linguistic behavior be assessed?
4. How can speaking behavior be assessed?
5. How can abilities related to speech be assessed?

The assessment of the adequacy of speech is basically an assessment of its effectiveness in communication. Speech is a primary tool for denoting to the listener a set of relations expressed by the speaker. This function is achieved by the formal structure of language. The relation of objects and conditions to abstract classes is the semantic problem; this relation is specified in dictionary definitions. The relation of classes to each other is the grammatical problem; this relation is specified by morphophonemic and syntactic rules by which a subject idea is related to a predicate idea in a complete sentence. Phonation, articulation-resonance, and temporal aspects of speaking contribute to these relations as they affect semantic and morphophonemic recognition of the word (was the word "four," "for," or "fort"; was it singular "light" or plural "lights"). The assessment of linguistic dimensions of speech involves testing their adequacy for communicating *content* of the message.

Yet speech that will be assessed will reflect *intent* at work. Linguistically, intent will be revealed metaphorically in the overtones of the content of logical discourse, in what the psychotherapist listens to with his "third ear." Even more, it will be signaled by "tone of voice," prosody, fluency, manner of articulation, and other aspects of the speaking process (Chapter 10). The less able a speaker is to communicate his intent through message content, or the greater the disparity between linguistic content symbols and nonlinguistic intent signals, or the heavier the speaker's reliance on nonlinguistic signals to influence his listeners, the greater will be his need to retain his signal system. Assessment that will reveal why a disorder is maintained as well as the prognosis for rehabilitation must include examination of impaired speech behavior as it signals intent as well as symbolizes message content.

PRINCIPLES OF ASSESSMENT

What is the speech pathologist attempting to accomplish when he examines defective speech? What principles guide inquiry? Basically, he follows the precepts of science as he attempts to describe the problem accurately, determine conditions that produced and maintain it, and plan objectives to be achieved in rehabilitating it.

Purpose

Information can be gathered in an examination of defective speech for three purposes: *description*, *assessment*, and *diagnosis*. Not just speech but behavior that reveals disabilities that could contribute to defective speech must be examined to meet these purposes.

Description. Description is fundamental. It is the fact-finding task. It corresponds in the method of science to observation. Just as science proceeds by measurement of observations, so does description. The degree of certainty of knowledge is related directly to the precision of measure. Too, we can have greater confidence in events tested here and

now than in those reported as past history. Still, since problems have a history, the speech pathologist has little choice—he must use two tools for description: tests and case history.

Testing. Testing involves direct observation of behavior, usually under specific conditions. Tests are structured ways of observing. They are devices interposed between examiner and subject to improve the reliability of observation. The stimuli presented may range from an audiometric test tone to an intelligence test question to a personality test inkblot. The more formal and standardized the test, the more specific are the conditions under which responses are observed.

Control of stimulus conditions contributes to the reliability of a test, but not necessarily to its validity. The once sacrosanct IQ test, for example, has come under fire, not because it is unreliable but because of growing doubt that it is a valid measure of whatever is meant by intelligence. At present, testing in many speech-related areas is in limbo. With language, with phonation, with speech-flow processes, as with intelligence, our conception of behavior that needs to be tested has in some ways changed considerably. Consequently, in many instances formal tests of such behavior are not yet available. In these instances the speech pathologist must rely on ingenuity and do the best he can to quantify informal observations.

Although conditions for testing can range from the most formal to informal, all must permit some type of quantification even if it is nothing more than ranking one performance as better than another on an ordinal scale, or at worst assigning behavior to one class or another on a nominal scale. Generally, when instrumentation can be used to measure performance, one can go considerably beyond merely saying what is being observed; he can say how much there is of each type of response. Unfortunately, since not many instrumental measures of speech behavior have been devised, we are better able to talk sensibly about the different types of speech responses than to compare the amounts of each type. What this means in practice is that we can identify classes of speech disorders of such types as voice, language, and stuttering more accurately than we can measure the degrees of severity of each type.

Case history. Information about how a speech problem came to be as it is cannot be obtained from testing alone. A case history will be needed. Good case histories should be tailored to the specific needs of individuals; thus they will be as unique as people themselves. Regardless of who the informant is, whether it be parent, friend, or the

---

What suggestions do Johnson and his colleagues (1963) have for the types of questions that should be included in a case history? How do they recommend conducting an interview?

---

speech-handicapped person, the information provided is a product of memory, with all the filterings and distortions attendant thereunto. Even if a questionnaire or rating scale is used that can help to structure and quantify recollections, such as the Vineland Social Maturity Scale developed by Doll (1946), it still cannot alter the inherent weakness of recalling information from memory.

Nonetheless, a case history can be revealing and helpful, especially if the examiner knows the kind of information needed. For example, for an understanding of the problems of a cleft-palate child, including the physical disabilities with which the child has struggled in his efforts to acquire speech, a *medical* and *dental history* will be necessary. A *developmental history* will be required to spot significant departures from the normal course of development of speech, personality, intelligence, educational achievement, and social relations with family and friends. From such inquiry come many details that, when organized in chronologic sequence particularly, reveal impressions of patterns suggestive of how the defective speech came about. More importantly, these patterns can be indicative of the person's past and current needs that find expression in both normal and defective aspects of speech.

Assessment. With the examination com-

pleted, the question arises: "What do you do with all this information?" The answer depends on whether your purpose is assessment or diagnosis. Although these two purposes are accomplished in much the same way, they are nevertheless distinctly different in objectives to be achieved and in types of information utilized. These differences will usually be reflected in the report of examination results. We will begin with the purpose of assessment.

Does Darley (1964) make similar distinctions in purpose? What terms does he use for different purposes?

Objectives. Assessment is the speech pathologist's primary purpose. The objectives are as follows:

1. To determine the nature and severity of the speech defect
2. To determine the prognosis
3. To determine appropriate therapeutic strategy

Thus assessment is done for a practical purpose: to determine what the speech pathologist should do to assist in the improvement of speech.

The first objective is to determine whether the suspected defect is in fact a defect, and if so, how severe it is. Two types of information will be needed to meet this objective: the results of the examination of speech behavior, and the criteria against which these results can be compared. A report of the speech examination should provide a detailed description of the linguistic and speaking performance. This, however, is a report of first-order facts. It does not interpret them. It does not evaluate, for example, whether the vocal performance described is normal or abnormal. An evaluative judgment of this description is the first objective of assessment. For it, criteria are needed.

The criteria can be objective or subjective. Objective standards include *linguistic* and *nonlinguistic criteria.* Linguistically, speech that violates grammatical rules or that is unintelligible is defective by adult standards. Obviously, a 3-year-old child who does not meet this standard would not be considered defective; thus a *developmental criterion* must be added. Developmental norms and linguistic standards provide the most objective criteria against which to assess most aspects of speech (Chapters 11 and 12).

Fluency and voice, however, particularly defy adequate assessment in a linguistic framework. The listener applies two nonlinguistic criteria to determine adequacy of fluency. First, he decides whether the speech he hears is fluent or disfluent. If it is the latter, then he must decide whether the disfluency is normal or abnormal. If the disfluency is abnormal, then he reaches the judgment that it is stuttering. These decisions are based on some very complex, subtle, and personal preferences about fluency.

As for voice, *cultural standards* dictate, for instance, that men sound like men, women like women, and children like children. When a person's voice that violates these standards can be brought comfortably within them, everyone is likely to be happier. The more important nonlinguistic criterion for voice, however, is *vocal hygiene*. Vocalization that abuses the larynx involves defective production. Highest priority, then, in evaluating vocal production must be given to assessing it against a *criterion of optimal production* (Chapter 13).

A *speech defect* can be determined with relative objectivity, but a *speech problem* is necessarily a subjective judgment. A defect, to be a problem, must make a problem for either the speaker or the listener. In fact, speech can pose problems even when demonstrable defects cannot be found. Some people think they have a severe problem of stuttering even though the listener can detect nothing wrong with the speech. Anxious parents often hear problems in their child's speech where no defect can be found. Conversely, one can have a speech defect about which he has little concern, so that a speech defect is not tantamount to a speech problem, or vice versa. Criteria for determining the magnitude of problems are nebulous.

The second objective of assessment is to determine the prospect for recovery from a speech defect. For this objective, information about conditions that can disable speech will be needed, in addition to the report of the speech examination. Here, the speech pathologist needs to know about sensory, perceptual, intellectual, motor, and learning abilities as well as about emotional, environmental, and personality conditions. This objective involves a crucial decision-making step in the assessment. It involves a determination of the extent to which a *speech impairment* may be a defect.

Let us say that you have seen a speech-handicapped child. Assessment of your descriptive findings shows that by linguistic standards speech is defective in grammar, vocabularly, and articulation; it is characteristic of a 3-year-old child. Because the child is 6 years of age, his speech is also defective by developmental standards. The child is unconcerned about his defect, but the parents are distraught, so that for them it is a problem. Knowing this much, however, does not tell you the extent of impairment or what to do about it. If, after considering various tests or related abilities and the developmental history, you are confronted with a monolithic picture of retardation, you would probably conclude that the impairment is severe, the prognosis poor, and the value of a program of speech therapy limited. On the other hand, if the picture is one of nearly normal physical development, you might well reach quite a different conclusion about the severity of impairment, the prognosis, and the value of therapy.

The third objective of assessment is to determine appropriate forms of therapy to assist in recovery. Information for this objective will be needed from the first two objectives about the defect, the problem, and the impairment. It will be needed from the behavioral examination of speech skills of which the person is capable, as distinct from what he normally does. It will also be needed from an assessment of the individual's needs as they determine his intent, which may be reflected in his speech disorders. An evaluation of speech-skill capability is necessary to determine where therapeutic progress is most likely to be expected, or where spontaneous recovery is possible. An evaluation of intent is necessary to determine the function that a speech disorder may serve. A person who uses defective speech to express intent will probably need to learn more effective ways of communicating this intent before permanent modification of his abnormal speech can be accomplished.

Information utilized. You may have noticed that all abilities and conditions essential to a speech pathologist's decisions can be observed in overt or covert behavior. Knowledge of the person's ability to perform essential skills of speech is more relevant to assessment than knowledge of anatomic or physiologic conditions. The anatomic fact of aglossia (no tongue), for example, does not necessarily doom one to defective speech. This principle holds even with the apparent exception of voice disorders in which feasibility of voice therapy may be contraindicated by the laryngeal condition. Here, the decision as to whether or not therapy might exacerbate laryngeal pathology is made by the physician. Once the speech pathologist has medical clearance, however, he proceeds on the basis of his behavioral assessment.

Although formal testing of speech-related behavior such as personality or intelligence is desirable (if not sometimes essential), and for some tests may require the service of a psychologist, informal testing by the speech pathologist will usually provide sufficient information for preliminary planning. In point of fact, any rehabilitative plan or prognosis is held tentatively, subject to revision as additional evidence becomes available. If, for instance, the prospect of spontaneous recovery seems good, and yet after a reasonable trial no improvement was observed, then the plan would be reevaluated. Too, responses may become available as therapy progresses that will alter plans and goals formulated originally. Therapeutic assessment and science progress by the same process: observe, formulate a tentative explanation, test its accuracy, and modify it as new evidence may require.

The basis for primacy of behavioral information is both pragmatic and philosophic.

Pragmatically, possibilities for compensatory adjustments are infinite; thus the speech pathologist does not know what a physically handicapped person can or cannot do until behavioral performance is tested. Philosophically, prediction of behavior from anatomic or physiologic evidence poses a similar dilemma for speech pathology as Feynman, the Nobel physicist, described for physics*:

> Had you never visited earth, could you predict the thunderstorms, the volcanoes, the ocean waves, the auroras, and the colorful sunset? . . . The next great era of awakening of human intellect may well produce a method of understanding the *qualitative* content of equations. . . . Today we cannot see whether Schröedinger's equation contains frogs, musical composers, or morality—or whether it does not.

Diagnosis. Where assessment is the province of the speech pathologist, diagnosis is accomplished by the physician. The speech pathologist seeks to understand the disabilities that produce and maintain the speech disorder. The physician seeks the etiology of these disabilities. He seeks diseases and lesions that disable functions of the apparatus required for speech. The speech pathologist can often aid in this task. A behavioral analysis of speech recognition, linguistic formulation, and spoken expression can provide crucial diagnostic differentiations among locations of lesions that produce deafness, agnosia, aphasia, apraxia, and dysarthria. Similarly, a hoarse voice is one of the earliest diagnostic signs of laryngeal pathology, just as hypernasality is a primary indicator of velopharyngeal incompetency. Thus the speech pathologist contributes vital information about speech skills to the diagnosis.

Because the speech pathologist is interested in the biologic correlates of these skills, he may study them anatomically and physiologically. He may, if asked, be able to venture an informed opinion about the neurologic, laryngeal, respiratory, or orofacial condition of a speech-handicapped patient.

---

*From Feynman, R., Leighton, R., and Sands, M., *The Feynman Lectures on Physics*. (Vol. 2) Reading, Mass.: Addison-Wesley Publishing Co., Inc. (1964).

But if he is not asked, he will be well advised to limit his contributions to diagnosis to a report of information about which he has special competence: speech behavior. To venture unsolicited observations about the physical status of a patient can be construed by a physician as a novice telling a professional about his own specialty.

METHODS OF ASSESSMENT

Application of the foregoing principles of assessment requires three types of information: delineation of behavioral skills to be examined, methods of examining them, and criteria for assessing their adequacy. We will look closely at speech behavior about which the speech pathologist is expected to have expert knowledge. We will look briefly at the speech-related behavior with which he is concerned but for which he shares responsibility with other professions. We will obtain an overview of formal and informal methods of testing this behavior (to catalog all relevant tests and to describe testing procedures in much detail would go far beyond the limits of this text). We will also look at the criteria by which speech behavior in particular can be assessed.

Assessment of language behavior

Language abilities to be examined. Three basic types of linguistic abilities should be examined: vocabulary, grammar, and the functional use of language. A test of vocabulary is a test of *semantic* ability: How many words can the person recognize and understand as a listener? How many words can he use meaningfully as a speaker? A test of grammar is a test of one's knowledge of how language works: *Phonemically*, how well is he able to recognize that words with different speech sounds have different meanings? *Morphemically*, how well is he able to understand and produce words of the appropriate grammatical category from a vocabulary pool of morphemic units? *Syntactically*, how well is he able to recognize and produce phrase-structure units organized to make grammatical sentences? *Transformationally*, how well is he able to understand and produce the various transformations of basic kernel sentences? Finally, a test of the functional use of language, though not involving structural units, examines *pragmatically* how speech is used for communicative purposes.

Methods and criteria for assessing language development. The concepts of generative grammar especially applicable to language acquisition have not yet culminated in a set of standardized tests of functional units of language behavior. Beyond vocabulary, formal tests currently available approach linguistic ability tangentially more than directly. First, let us look at the types of formal tests available and then consider some useful informal evaluations.

Vocabulary tests. Two frequently used tests of recognition vocabulary are the *Full-Range Picture Vocabulary Test* developed by Ammons and Ammons (1948) and Dunn's (1959) *Peabody Picture Vocabulary Test.* These require only that the child point to a picture that best illustrates the meaning of a word spoken by the examiner. Other vocabulary tests, such as that developed by Bangs (1961, 1968), utilize norms and procedures that have been reported in the literature but that are not available commercially.

Some of the shortcomings of "pure" vocabulary tests are met by the *Assessment of Children's Language Comprehension* (ACLC) (Foster, Giddan, and Stark, 1969). This instrument tests four levels of contextual complexity in which words are used. Although still in the developmental stage, it at least takes cognizance of the fact that comprehension of vocabulary requires understanding of the grammatical structure within which the words are packaged (Emerick and Hatten, 1974).

Comprehension and expression tests. Perhaps the most comprehensive and widely used commercial test is the *Illinois Test of Psycholinguistic Abilities* (ITPA), by Kirk, McCarthy, and Kirk (1968). Included are nine subtests of language reception and expression that examine the ability to assign meaning to linguistic symbols (vocabulary) and to hold symbols in memory long enough to arrange them in sequence (grammar). As

Spradlin (1967) points out, however, a child can master the tasks with one-word responses; thus the ITPA is a dubious test of knowledge of grammar. For that matter, Spradlin has essentially the same criticism for the *Parsons Language Sample*, a test he constructed several years earlier that is based on a skinnerian concept of language functions (Spradlin, 1963). The same limitation applies to the *Picture Language Inventories* designed by Lerea (1958) to measure a child's ability to comprehend and express vocabulary and language structure.

For children who can write, the *Picture Story Language Test* by Myklebust (1965) is a useful instrument for measuring language productivity, syntactic correctness, and abstractness or concreteness of meaning. Too, it is a test on which quantitative data have been obtained to provide norms for evaluating a child's performance. Such a test is of limited value, however, for assessing the adequacy of speech development. Carrow (1968), on the other hand, has developed an experimental test of the comprehension of linguistic structure with which various age groups have been tested. More recently, the *Northwestern Syntax Screening Test* (Lee, 1969b) of receptive and expressive grammatical ability has become available. Bzoch and League's (1971) *Receptive-Expressive Emergent Language Scale* (REEL) is of greatest value in revealing language disorders and the level of linguistic functioning of the young child from birth to 3 years of age. It can be administered in a single interview, but it is best used with extended observation of the child. Such tests as these are steps in the direction of broad assessment of implicit knowledge of the basic rules of language.

Language usage test. An instrument that extends the communication portion of the *Vineland Social Maturity Scale* is the *Utah Test of Language Development*, constructed by Mecham, Jex, and Jones (1958). Only indirectly a test of language per se, it is a scale of the number and levels of complexity of social circumstances in which spoken and written language are used for communication. Underlying it is the idea that as a child's knowledge of language develops, so do communicative functions of speech. Thus the scale not only provides an overview of situations in which speech can be used and reinforced but also provides a score that can be converted to the child's language usage age.

Informal measures of language. A procedure still frequently used as a standard method of evaluating language development was originated by McCarthy (1930) several decades ago and has gone through numerous revisions. As described by Johnson, Darley, and Spriestersbach (1963), complete with norms by which various measures from the language sample can be evaluated, at least fifty spontaneous utterances are obtained from the child. These utterances can be measured for length of response, grammatical complexity, useful vocabulary, and functional use of language. Many have agreed with McCarthy that the best single measure of language maturity is the mean length of response; measures of sentence completeness and grammatical complexity have not been as reliable, and vocabulary, of course, reveals nothing about knowledge of the structure of language.

Berry (1969) provided as complete a system for longitudinal study of language development as is available. It is designed to explore and evaluate normal and deficient verbal and language-pertinent nonverbal behavior. Not diminishing the value of standard tests, Berry stresses the need to evaluate objective measures against longitudinal observation: more can be learned by watching a child in his normal habitat than in formal test situations. She provides case history forms, exploratory materials, inventories, and developmental tables to guide longitudinal studies of comprehension and use of speech, sensorimotor and general motor development, socioemotional behavior, and attitudes in learning.

As for functional measures, they can be analyzed by Piaget's (1926) system for determining how much the child ignores his listener and uses speech egocentrically or, by contrast, uses it socially with consideration for the point of view of his listener. Clearly, if one follows Piaget's thinking in search of conditions that reinforce language acquisition, the same motives would not be sought for speech when it is used egocentrically as when it is used socially. The child apparently obtains very different satisfactions in talking to himself from those he obtains in talking to a listener.

What behavior would Schiefelbusch (1967) examine in assessing a child's development of functional uses of language and communication? What four functional stages of development does he propose?

Critique of language assessment procedures. In an analysis of strategies for evaluating language, Spradlin (1967) has made several points relevant to the concept central to this book. He sees language assessment as the initial step in a program of language therapy, a step that provides a basis for deciding the type of treatment needed to bring a child toward the language behavior of normal members of his community. With these community language goals specified as the terminal behavior to be achieved, the next requirement would be the specification of intermediate steps a child must take en route to normal language. With the goal and intermediate steps delineated clearly, what remains would be implementation of each step with a therapeutic program of systematic behavior modification.

A method of assessment that would provide the clinician with the essential information to initiate help would involve a test that samples language behavior at these intermediate steps. The point in the test at which the child fails would be the point at which therapy would begin. Preliminary work along these lines is underway. Menyuk (1964) has analyzed deviant and normal speech development by means of a generative model of grammar. She found that children with normal speech formulate sentences with increasingly differentiated rules of grammar, whereas those with infantile speech cling to general rules used crudely. Lee (1966, 1969a) has pursued this lead by devising *developmental*

sentence types that, though not a standardized scale, are a big step in the direction of testing intermediate steps of language acquisition.

The problem in accomplishing a therapeutically useful purpose with existing standardized tests is that they do not require responses that are adequate samples of normal language (normal speech usually requires more than one-word responses), they do not indicate the point in behavioral development at which training should begin, and they do not differentiate between persons who could profit from one type of treatment or another. Furthermore, they vary in the scope of language sampled, in the precision and reliability of measures used, and in the naturalness of the environment in which speech is tested. Unfortunately, a dilemma exists here that will be difficult to resolve. Precise reliable measures usually are gathered by trained observers in well-equipped laboratories. Generally, the shorter the response, the more accurate the measure—and the more atypical the speech that is sampled. Normal speech under normal conditions is available mainly to untrained observers (such as parents), who are poorly equipped to record their impressions.

Still, available standardized procedures do provide, in various ways, tests of receptive and expressive linguistic discriminations at semantic, grammatical, and phonemic levels. The ability to make these discriminations seems to be an integral part of the ability to use language. Too, since these discriminations seem to develop, the level of language maturation can be revealed by testing them, even though the behavioral processes by which different stages of language are mastered remain obscure.

The construction of tests that will reveal these processes, which make up the intermediate steps of language acquisition, will be a long, arduous task. We are not even certain yet of the different types of abilities required for language, let alone how much of each is necessary. How much of what type of information retrieval and memory storage capacity is essential to echo what is heard? To understand what is heard? To relate a subject idea to a predicate idea in a simple kernel sentence? To expand the phrase structure of either subject or predicate? To convert a kernel sentence into any of its transformations? What cognitive operations are required to detect relations in the environment (such as cause and effect, negation, absence, need for more information) that provide the basis for symbolizing experience? What ability to detect temporal order is necessary to detect phonemic sequence? What auditory abilities are needed to discriminate phonemes? Morphemes? Intonation patterns? Stress patterns? And what communicative functions are most likely to provide reinforcement of those skills that will lead, step by step, to the achievement of mature language? Answers to such questions will enhance the development of better procedures for assessing language acquisition.

Methods and criteria for assessing adult aphasia. Although the goal of achieving speech that is normal for the community is as applicable for the aphasic person as for the child with delayed language, the problems are different, as are the procedures for assessing them. Whereas the child has not yet figured out how language works, the person with aphasia knew, but his ability to utilize whatever linguistic knowledge he retains has been impaired by brain injury. Because aphasia is as much a neurologic as a psycholinguistic concern, tests of it reflect these orientations.

Until recently, two tests predominated in the examination of aphasia, the *Minnesota Test for Differential Diagnosis of Aphasia* (MTDDA), developed by Schuell (1965b), and the *Language Modalities Test for Aphasia* (LMTA), designed by Wepman and Jones (1961, 1966). Both have been shown in quantitative studies to be stable and reliable, and both provide a balanced set of tasks across a wide range of linguistic abilities. Rapidly gaining in popularity, however, are the *Porch Index of Communicative Ability*, or *PICA* (Porch, 1971) and the *Boston Diagnostic Aphasia Examination* (Goodglass and Kaplan, 1972), both standardized on large samples of aphasics with typical types and severities of problems.

The Minnesota Test has been subjected to extensive investigation and modification in the course of its development. Requiring about 3 hours to administer (a major weakness), the test includes items of varying complexity and difficulty that measure five areas of disturbance: audition, vision and reading, speech and language, visuomotor skills and writing, and numerical relations and arithmetic processes. One of its chief merits is its prognostic capacity. By following the performance of large numbers of patients, Schuell (1965a) has found that the overall pattern of aphasia impairment is a better predictor of recovery than is age, educational or occupational level, extent of neurologic involvement, or initial severity of aphasia. Accordingly, she has described five major and two minor categories of aphasia, each with its pattern of discriminating tests, clinical signs, and prognosis.

As with the Minnesota Test, the Language Modalities Test is intended to provide the clinician with a point of departure for therapy. Beyond this, the two tests differ considerably. Whereas Schuell has approached aphasia as a neurologic impairment that results in unitary loss of language ability in all verbal dimensions, Wepman has approached it as a psycholinguistic problem consequent to brain injury that involves different aspects of language. Too, Wepman's conception of aphasia, as well as the method of developing his test for it, has more clearly differentiated it from input and output transmission problems of agnosia and apraxia.

The assessment of behavioral effects of brain damage is a major concern of psychologists. Do they use such tools as the Wechsler Adult Intelligence Scale (WAIS) or the Bender Visual-Motor Gestalt Test for the same purpose as speech pathologists use language tests? Would neuropsychologic testing techniques and concepts such as Burgemeister (1962) and Smith and Phillippus (1969) describe be helpful to speech pathologists?

The PICA has attracted considerable clinical interest since its development. It utilizes responses to ten common objects in 180 test items to assess and quantify verbal, gestural, and graphic abilities. Extent of recovery can be predicted based on the patient's status one month after onset of aphasia. It also provides an explicit method for determining the point at which therapy should begin and for recording therapeutic progress. It can be administered in approximately an hour, although clinical skill is required to score items quickly and appropriately for response accuracy, completeness, responsiveness, promptness, and efficiency.

The Boston Diagnostic Aphasia Examination is designed to detect type of aphasia and location of lesion. This goal is accomplished by evaluating articulation, fluency, word-finding ability, syntax, speech retention span, serial speech, paraphasias, auditory comprehension, reading, and writing. The major value of the test is for diagnosis rather than for prognosis or guidance of treatment.

Shorter tests, less taxing of aphasic persons, are available to provide a gross overview of primary areas of difficulty. The *Short Examination for Aphasia* is Schuell's (1957) screening version of her Minnesota Test; it consists of subtests with the greatest prognostic value. The initial items of the Language Modalities Test are used for screening to determine the severity of impairment and the feasibility of further testing. Other tests are available, such as Eisenson's *Examining for Aphasia* (1954, 1973), Sarno's *Functional Communication Profile* (1969), and Sklar's *Aphasia Evaluation Summary* (1963). Eisenson's test includes items for appraising evaluative and receptive disturbances and productive and expressive disturbances. Although the test has been criticized for not being standardized and therefore not permitting a meaningful quantitative score, Tikofsky (1966) sees it as a most useful instrument in the hands of a skilled clinician. The Functional Communication Profile is not a traditional test but rather a method of measuring forty-five everyday communication behaviors. It yields a profile that can be compared with "typical" profiles of patients with right or left hemiplegia. Sklar's Aphasia Summary, constructed to yield a score for severely involved patients, includes speech and reading comprehension items and oral and graphic formulation tasks.

Assessment of speaking behavior

The speech pathologist should be skilled in examining the three behavioral processes of speaking: articulation-resonance, phonation, and speech-flow. Again the recurring theme: these are behavioral processes. Interesting as the speech pathologist may find anatomic or physiologic information about respiratory, laryngeal, and orofacial structures and functions, he does not examine them directly—if for no other reason because of the medical liability risks he would run. In some speech research laboratories, no instrument regardless of how innocuous is placed in a subject's mouth without the presence of a licensed physician. As you can see, application of this restriction to the clinical setting would preclude exact instrumental measurement of any aspect of speech production other than acoustical output. As we develop more precise methods of measuring speaking processes, this restriction will probably bind more tightly, possibly forcing speech pathologists to become licensed for self-protection when they utilize all the tools for measuring speech physiology available to them. In the meantime, examination and assessment of speaking behavior is our concern.

Articulatory-resonatory processes. Perhaps no activity has dominated the clinician's attention historically more than the assessment of articulation disorders. Three out of four speech disorders found in schoolchildren are of this type. Courses in phonetics have been justified in years past as providing the necessary skills for learning to test articulation. Yet only recently have we recognized clinically that articulatory disorders involve more than auditory and motor inability to hear or produce isolated speech sounds correctly, that connected speech involves the most complex sensorimotor coordinations, that these coordinations are the phonologic aspect of linguistic decision-making processes, and that resonance is not a separate process but an integral part of articulation (Chapter 3).

Articulatory-resonatory behavior to be examined. Articulatory skills seem so easy to examine that their linguistic and sensorimotor complexity is often not apparent. We tend to think of speech as a string of separate sounds joined together to make words. This idea is strengthened when speech is transcribed phonetically on the principle that each sound is represented by a separate symbol. From the standpoint of speech perception, this idea is valid. Phonemes have linguistic reality; they are what the listener perceives and discriminates to detect different words in a message. But phonemes are abstract classes of sounds. They are linguistic categories into which the listener sorts the specific acoustical events articulated by the speaker. Articulatory-resonatory behavior involves the skills by which these acoustical events are produced, but it would be uneconomical if not impossible to record in writing the uniqueness of each specific sound. We compromise by recording with phonetic symbols the linguistic classes into which the sounds fall.

Years ago, Stetson (1951) pointed out a fundamental problem for an analysis of articulation: we identify the individual consonant or vowel as the unit of articulation, and yet the basic unit of speech production is the syllable. The contrast between vowels and consonants has never been adequately defined, except when described in terms of the function of a sound as *syllabic* or *nonsyllabic*. The consonant, with which articulation tests are mainly concerned, occasionally functions as the core of a syllable. As such, it is a semivowel produced by the syllabic pulse of breath pressure that is the basic movement of speech production. More typically, the consonant functions nonsyllabically as the sound produced by rapid auxiliary vocal tract movements accompanying respiratory movements that release or arrest the syllabic breath pulse. Thus four types of syllables can be produced in isolation:

1. -V- (a syllabic vowel released and arrested by chest muscles alone: "a")
2. CV- (a syllable released by a nonsyllabic consonant and arrested by chest muscles: "the")
3. -VC (a syllable released by chest muscles and arrested by a consonant: "up")
4. CVC (a syllable released and arrested by consonants: "cup")

Because speech is a series of respiratory–vocal tract movements made audible, we can only agree with McDonald (1964) that a test of articulatory behavior must, in the final analysis, be a test of the adequacy of speech movements. Although in very slow speech or in singing, the movements may be *fixed* (a sustained, steady state of sound) or *controlled* (a voluntarily controlled transition, as in a diphthong), the typical type of speech movement is *ballistic*. The reason is that the normal rate at which speech flows, about fourteen phonemes per second, is too fast to permit volitional direction of movement. Too, ballistic articulatory movements must overlap to produce sounds at such rates. Acceptable articulation is achieved when one learns to direct these movements successfully to the articulatory postures required to produce the phonemes of normal speech.

Thus two skills are involved in articulatory-resonatory behavior to be examined: the ability to direct specific ballistic movements at phonemic targets, and the ability to differentiate all the phonemic targets normally used in the community. Defective articulation will be the result of a breakdown in either skill: dysarthria in an adult who once had normal speech being an example of the former, and a normal child who lisps exemplifying the latter (Chapter 12).

Methods of assessing articulatory skills. Methods of testing articulation will vary with the purpose. A linguist or experimental phonetician attempting to investigate the sound production of infants, for example, would probably need a system for testing and recording results that, in detail and concept, would be different from the tests for older children needed by a speech clinician. We will limit our concern to clinical tests, of which we now have four types. *Screening tests* and *diagnostic tests* are mainly concerned with detecting the ability to differentiate phonemic targets: *deep tests* emphasize the ability to produce necessary articulatory movements; and *phonologic tests* provide an analysis of articulatory errors as evidence of failure to complete mastery of phonologic rules.

Traditional methods of examining articulation have included screening and diagnostic tests. Screening examinations are utilized when a quick decision must be made about the general adequacy of articulation. Such tests are used extensively in public schools at the beginning of the year to locate children who have defective speech. Since screening tests are necessarily gross in the abilities they test, their major value is in separating those who may need help from those who probably do not. Frequently, these tests are constructed by the individual clinician for his own specific needs, although they are available in standardized form, such as the fifty-item version of the 176-item *Templin-Darley Tests of Articulation* (1970). Also available is the *Predictive Screening Test of Articulation* (Van Riper and Erickson, 1969) that is the most appropriate test for predicting which first-graders will outgrow their misarticulations and which will not.

Diagnostic examinations (the longer version of the standardized Templin-Darley Tests being one) are used to make clinical decisions about the need for therapy, about which sounds should be treated therapeutically and in which order, and about the assessment of therapeutic progress. A similar instrument, also popular, is the *Goldman-Fristoe Test of Articulation* (1969). As with screening tests, clinicians often design their own diagnostic examinations. Johnson, Darley, and Spreistersbach (1963) provide detailed instructions for preparing and administering them. Traditionally, these tests in-

---

How does Milisen (1954), a leading authority on articulation disorders, go about an examination? Why does he stimulate the sound in isolation and in nonsense syllables as well as in key words?

---

volve certain common features for eliciting and recording articulatory behavior:

1. Consonants, and often vowels and diphthongs, are tested in the positions in which they occur in words: *initially* (first sound in a word), *medially* (middle sound), and *finally* (last sound). Since vowels, diphthongs, and the consonants that normally develop early are rarely defective, tests are usually slanted toward items that will elicit the more frequently troublesome consonants, such as /s/, /r/, and /l/ and their various blends.

2. Sounds are tested in single words and often in nonsense syllables, in isolation as separate sounds, in sentences, and sometimes in reading and conversation.

3. Either the presentation of stimulus words is done with pictures that will elicit the test word, or the key word is spoken by the examiner. Elicitation by pictures is sometimes called the *spontaneous method,* and by oral presentation the *imitative method.* Some evidence indicates that both methods produce about the same results (Templin, 1947). Since other studies show that children improve their performance with the imitative method, most examiners prefer the spontaneous method (Snow and Milisen, 1954b).

4. A system is used to record the type of error for each sound tested and the stimulus condition for eliciting it. Usually a means of indicating the variability of the error is also provided, especially when an opportunity is given to improve the response by imitating the examiner's example.

5. Procedures for testing the ability to discriminate key sounds as a listener are sometimes included. Such examinations involve pairing words that depend for correct identification on the discrimination of test sounds.

Traditional tests have been criticized by McDonald (1964) as being inadequate in several respects. Sounds are tested mainly in single words, but single words rarely occur in speech as separate entities. Since consonants are produced by auxiliary movements that function to release or arrest syllables, testing them initially, medially, and finally in words serves no functional purpose. Also, the sampling of phonetic contexts for the different overlapping ballistic movements of articulation is random rather than systematic. To rectify these weaknesses, McDonald has devised a *deep test* of articulation, the strength of which, by virtue of attempting to test each sound in all possible syllabic combinations, proves to be its limitation: it is too long for the practical purposes of some clinicians with some types of patients.

As Winitz (1975) recommends, articulatory testing should be a continuous process of hypothesis testing. The initial hypothesis should be formulated after examining conversational speech. Thereafter it can be tested with such formal instruments as we have just discussed. An ongoing process of hypothesis testing will permit a differential assessment of the skills that are disabled. Is the difficulty one of differentiating phonemic targets or one of being unable to direct ballistic movements to the targets? If all necessary movements can be produced in some phonetic contexts but are not used in others, differentiation of the sounds would be suspected. If some necessary movements are not achieved in any phonetic context, neuromuscular control would be suspected. Clues to specific disabilities can be detected in the same way. A pattern of hypernasality, nasal air emission, compensatory glottal stops, or abnormal tongue postures against the pharyngeal wall is indicative of velopharyngeal incompetence to impound intraoral breath pressure for normal articulation. Furthermore, from these assessments of articulatory patterns, valuable information can be contributed to the differential diagnosis of pathology underlying the disability, possibly to the extent of diagnosing psychologic disturbance (Rousey, 1974).

With growing awareness that the majority of articulatory disorders are problems of phonologic development has come a linguistically sophisticated instrument, *The Fisher-Logemann Test of Articulation Competence* (1971). It requires as much clinical skill to administer as a deep test, and considerably more knowledge of phonology and distinctive feature theory to interpret. When the test is used skillfully, however, the results can be therapeutically rewarding. With discovery of underlying phonologic rules that govern the child's selection of distinctive features, the pattern of his articulatory errors can be revealed. From this pattern, his erroneous rule system becomes apparent. By correcting a few phonologic rules, multiple misarticulations can often be corrected.

Phonatory processes. The clinician is mainly on his own when he assesses vocal production. No standardized tests are available to guide him. Perhaps this paucity of formal examinations for voice reflects the difficulty of establishing norms for evaluating the adequacy of vocal production. When is pitch too high or too low? When is the voice too loud; too soft? What is good quality; bad quality? No linguistic rules provide firm standards. Society, too, is lenient and variable in its tastes in these matters; they vary not only from culture to culture but from one socioeconomic level to another (Miller, 1957). Does it make any difference, then, how voice is produced? The answer proposed is "Yes. But the primary standard against which vocal production should be assessed is vocal hygiene."

Phonatory behavior to be examined. No one quarrels with pitch and loudness as two of the behavioral dimensions of voice to be examined. Each is a single parameter that can be measured along a continuum. Clinically, a pitch pipe or piano serves admirably for pitch; for loudness, the clinician's ear is generally used. For more exact measurements, such as are required for research, various instruments are available. The information about pitch that should be measured

---

Do Hanley and Peters (1971) describe the instruments that can measure all forms of vocal behavior?

---

includes highest and lowest notes possible, pitch level used habitually, and pitch levels at which the voice functions smoothest and with least effort. Important aspects of loudness to be examined are its appropriateness to needs of various speaking situations and the level of loudness that can be maintained comfortably.

The measurement of quality is altogether different. It has been described perceptually with dozens of terms—"hoarse," "harsh," "strident," and "breathy" being favorites—and acoustical correlates of these ambiguous perceptions have been measured. The problem is that, being multidimensional, the production of quality has defied quantification in a fashion comparable to pitch and loudness. The solution proposed is to describe the four independent dimensions (voicing, vocal constriction, vocal focus, and vocal mode) and two dependent dimensions (vocal effort and vocal smoothness) of quality production that can be identified as separate elements. The quality of each vocal sound is conceived as being a product of some combination of all these elements, plus pitch and loudness. Each of these dimensions is therefore assessed as an integral component of any vocal sound, normal or abnormal (Chapters 3 and 13).

Methods for assessing vocal production. Traditionally, the methods for assessing elements of vocal production are available mainly for pitch. Based on the idea of *optimal pitch*—a notion that seems to have clinical validity but persistently escapes scientific verification (Thurman, 1958)—Fairbanks' (1960) method of assessing it is to compare *habitual* with *natural pitch*. Habitual pitch is the one around which voice is typically produced; natural pitch is the one at which the voice functions most efficiently, presumably near the lower fourth of the total range.

Utilizing the basic idea of this approach, Fig. 15-1 provides a method for assessing all vocal elements. For each dimension on the left, habitual performance can be marked, for example, with "H." Similarly, optimal performance as determined by criteria specified in Chapter 13 can be marked, for example, with "O." Each vocal element would thus be provided with a description of what is being done, in contrast with what should be done. Not only does this method point up deviant vocal dimensions, but it also indicates the direction and extent of deviation for each element. The goal of therapy would be to bring all "H's" into as close congruence with

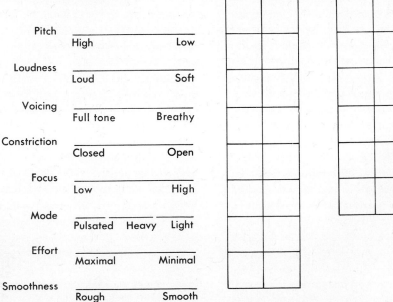

Fig. 15-1. Vocal performance assessment chart.

"O's" as would be deemed necessary for the individual.

Whereas the scales to the left of Fig. 15-1 are for describing vocal performance, the boxes to the right are for indicating judgments of adequacy. The need for optimal production in conversation varies, depending on such factors as the conditions under which voice is required, personal preference, and so forth. An athletic coach may be more distressed by lack of power than by the esthetics of a hoarse voice, a society matron's concern may be just the reverse, and a recluse may not speak often enough for vocal performance to be of much consequence regardless of inadequacy. Such considerations enter into judgments of conversational adequacy of each dimension. As for the adequacy of voluntary control, this determination is important to therapy. It concerns the ability to regulate each independent vocal dimension separately, as in an exercise, for instance. The assumption is that ability to control the elements of voice will facilitate vocal modification.

The two dependent vocal dimensions, effort and smoothness, are much like vocal barometers. When the independent dimensions are produced optimally, the amount of effort required for loudness is minimal, and the voice sounds smooth rather than rough. Observation of the combination of independent dimensions that results in the smoothest, most effortless voice is important for therapy. Usually a soft, breathy tone at a moderately low pitch, such as one might use when speaking confidentially, is easiest to achieve hygienically in heavy voice. Additionally, observation of smoothness is important for diagnosis. As Darley (1964) points out, tremors of pitch and loudness can be indicative of neurologic disabilities associated with cerebral palsy, cerebellar disease, and advanced Wilson's disease.

Medical diagnosis is particularly relevant to the assessment of disorders of voice for two main reasons. First, hoarseness is often the earliest evidence of laryngeal pathology. When a lesion is malignant, early detection is paramount. Second, the speech patholo-

gist is in no position to determine the basis of any hoarseness he may detect. It can result from inefficient use of normal vocal cords. It can also result from any form of laryngeal disability that involves asymmetric vibration of the cords. Until a speech pathologist has medical clearance for voice therapy, he risks initiating treatment that can harm rather than help. Furthermore, medical information is needed on the metabolic status of a patient as well as on the condition of the vocal tract. Velopharyngeal dysfunction or obstructions in nasal or pharyngeal cavities can not only alter resonance, but as West and Ansberry (1968) indicate, resonator shapes that reflect pressure waves that impede release of glottal pulses will also result in inefficient phonation.

Finally, a case history is a necessity in the assessment of voice disorders, which can result from and be maintained by a variety of conditions: chronic abuse such as public speaking, singing, or talking over the noise of traffic or cocktail parties; chronic infection or inflammation as with a persistent postnasal drip; allergy; smoking; yelling; injury and so on and on. Therapeutic progress can be easily undone if the maintaining conditions are not altered. Moore (1971), Boone (1971), Murphy (1964), and Johnson, Darley, and Spriestersbach (1963) have specific suggestions about background information needed to assess vocal functioning with a view to modifying it.

Speech-flow processes. The five elements of speech-flow (sequence, duration, rhythm, rate, and fluency) differ in ease of measurement and in criteria by which their adequacy can be assessed. No general statement will suffice. No standard tests are available that will reveal defectiveness of these elements. Yet each element can be delineated behaviorally, and criteria for the assessment of each can be described (Chapter 14).

Assessment of speech-flow behavior. The first three elements can be assessed linguistically. *Sequence* is the temporal arrangement of phonemes in proper order for pronunciation. *Duration* is the time spent articulating a phonetic segment. It contributes to articulation, rate, and prosody. *Rhythm* is the pattern of timing of phonetic events. As such, it includes durations of syllables and pauses as they contribute to English as a stress-timed language. Since these three elements can be affected by the length and type of speaking situation, they should be observed for adequacy in terms of pronunciation, phonetic intelligibility, and stress in words, sentences, contextual reading, and conversation. When word, phrase, and sentence stress are inadequate, speech is generally monotonous. Prosodic disturbances, as Darley (1964) points out, are diagnostic clues for deafness and for neurologic disorders such as Parkinson's disease, ataxia, and pseudobulbar palsy.

Rate and fluency have no linguistic effects normally. *Rate* is the speed of utterance. It can be measured directly, and has been measured for words per minute particularly. For special purposes, such as determining the maximum rate at which sounds can be articulated, a test of syllable rate would be more useful (MacKay, 1968). Rate is not apt to be considered defective unless it interferes with intelligibility or contributes to disfluency. Although norms are available for different groups speaking under different conditions (Fairbanks, 1960; Johnson, Darley, and Spriestersbach, 1963), one's rate can vary widely from average without being a disorder. Rates that are too fast or too slow are often found in central nervous system diseases, whereas erratic bursts of excessive rate are a predominant characteristic of cluttering and are also characteristic of anxiety reactions and the manic phase of manic-depressive psychosis.

Fluency is the smoothness of speech sound initiation and articulatory transition from one phonetic position to another. It has been measured indirectly by quantifying the frequency of occurrence of various types of disfluency (repetitions, prolongations, hesitations, and interjections) as they occur at sound, syllable, word, phrase, and sentence levels. Johnson's (1961) system of classification is used frequently. Several indexes of disfluency have been devised to display these

results and to provide a method of comparing individual performance against norms (Johnson, Darley, and Spriestersbach, 1963; Sander, 1961; Young, 1969). Still, these systems leave unquantified such factors as the duration and intensity of disfluencies and the general level of strain and struggle to speak. These factors may weigh heavily in judgments of severity of disfluency. Riley (1972) has devised a scale reported to be a valid and reliable measure of factors that bear on judgments of severity of stuttering in children and adults. In addition to scoring severity of disfluencies, it also permits scoring of struggle behavior associated with stuttering.

Fluency is usually not judged defective unless speech sound initiations are abnormal; this type of disfluency is identified as stuttering. As with rate, norms do not provide an unambiguous basis for evaluating fluency. Listeners may tolerate endless word and phrase repetitions as normal, and yet judge a single instance of excessive phonetic prolongation as stuttering. Assessment of disfluency should consider type, size of speech unit, frequency, duration, general level of struggle to speak, and the speaker's reputation for fluency (or stuttering).

Assessment of speech-related abilities

The speech pathologist does not examine speech mechanisms to evaluate disease conditions. Within the limits of his competence, he does examine respiratory, phonatory, and orofacial structures for speech adequacy; motor, sensory, perceptual, intellectual, and learning abilities; personality and emotional characteristics; and environmental conditions. He may enlist the assistance of specialists to examine these abilities, but it is his responsibility to assess their relation to speech. The fact of obvious disabilities such as accompany cerebral palsy, aphasia, or cleft palate permits no certain conclusions about speech defects.

Assessment of speech mechanisms
Breath stream management. Respiratory and phonatory processes interact to produce the breath stream of speech. Required are the abilities to inhale and maintain an ade-

quate air supply (for vital capacity), to compress air appropriately with respiratory muscles and resist air flow with laryngeal adjustments (for subglottal pressure), to regulate the type and rate of airflow (for voiced or voiceless breath stream), to regulate the mode of laryngeal vibration (for pitch), and to regulate the opening-closing rate and symmetry of movement of the cords within a vibratory cycle (for loudness and quality). All these abilities can be observed and measured with instruments, and some can be observed by eye, ear, or hand. The ultimate test clinically, however, is the ability to coordinate these respiratory-phonatory processes for acceptable breath stream production (Chapter 7).

When any dimension of vocal production is inadequate, disabled management of the breath stream can be a basic problem. But different disabilities can yield similar results. For example, quavering voice can reflect tremors in respiratory muscles, laryngeal muscles, or both. Gasping for breath after short utterances may be a sign of inadequate vital capacity or of inefficient management

---

Which speech disorders does Darley (1964) associate with respiratory deviations? What respiratory problems for speech has Hardy (1961) found among cerebral-palsied persons?

---

of an adequate air supply. The clinician should know specifically the disability that limits adequate speech if corrective efforts are to be profitable.

Because speech utilizes mechanisms that serve more basic biologic functions, such as breathing and eating, these primitive movements are sometimes used as tests of the adequacy of speech movements. The value of this procedure is becoming increasingly dubious. These tests may effectively determine whether muscles are at all capable of contracting, but they in no way test muscular coordinations in the incredibly swift movements of speech. As Noll (1968) observed, commenting on the clinical implications of Hardy's (1968) research on respiration in dysarthric patients, the value of focusing on

breathing exercises, respiratory synchrony, prolongation of expiration, and breath control is probably slight. Instead of the reflexive level, therapy should begin with voluntary learned movements of speech; physiologic breathing and speech breathing may not be comparable. The same could be said for all other processes of speaking. Instead of attempting to improve respiration as a means of facilitating articulation, research points to improvement of articulation as a means of facilitating respiratory efficiency.

Mason (1975) has prepared a description of principles and guidelines for the systematic and efficient examination of the structure and function of the face and intraoral mechanisms. By knowing what to look for and why, the clinician can follow a logical progression of observations that reveal interactions of form and function in the facial area, oral cavity, and pharynx. From these observations, accurate identification of orofacial pathology and malfunction can be accomplished quickly with minimum equipment.

Similarly, most respiratory-phonatory functions for speech can be assessed by the clinician without instruments. How long can a person hold his breath after deep inhalation? How slowly and smoothly can he blow it out on exhalation? Are abdominal or thoracic tremors felt during phonation? Is vocalization initiated at the beginning of, prior to, or near the end of exhalation? Answers to such questions will reveal much about vital capacity and respiratory control. The testing of laryngeal control necessitates other questions. Can the person breathe without stridor? Can he whisper? Can he sigh to terminate a yawn? Can he laugh with a clear voice? Does tone become breathier, louder, or more constricted as vocal effort is increased? Can he shout? Can he speak confidentially? Can he hum? Can he sing? In heavy voice? In light voice? The answers can be analyzed for the ability to abduct and adduct the vocal folds, to achieve cord closure for full voicing and loudness, to vary glottal pulse rate for pitch, to phonate in optimal vocal mode, and to achieve clear tone.

With instrumentation, clinical impressions

of respiratory-phonatory functions can be quantified. Respiratory movements of the thorax and abdomen can be measured with a *pneumograph*, visualized with a *fluoroscope*, or photographed with *cinefluorography*. Electrical activity in respiratory muscles can be recorded with *electromyography*. Vital capacity can be quantified with a *spirometer*, air volume used during speech with a *body plethysmograph*, airflow rate with a *pneumotachograph*, and subglottal pressure with a *tracheal needle* attached to a *pressure transducer* or with a *miniaturized pressure transducer* placed directly in the trachea. As for the larynx, electrical activity in any of the muscles can be measured by *electromyography*, cord length by *photography* and *lateral x-ray*, cord thickness by *laminagraphic x-ray*, and vibratory movements of the cords by *high-speed cinematography* or, somewhat

---

A state-of-the-art review of many of these measures along with acoustic measures, especially as they are used for detection and diagnosis of laryngeal dysfunction, has been provided recently (Perkins, 1975).

---

less adequately and less expensively, by *stroboscopy* or *glottography*. Those procedures that require x-ray examination, anesthesia, or needle insertion must, of course, be administered by a licensed physician.

Breath stream modulation. Articulatory-resonatory processes by which the breath stream is modulated for intelligible speech can be impaired by orofacial disabilities (Chapter 8). The tongue can be immobile, too small, or too large; dentition can be inadequate; lips can be immobile; the palatal vault can be too high, too low, or cleft; tonsils can protrude into the oropharynx; the nose can be occluded; and velopharyngeal sphincter control can be incompetent by virtue of velar cleft, paralysis, or insufficient tissue. Although remarkable compensatory adjustments are possible, the ability to adjust vocal tract constrictions, occlusions, and cavity sizes and shapes rapidly remains as the minimum articulatory requirement.

The clinician can observe most of these structures and movements by visual inspec-

tion; Darley (1964) and Emerick and Hatten (1974) describe what to look for, how to find it, and why. Johnson, Darley, and Spriestersbach (1963) provide what norms are available for evaluating the adequacy of the rate at which oral structures can be moved. Failure to achieve these norms suggests that the person would have to speak at a slower-than-average rate to articulate intelligibly. Assessment of velopharyngeal competence, however, requires radiography to visualize palatopharyngeal action directly. Oral and nasal air pressure and airflow measures during speech, nasal sound pressure measures, and manometric measures of oral breath pressure are valuable procedures for determining the adequacy of velopharyngeal closure (Netsell, 1969; Shelton, Diedrich, and Youngstrom, 1961; Shelton and others, 1969). An obturator is sometimes fit on a diagnostic basis and systematically reduced in size until articulation is affected (Shelton and others, 1968). No single clinical measure of palatopharyngeal closure is entirely satisfactory. The clinician must observe articulation, administer whatever closure tests are possible,

---

Bzoch (1972), Wells (1971), and Shelton, Hahn, and Morris (1968) provide thorough discussions of the diagnostic considerations of speech effects of orofacial disabilities.

---

consider the patient's history, and then make the best decision possible.

Assessment of general cognitive and motor abilities

Sensory and perceptual abilities. Auditory and somesthetic abilities are especially vital to speech. They are the modalities by which speech production is monitored. Other sensory avenues, of course, contribute information about the environment important to speech development, but even in this regard hearing is supreme (Chapters 5 and 6).

Crucial auditory abilities to be assessed include acuity, discrimination, and memory for speech sounds. Most tests of acuity require audiometric equipment. *Identification* or *screening audiometry* provides a relatively quick gross test of auditory acuity for pure tones; usually four or five are tested between 500 and 6,000 Hz. Screening standards range from a 10 to 20 dB loss at any frequency. Those who fail are generally referred for *diagnostic audiometry*, in which, beyond testing pure tones by air and bone conduction at many frequencies from 125 to 8,000 Hz, *speech reception threshold* and *discrimination score* or *articulation index* are examined. The acuity level at which half of a group of test words can be repeated correctly determines the speech reception threshold; the percentage of relatively loud phonetically balanced words repeated correctly deter-

---

Audiometric procedures and bases for evaluating various hearing test results are described by audiologists and otologists such as Davis and Silverman (1970), Newby (1964), Jerger (1963), and O'Neill (1964).

---

mines the discrimination score. Audiologists have a battery of sophisticated audiometric tests available to help speech pathologists determine the adequacy of hearing for speech. Furthermore, by differentiating lesions in the middle or outer ear from those in the inner ear, or ones in the cochlea from ones in the auditory neural pathway, the audiologist can distinguish peripheral disabilities from perceptual auditory agnosia. Whether a hearing disability that affects speech is peripheral or central will probably make considerable difference in the corrective treatment required.

Perceptual tests of discrimination for speech are also available that do not require audiometric equipment. All tests of discrimination pair similar and different sounds. Wood (1971) has shown, though, that auditory discrimination is a complex response that is far from being adequately tested by a decision of "similar" or "different." Some standard tests require only that a child point to a picture of the paired word spoken by the examiner (Templin, 1957; Pronovost and Dumbleton, 1953). Others require an indication of whether selected sounds in paired words or nonsense syllables are the same or different (Templin, 1943; Wepman, 1958), a concept that the child may or may not have.

A more recent standardized instrument, the *Goldman-Fristoe-Woodcock Test of Auditory Discrimination* (1970), also available commercially, is an attempt to minimize weaker features of such tests. Instructions are also available for tailoring discrimination tests to individual needs (Johnson, Darley, and Spriestersbach, 1963).

Auditory memory, an ability apparently more crucial for language than articulation, should receive special attention when brain injury or mental retardation is involved. Schuell's (1965b) aphasia test contains phrase-repetition tasks, and Kirk, McCarthy, and Kirk's (1968) ITPA and the Wechsler Adult Intelligence Scale (1955) provide tests of digit span. A subtest of Carroll and Sapon's

---

What auditory memory and discrimination abilities are tested with materials in appendixes of texts by Van Riper (1963) and Berry and Eisenson (1956)?

(1959) Modern Language Aptitude Test that is predictive of language learning ability is the Phonetic Script Test. A test of the ability to hold sound sequences in memory during shifts of attention, it requires repetition of nonsense syllables after performing a different task.

Clinical testing of somesthetic abilities for speech is a relatively recent development. Rutherford and McCall (1967) have identified several tactile and kinesthetic skills deemed necessary for speech and, along with others, have devised tests of tactile acuity, localization, and pattern recognition; of kinesthetic pattern recognition; and of two-point discrimination (Ringel and Ewanoski, 1965), mandibular kinesthesia (Ringel, Saxman, and Brooks, 1967), and texture discrimination (Ringel and Fletcher, 1967). Tests of oral stereognosis have been used frequently as measures of oral sensory function (McDonald and Aungst, 1967; Shelton, Arndt, and Hetherington, 1967). With them, differences in oral perception of form have been found among normal speakers and those with various types of speech handicaps (Baker, 1967; Moser, La Gourgue, and Class, 1967).

Intellectual, learning, and motor abilities.

Tests of learning and intelligence range from motor development scales to vocabulary tests. As far as speech is concerned, a mental age of 5 years is sufficient for mastery (Chapters 9 and 11). Nonverbal tests that will reach into infancy are therefore of special relevance. The Gesell developmental schedules (1947) and the Vineland Social Maturity Scale (Doll, 1946) provide norms for development of early motor, self-help, and socialization skills. As Darley (1964) indicates, however, schedules of physical maturation do not reliably predict later intellectual achievement. Too, the Vineland Scale is a report often filled out by parents that may reflect the bias of their hopes more than the reality of their child's condition. Criticism of these measures should be heeded when prediction of intellectual functioning is the issue.

On the other hand, when prediction of speech development is the concern, Lenneberg (1969) argues that motor milestones, such as those in Table 15-1, are the best index of language capacity. He maintains that tests of vocabulary, grammatical complexity, and other aspects of verbal performance reflect limiting conditions of disabilities and obscure the child's potential for language. His position is based on strong evidence of a biologic foundation for language acquisition that is reflected in close correlation between stages of motor and language development. The value of motor development scales such as the Oseretsky Tests of Motor Proficiency (1946) and the Heath Rail-Walking Test (1942) is limited for assessing speech acquisition mainly by applicable ages for the tests: the lowest age they reach is 4 years, an age at which language is normally well established.

Because motor and speech development are related to lateralization of cerebral function, tests of dominance are of interest, too.

Berry and Eisenson (1956) present several tests of dominance in the appendix of their book.

Evidence indicates that the establishment of dominance is a brain maturation function that begins about 2 years of age. It can be shifted early without permanent speech effects by lesions in what would normally become the dominant hemisphere (Lenneberg, 1967). Whether it can be shifted by changing handedness or any other form of training, especially after lateralization is completed at puberty, is another matter. Theoretically, success would require that stimuli be directed exclusively to the hemisphere to be trained, a virtually impossible situation to achieve.

Because intelligence is what intelligence tests measure, and what they measure main-

Table 15-1. Correlation of motor and language development*

Age (years)	Motor milestones	Language milestones
0.5	Sits using hands for support; unilateral reaching	Cooing sounds change to babbling by introduction of consonantal sounds
1	Stands; walks when held by one hand	Syllabic reduplication; signs of understanding some words; applies some sounds regularly to signify persons or objects, that is, the first words
1.5	Prehension and release fully developed; gait propulsive; creeps downstairs backward	Repertoire of 3 to 50 words not joined in phrases; trains of sounds and intonation patterns resembling discourse; good progress in understanding
2	Runs (with falls); walks stairs with one foot forward only	More than 50 words; two-word phrases most common; more interest in verbal communication; no more babbling
2.5	Jumps with both feet; stands on one foot for 1 second; builds tower of six cubes	Every day new words; utterances of three and more words; seems to understand almost everything said to him; still many grammatical deviations
3	Tiptoes 3 yards (2.7 meters); walks stairs with alternating feet; jumps 0.9 meter	Vocabulary of some 1000 words; about 80 percent intelligibility; grammar of utterances close approximation to colloquial adult; syntactic mistakes fewer in variety, systematic, predictable
4.5	Jumps over rope; hops on one foot; walks on line	Language well established; grammatical anomalies restricted either to unusual constructions or to the more literate aspects of discourse

*From Lenneberg, E., On explaining language. *Science*, **164**, 636 (1969). Copyright © 1969 by the American Association for the Advancement of Science.

ly is verbal ability, measured intelligence and language are necessarily linked closely. We have already looked at tests appropriate for multiply handicapped persons who understand language but do not use it: for example, the Full-Range Picture Vocabulary Test, by Ammons and Ammons (1948), and the Peabody Picture Vocabulary Test. Others include the Cattell Infant Intelligence Scale (1947), the Columbia Mental Maturity Scale, by Burgemeister, Blum, and Lorge (1953), the Arthur Adaptation of the Leiter International Performance Scale (1952), and Raven's Progressive Matrices (1947).

Understanding of language is required, too, for performance tasks of the most widely used and best standardized tests of intelligence, the Wechsler tests (WISC for children, WAIS for adults) and Terman and Merrill's Revised Stanford-Binet (1960). The IQ scores based on the full tests reflect language expression as well as understanding. A test that can be used to detect intellectual deterioration is the Shipley-Hartford Scale for Measuring Intellectual Impairment (1946). Based on evidence that abstract thinking is more severely affected by mental decline

---

What evidence does Harris (1963) offer that children's drawings can be used as measures of intellectual maturity? Are special considerations needed to test for mental retardation in brain-damaged children (Khanna, 1968)?

---

than is vocabulary, the differential in subtest scores for these two abilities serves as an index of deterioration.

Thus intelligence tests depend minimally on understanding of speech, but they probably do not provide the best determination of potential for language. Scales of early physical maturation seem better. In fact, if Guilford's (1967) structure-of-intellect theory is accepted, traditional tests of intelligence emphasize only about one fifth of the 120 abilities he has identified so far (Chapter 9). Such tests stress cognitive decoding operations and touch lightly the memory operations of learning and the information retrieval and evaluation operations required for decision making. Probably all these abilities are required for speech. When tests for them be-

come available, relations between intelligence and speech may be found that are not currently apparent.

Personality and emotional characteristics. Whereas we must assess speech mechanism, motor, and cognitive disabilities as they may interfere with intelligible utterance of message content, we must assess personality and emotional characteristics for needs underlying message intent. What needs press for expression? With what force? How are they managed? Answers are vital to understand how speech-handicapped persons cope with their defects, sometimes by compensation, sometimes by ignoring them, and sometimes by preserving them as covert expressions of intent. Too, assessment of emotional needs can reveal motivational clues around which therapy can be tailored to the individual.

This frame of reference puts emphasis on a psychodynamic assessment rather than on psychometric measurement of personality traits. Although an abundance of psychodynamic projective tests and psychometric inventories of personality characteristics are to be found, none was designed to reveal, nor has any revealed, consistent differences among speech-handicapped children or their parents (Goodstein, 1958a, 1960; Sheehan, 1958). Although alike in failure to produce discriminating results, they differ considerably in validity, reliability, objectivity, and standardization. The Minnesota Multiphasic Personality Inventory (MMPI), developed by Hathaway and McKinley (1951), comes closest to meeting psychometric standards, but its major merit is for differentiating among psychiatric groups; it, too, has been of little help with the speech handicapped (Goodstein, 1958b).

The classic projective instruments, Rorschach's Inkblot Test (1942) and Murray's Thematic Apperception Test (1943), fall short on validity. Not that they have been proved invalid, but because they can presumably reveal as much about the examiner as the examinee, they have yielded confused and contradictory results (Goodstein, 1958b). As confidence in the Rorschach and the TAT has waned, merits of the Kahn Test of Symbol Arrangement (1955) have grown. It requires little training to administer, it can be given and scored in less than half an hour, and the meanings a subject projects onto the symbols are not interpreted in terms of prior assumptions by the examiner. It seems to tap creativeness and loss of function consequent to stress (Ruch, 1967). Whether it would be as useful with speech as with psychiatric problems remains to be seen.

All in all, the assessment of psychodynamic conditions that may affect speech can tax a clinician's ability to the limit. As we have seen, formal tests provide little guidance. That such connections exist, however, is best shown by Rousey's work (1974). From his research and that of his colleagues at the Menninger Clinic has come the most persuasive evidence that certain problems of personality development can be determined by speech sound analysis (Chapter 10). If his conception proves valid, a standardized test of speech may become available for specifying personality disturbances.

Meanwhile, to proceed solely by clinical intuition offers little assurance of valid conclusions. An ingenious compromise devised by Haney (1969) that he calls Assessment by Developmental Signs is an informal system of psychodiagnosis designed specifically for speech clinicians. He traces personality and emotional development from infancy through the periods of muscle training, identification, latency, puberty, adolescence, and adulthood, to senescence. For each stage, he correlates signs of conflict, ego defense, and ego maturity with general developmental signs normally found. Then, from ages 3 to 11 years he utilizes work of Tobisman (1968) to trace speech and language development in relation to sensory, motor, perceptual, intellectual, personal, and social factors. Because formal testing in all these areas is generally impractical, Haney's system offers an invaluable method of screening a wide range of abilities for those which need probing in depth.

Assessment of environmental conditions. Speech is molded by the environment in which it develops. It produces social consequences that affect the form in which it is learned. It will reflect influences of culture, family, school, and job. Since interaction with parents is, of course, predominant during speech-learning years, parental attitude scales abound. Typical are the self-administered MMPI, and Schaefer and Bell's *Parental Attitude Research Instruments* (PARI). Interview and rating scales are also in good supply. Too, for the specific problem of stuttering, scales are available for rating listener attitudes toward stuttering and the stutterer's reactions to speech situations (Johnson, Darley, and Spriestersbach, 1963; Erickson, 1969). These instruments involve much the same problems as do those that measure personality. None has revealed consistent attitudes related to specific problems of speech; yet they can offer the clinician valuable guidance to attitudes, feelings, and reactions that should be explored.

Considering the limitless environmental conditions that could affect speech, the clinician's judgment of important areas to pursue by interview is likely to be his most productive guide. Is the child from a broken home; from a bilingual family? How does he relate to peers, at home, at school? With whom does he identify? Who teases him? How noisy is his speaking environment? Does the mother work? What is the socioeconomic status? Is the aphasic person's family willing to actively help in therapy? Are the stutterer's parents covertly rejecting? Is the child with cleft palate or cerebral palsy overprotected? These among endless other questions may hold crucial clues to a speech defect, or they may be irrelevant.

With so many possibilities available, the clinician must guard against post hoc reasoning: chance alone will probably produce some suspicious environmental conditions that could be blamed for speech difficulties even though unrelated in actuality. The nature of the problem, the physical disabilities involved, the meaning of the defect to the speaker as well as to the listener, and the overt and covert social pressures must all be weighed if environmental influences on the speech handicapped are to be assessed judiciously.

The answers—résumé

1. What is the purpose of examining language and speaking behavior?

Speech is examined for three purposes: description, diagnosis, and assessment. Description is fundamental. It is the fact-finding task of measuring test performance and gathering case history. Information gathered can be used for diagnosis and assessment. In diagnosis, the physician seeks etiology, the lesion or disease that disables skills required for speech. The speech pathologist can aid diagnosis with speech examination information that can help differentiate one disability from another. In assessment, the speech pathologist holds the primary responsibility for determining the nature and severity of the speech defect, prognosis, and appropriate therapy. In addition to information about language and speaking skills, descriptions of relevant sensory, perceptual, intellectual, motor, and learning abilities and of emotional, personality, and environmental conditions are needed for assessment.

2. What principles guide the assessment of disorders of speech?

The speech pathologist follows the principles of science in differential assessment: he observes and describes speech behavior and related disabilities as accurately as possible, formulates a tentative explanation of conditions that produced and maintain the disorder (from which he constructs a therapeutic plan), tests effectiveness of the plan, and modifies it and his assessment as new evidence may require. At all stages of assessment he will need criteria for determining the adequacy of performance observed. Too, he will be mindful that a speaker's message must be evaluated for the signal system of covert intent as well as the symbol system of overt intelligible utterance of content.

3. How can linguistic behavior be assessed?

Semantic, phonemic, morphemic, syntactic, and transformational skills of language and its functional uses can be assessed developmentally in part by formal tests of vocabulary, grammar, and usage. Methods of assessing development that provide clinical guidance for the initiation of therapy are incubating. Until they are hatched as standardized tests, informal examination of language in natural settings will be needed.

Tests of aphasia have evolved along neurologic and psycholinguistic lines. From extensive investigations of brain-injured patients, major tests provide reasonably accurate prognoses and guidance for therapy. Shorter screening tests, less taxing of aphasic patients, are available to provide a gross overview of primary areas of difficulty.

4. How can speaking behavior be assessed?

Articulatory-resonatory behavior can be assessed against standards of intelligibility and developmental norms for the ability to differentiate all the phonemic targets normally used in the community, and to direct ballistic movements of speech structures at these target positions. Screening, diagnostic, phonologic, and deep tests of articulation are available for this purpose.

Phonatory behavior can be assessed against the primary criterion of vocal hygiene for the ability to produce voice of socially acceptable pitch, loudness, and quality. Vocal production of quality is multidimensional; in addition to effects of pitch and loudness, it is controlled by independent dimensions of voicing, vocal focus, vocal constriction, and vocal mode that affect the dependent dimensions of vocal effort and smoothness. Since constriction is the key to vocal abuse, adjustment of any independent dimension of vocal production that interacts minimally with constriction is optimal.

Three elements of speech-flow behavior—sequence, duration, and rhythm—can be assessed linguistically: phonetic sequence by pronunciation, phonetic duration by articulatory and prosodic intelligibility, and rhythm by prosody. Rate must interfere with intelligibility or contribute to disfluency to be considered defective. Fluency is considered normal unless disfluencies involve abnormal speech sound initiations; then, a judgment of stuttering is probable.

5. How can abilities related to speech be assessed?

Speech mechanism abilities to develop subglottal pressure, manage its glottal release as a voiced breath stream of speech, and modulate it in the vocal tract for intelligible utterance can be assessed for most clinical purposes by eye, ear, or hand. For research, instrumentation is available for relatively exact measurements of physiologic, anatomic, and acoustical correlates of speaking behavior.

Sophisticated methods for assessing the status of the auditory system have been developed. For quick gross tests of hearing acuity, screening audiometry is available; for detailed measures of acuity and speech discrimination, and for differentiation of sensory from perceptual losses, diagnostic audiometry can be used. Formal testing of somesthetic abilities for speech is in its infancy but shows promise.

Of the many tests of intellectual, learning, and motor abilities, those that examine physical maturation are probably most predictive of language capacity, since speech and motor development appear to be biologically based activities that unfold together with physical maturation, especially of the brain. Standard tests of intelligence require, minimally, language comprehension even for performance scales. Too, they measure only a fraction of the intellectual abilities that have been identified and that are probably required for speech. Thus they test language achievement but not speech potential.

Whereas other speech-related abilities are assessed for their interference with intelligible utterance of message content symbols, personality and emotional characteristics are assessed for the needs underlying message intent that speech defects can signal. Although a psychodynamic analysis is more profitable for clinical modification of speech than for psychometric measurement of personality traits, the validity of classic projective tests is becoming increasingly suspect. Thus increased responsibility is placed on the clinician for knowledge of what to observe in the assessment of psychodynamics. Diagnostic tools are being developed to assist in this task.

Much the same problem exists for assessing environmental effects on speech: attitude, interview, and rating scales abound, but they have proved of more value in suggesting areas of inquiry for clinicians to pursue than in demonstrating environmental conditions that affect speech. The nature of the disorder, the physical disabilities involved, the meaning of the defect to speaker as well as listener, and overt and covert social pressures must all be weighed if environmental influences on speech-handicapped persons are to be assessed judiciously.

REFERENCES

Ammons, R., and Ammons, H., *The Full-Range Picture Vocabulary Test*. Missoula, Mont.: Psychological Test Specialists (1948).

Arthur, G., *The Arthur Adaptation of the Leiter International Performance Scale*. Washington, D.C.: Psychological Service Center Press (1952).

Baker, D., The amount of information in the oral identification of forms by normal speakers and selected speech-defective groups. In Bosma, J. (Ed.), *Symposium on Oral Sensation and Perception*. Springfield, Ill.: Charles C Thomas, Publisher (1967).

Bangs, T., Evaluating children with language delay. *J. Speech Hearing Dis.*, **26**, 6-18. (1961).

Bangs, T., *Language and Learning Disorders of the Preacademic Child*. New York: Appleton-Century-Crofts (1968).

Berry, M., *Language Disorders of Children*. New York: Appleton-Century-Crofts (1969).

Berry, M., and Eisenson, J., *Speech Disorders*. New York: Appleton-Century-Crofts (1956).

Boone, D., *The Voice and Voice Therapy*. Englewood Cliffs, N.J.: Prentice-Hall, Inc. (1971).

Burgemeister, B., *Psychological Techniques in Neurological Diagnosis*. New York: Harper & Row, Publishers (1962).

Burgemeister, B., Blum, L., and Lorge, I., *Columbia Mental Maturity Scale*. New York: Harcourt, Brace & World (1953).

Bzoch, K., *Communicative Disorders Related to Cleft Lip and Palate*. Boston: Little, Brown & Co. (1972).

Bzoch, K., and League, R., *Assessing Language Skills in Infancy*. Gainesville, Fla.: Tree of Life Press (1971).

Carroll, J., and Sapon, S., *Modern Language Aptitude Test, Form A*. New York: Psychological Corp. (1959).

Carrow, M., The development of auditory comprehension of language structure in children. *J. Speech Hearing Dis.*, **33**, 99-111 (1968).

Cattell, P., *The Measurement of Intelligence of Infants and Young Children*. New York: Psychological Corp. (1947).

Darley, F., *Diagnosis and Appraisal of Communication Disorders*. Englewood Cliffs, N.J.: Prentice-Hall, Inc. (1969).

Davis, H., and Silverman, R., *Hearing and Deafness*, New York: Holt, Rinehart & Winston, Inc. (1970).

Doll, E., *The Vineland Social Maturity Scale*. Philadelphia: Educational Test Bureau (1946).

Dunn, L., *Peabody Picture Vocabulary Test*. Circle Pines, Minn.: American Guidance Service, Inc. (1959).

Eisenson, J., *Examining for Aphasia*. New York: Psychological Corp. (1954).

Eisenson, J., *Adult Aphasia: Assessment and Treatment*. New York: Appleton-Century-Crofts (1973).

Emerick, L., and Hatten, J., *Diagnosis and Evaluation in Speech Pathology*. Englewood Cliffs, N.J.: Prentice-Hall, Inc. (1974).

Erickson, R., Assessing communication attitudes among stutterers. *J. Speech Hearing Res.*, **12**, 711-724 (1969).

Fairbanks, G., *Voice and Articulation Drillbook*. New York: Harper & Row, Publishers (1960).

Feynman, R., Leighton, R., and Sands, M., *The Feynman Lectures on Physics*, (Vol. 2) Reading, Mass.: Addison-Wesley Publishing Co., Inc. (1969).

Fisher, H., and Logemann, J., *The Fisher-Logemann Test of Articulation Competence*. Boston: Houghton Mifflin Co. (1971).

Foster, R., Giddan, J., and Stark, J., *Assessment of Children's Language Comprehension*. Palo Alto, Calif.: Consulting Psychologists Press, Inc. (1969).

Gesell, A., and Amatruda, C., *Developmental Diagnosis*. New York: Harper & Row, Publishers (1947).

Goldman, R., and Fristoe, M., *Goldman-Fristoe Test of Articulation*. Circle-Pines, Minn.: American Guidance Service (1969).

Goldman, R., Fristoe, M., and Woodcock, R., *Goldman-Fristoe-Woodcock Test of Auditory Discrimination*. Circle Pines, Minn.: American Guidance Service (1970).

Goodglass, H., and Kaplan, E., *Boston Diagnostic Aphasia Examination*. Philadelphia: Lea & Febiger (1972).

Goodstein, L., Functional speech disorders and personality: a survey of the research. *J. Speech Hearing Res.* **1**, 359-376 (1958a).

Goodstein, L., Functional speech disorders and personality: methodological and theoretical considerations. *J. Speech Hearing Res.* **1**, 377-382 (1958b).

Goodstein, L., MMPI differences between parents of children with cleft palates and parents of physically normal children. *J. Speech Hearing Res.*, **3**, 31-38 (1960).

Guilford, J., *The Nature of Human Intelligence*. New York: McGraw-Hill Book Co. (1967).

Haney, R., *Assessment by developmental signs. Unpublished clinical manual of the University of Southern California Center for the Study of Communicative Disorders* (1969).

Hanley, T., and Peters, R., The speech and hearing laboratory. In Travis, L. (Ed.), *Handbook of Speech Pathology and Audiology*. New York: Appleton-Century Crofts (1971).

Hardy, J., Intraoral breath pressure in cerebral palsy. *J. Speech Hearing Dis.*, **26**, 309-319 (1961).

Hardy, J., Respiratory physiology: implications of current research. *Asha*, **10**, 204-205 (1968).

Harris, D., *Children's Drawings as Measures of Intellectual Maturity*. New York: Harcourt, Brace & World (1963).

Hathaway, S., and McKinley, J., *Minnesota Multiphasic Personality Inventory: Manual*. New York: Psychological Corp. (1951).

Heath, S., Rail-walking performance as related to mental age and etiological type among the mentally retarded. *Am. J. Psychol.*, **55**, 240-247 (1942).

Jerger, J., *Modern Developments in Audiology*. New York: Academic Press, Inc. (1963).

Johnson, W., Measurements of oral reading and speaking rate and disfluency of adult male and female stutterers and nonstutterers. *J. Speech Hearing Dis., Monogr. Suppl.* 7, pp. 1-20 (1961).

Johnson, W. Darley, F., and Spriestersbach, D., *Diagnostic Methods in Speech Pathology.* New York: Harper & Row, Publishers (1963).

Kahn, T., Personality projection on culturally structured symbols. *J. Project. Techniques*, **19**, 431-442 (1955).

Khanna, J., *Brain Damage and Mental Retardation.* Springfield, Ill.: Charles C Thomas, Publisher (1968).

Kirk, S., McCarthy, J., and Kirk, W., *Illinois Test of Psycholinguistic Abilities.* Urbana: University of Illinois Press (1968).

Lee, L., Developmental sentence types: a method for comparing normal and deviant syntactic development. *J. Speech Hearing Dis.,* **31**, 311-330 (1966).

Lee, L., Recent studies in language acquisition. *Asha*, **11**, 272-274 (1969a).

Lee, L., *Northwestern Syntax Screening Test.* Evanston. Ill.: Northwestern University Press (1969b).

Lenneberg, E., *Biological Foundations of Language.* New York: John Wiley & Sons, Inc. (1967).

Lenneberg, E., On explaining language. *Science*, **164**, 635-643 (1969).

Lerea, L., Assessing language development. *J. Speech Hearing Res.*, **1**, 75-85 (1958).

MacKay, D., Metamorphosis of a critical interval: age-linked changes in the delay in auditory feedback that produces maximal disruption of speech. *J. Acoust. Soc. Am.*, **43**, 811-821 (1968).

Mason, R., Principles and methods of orofacial examination. Unpublished educational manual. Lexington: University of Kentucky (1975).

McCarthy, D., The language development of the preschool child. *Child Welfare Monogr.*, No. 4. Minneapolis: University of Minnesota Press (1930).

McDonald, E., *Articulation Testing and Treatment: a Sensory-Motor Approach.* Pittsburgh: Stanwix House, Inc. (1964).

McDonald, E., and Aungst, L., Studies in oral sensori-motor function. In Bosma, J. (Ed.), *Symposium on Oral Sensation and Perception.* Springfield, Ill.: Charles C Thomas, Publisher (1967).

Mecham, M., Jex, J., and Jones, J., *Utah Test of Language Development.* Minneapolis: American Guidance Service (1958).

Menyuk, P., Comparison of grammar of children with functionally deviant and normal speech. *J. Speech Hearing Res.*, **7**, 109-121 (1964).

Milisen, R., A rationale for articulation disorders. *J. Speech Hearing Dis., Monog. Suppl.* 4, pp. 5-18 (1959).

Miller, R., An experimental study of the evaluations by untrained listeners of efficient and inefficient voice production as to quality. Doctoral dissertation. University of Southern California (1957).

Moore, P., Voice disorders organically based. In Travis, L., (Ed.), *Handbook of Speech Pathology and Audiology.* New York: Appleton-Century-Crofts (1971).

Moser, H., La Gourgue, J., and Class, L., Studies in oral sterognosis in normal, blind and deaf subjects. In Bosma, J. (Ed.), *Symposium on Oral Sensation and Perception.* Springfield, Ill.: Charles C Thomas, Publisher (1967).

Murphy, A., *Functional Voice Disorders.* Englewood Cliffs, N.J.: Prentice-Hall, Inc. (1964).

Murray, H., *Thematic Apperception Test.* Cambridge, Mass.: Harvard University Press (1943).

Myklebust, H., *Development and Disorders of Written Language.* (Vol. 1) *Picture Story Language Test.* New York: Grune & Stratton, Inc. (1965).

Netsell, R., Evaluation of velopharyngeal function in dysarthria. *J. Speech Hearing Dis.* **34**, 113-122 (1969).

Newby, H., *Audiology.* New York: Appleton-Century-Crofts (1964).

Noll, J., Discussion of respiratory physiology: implications of current research. *Asha*, **10**, 205-206 (1968).

O'Neill, J., *The Hard of Hearing.* Englewood Cliffs, N.J.: Prentice-Hall, Inc. (1964).

Oseretsky, N., *The Oseretsky Tests of Motor Proficiency.* Minn.: Educational Test Bureau (1946).

Perkins, W., Normal vocal tone generation: detection, diagnosis, and management of abnormal vocal tone generation. In Tower, D. (Editor-in-chief), *The Nervous System.* (Vol. 3) *Human Communication and Its Disorders.* New York: Raven Press (1975).

Piaget, J., *The Language and Thought of the Child.* New York: Harcourt, Brace, & World (1926).

Porch, B., *Porch Index of Communicative Ability.* Palo Alto, Calif.: Consulting Psychologists Press, Inc. (1971).

Pronovost, W., and Dumbleton, C., A picture-type speech sound discrimination test. *J. Speech Hearing Dis.*, **18**, 258-266 (1953).

Raven, J., *Guide to Using Progressive Matrices.* London: H. K. Lewis and Co. (1947).

Riley, G., A stuttering severity instrument for children and adults. *J. Speech Hearing Dis.*, **37**, 314-322 (1972).

Ringel, R., and Ewanoski, S., Oral perception. I. Two-point discrimination. *J. Speech Hearing Res.*, **8**, 389-398 (1965).

Ringel, R., and Fletcher, H., Oral perception. III. Texture discrimination. *J. Speech Hearing Res.*, **10**, 642-649 (1967).

Ringel, R., Saxman, J., and Brooks, A., Oral perception. II. Mandibular kinesthesia. *J. Speech Hearing Res.*, **10**, 637-641 (1967).

Rorschach, H., Psychodiagnostics: a diagnostic test based on perception. Berne: Hans Huber Medical Publisher (1942).

Rousey, C., *Psychiatric Assessment by Speech and Hearing Behavior.* Springfield, Ill.: Charles C Thomas, Publisher (1974).

Ruch, F., *Psychology and Life.* Glenview, Ill.: Scott, Foresman & Co. (1967).

Rutherford, D., and McCall, G., Testing oral sensation and perception in persons with dysarthria. In Bosma, J. (Ed.), *Symposium on Oral Sensation and Perception.* Springfield, Ill.: Charles C Thomas, Publisher (1967).

Sander, E., Reliability of the Iowa Speech Disfluency Test. *J. Speech Hearing Dis., Monogr. Suppl.* 7, pp. 21-30 (1961).

Sarno, M., *The Functional Communication Profile.* Rehabilitation Monograph 42. New York: Institute of Rehabilitation Medicine, New York University Medical Center (1969).

Schaefer, E., and Bell, R., *Parental Attitude Research Instruments: Normative Data.* Bethesda, Md.: National Institutes of Mental Health (undated).

Schiefelbusch, R., Language development and language modification. In Schiefelbusch, R., Copeland, R., and Smith, J. (Eds.), *Language and Mental Retardation.* New York: Holt, Rinehart & Winston, Inc. (1967).

Schuell, H., A short examination for aphasia. *Neurology*, **7**, 625-634 (1957).

Schuell, H., *Differential Diagnosis of Aphasia With the Minnesota Test.* Minneapolis: University of Minnesota Press (1965a).

Schuell, H., *The Minnesota Test for Differential Diagnosis of Aphasia; Administrative Manual and Card Materials.* Minneapolis: University of Minnesota Press (1956b).

Sheehan, J., Projective studies of stuttering. *J. Speech Hearing Dis.*, **23**, 18-25 (1958).

Shelton, R., Arndt, W., and Hetherington, J., Testing oral stereognosis. In Bosma, J., (Ed.), *Symposium on Oral Sensation and Perception.* Springfield, Ill.: Charles C Thomas, Publisher (1967).

Shelton, R., Diedrich, W., and Youngstrom, K., The evaluation of speech mechanisms. *J. Kan. Med. Soc.*, **62**, 396-399, 403 (1961).

Shelton, R., Hahn, E., and Morris, H., Diagnosis and therapy. In Spriestersbach, D., and Sherman, D. (Eds.), *Cleft Palate and Communication.* New York: Academic Press, Inc. (1968).

Shelton, R., and others, Effect of prosthetic speech bulb reduction on articulation. *Cleft Palate J.*, **5**, 195-204 (1968).

Shelton, R., and others, The relationship between nasal sound pressure level and palatopharyngeal closure. *J. Speech Hearing Res.* **12**, 193-198 (1969).

Shipley-Hartford Scale for Measuring Intellectual Impairment. Hartford, Conn.: Neuro-Psychiatric Institute of the Hartford Retreat (1946).

Sklar, M., Relation of psychological and language test scores and autopsy findings in aphasia. *J. Speech Hearing Res.*, **6**, 84-90 (1963).

Smith, W., and Phillippus, M., *Neuropsychological Testing in Organic Brain Dysfunction.* Springfield, Ill.: Charles C Thomas, Publisher (1969).

Snow, K., and Milisen, R., The influence of oral versus pictorial presentation upon articulation testing results. *J. Speech Hearing Dis.*, *Monogr. Suppl.* 4, pp. 30-36 (1954a).

Snow, K., and Milisen, R., Spontaneous improvement in articulation as related to differential responses to oral and picture articulation tests. *J. Speech Hearing Dis.*, *Monogr. Suppl.* 4, pp. 45-50 (1954b).

Spradlin, J., Assessment of speech and language of retarded children: the Parsons Language Sample. *J. Speech Hearing Dis.*, *Monogr. Suppl.* 10, pp. 8-31 (1963).

Spradlin, J., Procedures for evaluating processes associated with receptive and expressive language. In Schiefelbusch, R., Copeland, R., and Smith, J. (Eds.), *Language and Mental Retardation.* New York: Holt, Rinehart & Winston, Inc. (1967).

Stetson, R., *Motor Phonetics.* Amsterdam: North-Holland Publishing Co. (1951).

Templin, M., A study of sound discrimination ability of elementary school pupils. *J. Speech Dis.* **8**, 127-132 (1943).

Templin, M., Spontaneous versus imitated verbalization in testing preschool children. *J. Speech Dis.*, **12**, 293-300 (1947).

Templin, M., *Certain Language Skills in Children.* Institute of Child Welfare Monograph Series, No. 26. Minneapolis: University of Minnesota Press (1957).

Templin, M., and Darley, F., *The Templin-Darley Tests of Articulation.* Iowa City, Iowa: Bureau of Educational Research and Service, University of Iowa (1970).

Terman, L., and Merrill, M., *Stanford-Binet Intelligence Scale: Manual for the Third Revision, Form L-M.* Boston: Houghton Mifflin Co. (1960).

Thurman, W., Frequency-intensity relationships and optimum pitch level. *J. Speech Hearing Res.*, **1**, 117-123 (1958).

Tikofsky, R., Language problems in adults. In Reiber, R., and Brubaker, R. (Eds.), *Speech Pathology.* Amsterdam: North-Holland Publishing Co. (1966).

Tobisman, K., Evaluation of the behavior of children by developmental signs. Unpublished research, University of Southern California (1968).

Van Riper, C., *Speech Correction: Principles and Methods.* Englewood Cliffs, N.J.: Prentice-Hall, Inc. (1963).

Van Riper, C., and Erickson, R., A predictive screening test of articulation. *J. Speech Hearing Dis.*, **34**, 214-219 (1969).

Wechsler, D., *Manual for the Wechsler Adult Intelligence Scale.* New York: Psychological Corp. (1955).

Wells, C., *Cleft palate and its Associated Speech Disorders.* New York: McGraw-Hill Book Co. (1971).

Wepman, J.., *Auditory Discrimination Test.* Chicago: Language Research Association (1958).

Wepman, J., and Jones, L., *Studies in Aphasia: an Approach to Testing: Manual of Administration and Scoring for the Language Modalities Test for Aphasia.* Chicago: Education-Industry Service (1961).

Wepman, J., and Jones, L., Studies in aphasia: a psycholinguistic method and case study. In Carterette. E. (Ed.), *Brain function. (III) Speech, Language and Communication.* UCLA Forum in Medical Sciences No. 4. Los Angeles: University of California Press (1966).

West, R., and Ansberry, M., The Rehabilitation of Speech. New York: Harper & Row, Publishers (1968).

Winitz, H., *From Syllable to Conversation.* Baltimore: University Park Press (1975).

Wood, N., Auditory perception in children. Final report, Social Rehabilitation Services research grant No. RD-2574-S (1971).

Young, M., Predicting ratings of severity of stuttering. *J. Commun. Dis.*, **2**, 174-189 (1969).

Chapter 16

Therapy of disorders of speech

Questions

1. What assumptions underlie the therapy of disorders of speech?
2. What modes of therapy are applicable to disorders of speech?
3. What therapeutic methods will modify disorders of speech?

ASSUMPTIONS OF THERAPY

Practitioners of therapy often work from a hidden agenda. The intervention of one person, the clinician, in the life of another, the client, is sufficiently sanctified when done in the name of therapy that motives, reasons, and effects are rarely examined. Ostensibly, clinicians work from noble motives to help relieve the handicapped of defective speech. But this is more a statement of hope than a prescription for solid achievement. The therapeutic process is immensely complex in ways that go far beyond the scope of what we can cover here. Still, a glimpse of some frequently unrecognized fundamental assumptions must be a prelude to the consideration of therapeutic methods.

The hidden agenda

The speech pathologist reveals his agenda of assumptions by what he does in each therapeutic encounter. To the extent that he is aware of his assumptions, his agenda is open to inspection. Like it or not, wittingly or blindly, he cannot avoid assuming answers to the following questions:

1. Is he responsible for the client's functioning as a whole, or for only the part-functions of speech?
2. Should he view man behaviorally, as scientifically knowable, or phenomenologically, as unique and free, and hence unpredictable?
3. For whose benefit should he modify behavior—the client's, the parent's, or society's?
4. Whose value system should he follow in setting therapeutic goals—the client's or his own?
5. For what motives should he offer therapy—money, power, altruism, or the solution of his own problems?
6. Should he persist with methods of therapy in which he is trained that prove unsuccessful or experiment with new methods?

The answers assumed to this agenda have far-reaching consequences. These assumptions should be recognized explicitly and weighed deliberately. The following are some guides to consider in selecting answers for these six issues:

1. To limit responsibility to the modification of deviant speech behavior is superficially a straightforward, simplifying choice. What it ignores is the significance of that behavior to the client. More subtly perhaps than anything else one does, the manner of speaking can signal message intent of which even the speaker may be unaware. Too, attempts to modify behavior that signals intent, without developing alternate methods of expressing it, ignore motivation. For example, dependent needs and aggressive feelings, which presumably can be signaled covertly through speech defects, would not evaporate if the defect were altered. More likely, the defect would resist permanent modification until methods of coping with the pressing needs of the whole person were considered.

Extending the responsibility to these needs, attractive as that solution may be for some, involves speech pathologists in problems for which they will not be prepared without extensive additional training in psychotherapy and personality theory. The object of the therapist here, as London (1964) says, "is grand and dangerous, demanding of him at his moral best the utmost in discretion and circumspection—he aims toward the core of meaning of his patient's life, prepared to reshape and mold it to new designs whose implications, though unknown, must be great indeed." The risk of success is awesome, so much so that traditionally the psychotherapist, assuming a gentle stance, exerting no direct control, but reflecting realities of the world, works toward insight that will free the patient to live more successfully with his fellowman.

A middle course strikes a balance that avoids assuming responsibility for all areas of a client's life, and yet copes with those covert needs that thwart permanent modification of impaired speech—a balance easier to maintain in principle than in practice. Those who see all behavior as a manifestation of some central meaning around which life is organized would argue that changing a segment of a client's life necessarily leaves the clinician responsible for whatever effects may reverberate throughout the personality. If buried beneath symptomatic speech disorders are truer miseries, how can the speech pathologist disclaim them as his doing when he is the agent of their revelation? Still, others of behavioral persuasion have found no evidence of debilitating side effects by direct removal of psychologic symptoms (Wolpe and Lazarus, 1966). If the same applies to speech symptoms, a middle course appears feasible.

2. The existential psychologist's view of man as a phenomenon is compelling for humanists concerned with experiencing the rich texture of life, with preserving the sanctity of the person, and with according recognition to consciousness of the subjective condition of being. An existential view accords with our inside certainty that we are not pawns in the hands of circumstance subject to external control, that we make our own destiny, that we are unique, and that we are free to do the unpredictable.

For the speech pathologist concerned with modifying discernibly maladaptive, explicitly identified segments of speech, the behaviorist's view of man, unattractive as it may be personally, has vast practical advantages professionally. Without its "tough-minded" as-

---

These opposing views of man were the subject of a symposium reported by Wann (1964) and discussed by Hitt (1969).

---

sumption that speech behavior can be studied scientifically, understood, predicted, and controlled, clinicians could offer the speech handicapped little assurance of help.

3. Ideally, everyone benefits from correction of defective speech. But this is not always true. To whom is the speech pathologist responsible when parents bring a child for correction of defective articulation about which the child is unconcerned; when a college student is required to have therapy for his stuttering if he is to receive a teaching credential; when a foreign student's continuation in professional studies depends on enrollment in a speech clinic? Answers are not

clean; they are muddied by contingencies. Do parents know best? When personal and social considerations are at odds, which should prevail? Would it be in a client's best interest to persuade him that he has a problem? By whose judgment? These questions are difficult enough when responsibility is limited to part-functions of speech; they are much more troublesome when extended to the whole person.

4. Whether the client's or the clinician's value system should prevail in determining behavioral modification seems, at first glance, a rhetorical question. It is the client's speech to do with as he will. The criteria by which it could be judged as a problem are open to him. If in his judgment his speech does not interfere with communication, is not esthetically unpleasant, is not damaging to his speech mechanism, or is not personally distressing, he is free to not choose therapy, or, if it is forced on him, to resist it.

If he does elect help, however, especially with someone whose broad concerns reach beyond speech, then the therapist's

---

London (1964) deals eloquently with the problem of the psychotherapist as a moral agent in the *Modes and Morales of Psychotherapy.*

---

values, even on moral issues, will necessarily tend to predominate. No one is free of personal values, clinicians included. Client selection of a therapist is tantamount to selecting a set of values ranging from speech to life-style to religion. The clinician is professionally obligated to reinforce that behavior that he judges to be in the best interest of the client. Client preference, however, affects reinforcement only after filtering through a clinician's judgment. Even when therapy is limited to speech, the clinician's values affect more than articulation, fluency, voice, or language. By what he does and by being what he is, the therapist provides a model for the client to emulate in all dimensions of life. For the clinician to reinforce desired speech responses effectively, his approbation must be of value to the client. For the same reason the clinician's example will implicitly shape the client in areas beyond therapeutic concern.

5. Motives for offering therapy are easily and unnecessarily whitewashed. The best clinicians are likely to have a realistic view of reasons for their professional choice. Probably the most suspect is the most obvious motive: altruistic dedication. Genuine concern for the handicapped is, ideally, a major component of any therapist's motivation. Unless it is tempered by other, tangible satisfactions, however, it may cloak two good reasons for not being a clinician: the desire to exercise the power built into the client-therapist relation, and the desire to solve one's own problems through another. Granted that the therapist's value system cannot be avoided, still, it should distort client needs and perceptions minimally. Therapy should be mainly for the client's benefit, not the clinician's.

6. How long therapy that is supposed to produce eventual effects should be continued without evidence of those effects is one of a clinician's most difficult problems. Therapeutic failure can be attributed to the method itself, to lack of skill in applying it, or to inappropriate application. Methods of successful therapy are as difficult to define as methods of successful parenthood, and for similar reasons. The variables involved and their interactions are staggering in number. Despite extensive investigations of psychotherapy, Raimy's facetious definition of it as "an

---

Does Strupp (1962) conclude from his review of studies of the psychotherapeutic process that the method or the therapist is of primary importance to effective treatment?

---

unidentified technique applied to unspecified problems with unpredictable outcomes" has uncomfortable ingredients of truth. The effects of speech therapy, though rarely studied, are thought to be more certain, primarily because the behavior to be modified can be made relatively explicit. Currently, though, no therapeutic prescription is available with which a clinician could persist with solid expectation of eventual

success. The alternative to giving each method a thorough trial is to flit from one to another, a procedure likely to produce even fewer results. The dozens of techniques used for disorders of stuttering and voice attest to dissatisfaction with results of any one or group of them for these difficult problems.

Pointed up by this dilemma is the need to fit treatment to the client. Therapy can thus be approached as a scientific inquiry in which the theory to be tested is the clinical assessment of the problem. From the assessment, effects of specific treatment procedures are predicted. Included must be the expected effects in a therapy session, each session being a test of a clinical hypothesis. When predicted results are not found, the clinician must interpret the failure. Were the wrong effects predicted? Were treatment procedures implemented improperly? Were uncontrolled variables obscuring hypothesized results? When such questions do not answer predictive failure, then doubt of the general assessment must be entertained. Approached in this manner, lesson plans become more than rote exercises in stating steps of therapy; they become exacting tests of understanding of each client's particular problem.

Therapy does not proceed from absolutes. No eternally "right" assumptions exist. Therapists are strategists who utilize clinical

---

Schulz (1972) has done an extensive analysis of the clinical decision-making process. He provides a general model to guide the therapist in reaching treatment as well as assessment decisions.

---

judgment to make the best decision possible from limited evidence in the face of uncertain outcomes. The challenge is exacting, the responsibility sobering, and the reward mighty.

MODES OF THERAPY

If we start from the premise that the speech pathologist's primary concern is with modification of defective speech, we have a firm basis for evaluating the relevance of different modes of therapy. The two major modes, following London's (1964) analysis, are *action,* or *behavior, therapies* and *insight therapies.* Comprising the former are those that *reduce anxiety* and those that *modify explicit behavior,* the category into which most of *speech therapy* fits. Comprising the latter are *nondirective* and *psychoanalytic therapies* designed generally to arouse and extinguish unrealistic anxieties. An additional mode, *directive counseling,* is best considered separately.

Models for therapy

Conceivably, speech pathologists may cope with four combinations of conditions to modify defective speech permanently. Speech clinicians, tacitly or by explicit design, work from these combinations. Derived from clinical observation and speculation, they are theoretical distinctions that may not exist in fact. Rather than argue the issue, let us assume their merits in principle and, to keep the distinctions anchored empirically, set up operational specifications by which each combination could be identified if, indeed, it does exist.

The first combination is the simplest. It could be considered the "bad habit" model: for whatever causes, the wrong pattern of speech was learned and persists only because the correct pattern has not been learned. The second is the "vicious circle" model: the wrong pattern was learned and persists in part because the speaker's struggles to avoid defective speech exacerbate his problem. The third could be called the "bad habit with benefits" model: for whatever causes, the wrong pattern was learned and persists in part because of reinforcing secondary benefits from it. The fourth is the "symptomatic disorders" model: the disorder was acquired and is maintained as a psychoneurotic symptom of personality conflict. For each model, a different rationale for therapy would be required.

The "bad habit" model. The bad habit model, most typically invoked for disorders of articulation, can apply to any defective speech behavior that can be permanently altered with little resistance or anxiety. The

original and maintaining causes are irrelevant to the rationale for modification of the disorder in this model. Even with mongolism, an unrepaired cleft palate, dysarthria, or a hemilaryngectomy, the issue is not how these disabilities limit capacity for normal speech. Rather, it is the client's ability to alter his behavior to whatever goal is feasible. The making of necessary changes with minimal difficulty and disturbance constitutes operational evidence that the bad habit model is an appropriate rationale for therapy designed to modify explicitly identified defective elements of speech.

The "vicious circle" model. The idea that the greater the struggle to avoid a defect, the more the performance deteriorates has been applied frequently to stuttering: the "anticipatory struggle" theory is a widely held example. The same idea is probably applicable to a wide range of problems, from the aphasic patient's "catastrophic" reaction to failure to the dysphonic patient's struggles to be heard. Whether original causes continue or not, anxiety about the problem helps to maintain it, primarily because it interferes with the acquisition of a correct response that could replace defective behavior. Operational evidence that the vicious circle model is a fitting rationale for therapy is found when the reduction of struggle permits evoking of desired behavior that subsequently can be permanently established with appropriate schedules of reinforcement.

The "bad habit with benefits" model. Punishing as maladaptive speech can be—it is advertised with every utterance—humans seem inclined to make the best of bad things, speech defects included. Girls can discover that a lisp is cute, a breathy voice sexy; aphasic persons can vegetate in dependency, supported by an overly solicitous family; stutterers can attribute social failures to their inability to speak normally; and so on and so on. For some, secondary benefits assume primary proportions sufficient to disrupt, bluntly or subtly, direct corrective efforts. The operational test of this bad habit with benefits model as a rational basis for therapy is resistance to modification of the defect or, if it does yield, disturbance that could be attributed to deprivation of secondary gains.

The "symptomatic disorder" model. In practice, the observable effects of the symptomatic disorder model are virtually indistinguishable from those of the bad habit with benefits model. In theory, psychodynamic conflict is a primary cause of symptomatic disorders in the fourth model, whereas it is the basis for secondary gains in the third. Aphonia can illustrate the similarities and theoretical difference. A woman with strong dependency needs retained her voice through years of teaching to support an alcoholic husband. After surgical removal of a nodule that required sick leave to permit vocal rest, aphonia persisted that prevented her return to work—a secondary gain neatly tailored to her need to retaliate and yet remain passive. Another woman, similar psychodynamically, became aphonic after being deserted by her husband and returning to live with her domineering mother: a primary symptomatic expression of helpless despair and defense against indignant rage—presumably a psychoneurotic conversion reaction (Chapter 10). Despite such differences in origin, unconscious needs are expressed symptomatically in both models. Therefore the important operational feature for therapy that we will use to distinguish the symptom model is modification of defective speech by resolution of psychodynamic conflict without direct attention to the symptom.

Summing up therapeutic needs. The operational specifications of each model present a characteristic set of therapeutic problems. Educational strategies, such as behavioral modification procedures designed specifically for speech, are especially appropriate for the bad habit model. Additionally, counseling would be helpful for client, family, and teachers regarding the nature of the problem and the necessary conditions for permanent correction. The vicious circle model requires therapy for speech, counseling, and anxiety-reduction procedures to help obtain desired responses for subsequent reinforcement. The bad habit with benefits model, in addition to therapy for speech (and possible anxiety-reduction techniques to help establish desired responses and counseling to help make them permanent), would require insight therapy to resolve conflicts basic to secondary gains from maladaptive speech. The primary requirement of the symptomatic disorders model is resolution of psychodynamic conflict. Counseling, therapy for speech, and anxiety-reduction procedures could be utilized as needed. Major therapeutic requisites for these models are summarized in Table 16-1.

Speech pathologists are not necessarily proficient in insight therapies nor in all forms of behavior therapy. Therefore we will discuss only those psychotherapeutic rationales and procedures particularly relevant to correction of speech for this mode of therapy. Since knowledge of conditions for behavioral

Table 16-1. Models of therapy

Type of therapy required	Model of therapy			
	I Bad habit	II Vicious circle	III Bad habit with benefits	IV Symptomatic disorders
Behavior therapy Speech therapy Anxiety reduction	Essential	Essential Important	Essential Use if needed	Use if needed Use if needed
Counseling	Important	Important	Important	Important
Insight therapy			Essential	Essential

modification of speech, however, is a primary obligation along with counseling objectives and methods, we will explore them closely.

Insight therapies

"Insight" identifies the traditional purpose of therapies in this mode. We will persist with the term as a convenient label, not as an explanation of why these therapies can be effective. In point of fact, insight is more likely to be a by-product of therapeutic change than a basic cause (Hobbs, 1962). Doubly valued, its moral good dates at least from Socrates ("an unexamined life is not worth living") and its therapeutic value, now in doubt, from Freud. With insight presumably comes relief from symptoms and greater self-control. Some think that this concept is a fiction preserved by psychotherapists who have historically filtered clinical impressions through theories of personality and social philosophy that have more pretension than title to scientific status (London, 1964). What has become abundantly apparent in the cold, empirical light of actuarial evaluations is that insight works no necessary effects on behavior (Eysenck, 1961). It can be valued for itself, but not as a certain agent of therapeutic change.

Why, then, bother with a mode of therapy held in such scientific jeopardy? The answer is that within this mode of therapy there are techniques of demonstrated value to speech pathologists charged with effecting permanent improvement of speech. Also, no alternate mode of therapy exists for those troubled by the idea that man is no more than the sum of his parts, which, when repaired, make him whole again. Nor does an alternative exist for those who see all behavior, normal and disordered, as an extension of a personal system of meaning. As Haney (1971) says of therapy for the child with communicative problems*:

---
*From Haney, R., Child therapy: relationship and process. In Travis, L. (Ed.), *Handbook of Speech Pathology and Audiology*. New York: Appleton-Century-Crofts (1971).

The purpose is to provide him with increasing appreciation for the uses of verbal communication in securing his needs, in mediating anxiety and in identifying the rights, significance and interdependence of himself and others. Children need to be in a relationship that is warm and deeply believing, with a person who is patiently willing to search and be open and communicative with respect to his own nature. Children need to be in a therapeutic setting with people who are capable of recognizing growth signs and carefully selective in the responses they offer. . . . Child therapy is, indeed, a matter of searching and sharing—a matter of careful receiving and thoughtful giving.

Need for insight therapy techniques: instigation of anxiety. The ways in which therapeutic progress can be sabotaged are infinite. If we assume that disorders of speech can yield secondary gains, that they can serve as neurotic symptoms, that they can signal unconscious intent more readily or effectively than can symbolic content, then we must assume that they can serve functional purposes. Reasonably, a disorder from which a client can depart easily and comfortably can be assumed to have had little personal value. Conversely, the greater its functional importance, the more we would expect its alteration to be vigorously resisted and, its defense failing, the more anxiety we would expect to accompany its demise.

What do Goldstein and his co-authors (1966) say of resistance to behavior change?

In practice, resistance is often obvious in children. For example, a child may want no one tampering with his speech in or out of the clinic, no matter how gross the defect. Head-on resistance invites head-on attacks by parents, teachers, and other forces of society with sufficient power to enforce overt compliance. But like the small boy who, ordered to stand in the corner, preserved his autonomy by announcing, "It's not the same corner," children may lose "speak up"— "slow down"—"don't mumble" battles but win their wars by never effecting overall permanent improvement of speech.

Therapists, too, join the encounter, but

they are usually more circumspect: they first establish *rapport*. By demonstrating acceptance and goodwill, they hope to enlist the client's cooperation in correcting his defective performance, all in his best interest. This clinical strategy can be successful. Ironically, though, short-term success seen in the clinic contrasted with failure in *carryover* to daily life is likely to reflect escalated complexity of the resistance problem. Caught between the Scylla of relinquishing his psychically necessary speech disorder and the Charybdis of impairing the good opinion of his revered clinician, the child may pay lip service, even convincing himself, to the fiction that he wants improved speech. Only the blunt fact that he does not take the necessary steps outside of the clinic to make corrections permanent gives the lie to rapport as being enough.

In adults, resistance that preserves disorders for psychic reasons is especially difficult to trap. Enshrouded in layers of conflicting motives, the summation of a speaker's divergent intent is best seen in the pattern of what he does; when deeds diverge from words, the disparity reveals the regions of conflict. The socially inclined woman who, by persistent vocal abuse, faces a fourth round of laryngeal surgery that she professes she will do anything to avoid exemplifies such divergence. She will enter into therapy with apparent determination, demonstrate the ability to perform necessary vocal skills during clinical sessions, and yet comply hardly at all with outside assignments: she persists in addressing social groups and speaking over the noise of garden parties and cocktail parties. When confronted gently with the necessity of complying with clinical directions, she demures coyly. When confronted firmly, she trades in her clinician for one less demanding. She is continuously in treatment and yet continuously resists it with strategies and explanations for failure that absolve her of responsibility, at least in her own eyes.

Evidence of successful penetration of resistance is seen in arousal of anxiety. Curiously, such evidence is the most hopeful sign of progress when resistance is a problem. Conversely, permanent modification of speech without disturbance indicates that suspected resistance was either nonexistent or has already been resolved. Stutterers who assign most of their woes to speech often exemplify problems of resistance and disturbance. Their problem is sufficiently maladaptive in reality that everything from scholastic difficulties to social isolation can be attributed to it. One stutterer who had a host of complaints all laid to his speech disorder made no progress in more than a year of psychotherapy until stuttering was removed for 6 months with rate control procedures. During this period of stutter-free speech, he could not avoid recognizing that his other complaints persisted. Although his speech relapsed temporarily, he at least was able to progress in psychotherapy.

Another stutterer, a bright, handsome young adult, was so sorely afflicted that after 5 years of speech therapy and psychotherapy, he averaged only 50 to 200 words per hour. One morning after a session in which the protective value of his stuttering had once again been placed before him, he awoke unable to stutter. When he arrived 4 days later for his next session, he was haggard, unshaven, and still fluent. He felt "raw, exposed, and miserable"; he protested that he would "do anything to stutter again" during his first month of fluency. Subsequent social behavior was as different as his speech. Previously shy and retiring, he became verbally aggressive; never having dated before, he became a veritable Lothario complete with sports car. Why, after years of resisting therapy, he was suddenly able to change drastically overnight is a matter of conjecture. What is apparent was the inverse relation between resistance and anxiety.

Insight therapy techniques. The plentitude of systems of psychotherapy and psychoanalysis designed to cure ignorance of self (plus related symptoms) attests to varieties of personality theories more than of techniques (Harper, 1959; Munroe, 1955; Ford and Urban, 1963). Most systems are all-purpose; they do not constitute a battery from which the clinician can select the one most appropriate for a specific problem. Adherents of most systems treat most people for most problems for which most advocates of most other systems would offer treatment (London, 1964).

Wolpe (1957) describes play therapy and psychodrama as more accessible routes than dream analysis to the fantasy life of speech-handicapped children. Do these methods adapted to children differ mainly in principle or in technique? Do they require any less skill or training than is required for adult psychotherapy?

Not therapists' beliefs but what they do in exercising their beliefs can be studied scientifically. Differences in technique among insight therapists, except for adaptations to children or to groups, virtually vanish when viewed directly rather than through the filters of their theoretical systems. Even what seem to be major technical differences between nondirective and psychoanalytic therapy are more apparent than real. The freudian analyst *interprets* implied feeling in his search for the roots of a symptom, whereas the rogerian therapist *reflects* implied feeling in his effort to understand and accept. Skill in detecting feelings that patients will profit from recognizing keeps freudians and rogerians at about the same inferential "depths." If interpretations are too deep, they are meaningless; if reflections are too shallow, they are mimicry, not empathy. Similarly, presumed differences in directiveness are specious. The nondirective rogerian, by selectively reflecting some responses and not others, subtly steers his client as surely as does the more obviously directive analyst (London, 1964).

If procedural commonalities tie insight therapists together, what must a clinician do to produce psychotherapeutic changes? Rogers (1957) proposed what he considered to be the six necessary and sufficient conditions for constructive change with his system:

1. Two persons are in psychologic contact.
2. The client, vulnerable or anxious, is in a state of incongruence.
3. The therapist is integrated and congruent in the relation.
4. The therapist experiences unconditional positive regard for the client.
5. The therapist experiences and communicates empathic understanding.
6. The client perceives the therapist's empathic communication.

Hobbs (1962), viewing all types of psychotherapy, identified five common sources of gain within which Rogers' conditions would fit:

1. The therapeutic relationship itself. The client, fearful of personal involvement, is afforded a sustained intimate experience without being hurt.
2. Divestment of symbols of their anxiety. The most private concrete verbal and nonverbal symbols with which the client thinks about his problems are uttered openly until they cease to be disturbing.
3. Practice in decision making. The client is afforded abundant opportunities to assume responsibility for managing his own life.
4. Repair of personal cosmology. Man imposes a conception of order on the world to provide a feeling of control of his destiny. Anxiety resulting from loss of control of maladaptive behavior is resolved by helping the client erect a cognitive structure from which he can predict consequences of his performance more accurately.
5. Resolution of the transference relationship. Clients are confronted directly with the irrationality of their maladaptive, neurotic methods of relating to the therapist.

Whether or not Rogers or Hobbs has offered a definitive analysis of the conditions required for psychotherapy, they have at least isolated, in relatively explicit terms, major dimensions of therapy for the whole man.

Applications to speech. Which of these techniques have special value for modification of defective speech? None are excluded

Travis (1971a) describes the psychotherapeutic process as it can be applied to speech-handicapped persons. Is his goal resolution of neurosis in the whole person or modification of a part function of speech?

as sacrosanct procedures in which speech pathologists should not participate. Most speech clinicians use them for a different purpose, however. Since they use them to facilitate correction of speech, they stop short of the psychotherapist's goal of resolving neurosis in all areas of the client's life that are being disabled.

Applying Hobb's five sources of gain to therapy for speech, let us see how they would help resolve resistance to permanent improvement.

1. The therapeutic relationship would be one in which the client as a person would be accepted unconditionally. His speech performance, however, would be evaluated and appropriately reinforced.

2. Feared words and situations would be exposed and practiced openly until they were cleared of anxiety, a long-established procedure for therapy with stutterers.

3. All decisions that test motivation for therapy would be made by the client, such as day-to-day and overall goal setting, frequency and length of practice periods, and any other decisions that would make therapy something the client does for himself.

4. Resistance and disturbance bespeak the significance of a speech disorder in the client's conception of how he can cope with his world. That conception would be altered as speech is altered if progress is to be minimally distressing. A client who feels helpless, for example, may cling tenaciously to a disorder that offers the slightest excuse for demanding a dependent relation. Repair of the client's cosmology is vital when resistance has been penetrated and anxiety released, as, shorn of a crutch, he feels his ability to cope weakened.

5. The technique of *confrontation* in the resolution of transference is a powerful tool that could be used for resistance. Where the psychotherapist must confront clients with

relatively nebulous patterns of neurotic behavior that have transferred to therapy, the speech pathologist has more tangible evidence available.

This final point deserves elaboration. Rarely with adults will resistance be obvious. It can be trapped only when squarely opposed to reality. Before a speech pathologist can discount client failure as resistance, the steps to be taken toward recovery must be clearly identified. If the client takes the steps and does not improve, the clinician has failed to provide the proper treatment. But if the client fails to take what are presumed to be necessary steps, then he can be confronted with the incongruity of his position: he ostensibly wants help for his speech; he continues to invest time and money in therapy; yet he does not partake of the help for which he is paying. If he rationalizes that the prescribed steps would not help, he can be confronted with the question of why he persists in therapy if he has little confidence in the treatment. If he rationalizes that he did not have time or opportunity, the strength of his desire for help can be questioned.

Strengths and limits. Insight therapy techniques are addressed more explicitly than any other procedures to alignment of motives into a congruent whole. Whereas the speech pathologist can directly facilitate speech discriminations to be learned, he has no direct access to the biologic process by which stimuli are tested for novelty, for relevance to goal-directed behavior, for visceral appetitive significance, or for instinctual needs. Only stimuli judged to be of significance by this biologic test seem to be preserved in memory, that is, learned (Livingston, 1967). But one is not necessarily aware of all motivational elements involved in this test of significance—hence the basis for divergence of a speaker's implicit intent from the explicit content of his message. What one wants is spoken louder by deeds than words. When deed and word are congruent, the speech clinician can proceed successfully with straightforward behavioral modification of speech. When they are incongruent, concepts and techniques of insight therapies may be essential to resolve resistance and disturbance.

In dedication to gut issues of existential meaning, morality, and the like, however, lies the flaw of insight therapies. These issues cannot be captured within explicit definitions, and insight into these problems offers little certainty that helpful changes in behavior will necessarily follow. Insight therapies, long on humanistic concerns, are short on prediction and control of behavioral consequences. Not wishing to direct a client's life, psychotherapists avoid blueprints of the final model of humanity they hope to produce. Lacking precise specifications of the performance they seek, and hopeful in their assumption that with "real" insight (as distinct from "intellectual" insight) a splendid specimen will emerge from the therapeutic cocoon, they exert little control over the behavior explicitly reinforced. The speech pathologist, responsible for effecting specific changes in specific directions for specific dimensions of speech, will probably be disappointed if he relies solely on insight therapies as his therapeutic tool.

Behavior therapies

Behavior therapists, or *action therapists* as London (1964) calls them, are not concerned directly with the nebulous substance of personality, meaning, self, and other such constructs of insight therapists. It is enough for them to shape behavior, excising defective in favor of normal components. If in the process behavior therapists exert intense control of clients much as a surgeon would to relieve physical complaints, the price in momentary loss of autonomy is considered small when measured by lasting improvement. Applying principles of learning systematically, they have built technologies for modifying behavior with which they can produce remarkably predictable results. The more explicitly the behavior to be altered can be controlled, the more impressively they can display effectiveness of their therapeutic wares.

Growth of behavior therapy in the last decade has exploded into almost every area of clinical concern. This wave of the future has reshaped treatment methods, especially in psychiatry and clinical psychology, for problems ranging from psychosis to smoking reduction. Because speaking processes are observable and relatively controllable, speech pathologists have been particularly receptive to various forms of behavior therapy. Interest has ranged from methods designed to reduce anxiety to methods for the explicit modification of speech.

Anxiety-reduction therapies. Perhaps the most popular anxiety-reduction method is the reciprocal inhibition technique devised by Wolpe (1962, 1969) and developed by Wolpe and Lazarus (1966). A systematic procedure for desensitizing anxiety, it first requires the establishment of deep relaxation as the polar opposite of anxiety. Then, working from the weakest to the strongest items from a list of anxiety-provoking situations, the patient is asked to imagine each item as vividly as possible. If relaxation is unimpaired, therapy progresses through the hierarchy until an imagined situation disturbs relaxation. Imagining is then stopped, relaxation is reestablished, and the situation is reimagined. This process of reciprocally inhibiting (not extinguishing) anxiety with relaxation is continued systematically until all items can be imagined without anxiety. These effects apparently carry over from imagery to life situations with few side effects or relapses; recovery rates of 80% to 90% have been reported (Wolpe and Lazarus, 1966).

Also based on learning theory is a method of anxiety extinction created by Stampfl called *implosion therapy* (London, 1964). Although anchored to the same theoretical moorings as the systematic desensitization method that inhibits anxiety, the approach of implosion therapy is diametrically opposite: Stampfl arouses anxiety as high and as long as possible in order to extinguish it by nonreinforcement as quickly as possible. Since its success rests heavily on the clinician's ability to frighten a patient with vivid verbal imagery, it is especially taxing of therapeutic skill.

Applications to speech. These anxiety-reduction procedures are well adapted to achieve the second of Hobbs' sources of gain in psychotherapy: divestment of symbols of anxiety. Stuttering has seemed to be the most relevant problem for use of these methods—many presume that anxiety is the intervening variable that elicits stuttering. Gray and England (1972), using reciprocal inhibition procedures, have put this idea to its most extensive test. They found that this method did indeed reduce anxiety responses quickly and effectively, but that the prevailing clinical impression of a one-to-one relation between anxiety and stuttering is apparently more fiction than fact. Stuttering improved at about the same clinical cure rate, around 30%, as has been reported for other types of therapy.

The appropriateness of anxiety-reduction methods need not hang on direct speech effects. Reduction of tension may not automatically improve a voice, language, articulation, or speech-flow problem, but it can enable a client to attend to skills to be learned. Compared to insight therapy techniques, anxiety-reduction methods produce relatively quick and certain relief. Compared to operant procedures, these methods are imprecise: they are attempts to manipulate unobservable imagery to effect an unobservable variable, anxiety. A clinician has no assurance that the client is imagining the proper image or that he is feeling anxious or relaxed. Gray and England (1969) attempted to solve part of this problem by using *electroskin conductance* (ESC) and *evaporative water loss* (EWL) techniques as operational measures of anxiety. Even this expensive solution presumes that these techniques are valid physiologic measures of anxiety, a shaky premise. Still, for specific fears, these methods are the most effective available.

Operant therapy (behavior modification). The *experimental analysis of behavior*, better known as *operant conditioning*, has no peers as a technology of learning (Chapter 2). Not a theory of learning so much as a demonstration of conditions under which learning occurs, it permits greater prediction and control of behavior that can be identified than any other approach. Proceeding from the principle that the future of all behavior is determined by its consequences, it has been sharply criticized as inadequate to explain higher-order human functions such as language and thought (Chomsky, 1968). To the extent that deviant speech can be identified and measured, however, such criticisms, appropriate as they may be, need not impair the therapeutic effectiveness of this approach (Peterson, 1968).

The fundamental requirements for operant therapy are that goals to be achieved be clearly specified and that all behavior of interest, desired and undesired, be reliably measurable. *Operant therapy* is not a scatter-

---

Johnston and Harris (1968) discuss in detail procedures for observing and recording verbal behavior.

---

shot approach in which the clinician, armed with a quiverful of techniques, shoots in a general direction with hope of hitting a profitable target. The therapist must know his aiming point exactly. Abstract goals are not enough. Terms such as "fluent" speech, "good" vocal quality, and "intelligible" speech are too vague to be useful. They do not specify in measurable form what the client is to accomplish. Clearly, operant therapy requires that clinician and client agree on precisely where they are going before they start. Once the client is satisfied with the destination, the clinician assumes full responsibility for directing the therapeutic trip (Kanfer, 1968).

The three types of procedures used in operant conditioning—measurement of response frequency *base lines*, *modification of behavior*, and extension of *stimulus control* of responses—are analogous to the clinical processes of assessment, treatment, and carryover.

Measuring base lines. Of these operant procedures, measurement of stable base lines tests observational rigor and is the backbone for obtaining predictable therapeutic results. As the assessment procedure prior to treatment, three payoffs follow base-line measures of rate of responses to be modified. The first payoff is unambiguous recognition of behavior to be modified. Responses change most predictably as their consequences follow consistently and immediately. Clinicians who have only vague impressions of responses they are to reinforce or punish are likely to be neither consistent nor immediate.

The second payoff is a basis for determining stimulus conditions that control responses. On this foundation can be erected a scientific approach to therapy. By systematically arranging the contingencies of reinforcement and punishment under specific stimulus conditions as the independent variable, and by observing changes from the base line of response frequency as the dependent variable, therapists can promptly test the accuracy of their clinical hypotheses.

The third payoff is a basis for measuring therapeutic progress. Frequency of occurrence of desirable and undesirable responses at various stages of treatment can be compared with initial base-line frequencies.

Modification of behavior. Modification of behavior, the clinical treatment phase of operant therapy, can be approached three ways: by altering *rate of responding*, by *shaping* new responses, and by manipulating responses with *stimulus control*. Changing the rate of responding is easiest; undesirable responses are punished, desirable ones reinforced. For example, when a small boy with vocal nodules speaks softly, an M & M candy is awarded immediately; when he speaks loudly, a candy is promptly forfeited.

Shaping new responses is more complicated, but with this tactic remarkable results are possible: witness animal acts in circuses

---

Brookshire (1967) offers a succinct, lucid description of how principles of operant conditioning can be applied clinically by speech pathologists.

---

and pigeons that play baseball. The idea is to select an available response with some characteristics in common with the desired *terminal behavior;* a belch is frequently used for newly laryngectomized patients who are to learn esophageal speech. By selectively

reinforcing closer approximations of the terminal goal, that is, by *successive approximations*, the desired new responses are achieved. Finally, stimulus control is a technique applicable to responses that occur in some situations but not others, such as stuttering. Stutterers are typically more fluent under some conditions than others. For them, fluency can be used as a *competing response* to stuttering. It can be extended gradually to all speaking conditions by selectively reinforcing it in situations that successively approximate those in which stuttering occurs.

Many responses are built on previously established behavior and therefore are part of a *systematic sequence*. Children do not learn prepositions and articles, for example, until they have mastered subject-predicate relations of grammar. A major challenge for speech pathologists is the determination of the systematic sequence by which speech skills are learned initially and by which defects can be corrected subsequently.

With the establishment of individual terminal responses, they can be *chained* into appropriate series. As an illustration, an aphasic patient may use only one-word responses. To successively approximate complete sentences, he would be reinforced first at the end of appropriate two-word phrases, then for syntactic three-word combinations, and so on until normal phrasing is achieved. The principle followed in chaining is to withhold reinforcement until the final response, along with the entire sequence, is produced properly.

Carryover. Carryover, the nemesis of many therapists, is essentially a problem of extending stimulus control over desired speech responses to daily life. Like it or not, the contexts within which responses are learned tend to control their emission. Therapists are constantly plagued with desirable responses that occur only in the clinic. Systematic manipulation of stimulus control is important for initiating as well as for terminating therapy. The less resemblance between clinical and daily life conditions at the outset of treatment, the less likelihood that undesirable responses will be carried into the clinic setting. Conversely, toward the end of treatment, clinic conditions should resemble the client's normal environment as closely as possible. The clinic situation can be altered gradually after terminal behavior is established by changing settings and social complexity. A particularly effective tactic, when possible, is to bring crucial persons in the client's life—spouse, friends, parents—into the clinic. Their presence then exerts stimulus control over the speech improvements at home, school, and work.

Contingencies of reinforcement. All procedures for modifying behavior and making it permanent are accomplished by management of contingencies of reinforcement. These contingencies have two dimensions, both of which therapists must manage in controlling the consequences of client behavior. One is *types of reinforcement,* the other, *schedules of reinforcement.*

Because one man's reward is another's punishment, the types of reinforcement are defined by their consequences. Conditions following a response that increase its frequency of occurrence are reinforcing; those that decrease its frequency are punishing. By this operational test of stimulus value, personal variations are accommodated without becoming hopelessly entangled in trying to prove an individual's taste for a particular stimulus at a particular time.

Reinforcement comes in two forms, as does punishment. Stimuli that are rewarding, that are sought, characterize *positive reinforcement;* those that offer escape or avoidance of noxious conditions are *negatively reinforced.* Both increase the frequency of response—one of approach, the other of avoidance behavior. As for the two forms of punishment, one decreases response rate because contingent stimuli are aversive, the other because positive reinforcement is withheld (Brookshire, 1967).

Although punishment can be used to decrease error responses and sharpen discriminations, positive reinforcement is essential to establish desired responses in the first place, if for no other reason than to avoid the possibility of negative side effects from noxious consequences of punishment (Kanfer, 1968). This approach is in one way easier and in another more difficult with children than adults. Positive reinforcement for children is easier because they want so many things. Candy, pennies, and intriguing toys can all be rewarding, especially if linked to what the child wants at the moment. This idea has been systematized by Addison and Homme (1966) in what they call "the reinforcing event (RE) menu." It consists of a "menu" of stick drawings of available RE. Before the desired task is performed the child selects the event he would prefer; he then completes the task and, if it is satisfactory, receives his reinforcement immediately. Adults, on the other hand, are not apt to exert themselves mightily for trinkets and tidbits. Still, for those who are good candidates for therapy, improved performance has intrinsic rewards.

An approach to reinforcement applicable to children and adults is based on work by Premack (1959, 1961, 1963a,b) and has been elaborated by Homme (1965, 1966). The basic conception of this differential probability hypothesis, sometimes called the *Premack principle,* is that for any pair of responses, the more probable one will reinforce the less probable one on which it is made contingent. This principle takes cognizance of the tendency for motivations to fluctuate; what is reinforcing one minute may be neutral or aversive the next. Restated, what is high in probability one minute may be low the next. For example, the speech pathologist, ever alert for high-probability behavior to be made contingent on desired speech performance, may observe a child sneaking glances at construction work next door—high-probability behavior. By making a half-minute view of construction contingent on the low-probability speech response, the speech pathologist uses the former to reinforce the latter. This principle seems too simple to be effective, but effective it seems to be.

Schedules of reinforcement, each yielding a characteristic response pattern, are plentiful; they range from variable and fixed interval and ratio schedules to schedules for differential reinforcement of high and low rates. Of particular clinical relevance are schedules to initiate and terminate therapy. Generally, *continuous reinforcement* (crf) should be used early in treatment, when the rate of correct speech response is low. Although most effective for increasing the frequency of occurrence, this schedule does not make a response resistant to *extinction*. Therefore, once an adequate response rate is achieved, large *variable ratios* (VR) and *variable intervals* (VI) are preferred. These schedules make the sequence of reinforcements and intervals between reinforcements unpredictable; the result is steady *emission* of the response in expectation of eventual reinforcement. Variable schedules not only build permanence of response; they also are more typical of reinforcement conditions found in everyday life (Brookshire, 1967).

Speech therapy. Speech therapy has evolved for the most part from useful techniques for modifying speech. Unlike operant therapy that is an applied form of operant conditioning principles, speech therapy has grown largely by pragmatic trial and error. Attempts to fit it within a theoretical framework have come from two directions. Backus (1957), drawing heavily from field theory, general semantics, interpersonal theory, and client-centered therapy principles, devised a system of group therapy within which psychotherapeutic objectives could be met while achieving specific alterations in speech. On the other hand, Van Riper and Irwin (1958), using Fairbanks' (1954) model of the speech mechanism as a servosystem, conceive of the *feedback theory* as the rationale for the corrective process.

Backus and Beasley (1951) hold that the greatest potential for speech therapy is in the use of speech for creating significant and satisfying interpersonal relationships. To this end they recommend working from conversational speech to facilitate the following:

1. The principle that learning proceeds by differentiation from whole to parts
2. The principle that learning involves perceptual organization of new wholes
3. Changes in self-image, social skills, and speech production
4. Handling the problem of transfer of training

Seeking much the same destination from the opposite direction, Van Riper (1972), by implementing the feedback theory of speech therapy, isolates and corrects defective parts of speech before attempting to incorporate them within a conversational context. The corrective process, by analogy to automatic control systems, includes three basic functions: *scanning, comparing,* and *correcting.* What is scanned by the client in speech therapy is auditory and somesthetic feedback from his own speech output. This feedback is then compared with the pattern to be achieved. If a discrepancy exists, output is corrected until feedback matches the desired pattern. Normal children, presumably following some such sequence to acquire intelligible speech, scan their own efforts, compare how they sound with how adults sound, and gradually correct their output to adult standards, at which time speech is *stabilized* and becomes automatic. The child no longer need compare his performance by ear with external standards; he now has "built-in" criteria for how his speech should sound and feel, either or both of which he can use for automatic control.

The person who stabilized defective speech has apparently stopped listening to himself in comparison with a normal model. Therefore, speech therapy, as Van Riper and Irwin (and probably the majority of speech clinicians) conceive it, is designed first to reacquaint the client with the sound of appropriate speech to be achieved, a process called *ear training.* With the speech pattern to be produced identified, the defective segment is scanned and compared, varied and corrected, and finally stabilized in isolation and then in progressively more complex contextual settings. Shelton (1968) and his associates are finding that this sequence involves distinct learning phases. Drawing heavily from motor learning, they have schematized permanent mastery of a skill into acquisition-generalization-automatization phases of remediation.

Speech therapy vis-à-vis operant and insight therapy. Casting speech therapy in the larger context of operant therapy derived from learning principles and of insight therapy derived from personality theory, Van Riper and Irwin's system fits within the former, whereas Backus' approach is closer to the latter. These divergent forms of speech therapy are complementary: the strength of one is the weakness of the other.

Backus strives to maintain the integrity of the whole person by working on speech in conversational contexts. This approach accords well with the insight therapist's concerns but poses a distinct problem for correction of specific defects, the forte of operant therapy. Efficient modification of behavior requires that reinforcement or punishment be immediately contingent on the behavior to be altered. Not only does conversation complicate the clinician's effort to administer contingent consequences promptly, but use of groups makes necessary attention to any one group member for effective correction of his speech virtually impossible.

By contrast, Van Riper and Irwin's principles of speech therapy translate into operant therapy with little difficulty. They, along with most other speech pathologists who write about the treatment of articulation disorders especially, identify in detail the segments of speaking behavior to be corrected and how they should sound. These basic requirements are essential for obtaining operant base-line measures and for determining terminal behavior toward which defective speech can be shaped. They also detail the steps by which isolated speech segments, once corrected, can be extended systematically to daily conversation—a close parallel to the operant extension of stimulus control of responses. They have little to say, however, about the vital issue of contingencies of reinforcement, and even less to say about problems of resistance, disturbance, and other humanistic concerns of insight therapists.

All in all, speech therapy is long on

identification of standard and defective articulatory behavior, probably because of detailed phonetic descriptions available from linguistic studies. Descriptive precision of behavioral dimensions of language, voice, and speech-flow drops off sharply. Notably lacking, too, considering the speech pathologist's reliance on the learning process as his sole tool of therapy, is a theoretical grounding of speech therapy in principles of learning. It does not regularly violate these principles, but neither does it profit from them maximally.

Counseling

Counseling has many facets. It can be used to resolve psychodynamic conflicts. Z. Wolpe (1957), for example, describes a form for parents designed to resolve conflicts in themselves that they have visited on their children. Counseling can be used to help the handicapped live gracefully and effectively with a speech impairment so long as it persists (Johnson and others, 1967). It can be used to instruct clients, parents, spouses, teachers, and friends in the ways in which they can facilitate rehabilitation (Webster, 1966). We will consider the latter forms of counseling. The first, important as it can be for symptomatic disorders (therapy Model IV), involves a psychotherapeutic relation for which the speech pathologist is likely not to be prepared.

Johnson and his associates (1967) described several tactics by which the speech handicapped can be helped to live with their problems, a type of counseling especially relevant for clients caught in the vicious circle of therapy Model II. Foremost is acceptance of one's best without resentment or apology—provided it is the best that can be accomplished currently. Too, shortcomings are more palatable when kept in perspective, a matter of according full value to one's assets and of weighing judiciously the realistic consequences of one's disorders. Another antidote to the potential devastation of defectiveness is the freedom to talk about it impersonally, objectively, and intelligently. Handicapped persons who, by silence, hope that their impairment will pass unnoticed trap themselves coming and going. If they fail, the importance of their obvious difficulty is escalated to the status of "touchy subject." If they succeed, they are in worse trouble: they put themselves under constant pressure to maintain the deception of the first impression, thereby magnifying what may be a small defect into a mountainous difficulty.

Instructional counseling is particularly relevant to therapy Models I, II, and III, in which direct correction of impaired speech is a primary objective. The clinician cannot hope to effect permanent improvements by his direct efforts alone: 1 or 2 hours out of the 168 of each week afford small leverage for the modification of behavior. The client and his spouse, parents, teachers, or friends will have to cooperate, even to the extent of administering contingencies of reinforcement. To be of help, they must be instructed in exactly what to do, and why. The more they understand the nature of the problem, the more sensible assistance they can offer, not only in carrying out schedules of reinforcement, but also in modifying the client's environment where it may be a major factor: a child with vocal nodules in a family of "screamers" is unlikely to improve until the decibel level at home is lowered.

Role playing, as described by Webster (1968), can be a particularly useful counseling tool for speech pathologists. Cooperation outside the clinic is particularly essential for carryover. A major reason for the difficulty of this phase is that stimulus control established in the clinic is not successively approximated to daily living conditions. Clinical sessions can be used, then, for demonstration and instruction in procedures to follow until the next session.

METHODS OF SPEECH REMEDIATION

Speech pathology is showing a major sign of maturation. Its members are shifting their emphasis to evaluation of the effectiveness of their clinical procedures. The first questions that skilled clinicians ask these days about techniques are: "How well do they work?" "How thoroughly have they been tested?" If

the answers are satisfying, then they return to their favorite question of earlier years: "How do you do it?"

This author feels that he would be remiss to present detailed accounts of how he does therapy. Were space in this text unlimited, he would probably be unable to avoid the temptation. Therapy is a personal encounter of a clinician with his clients. This encounter is fraught with pitfalls that resist measurement and documentation. Fortunately, since seasoned clinicians such as Blakeley (1972) and Van Riper (1972) have published personal accounts of their therapeutic experiences with a multitude of persons having a wide range of communication disorders, the need for another personalized account is not pressing.

The purpose of this book is to present an evenhanded account of the best information available to the profession. The mature student, then, needs the answers to the following questions concerning clinical procedures for a particular problem: What methods are available? How reliable are they? Where can I find out how to administer them?

Most of the methods used for remediating communicative disorders fit under one of three banners these days: psychotherapy, behavioral modification (operant therapy), and speech therapy. How does a clinician evaluate the relative merits of each? If one assumed equal reliability of results, the procedure of choice would best meet the following criteria:

1. The changes produced would be relevant to those sought by the handicapped individual.
2. Observable and measurable behavior would be modified, thereby permitting prediction and control, plus evaluation, of therapeutic effects.
3. Applications of demonstrated principles of learning would be logical.
4. The approach to therapy would be feasible for use by virtue of the clinician's training.

Psychotherapy is for the most part beyond our consideration by the fourth criterion: most speech pathologists are not trained to use it as a primary therapeutic tool. Certainly they may use its procedures as adjuncts to therapy, as E. Cooper (1965) has done with

---

Travis (1971a,b) offers a vivid description of how the psychotherapeutic process operates and how it can be applied successfully to adults who stutter; Z. Wolpe (1957) and Haney (1971) describe its application to children. Many others have written about this approach (Barbara, 1962; Hejna, 1963; Murphy and FitzSimons, 1960).

---

his interpersonal communication therapy, and certainly they should understand its principles, but most will not be prepared to rely on it as the major method of effecting therapeutic change. They must recognize, though, that it will often be needed in large measure with problems such as autism, infantile speech, functional dysphonia and aphonia, and some cases of stuttering. Its need in small measure is likely to be present with most disorders of speech, if only to cope with the resistance and disturbance that often accompany efforts to alter personally important behavior. But adequate discussion of psychotherapeutic procedures would take us too far afield, so we will focus on procedures for modifying speaking behavior and language.

Because speech therapy is just as behavioral as behavioral modification (the former derived pragmatically, the latter from operant learning principles), the same general therapeutic considerations underlie most of the methods for remediating speech that will be considered. From assessment the speech pathologist determines dimensions of the problem as exactly as possible. He makes this determination by comparing what the client does with what he should be able to do (Chapters 11 to 15). Holding this goal as the terminal behavior to be achieved, the clinician is ready to undertake therapy. He must now find responses that can be systematically modified to the desired form; the closer they approach terminal behavior, the less difficult the therapeutic task will be. If the response already exists but occurs too infrequently, its rate can be increased. If it exists but in the wrong context, its occurrence can be ob-

tained under appropriate conditions by stimulus control. If only segments of it are available, they can be shaped by successive approximation to their terminal form. If it is part of a systematic sequence, prerequisite abilities can be established prior to obtaining the desired response. If it exists in isolation but is needed in a larger context, it can be chained with other responses into an appropriate series.

In a word, the clinician must begin where his client can perform without failure and, by careful selection of types and schedules of reinforcement, move step by step to the terminal goal. No step is taken until its success is assured. At the first sign of failure the therapist mounts a strategic retreat to a point at which successful performance can be reestablished.

Therapy of language disorders

Disorders of language may involve vocabulary, grammar, and functional use of speech for communication. Although these aspects, singly or in combination, characterize any linguistic deficit, remedial methods reflect the nature of the disorder. Programs for cognitively impaired children who are profoundly retarded are somewhat different from programs for those who are moderately retarded. Treatment of the aphasic child may differ from that of the autistic child or the child with a learning disability; for that matter, it may also differ from treatment of the aphasic adult. As for persons who speak nonstandard English, their problems are entirely different. This discussion will reflect these differences.

Remediation of delayed language development. Without doubt mute, unresponsive children, whether severely retarded or psychotic, can be taught imitative speech. They can even be taught to use these responses to label concrete events and express simple demands—that is, they can make and use vocal utterances functionally. Herein lies the crucial reservation—are these responses clever imitations such as might be taught to "talking animals," or do they indeed constitute meaningful speech? Of course, for behaviorists, meaning is mentalistic, unmeasurable, and hence meaningless. Theirs is a functional test: if imitative vocal responses do everything that "meaningful speech" does, then by functional definition it is speech. In any event, the following practical questions are relevant: "How far toward normal conversational speech can these cognitively impaired children progress?" "How far back must the therapy program reach to maximize a child's chances for language development?"

To begin, if more than imitative utterances are sought, therapeutic conditions must facilitate a child's insight into how language works. We should seek procedures that can, by starting where the child is in his development, aid him in progressively unfolding, layer by layer, the various stages of language acquisition. By analyzing functional units of

---

How does this approach compare with that of Wood (1964), who has pioneered in the language problems of children?

---

language behavior, and by knowing the normal sequence in which these units develop, we should eventually be able to make

---

Lee (1969), noting that transformational complexity, more than sentence length, is important to language acquisition, has provided a lucidly detailed example of how a clinician could help a child progressively unravel linguistic confusion by first recognizing basic kernel sentences and then building a set of transformational operations that could be applied to them.

---

explicit for any child the linguistic behavior that he would have to acquire as his next step. By arranging contingencies of reinforcement for each step, we should be able to make maximum use of whatever capacity he has to move along the route to normal language.

This rosy glow of what could be accomplished is clouded mainly by conditions of readiness for language. Their exact dimensions are still fuzzy, but we can see them clearly enough to have a good suspicion of those that will foster linguistic growth.

Anything that will aid motor development and maturation of the brain should help. Anything that will aid sensory input, auditory input especially, should help. Anything that will aid perception and the temporal organization of sound sequence should help. Anything that will aid in the storing and retrieving of perceptual discriminations should help. And anything that will aid in social use of language should help.

Here again, a vista of opportunities spreads before us, few of which have been thoroughly explored. Richardson (1967), for instance, has described methods based on the Montessori approach for early sensorimotor training as preparation for language learning. Equipment and techniques are available for selective amplification of auditory sensory input; other sensory inputs can be masked if they are confusing. Speech can be spoken slowly or recorded and played back slowly to help the child who has difficulty sorting out the temporal order of speech events. Then, as Luria (1961) and the Russian investigators have shown, memory functions and transfer of learning can be facilitated by enlarging a child's vocabulary of meaningful words.

Too, Schiefelbusch (1967), analyzing the role of language in the child's interaction with his environment, has shown how feedback of effects produced with speech help to guide the course of language development. More recently, Muma (1975) has analyzed communication as a game involving "dump and play" operations used to achieve effective and efficient interpersonal communication. This type of analysis points up the nuances involved in adapting the sending and receiving of messages to ensure their reception. The development of skills on this level of communication, however, requires sufficient mastery of semantics and grammar to be able to shade the meaning of an idea one way or another.

Such leads as these are derived largely from principles of learning and from work in psycholinguistics. From them, and from applications of systems analysis and programming, have come the beginnings of systematic attempts to design, administer, and evaluate programs for children with language disorders.

Remediation of language disorders of mentally retarded children. Schiefelbusch (1972) reviewed the few longitudinal programs that have attempted to evaluate the effectiveness of teaching language to cognitively impaired children. A sampling of a couple of these programs gives an idea of the strategies used. Lent's group divide their program into a preverbal and verbal section. Attending behavior, motor imitation, and vocal imitation are stressed preverbally, whereas receptive language and a prelinguistic expressive repertoire are stressed in the verbal section. Each section is divided into phases, and each phase is divided into parts. The parts have initial inventories with which to assess those tasks the child can perform and those he cannot. He is trained to master all parts before proceeding to the next phase.

Spradlin, Baer, and Butterfield (1970) have devised a similar language-training strategy (shown diagramatically in Fig. 16-1). Their functional program is devised for teaching increasingly complex language. It requires sequential steps in which later linguistic forms are dependent on earlier achievements.

What can be accomplished with these and other training strategies? The answer, of course, depends on many considerations, not the least of which are the nature and extent of retardation. With the moderately retarded who have language, albeit not very intelligible, Lent (1968) has shown that operant procedures can be used successfully. Children in his Mimosa Cottage project not only improved articulation but also improved use of speech in facilitating social relations and preparing for return to the community. Success can also be achieved with disadvantaged children. Their langauge complexity and output of spontaneous speech can move in a year from the level of Head Start children to that of professors' children (Risley, Hart, and Doke, 1972).

With severely retarded children, improvement still seems possible, but it is far more modest. Imitative speech responses, even of some length, seem to pose no particular problem. How far they can reach in rule-governed language is another matter. As many as 25% of mute children have learned rudimentary language responses after herculean training efforts (Baer, Guess, and Sherman, 1972; Bricker, 1972). Clearly, children raised in institutions are more retarded in speech and language development than are those raised at home. Ironically, the institutional children are the ones who can make the greatest progress when placed in a residential family unit. Presumably, that part of their retardation which can be attributed to their deprived institutional life can be offset, at least in part, with an enriched environment (Lyle, 1960). That part of retardation, however, which reflects organic impairment does not seem much amenable to improvement (Kirk, 1958).

Remediation of language disorders of autistic children. The autistic child (a term generally used interchangeably with the psychotic child) exhibits a different pattern of disabilities from those of the mentally retarded child. Although the involvement affects many aspects of performance, from aloof interpersonal relations to impaired intellect to deviant language, still the nature of these disabilities appears to be different (Chapter 10).

The language impairment, for example, seems to be more deviant than delayed. Whereas the mentally retarded primarily show delay in acquiring linguistic rules of grammar and articulation, autistic deficits are characterized more by inability to analyze both verbal and nonverbal patterns in terms of functional relationships. Thus, the psychotic child can name objects, but he uses the name echoically rather than meaningfully to express an idea. These special problems probably must be considered in any language-training program for psychotic children.

Baltaxe and Simmons (1975) have reviewed these programs and report success ranging from minimal to moderate. The ma-

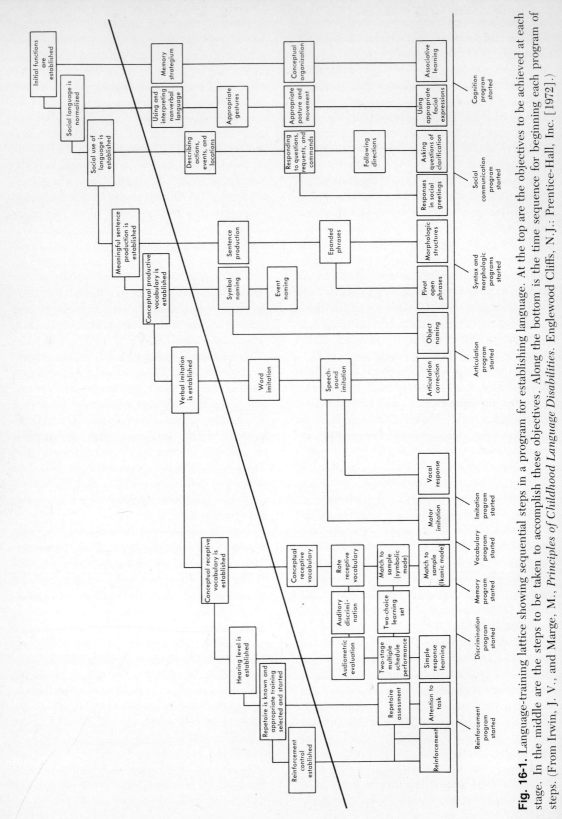

Fig. 16-1. Language-training lattice showing sequential steps in a program for establishing language. At the top are the objectives to be achieved at each stage. In the middle are the steps to be taken to accomplish these objectives. Along the bottom is the time sequence for beginning each program of steps. (From Irwin, J. V., and Marge, M., *Principles of Childhood Language Disabilities*. Englewood Cliffs, N.J.: Prentice-Hall, Inc. [1972].)

jority are based on a skinnerian model of language acquisition-by-imitation and reinforcement. The direction that they suspect is most profitable couples behavior modification techniques with psycholinguistic findings. Such behavioral interventions as Lovaas (1968) has described can presumably be used to assemble an efficient vehicle for establishing linguistic rules rather than imitative behavior.

Such an approach has been taken by Hirsch and Silvertson (1975). They have designed a comprehensive educational program for the schools, with heavy emphasis on language and individualized instruction. They used Eisenson's (1972) five stages of morphemic development in a highly structured framework. Their results are encouraging. Of fifteen children who had no functional language, twelve improved in comprehension and thirteen showed marked improvement in expression. Preschoolers outgained school-age children, which is an argument for early intervention. But older children did progress, even though not as much as the younger ones.

In London, a study of effects of three different educational approaches was made (Bartak and Rutter, 1971). One was psychotherapeutic, one was educational within a permissive environment, and one was a highly structured educational environment. In none of the environments were operant principles of reinforcement used optimally. Even so, effects of these different approaches were clearly discernible. Not surprisingly, austistic children in the highly structured approach showed the greatest progress (Rutter and Bartak, 1973). Still, all the approaches yielded significant gains, but more in mechanical skills than in understanding. When the children failed to understand what was said to them, they were apt to respond with echolalia and disruptive, stereotyped behavior—hence the importance of stressing cognitive operations of meaning and understanding rather than mechanical mastery of rote responses.

Remediation of language disorders of children with aphasia. Autistic children differ from aphasic children mainly in their need for greater structure in the treatment process. Both have a central language impairment that disrupts their ability to interpret their auditory environment. Accordingly, both have great difficulty in learning oral language, and because they do not learn language naturally by ear, their whole basis for learning to read and write and think abstractly is seriously affected. But this is the focus of the difficulty with aphasic children. With autistic children, the involvement is more profound (Churchhill, 1972). All their sensory channels seem to be affected. Their ability to organize perception of their world is therefore seriously impaired, whether by vision, touch, or audition (Wing, 1966). Probably for this reason, the autistic child must rely on the treatment program to provide structure for his perception that he is not innately equipped to provide for himself.

The aphasic child is more fortunate. Since his visual and auditory channels are largely uninvolved, he is able to establish a reasonably organized view of his world. His problem is how to make sense of the sounds he hears. What he needs is a program that gives him a chance to sort out his auditory environment, especially the speech aspects of it, and fit it with the cognitive structure he has already worked out through his visual and somesthetic senses.

Such programs can be considerably more flexible than for autistic children. Some utilize such a framework as Eisenson's (1972) stages of morphemic development. Some stress Myklebust's (1971) interpsychoneurosensory and intrapsychoneurosensory principles of learning. Some employ programmed materials available commercially (Gray and Ryan, 1971). Some are built around Piaget's concepts of language as it relates to cognitive development. And some combine these approaches in various ways. They all have in common a heavy emphasis on auditory stimulation and mastery of the perception and production of oral language.

Remediation of language disorders of children with minimal brain dysfunction and learning disabilities. Children with minimal brain dysfunction and learning disabilities do have language problems, but they mainly involve the visual system. Were the auditory system impaired, their innate capacity to acquire oral language would be affected; they would probably be aphasic. They have speech, however. Their language disorders are chiefly in the areas of reading and writing. Because these disorders are somewhat tangential to our major concern with oral language, we will sketch only briefly the special education programs designed for them.

Children with learning disabilities appear to be equipped to learn normally, but they do not do so. Their disturbance in cognitive processes is presumed to entail minimal brain dysfunction. The fact that the number of "hard" and "soft" neurologic signs seems to be roughly proportional to the amount of learning deficit supports this presumption (Myklebust, 1975). Thus minimal brain dysfunction and learning disabilities are not separate problems in reality, but, depending on the child's behavior, they may be dealt with differently in the special educational programs for them.

The hyperactive, distractible child, the so-called "brain-injured" child, who poses behavior problems as well as severe learning deficits will probably be placed in an educationally handicapped class (Wood, 1964). Such classes are typically all-day, self-contained units of six to eight children. Management of disruptive behavior is often a necessary prelude to educational endeavors.

Those children with learning disabilities who can function in a regular classroom are usually given an hour or two a day of special assistance, perhaps in specially equipped and staffed resource rooms. Such assistance may also be provided by itinerant consultants, who may work with the children or only with their teachers.

Approaches to treatment of these children vary. Some stress visual-motor capabilities and largely ignore auditory input. This emphasis is for the sake of developing reading and writing skills necessary for successful academic performance. Other approaches use a multisensory approach to accomplish the same objective. Auditory, tactile, and kinesthetic channels are used along with the visual (Gearheart, 1973). Among the most popular, though, are approaches that stress language acquisition (Kirk and Kirk, 1971; Johnson and Mykelbust, 1967), in which auditory functioning is as important as visual functioning.

Rehabilitation of aphasia in adults. Wepman (1969) observed that too many patients improve and too many fail without our knowing why. As he says, if we even knew the stages through which those who do recover progress, we might begin to understand why others do not improve. Scientific inquiry has been addressed more to the nature of aphasia than to recovery from it. This discrepancy led Holland (1969) to identify three cogent problems: first, we have more principles for aphasia therapy than specific implementations of those principles; second, lacking specific techniques to evaluate, we are woefully short of hard data on the efficacy of language therapy; and third, because aphasic patients are often not referred for treatment until the possibility of spontaneous recovery has been exhausted, they arrive in the speech pathologist's office after the period of maximum therapeutic effectiveness has passed with the first year after brain injury.

Clearly, the need for tangible therapeutic goals and methods of achieving them is urgent. We can look to three sources for guidance. Some clinicians have published procedures they use, presumably with reasonably good results (Longerich and Bordeaux, 1954; Agranowitz and McKeown, 1964). A few clinical programs have been developed and refined through research (Wepman, 1951, 1953, 1958; Eisenson, 1973, 1975; Sarno, Silverman, and Sands, 1970; Schuell, Jenkins, and Jiminez-Pabon, 1964; Luria, 1970), others through application of operant principles of learning (Holland, 1970). Finally, we can infer from knowledge of aphasia the goals that, logically, need to be achieved. From these sources, and particularly from Eisenson's (1973) rationale of recovery, the following picture of therapy for aphasic persons emerges.

Facilitation of language recovery. What conditions must a clinician consider to plan effective therapy for an adult with aphasia? First, recovery probably depends on neural reorganization. As Schuell, Jenkins, and Jiminez-Pabon (1964) observed, repeated sensory stimulation is essential for organization, storage, and retrieval of patterns in the brain under normal conditions. They concluded that it would be strange if the same requirement of sensory stimulation does not also apply to language and its recovery. As for the primary type of stimulation needed, it should probably be auditory. It is by these processes that language is acquired normally. They are the processes invariably impaired in aphasia, and it is retention span for auditory information that is invariably reduced in aphasia.

Another consideration is the likelihood that recovery of function involves neural reorganization that bypasses defective neural systems in favor of developing new circuitry. Luria (1970) is convinced that the only means of compensating for functions lost to cortical damage is the transferral of those functions to undamaged brain structures. This approach often involves learning to accomplish old functions in new ways. Such recovery rarely culminates in the reorganized function's becoming completely automatic, nor does it result in establishment of a function identical to the one that was lost. Whether aphasic language must be recovered by progression through stages is a moot question. Nevertheless, the need to pass through stages would not necessarily imply that the aphasic person must pass through each stage as he improves, nor would it imply that such stages are equivalent to those a child passes through as he learns language naturally.

The adult aphasic patient's innate capacity to acquire language has long since waned. Moreover, his once-mastered linguistic knowledge, though somehow impaired, is undoubtedly quite different from that of the child who is still figuring it out. Thus, in all likelihood, the clinician does not teach an aphasic patient something he does not already know. Rather, therapy helps a patient to retrieve what he knows more readily than if he were left to his own devices.

Whether therapeutic effectiveness is best served by programmed instruction or by conventional patient-clinician contact probably depends on the preference and training of the clinician. Eisenson (1973) prefers programmed instruction as an adjunct. Sarno, Silverman, and Sands (1970) used it and found no more improvement with severely impaired global aphasics than when they were treated conventionally.

On the other hand, taking the premise that aphasia rehabilitation is mainly a process of reestablishing a circumscribed basic vocabulary and grammar from which refinements can be generalized, Holland (1970) has demonstrated the effectiveness of programmed instruction. One program started with single sounds, moved to words, and then continued to syntactic phrases in regenerating the once-normal knowledge of language. Another program expanded auditory memory span and the ability to repeat spoken language, and still another extended the ability to retain meaningful material in complex sentences. Others dealt with senses other than hearing and with detecting and correcting spelling confusions. Such an approach furnishes measurable effects of clinical techniques, and it develops a close client-therapist interaction in which the programmer makes a series of "educated guesses." The learner tests their correctness by his performance, the program is revised accordingly, and then it is tried again.

That persons with aphasia can improve has been demonstrated repeatedly. Spontaneous recovery seems to be greatest during the first 2 months and then tapers off until 6 months have elapsed. That the speech pathologist can facilitate improvement has presumably been demonstrated in the thousands of hours of therapy with such patients. With rating-scale evaluations (Sands, Sarno, and Shankweiler 1969; Marks, Taylor, and Rusk 1957), as well as with quantitative PICA measures before and after treatment (Dabul and Hanson, 1975), significant improvement has been found from treatment begun one year after onset of aphasia. Dabul and Hanson discovered, however, that treatment beginning 6 months after onset is much more likely to be successful with patients above rather than below the 50th percentile on the overall PICA score. With early treatment, by contrast, low-scoring patients were likely to make large gains.

That anyone could say with assurance what problems have to be solved in what order to demonstrate improvement would, at this time, be problematic. The clearest fact is that aphasia, a disorder of untold magnitude psychologically as well as linguistically, can be helped significantly.

Nonlinguistic problems. Beyond the language deficit, a potential multitude of other problems may face the aphasic person. After injury, measured intelligence and educational achievement tend to be lowered, but fortunately the loss is frequently reversed with recovery. The abilities to discriminate, to make rapid judgments, and to plan effectively seem to be typically impaired. Behavioral aberrations and personality changes that exaggerate pretrauma characteristics are often observed, but they, too, can return toward normal as language and insight are regained. The ability to monitor and correct errors in one's own performance can provide an index not only of severity but also of recovery from aphasia as egocentric interest in only those concrete conditions of direct value to immediate needs gives way to broader interests. Impulsive "catastrophic" reactions are notorious, but they appear to be more related to frustration and stress than to inability to sustain a performance within reduced limits of the injured capacity. Conversely, euphoria is typical during the period after injury, and, although unrealistic, it can be utilized to facilitate early therapy. Perhaps the most disabling condition is withdrawal and loss of initiative as the aphasic patient, who fatigues easily, becomes convinced through repeated failures to communicate effectively that he is helpless and hopeless (Wepman, 1951, 1958; Spreen, 1968; Brookshire, 1968).

All these conditions at best are mild deterrents to recovery, but they can be devastating. Are they independent consequences of brain injury, of aphasic impairment, or of interacting effects that exacerbate linguistic and nonlinguistic problems alike? Probably the latter. With certainty, though, they must be considered in any program of rehabilitation. They must be considered by all who will be involved; seeds of recovery must be tended on a full-time basis. After injury, the physician and hospital staff will be of vital importance, not only for treatment of physical conditions that frequently include hemiplegia, convulsions, facial paralysis, and hemianopia, but, equally important, for coping with the inevitable psychologic problems and aiding in the rehabilitation of language. With return home, this burden shifts to the family, who can make or break prospects of recovery.

The speech pathologist's role. The speech pathologist will play a different, and in some ways more crucial, role. By virtue of his professional responsibility for the central area of concern, language disturbance, he finds himself, perhaps inadvertently, at the hub of recovery operations. For one thing, he cannot rehabilitate language in a vacuum. He must know how speech interacts with all facets of the aphasic patient's life. But even seeing the patient daily would not be often enough. In a sense, he must share the podium with the physician in conducting the psycholinguistic portions of the rehabilitation orchestra. Nurses and family members will play their tunes longer and often louder than will the speech pathologist. But if he has the whole linguistic and nonlinguistic score from which to conduct rehabilitation, he can obtain harmony where cacophony might otherwise prevail.

His overture to therapy must begin early for several reasons. The most urgent need is to head off the sense of devastation that can overwhelm the aphasic individual as he recuperates from his initial shock and physical debilitation. With dawning realization of the scope of damage, discouragement and frustration can be monumental. Paradoxically, at first he will probably be euphoric and unconcerned about his condition: a predictable consequence of brain injury. Too, whatever spontaneous recovery is possible will occur in the early months after trauma. These two conditions offer motivational leverage that can make the difference between successful and unsuccessful rehabilitation. Couple this advantage with the progress that can be achieved with therapy, and the need for initiating early training is apparent.

Equally as important as demonstrating concern and the prospect for improvement is the need to forestall the conviction on the part of the aphasic patient and his family that his condition is hopeless. The inclination on all sides will be either to overprotect or reject. Initially helpless, he is easy prey for either attitude. These attitudes can best be prevented by involving him as early as possible in active (as opposed to spectator) participation, first in the hospital and later at home. Too, a realistic evaluation of his prospects for recovery should reflect his pretraumatic condition as well as the extent of his injury. How closely he can approach his original intellectual and personality condition will depend heavily on his sense of hope and determination.

Treating language problems of disadvantaged children. A battlefront in President Johnson's War on Poverty was improvement of the verbal ability of the economically disadvantaged child. The task force assigned to this skirmish was the "Head Start" program. To some, success of such efforts must stem from recognition of two basic issues (Baratz, 1968). First, the language of the disadvantaged child's ethnic culture must be respected as his legitimate "native" language. Any other attitude devalues more than his speech; it devalues his culture, and it devalues him. Second, the need to learn standard English must be demonstrated as a need for a second dialect, not as a need to replace his nonstandard language with the standard version. In effect, the disadvantaged child, if he is to move beyond his ethnic culture and yet not deny it, will need to be bilingual in English.

Shriner (1971) takes issue with several of Baratz' assumptions and concludes his review of language skills of the economically deprived by citing Bereiter and Engelmann's (1966) controversial instructional program for such children. It probably stands at one end of the educational continuum as an effective method of filling the minds of these children with as many facts as are stuffed into the heads of their middle-class peers. The objection is that it utilizes repetitious rote learning with little attempt to facilitate thinking.

Unfortunately, the other end of the educational continuum for teaching oral standard English to disadvantaged children is so ill defined as to be nonexistent. Shuy (1972) tells of the difficulties he had tracking down such programs as could be found. They had, for the most part, been developed in total isolation from each other. Worse, the materials lean heavily on foreign language teaching techniques, with little input from linguistic research as to the nature of nonstandard English.

Therapy of articulatory-resonatory disorders

Articulatory disorders, being deviations from standard phonemes of the language, have been the traditional focus for speech correction, probably because desired terminal behavior can be specified explicitly. The problem seems simple: alter the sounds of speech produced improperly until they are aligned with linguistic norms. The clinician must resolve two basic issues to achieve this solution. First, he must decide what the goal he seeks will be. Will it be ability to discriminate perceptually all phonemes of the language, or will it be ability to produce distinctive features of all phonemes acceptably? Although interrelated, these skills are distinctly separate, the former involving input processes, the latter, output processes. For the second basic issue, he must select initial behavior to be modified into terminal form. Should therapy start with "ear training"—a perceptual skill—or with production skills as close to terminal form as possible? Let us consider the relative merits of both sides of these two issues.

Perception versus production: is ear training necessary? Perceptual differentiation of speech sounds can be a primary goal to facilitate understanding in disorders of language; it is a means to the end of intelligible speech in articulatory disorders. The following question is relevant in the achievement of normal articulation: How essential is awareness of differences among phonemes? Van Riper and Irwin (1958) argue cogently from their feedback theory premise that speech is learned by ear; only after articulation is stabilized— correctly or defectively—does one cease to monitor production by ear. Therefore, to improve defective articulation one must listen to the correct sound so that the error in what is done habitually can be detected—hence the necessity for beginning therapy with ear training.

Mowrer, Baker, and Schutz (1968) argue from learning principles that auditory discrimination may not, in fact, be the basis of improved articulation after ear training; other variables may account for both improved perception and production. Research from learning and speech laboratories favors their position. The efficacy of ear training is based on the assumption that the production of a desired response is a function of perception of the form that a response should take. The motor theory of speech perception turns the case around: speech is decoded in terms of equivalent motor speech patterns (Liberman and others, 1967). Furthermore, as Goldiamond (1962b) has demonstrated, perceptual responses are determined by their consequences. Perceptions, like motor responses, are differentiated as they are differentially reinforced. But differential motor responses are not established by reinforcing perception, nor vice versa. Although perception and production of speech are normally interrelated, each is a separate skill. Presumably, improvement of one does not automatically ensure improvement of the other.

The issue of ear training as a goal, then, depends on the issue of selecting auditory discrimination as the point of departure for the modification of articulatory behavior. In theory, ear training, as efficient application of learning principles, falls short if it does not contribute directly to the modification of articulation. In practice, it does no harm. The worst that could be said of it is that it may be inefficient, possibly to the extent of doubling the number of therapeutic steps.

Despite theoretical doubts, many speech clinicians have faith in the commonsense objective of ear training: the client should be able to recognize the standard sound he is to learn before he attempts to make it. They point to their success with clients who, thoroughly prepared with ear training, make the transition to correct sound production with ease. They also find merit in it as a starting point for shy children who will not produce vocal utterances. To these ends, Van Riper (1972) describes four sets of ear-training techniques in detail. The first begins with listening procedures that *isolate* the target sound from its confusing phonetic context. Then its auditory characteristics are *identified*, and the client is *stimulated* with the sound to ensure its recognition. The final step of *discriminating* correct from incorrect sounds should be relatively easy. This procedure is demonstrably effective for teaching auditory discrimination.

In the final analysis, however, the objective of articulatory therapy is correction of speech sound production; auditory discrimination is incidental to this goal. Conceivably, speech could be corrected without increased perceptual awareness of phonemic distinctions. After all, since most normal speakers are oblivious to these distinctions, we can legitimately question the value of auditory discrimination for its own sake (Milisen, 1966). On the other hand, Garrett (1968) reports the effects of programmed discriminative training of normal, aphasic, and retarded children that generalized to improved articulatory production, even though the procedures should have improved only sound discrimination—theoretically. Thus the question of whether or not alternate routes to improved articulation are more expeditious than ear training or some programmed-discrimination version of it remains unanswered.

Modification of articulation. Behavior modifiers would hold that application of operant learning principles through the technology of programmed instruction offers the most efficient means of correcting articulation. Mowrer, Baker, and Schutz (1968), who have demonstrated such a program for correcting a frontal lisp, stress two operant

---

Holland and Matthews (1968) describe the general application of teaching machine concepts to speech pathology, and McDearmon (1968) describes specific applications to phonics.

---

procedures: successive approximation and differential reinforcement. Because incorrect articulatory responses occur under stimulus conditions that would normally control correct responses, reinforcement of error sounds is likely to persist unintentionally. Extreme care is required in introducing stimuli under which only the correct sound is reinforced. This idea has been stressed in speech therapy for years: avoid beginning treatment with familiar words with which old articulation habits are strongest.

The same arguments that justify ear training are applicable to successive approximations of correct articulatory responses. By selecting behavior to modify that the client already produces, avoidance of failure is assured; it may be as far removed from the terminal goal of articulating /s/, for example, as putting the tongue behind the teeth. The point is that since speech is produced by movements of speech organs, it is the movements that must be controlled. Therefore existing movement patterns closest to the terminal form offer the obvious starting point. Because some part of any speech movement is available in anyone alive and breathing, behavior with which to start successive approximations always exists, rudimentary as it may be. In such cases, behavior must be shaped to its new form. Often, though, by careful articulation testing, the target sound can be found in certain phonetic contexts. Goda (1970) has developed drill materials to help the clinician locate and capitalize on these contexts. They are the

starting point for "integral stimulation therapy." Devised by Milisen (1954) prior to the advent of operant therapy in speech pathology, this approach utilizes procedures that are virtually indistinguishable from those of the behavior shapers. With the desired sound available, even though inconsistently, it need not be shaped. The problem is to extend its occurrence through the technique of stimulus control to replace error sounds.

Various pragmatic procedures from speech therapy can be adapted for use according to operant principles. In fact, similarities are so plentiful that differences between these two systems of therapy nearly vanish. Van Riper (1972), for instance, describes five tactics that could be considered variations of behavior-shaping procedures for obtaining target sounds: *progressive approximation*, in which the therapist joins the client in his error sound and then together they move through a series of transitional sounds, each closer to the standard sound; *auditory stimulation*, in which client imitates clinician; *modification of other sounds already mastered*, in which /s/, for example, can be reached by modifying /t/ or /θ/; and *phonetic placement* and *tongue exercises*—similar to the *moto-kinesthetic method* devised by Young and Hawk (1955)—in which the speech mechanism is moved into the positions needed for target sounds. Another tactic, *use of key words*, in which words containing the correct sound are used as reference guides for correction, resembles stimulus-control procedures of behavior modification.

The systematic steps recommended in speech therapy to reach the goal of normal conversational articulation also translate easily into operant terms. Mowrer, Baker, and Schutz (1968), as an example, recommend successive approximations starting with the sound in isolation, then in words and sentences, and eventually in free speech. Speech therapy follows the same sequence, but the steps are in smaller increments—an instance of outdoing operant therapists at their own strategy. Beginning with isolation (some prefer to start with the syllable as the speech unit), the sound is next ...ngthened and stabilized in unfamiliar nonsense syllables and words; then in short, simple familiar words, phrases, sentences, controlled conversation, and free conversation; and finally in situations outside the clinic by means of speech assignments. Limited nucleus situations are used in which correct speech is required, and in which parents, friends, and teachers are involved in the carryover process (Powers, 1971; Van Riper, 1972).

Given all these similarities, what, then, is the essential difference between speech therapy and operant therapy for articulatory-resonatory disorders? Aside from the fact that the former is largely pragmatically derived, whereas the latter is an application of learning principles, procedurally they overlap completely. To the extent that they differ, behavior modifiers are more systematic in their use of types and schedules of reinforcement, control of stimulus conditions, and planning of sequences of responses to obtain desired behavior.

Winitz (1975) has come as close as any to a successful marriage of traditional views of speech pathology with learning principles. But his is a ménage à trois; he also included phonologic theory in the wedding. What he offers is a sophisticated instructional model for the treatment of articulatory disorders. Grounded in distinctive-feature analysis, treatment proceeds from testing of articulatory production and paired-comparison discrimination, to use of acquisition principles (such as shaping procedures and facilitation of coarticulation), to transfer and recall of correct articulation in conversational speech.

Effectiveness of therapy: some comments. Which of these approaches to treatment is most effective? Surprisingly, we have little solid evidence with which to answer that question. Considering the high prevalence of articulatory disorders and their preponderance in the case load of most clinicians, one would think that we would be overrun with treatment effectiveness studies. Not so. The literature speaks loudly with descriptions of different versions of how to accomplish articulation therapy, but it is virtually silent about results the clinician can expect.

This dearth is regrettable, but it may speak more to the success rather than the frustrations of the therapeutic endeavor. Clinicians have traditionally viewed "simple" articulation disorders as relatively "easy" to treat. Many children outgrow these developmental disorders spontaneously. With improvement in much of one's case load assured by the maturation process, minimal dissatisfaction with therapeutic procedures would be expected. This spontaneous improvement may explain in part why we have not extensively explored this problem.

As we are increasing our knowledge of articulatory disorders and recognizing that they are intricately embedded in the complexity of language, we are shedding our notion that because they yield to treatment, they are simple. In fact, until we know how much of our success can be attributed to therapy rather than to spontaneous recovery, and how permanent are improvements that can be transferred from the clinic to everyday life, and which methods achieve the best results most efficiently, we cannot be certain which therapy does work and how well. Far from being simple, articulatory disorders may prove to be a new frontier in speech pathology.

Therapy of phonatory disorders

Therapy of vocal disorders has plagued speech pathologists more because we have known better what is wrong with a voice than how to make it right. Two approaches have prevailed. On one side, clinicians have worked with segmental elements that they could identify, mainly pitch and loudness. This approach has the merit of specificity. Techniques such as Fairbanks' (1960) for determining natural pitch level have been used extensively. Therapeutic procedures for measuring and modifying loudness have been less specific; for quality they have been vague. On the other side has been a holistic approach to treatment. Brodnitz (1965) and Murphy (1964), for example, stress that voice must be rehabilitated in relation to the needs of the whole person. Since the elements of voice interact in expressing these needs, they must be rehabilitated in a holistic context.

These approaches differ in emphasis; they are not mutually exclusive. Clinicians working either holistically or segmentally manipulate whatever vocal behavior they can control

---

Aronson (1969) describes interdisciplinary treatment of psychogenic aphonia. He illustrates the collaboration among psychiatry, laryngology, and speech pathology involved in successful remediation.

(usually pitch) and observe changes in other aspects of voice (usually loudness and quality). To this end Van Riper and Irwin's (1958) feedback theory of therapy applies: scan pitch, loudness, and quality feedback from one's own vocal performance, compare for differences with the vocal model to be achieved, correct vocal output to match the model, and stabilize the new voice. Taking this cybernetic tack, Shearer (1959) encourages trying a wide variety of pitches, loudnesses, and qualities in the search for combinations that will afford the best new base line for vocal production.

Establishing hygienic vocal production. Vocal rehabilitation would profit if the merits of segmental and holistic approaches could be merged. With delineation of vocal dimensions to be controlled, a clinician could recognize each component explicitly, understand how it contributes to the whole, and modify it appropriately. By contrast, when vocal elements appear indistinguishable in a symbiotic jumble of interrelations, he has no choice but to work either on isolated segments that can be identified or on the whole voice as an undifferentiated unit. With a holistic concept of optimal vocal balance as a goal, the clinician could unite independent components in the richly complex interactions of the normal voice that serve needs of the whole person. Recognition within this concept would be afforded the ease with which tension (emotional and otherwise) can pull voice out of balance. The objective of therapy, then, would be to provide the client

with tools with which to realign his voice easily, quickly, and surely.

The key to vocal hygiene and optimal balance is freedom from vocal constriction (Chapter 13). A variety of techniques is available to accomplish this end. Ear training can be used for self-listening, imitation, and comparison in the search for a new voice (Murphy, 1964; Cooper and Nahum, 1967). Breathing exercises can be used directly (Rubin and Lehrhoff, 1962; Greene, 1964; Berry and Eisenson, 1956) or indirectly (Brodnitz, 1965; Murphy, 1964). For some, relaxation is a by-product of correct pitch, breath control, and soft vocal attack (Moore, 1971). For others, it is a major emphasis—often incorporated with posture exercises (Van Thal, 1967; Greene, 1964; Rubin and Lehrhoff, 1962). Masking is suggested as a means of depriving a client of the sound of his defective vocal pattern while an improved voice is being established (West and Ansberry, 1968). Shaking of the jaw and rapid mandibular movement are recommended by Brodnitz (1965) and Palmer (1949) to counteract tightness. Briess (1959) works for restoration of normal dynamic laryngeal muscle balance. Actually, the list could be extended to include most of the forty techniques listed by Murphy (1964). Unfortunately, such an abundance of procedures bespeaks dissatisfaction with results achieved as much as it attests to clinical ingenuity.

Effectiveness of therapy. How can a clinician select from this plethora of tactics those most effective? Chances are that all have worked well with some clinician for some client at some time. What evaluations of clinical results are available offer limited help. Those few that are based on more than small samples of patients report their results in terms of subjective clinical impressions. These impressions are too easily inflated by the clinician's hope of what he has accomplished to place much confidence in them. Furthermore, little agreement exists among clinicians as to the mechanisms of vocal abuse to which the therapeutic endeavor is addressed. Voice therapy thus remains essentially an art (Perkins, 1975).

Determination of the effectiveness of various types of treatment of vocal disorders will require measurement, prediction, and control of the elements of vocal production. A significant breakthrough is not likely until vocal function yields to scientific analysis. Then, perhaps, evidence can supplant opinion, and progress can be made in the prevention of functional disorders comparable to that now being made in the detection and diagnosis of laryngeal dysfunction. Meanwhile, as far as practicing voice therapy is concerned, we have no alternative but to rely on clinical judgment and a clear rationale for achieving a clearly defined goal.

Goal of voice therapy: vocal efficiency. The proposed goal of voice therapy is to approach optimal vocal balance as closely as capacities and individual needs permit (Chapter 15). Its pursuit leads to vocal efficiency and to Greene's (1964) ideal of balanced tone. The basic concept is that balance is achieved only when the vocal dimensions are "tuned" to interact optimally for greatest efficiency—maximal output for minimal effort (Perkins, 1957). This is merely an extension to voice of a principle that applies to efficient operation of any functional system—human, mechanical, or otherwise. Any skilled performance, whether a golf stroke, tennis swing, or high-wire act, has a "grooved feeling" when it has been purified by maximal simplification. Perfection of technique always involves the removal of unnecessary elements. Hence, artistic performances of any skill tend to be basically similar; individual styles of the ablest performers vary only to the extent that ease and simplicity are unimpaired. The right way to produce complex acts is narrow; wrong ways permit infinite variety.

Applied to voice, the various disorders represent deviations from a single optimally balanced coordination of vocal dimensions (Chapters 3 and 13). The number of different disorders is as unlimited as the possible deviations from optimal. The goal of therapy, then, is to "tune" elements of vocal production much as a mechanic tunes the various systems in an automobile engine. Starting

with deviant dimensions of a particular disorder is not necessarily the most therapeutically productive point of departure; punishment would be required to reduce the frequency of undesirable vocal behavior. Deviant features tell the clinician how the voice is out of balance.

What is needed for therapy is specification of conditions under which the voice comes closest to being in balance. These desired conditions can be perfected by positive reinforcement to whatever level is feasible and necessary and then can be extended by stimulus control into normal speech. Experimentation with all six independent vocal elements can reveal combinations that yield clearest, smoothest, biggest, and most effortless voice. Therapy for a given individual should start with such combinations (Chapters 3 and 13).

Methods of obtaining vocal balance. In vocal behavior, as in articulatory behavior, modification is achieved most efficiently with operant therapy. Following this rationale, we must obtain the emission of desired vocal behavior with which therapy can begin and provide sequences by which it can be successively approximated to the terminal goal of optimal vocal balance in daily conversational speech. Emphasis would be on procedures for obtaining optimal production; operant procedures for strengthening and extension to daily life of desired vocal responses could be the same as those already discussed.

The *chewing method*, conceived by Froeschels (1952) over three decades ago, has been elaborated and used extensively by European phoniatrists for the most part (Brodnitz, 1965; Weiss and Beebe, 1951). Its proponents report excellent results in bringing vocal functioning into natural balance through the activation of a reflexive process. Recognizing that chewing and speech use primarily the same muscles, Froeschels reasoned that proper muscular balance for speech could be restored by extending the natural balance of chewing. First, the intent to chew breath is substituted for that of speaking. Then, after silent, vigorous chewing, phonation is added. Great variety is encouraged in uninhibited chewing of sound; the clinician joins in. Gradually, words are interspersed in the chewing, then alternate periods of chewing and talking, and then reading and conversation, until eventually chewing motions are faded, leaving naturally balanced phonation.

In the hands of a skilled clinician, the chewing method is probably an effective means to the end we have specified of optimal vocal balance. It would seem to be especially applicable to children, emphasizing as it does babbling types of vocalization in conjunction with chewing. Furthermore, it is a holistic approach that does not require specific attention to vocal details. Many adult clients resist it, however, probably because it embarrasses them. Murphy (1964) suggests that it works best with clients who need an authoritative clinician who can also provide psychotherapeutic assistance.

Cooper (1973) has raised his voice frequently in behalf of his conviction that raising pitch is most often the best antidote for vocal misuse. What he seems to work for, and to achieve with an impressive number of cases, is essentially what is being described here as vocal balance. Not many speech pathologists are convinced, though, that the simplistic procedure of merely raising habitual pitch accounts for his results.

Emphasizing the positive, Boone (1971) stresses a "can do" approach to voice therapy. His injunction, which is completely congruent with operant principles, is to search continuously for those hyperfunction-reducing vocal behaviors that the patient can do. They become the targets of voice therapy.

For clinicians who seek more explicit identification of the phonatory behavior they are managing, let us examine a method of utilizing the vocal dimensions we have proposed. Treatment begins by emitting and identifying the "feel" of the vocal elements of an optimally balanced voice—the terminal behavior. Curiously, how the voice feels provides much more certain guidance for its production than feedback of how it sounds. Listening to one's own voice can be mislead-

ing; a speaker can approach "objective" guidance of phonation better by feel than by ear. Two dimensions, constriction and focus, offer the crucial checkpoints. Along the constriction continuum, the desired response is an "open throat" that can be achieved adequately during quiet breathing. Awareness of the sensation by which this response can be controlled can be heightened by contrasting the constriction of a swallow with the expansion at the peak of a yawn.

To the extent that voice is unbalanced, it is out of focus; its effortless "projection" is impaired. It feels as though it were "manufactured" in the throat. When vocal focus is low, the voice is most susceptible to constriction and abuse. Although these consequences can be minimized by using a soft, breathy voice at comfortable pitches, they are not eliminated but merely masked. That constriction and vocal abuse are inherently present with low vocal focus is easily revealed by increasing loudness. As it increases, the voice becomes tighter and more strained, even when a comfortable pitch is used.

The clinical objective, then, is to raise vocal focus as high in the head as possible. When high enough, voice can be produced with maximal loudness without becoming constricted. The tone feels disconnected from the throat and seems to float effortlessly in the head, regardless of whether the pitch is high, low, or mid level. Some describe the feeling as being "like talking on a hum." Others say that the tone feels deep and long. Still others say that it feels big and effortless. Until these sensations are experienced, these subjective descriptions probably seem like so much mumbo jumbo. Once experienced, however, these sensations become stable guides to vocal efficiency.

Techniques for achieving high focus vary in power. Unfortunately, those easiest to describe and use are least powerful. Conversely, the most powerful procedure is almost certain to be misused if attempted without guidance. It involves use of the light voice (falsetto) and, unless done correctly, will result in vocal strain. Ironically, its merit lies in its ability to reveal constriction at any focal level that is not optimally high. This much description is given merely to indicate that such a technique exists.

Less powerful, but more easily described and mastered, is use of our ubiquitous soft, breathy tone. Softness is used to obtain the feeling of effortlessness. Any attempt to push or force the focus of the tone upward is doomed. Since a high focus feels effortless, the greater the effort to force it up, the farther it plunges into the throat. Breathiness is used to offset the tendency typical of a low focus to squeeze the tone from the neck. As the tone is "flooded with air," it feels as though it has floated into the head.

Still less powerful, but easiest of all to use, is a technique devised by Cooper (1973). Merely say "uh-huh" easily and note where the focal point of the tone seems to be located. If the tone is produced softly and without strain, it should seem to be centered in the nose. Although not optimally high for heavy vocal usage, it is still high enough to be helpful.

All persons capable of phonating can approach vocal balance, some closer than others. Although elements of constriction and focus offer the major checkpoints, other dimensions can be used to facilitate achievement of the goal. Only the optimal portions of each independent dimension are utilized at first: when a person is working in normal heavy vocal mode, pitch extremes are avoided, soft rather than loud tones are used, soft and breathy vocal attacks are sought, and partial voicing is preferred to full voicing. For dependent dimensions, production is checked for the adjustment of each element that requires minimal effort and yields maximally smooth tone.

Perkins (1971) has described other sequences of therapy for reducing constriction that utilize many of these vocal dimensions. Because he did not include the element of focus, these sequences do not lead specifically to optimal vocal balance.

Whatever therapeutic sequence is devised should be built on a common assumption: each step would presume the ability to perform the preceding ones. It is far better that each step be mastered well than that many be covered rapidly. Whenever the objective to be achieved at any step is missed, the client should, before attempting to reextend vocal balance farther through the sequence, back up immediately as many steps as necessary to establish performance at which he can succeed without exception. Because the voice tires, especially later in therapy when louder tones are used, short, frequent practice periods not in excess of 5 minutes are much preferred to longer sessions. Even this short a period should be curtailed when the objective cannot be achieved easily.

With vocal balance established and stabilized by this sequence of successive approximations, it can then be extended by operant procedures for stimulus control to conditions of daily living.

Meanwhile, the client will almost certainly need to talk, but his new voice is not yet ready for use. What is needed is a communicatively useful temporary voice that will not undo therapeutic effects faster than progress can be made. As successful a makeshift solution as any, to be used from beginning to end of therapy, is to have the client speak softly in daily life as if he were carrying on only confidential conversations. This strategy avoids the stress and abusive strain of loudness and the pitfalls of whispering, and yet retains the hygienic benefits of breathy production. As optimal balance is achieved it will tend to carry over easily and will eventually replace this interim voice.

Teaching esophageal speech. Most laryngectomees are past the prime of life. They face psychologic and social, to say nothing of physical, problems that go far beyond learning how to talk again. Perhaps we should not be surprised that available evidence points consistently to such psychologic factors as personality, motivation, family environment, and aspiration level having more to do with development of good esophageal speech than anatomic or physiologic factors (Gardner, 1951; Stoll, 1958; Hodson and Oswald, 1958; Diedrich and Youngstrom, 1966). It is not that these considerations are unique to laryngectomized individuals, but they are of such importance in teaching esophageal speech that successful progress through the following stages depends on them.

Various authorities organize the steps in acquiring esophageal speech somewhat differently, but the sequence is remarkably similar. Moreover, although not cast formally in the model of operant therapy, available speech therapy procedures are readily adaptable to that approach. Snidecor (1969), for example, describes nine levels of achievement, each of which presumably depends on preceding levels.

1. Quick intake and expulsion of air (Early success in producing any vowel, preferably during the first day's attempts, is important. A tongue-pumping injection technique may be easier to achieve initially than an inhalation technique.)
2. Ability to produce all speech sounds in at least rough form, with emphasis on plosives (*tea, bee, pet, cat, cow*)
3. Ability to articulate intelligible one-syllable words that can be used to communicate ("yes," "no," "hi," "please")
4. Ability to articulate useful two-syllable words
5. Ability to articulate simple phrases on one air-charge if possible with effective phrasing and clear tone preceding attempts to increase loudness
6. Adequately loud, clear, intelligible connected speech, with emphasis on careful articulation
7. Adequate prosody by varying loudness, pitch, quality, and duration
8. Ability to utilize esophageal speech in active conversation
9. Ability to speak at reasonably normal rates

Diedrich and Youngstrom (1966) describe essentially the same sequence but divide it into two stages: acquiring the first sound and developing efficient and intelligible speech. Between their detailed description of how to accomplish the first stage and Snidecor's of how to achieve the second, a clinician can find explicit guidance for teaching esophageal

speech. Of course, clinicians vary a bit in the procedures they prefer in accomplishing these goals. For instance, Moore (1971) recommends starting training as soon as possible after the decision to perform a laryngectomy is made, even before surgery. Too, he finds much early motivational value in presenting a good esophageal speaker to the new patient. He also prefers starting with the inhalation technique because, when it can be mastered, it offers the most normal-appearing method of insufflation.

Therapy of speech-flow disorders

Therapy of stuttering. Modification of the stutterer's speech to a goal of fluency would be unrealistic and, to a large extent, unnecessary: few of us speak fluently even most of the time, let alone all of the time. The aspect of normal speech of which the stutterer is capable—the essence of normal speech—is the ability to coordinate sound initiations and articulatory transitions easily, effortlessly, and automatically, even though disfluently. Desired modification is simplification of speech.

What the person who stutters needs to learn is how to do what he is attempting to do without including all of the interfering things that he does. To make speech flow freely, he must do so without pushing it, forcing it, struggling with it, or avoiding it; he must speak without tensing himself anywhere from scalp to toes to produce the words. He needs to obtain the feel of the easy rhythmic flow of automatically coordinated speech sounds. As Wendell Johnson might have put it, he needs to discover that he can speak without hesitating to hesitate.

Although authorities now agree reasonably well on what the stutterer does to earn him this label, they vary in recommendations for what will help him recover. The search for an all-purpose "cure" has, historically, yielded an unabated series of flops. Yet probably most techniques that have been tried have worked for some. If we knew with certainty why a person stutters, a specific treatment to meet his specific problem could presumably be devised. As it is, we have insufficient evidence to require support of one theoretical position over another (Yates, 1969). Hence major therapeutic approaches to stuttering reflect current conceptions of the problem that can be divided two ways: those that view it as behavior subject to direct modification by operant procedures, and those that view it as a function of internal intervening variables.

This latter conception encompasses the theories that traditionally have produced most of the recommendations for therapy. "Anticipatory-struggle" theories posit apprehensive anticipation of stuttering as the intervening variable. Conflict and anxious expectancy of stuttering is the central problem to be treated, in this view. "Repressed-need" theories, on the other hand, posit neurotic anxiety as the intervening variable of which stuttering is a symptomatic expression. Here, reduction of neurotic conflict is the core issue to be resolved. More than with most defective speech, a given problem of stuttering may be treated by speech therapy, psychotherapy, or operant therapy. Many confirmed stutterers have tried all three. Although we will not undertake a discussion of psychotherapy, elements of it will be found woven into traditional speech therapy for stuttering.

Speech therapy. A common bond linking various versions of speech therapy is the view that stuttering is learned in a milieu of interpersonal stress. Accordingly, two prongs of treatment are characteristic: one to cope with disrupted speech, the other with communicative fears. Speech therapy has been for years and still is largely the mainstream approach of speech pathologists in the United States.

A series of publications of the Speech Foundation of America (Memphis, Tennessee) reports conferences on stuttering of leading representatives of the speech therapy approach.

Those who hold this view pursue two main treatment objectives: help the stutterer to improve his attitude about himself and his speech, and help him to stutter effortlessly and fluently. Several approaches are taken to change attitudes. The stutterer is encouraged to examine his own and his listeners' reactions to his stuttering. He is urged to stutter openly and frequently, partly to increase opportunities for objective observation of his speech, and partly to desensitize his dread of stuttering. Striving for "false" fluency is deplored. Above all, he must learn to avoid avoidance of expected stuttering, even to the point of "faking" stuttering. To hide leads to deception, guilt, and shame.

As the stutterer discovers that he is not a helpless victim in the grip of stuttering, he becomes more adept at analyzing what he is doing that he need not do in order to speak effortlessly. Many clinicians use Van Riper's (1973) three procedures to achieve fluent stuttering: pullouts, preparatory sets, and cancellation. The stutterer uses *pullouts* to extricate himself from a block. Instead of struggling, he learns to ease himself out of difficulty with smooth, controlled prolongations. To replace anticipatory rehearsals of expected trouble, he moves the effortless pullouts forward and uses them as *preparatory sets* for easy speech initiation. Instead of preparing to struggle with an expected block in a "frozen" speech posture, he begins speech with relaxed movements. As he masters pullouts and preparatory sets, he is equipped to use them for *cancellation*. He does this by stuttering again after each block with which he struggles, but this time with his new modified version of stuttering that is simpler.

Are Johnson and his colleagues (1967), Van Riper (1973), Bloodstein (1975a,b), and Williams (1971) in basic agreement about how they would help stutterers simplify their speech?

Recently, efforts to conceptualize speech therapy objectives within the framework of learning theory have blossomed (Wischner, 1969). Brutten has been instrumental in what is perhaps the most rigorous example (Brutten, 1975; Brutten and Shoemaker, 1967). Taking the view that disintegration of speech is the consequence of emotional stress, he has analyzed stuttering in terms of disruptive instrumental responses and classically conditioned emotional responses. He then applies principles of learning theory to the extinction of these responses. Similarly, Gregory (1968, 1973) has applied concepts of extinction, counterconditioning, generalization, and discrimination to alterations of stutterers' perceptions, attitudes, and speech patterns, as well as to reduction of their fears, avoidances, and tensions.

As for treatment of communicative fears, changes are sought in two areas: in how the stutterer views his speech, and in how he views himself. The more confirmed the stutterer, the more likely his conviction that speaking is monstrously difficult, that it is an endeavor to be approached with apprehension and uncertainty, that it is a task with which he must struggle. To acquire the opposite view—that speech production is easy —is vital.

A characteristic of confirmed stutterers is avoidance of situations, words, and sounds that are likely to be difficult. Van Riper (1973), especially, has been prolific in devising techniques for helping stutterers face rather than flee from stuttering. Such procedures include assignments in which the stutterer confronts the scope of his problem. He identifies "Jonah" sounds that he attempts to sidestep with alternate words. He identifies feared words for which he develops an extensive vocabulary of synonyms. He identifies speaking situations, such as using the telephone, that he will sometimes literally walk a mile to avoid. Once he can recognize the conditions from which he attempts escape, he is then gradually toughened to them by *desensitization* techniques until he can face them squarely and devise more successful ways of coping.

Johnson and others (1967) and Williams (1957, 1968) have been especially concerned with how stutterers think about their problem. The essence of their point is that stuttering is not some mystical thing that happens; it is, instead, behavior that the stutterer is capable of managing and for which he is responsible. By describing to himself in objective terms what he *does* differently

when he stutters from when he speaks easily, the stutterer discovers that he can control stuttering instead of its controlling him.

Clinicians who see stuttering as the cause rather than the consequence of personality conflict will be inclined to alter the client's image of himself as a stutterer. Sheehan (1968, 1969, 1970, 1975) in particular has discussed this aspect of the problem as a role conflict. To change from a self-concept of being a stutterer to that of being a normal speaker requires a change of roles. Because stuttering begins at an early age and carries with it a social stigma, we should not be surprised by the extent to which a stutterer may build his life around his problem. To alter a self-concept of being a stutterer is frequently to alter an entire mode of living. Desirable as such alteration may be, its price can be high. Witness one severe stutterer who overnight became unable to stutter. The immediate consequence was a month of acute anxiety; the long-term consequence was a personality change from being submissively docile and sexually timid to being abrasively hostile and aggressively amorous.

Help for children. Should the therapist intervene in the life of a child in the early throes of stuttering? Does prudence dictate waiting to see whether the child will outgrow the problem, as Martyn and Sheehan (1968) have shown that possibly 80% of children who stutter will do? This course of action would be attractive if we could predict who will outgrow stuttering and who will not, as we may well prove able to do if Stromsta's preliminary findings hold up (Chapter 14). Should we undertake therapy directly with the child and risk enlarging his awareness that he has a problem? Should we, instead, work with the child's parents in an oblique effort to ameliorate stuttering? The goals of treatment for children who stutter hinge on answers to these questions.

Luper and Mulder (1964) and Johnson and others (1967) have wrestled with these issues. Have they arrived at the same conclusions?

Again, we find two approaches to treatment of the child that depend for their selection on the clinician's theoretical bias. Those who see stuttering as a neurotic symptom will seek to help the child find more direct and responsible ways of managing his feelings. They will work toward more mature forms of personal adjustment, and they will probably utilize play therapy to reach these goals. Because stuttering is only one of many possibly symptomatic expressions of neurosis, the objectives of such therapy are not as explicitly concerned with stuttering as they are with personal adjustment generally. Play therapy, such as used by those treating "neu-

---

What would Murphy and FitzSimons (1960) have to say about this point of view?

---

rotic stuttering," is not likely to be much different from what it would be for such problems as "neurotic articulation" or "neurotic voice."

Treatment of the child by clinicians who are attempting to head off development of full-blown struggle responses is often addressed to goals such as Luper (1968) and Williams (1971) propose. These goals include attempts to minimize those features of disfluency that increase the probability of its being judged as stuttering: that is, any form of tensing or forcing of speech sound production. The goal here is to help the child recognize his unnecessary efforts when they occur and to contrast and replace them with easy, normally flowing speech.

Other goals include helping the child avoid his avoidances, harmful generalizations, and secondary gains that can accompany stuttering. Whereas the child has found reinforcement by going around a hard word or sound, the clinician offers reinforcement for going straight through the stuttering. Whereas the child sees stuttering as a crippling handicap that limits him in what he can do, the clinician shows him that realistically he can stutter and still achieve whatever success he would otherwise attain, whether in school, on the playground, in sports, or even in such speaking activities as dramatics and public address (Williams, 1971).

As with therapy for children, so it is with

their parents, that treatment may be directed to their psyches or to their performances. Some who see stuttering as a neurosis view its roots in personality conflicts of the parents. The child's stuttering, therefore, is seen as an external manifestation of parental neurosis. Solve the parent's psychic distress, and the child will improve (Z. Wolpe, 1957). Those who counsel parents and teachers in ways of minimizing negative responses to disfluency will probably be influenced in their goals by Johnson's point of view more than any other. Having demonstrated that stuttering usually develops after rather than before parents or teachers diagnose it as such (this is the essence of his *diagnosogenic theory*), Johnson and others (1967) addressed recommendations to teachers as well as to parents. Over and above various specific admonitions, he offered the following general advice that is particularly relevant for all who would help young stutterers*:

Listen to the child well, to what he is saying, and almost saying, and not saying at all. He has something he wants to tell you, something that has meaning for him, that is important to him. He is not just being verbally frisky.

Respect him as a speaker. Listen to him enough to hear him out. It is wonderful for him as a growing person to feel that he is being heard, that others care about what he is saying. Assume he's doing the best he can and that it is more important for him to want to talk to you than to sound correct.

Behavior modification. As an approach to the remediation of stuttering, behavior modification, utilizing operant principles, differs from most speech therapy in four important ways: it is more consistently rigorous in identifying behavior to be modified; it requires no assumption about etiology; it requires no assumption about stuttering as a function of such intervening variables as anxiety, fear, or expectancy; and it emphasizes what the client does successfully rather than what he does defectively.

---

*From Johnson, W., and others, *Speech-Handicapped School Children*. New York: Harper & Row, Publishers (1967).

Despite dissimilarities, speech therapy as practiced by clinicians such as Williams (1968, 1971) is as much concerned with behavior as is operant therapy. In fact, the development of stuttering as anticipatory struggle behavior has been explained by Shames and Sherrick (1963) according to operant principles. More recently, operant approaches to accomplish two aspects of speech therapy have been formulated: modification of the form of stuttering by procedures based on Van Riper's cancellation techniques, and modification of positive and negative thematic content of language that seemed either beneficial to or incompatible with therapeutic progress (Shames, Egolf, and Rhodes, 1969; Shames and Egolf, 1976).

The success of many versions of speech therapy hangs on the validity of presuming that stuttering is a function of some form of negative emotion and that it develops as a consequence of punishment of disfluency. As Siegel (1969) indicates, these ideas are only assumptions; empirical evidence is not available to deny or affirm them definitively. Such research as has been done, however, stands directly opposed to them. Gray and England (1972), at the end of an extensive study of the effects of deconditioning anxiety in thirty stutterers by reciprocal inhibition, concluded that although speech and situational anxieties were effectively reduced, this reduction had no necessary relationship to the frequency or severity of stuttering. Perkins (1967) reached essentially the same conclusion in a smaller investigation.

Considerably more evidence has accumulated against the other assumption—that stuttering develops from punishment of fluency failures. Punishment has consistently reduced disfluency when made contingent on it, whether normal or stuttered (Goldiamond, 1965; Martin and Siegel, 1966a,b; Martin, 1968; Siegel and Martin, 1965, 1966, 1967, 1968). As Brookshire and Eveslage (1969) have shown, random punishment does augment disfluency, a fact that probably accounts for increases in stuttering after noncontingent punishment reported by Van Riper (1937), Hill (1954), and Stassi (1961).

Thus, unless punishment of disfluency and the effect of negative emotion on stuttering operate differently in children from the way they operate in adults (on whom the research has been done), the foundation on which much of speech therapy for stuttering is built is shaky. Nonetheless, it has provided many clinical successes.

Of the available approaches, behavior modification best meets the four criteria for rehabilitative methods with which this section was introduced. Goldiamond (1962a, 1965) pioneered the use of operant procedures for replacing stuttering with normal speech. Rather than punishing or calling attention to undesirable disfluencies, he obtained fluency in laboratory conditions by the use of delayed auditory feedback and rate control. Curlee and Perkins (1969) extended his work by devising a system of conversational rate control procedures that, utilizing stimulus control principles, carried over normal speech from the laboratory to daily life.

Until recently procedures to eliminate stuttering, such as speaking in rhythm to a waving finger, were viewed as the stock-in-trade of quack cures. They were thought to work temporarily as crutches, but when they ceased to distract the stutterer from expectancy of difficulty, they would wear out, leaving the victim more helpless than ever. With their use in research to establish fluency, and with recognition that stuttering can be eliminated and is not necessarily a condition of "foreverness" (four fifths of those who once stuttered may recover spontaneously), these fluency-producing procedures are becoming clinically respectable (Marks, 1969). The rationale for their use is that since fluency and disfluency cannot coexist simultaneously, rather than suppress stuttering by punishing its occurrence, conditions can be utilized under which fluency prevails as a competing response. With this approach fluent speech need not even be shaped; it is potentially available in probably every client's behavioral repertoire and can be extended to normal speech by stimulus control. Because this strategy holds the key to relatively efficient and certain elimination of stuttering, let us look at three techniques that consistently obtain fluent speech-flow, even if temporarily:

1. *Articulatory rate control* can be established with syllable prolongation. Delayed auditory feedback (DAF) provides a convenient means of establishing desired amounts of prolongation, but it is not essential to the achievement of successful results (Perkins, 1973a). With instructions to articulate slowly and to prolong vowels long enough that 250 msec delay will not disrupt speech, a rate of about 30 words per minute is established. This rate will free most stutterers from the behavior and feeling of stuttering. It can be increased gradually by reducing DAF in 50 msec steps until no delay remains. With attention to phrasing in conjunction with a slow-normal rate, fluent speech can be established in the clinic and then extended into everyday speaking situations. This technique is effective with conversation or reading and with stuttering of all degrees of severity (Curlee and Perkins, 1969).

2. *Auditory masking* also reduces stuttering for many, especially when the masking noise is loud enough to obscure most of the sound of the speaker's own voice (Trotter and Lesch, 1967; Perkins and Curlee, 1969; Cherry and Sayers, 1956). When masking is effective, and it usually is, it still has four typical problems: the ear plugs that must be worn induce partial hearing loss for another speaker's speech, the masking noise must be turned on to speak and off to listen (a cumbersome procedure), tolerance for the noise is limited, and most important, the achievement of fluency seems to be by "magic." Because the stutterer has no control over the process, he is helpless to recover fluency when he loses it. Some hearing-aid size masking units have been built, however, that are designed to minimize, if not eliminate, those problems.

3. *Rhythm*, among other procedures for instating fluency (Andrews and Harris, 1964; Brady, 1971; Meyer and Comley, 1969), has been investigated. Typically established by metronome, the rhythm of the fluent speech obtained is far removed from normal prosody. Rhythm therefore seems less desirable than rate as a means of obtaining the emission of fluency behavior that closely approximates the terminal form desired (Ingham, 1975).

Those who use behavior-shaping procedures have recognized that fluency is easy to establish but difficult to maintain if it is not incorporated into normally rhythmic speech. Without normal expressiveness, stuttering is usually preferred to fluent monotony. Accordingly, elaborately systematized programs have been designed for shaping an approximation of normal speech. Beyond achieving fluency, this goal also frequently requires the more difficult task of establishing normal rate, phrasing, phrase initiation, breath-stream management within the phrase, vocal production, and prosody. Once shaped, sometimes with a token economy, these skills are then generalized to daily life and stabilized for permanence (Andrews and Ingham, 1972; Brady, 1971; Ingham, 1975; Perkins, 1973a,b; Ryan, 1971; Shames, 1975, 1976; Webster, 1974).

Despite squabbles between traditionalists and "young Turk" behavior shapers, the objectives of these two views are not significantly different. Both attempt to improve the stutterer's attitude about himself and his speech, and both attempt to make speaking easier. Curiously, what the behavior shapers have devised goes a step beyond the traditionalists' efforts to establish fluent stuttering. Instead of simplifying the preparatory set, simplification is moved even farther forward to head off preliminary preparations for stuttering. Such "stickiness" is prevented by preserving the skills of normal speech.

Thus behavior modifiers do not suppress stuttering. They merely head it off before it begins. Whether stuttering is mild or severe is of little consequence, since struggle characteristics drop out with establishment of fluency. The focus, then, is not on how speech goes wrong during stuttering. Instead, it is on how to install and maintain essential elements of speech when it is right.

As for the stutterer's attitude, traditionalists attempt to change it as a prelude to making speaking easier. Behaviorists come at the same objective from the opposite direction. Proceeding on the assumption that nothing succeeds like success, they establish normal speech as the starting point and let change in attitude follow. To the extent that the stutterer convinces himself that he has the skill to control his speech normally—especially in feared situations he would usually avoid—his attitude will change.

Effectiveness of therapy. More work has been done on the effectiveness of treatment of stuttering than on any other speech disorder. The reason is not clear. Perhaps it is because of such widespread dissatisfaction with treatment results. Unlike articulation, stuttering is not regarded as simple. (In reality, it may prove to be no more complex.) Nevertheless, fifty-eight studies dating back to 1928 and showing the percentage of cases who improved have been summarized by Bloodstein (1975a). These studies are largely reports of subjective impressions of improvement. They do not provide a firm basis for comparing one result with another, or for knowing how long the improvement lasted.

Recently, though, attempts to obtain reliable and comparable measures of therapeutic effectiveness and efficiency have begun to appear. Ingham (1975) has provided an insightful review of much of this work. Perhaps because operant methods encourage accurate measurement of rate and disfluency, and perhaps stung by traditionalists' objections that quickly achieved fluency is temporary and will fade as novelty wears off, behaviorists have gone to considerable lengths to measure, test, and report the outcomes of their therapeutic procedures (Brady, 1971; Ingham, 1975; Ingham and Andrews, 1971, 1973; Perkins and others, 1974; Shames, 1975, 1976; and Webster, 1974).

They have demonstrated with direct observation that upwards of 60% of stutterers achieve normally expressive, fluent speech. Furthermore, approximately 90% retain some improvement on a long-term basis. Of these clients, more than 50% can remain virtually free of stuttering on a reasonably permanent basis. Lacking equivalent evidence, the best rating-scale studies of traditional

therapy suggest lasting improvement in 30% to 50% of the clients (Gregory, 1972; Prins, 1970).

Therapy of cluttering. Because cluttering is a term applied to a constellation of handicaps, we will forego discussing all the therapeutic goals that can be appropriate—they cover the scope of this book. Cluttering can include problems of language, of articulation, of voice, of fluency, as well as of rate and rhythm, to say nothing of reading, writing, music, and learning problems. Because it is so rare, or because it goes unrecognized, or for whatever reason, cluttering seems to be the stepchild of speech disorders in the United States. Few have studied its nature, fewer have even written about its treatment, and no one has evaluated the effectiveness of what can be done for people afflicted by it. From such descriptions of therapy as are available, let us look briefly at goals and techniques for management of rate and rhythm, problems not considered elsewhere.

Rate. The goal of treatment for the excessive speed of cluttering is mastery of a reasonable rate that is slow enough to permit intelligible speech and, with good fortune, accurate articulation. Among procedures for obtaining behavior that can be modified to this objective are some already described for stuttering: rate control with delayed auditory feedback, speech shadowing, and speaking in time with the slow beat of a metronome or waving finger. Other useful techniques have been described by Bradford (undated). Included are negative practice (speaking too rapidly on purpose is contrasted with slower speech), underscoring of the usually slurred final consonant in reading passages, and reading through a window card (the rate of exposure of words can be controlled).

Rhythm. Prosodic elements are distorted in the dysrhythmic "spurt-like" expulsion of cluttered speech. To achieve mastery of normal rhythm, a desirable goal, the clutterer needs to discover which of the prosodic features he is distorting, rhythm being a product of how syllables are timed, stressed, and inflected.

The first step in establishing control of

rhythm is work on syllabification: the number of syllables spoken can be counted, spoken slowly with equal stress, and then spoken slowly with normal stress. Next, timing of syllables in words and phrases is emphasized. Purposeful use of silence between short phrases, careful juncturing of sounds that join syllables together, marking of short phrases in reading material, and use of short phrases in conversation are available techniques.

The next steps can be intermingled. By following the tapped-out rhythm of poetry that has a simple beat, the clutterer automatically stresses the proper syllables. Even if such a technique does help to establish normal speech rhythm, it may still be inadequate for inflectional differences among questions, answers, and explanations or for clarification of meaning by emphasis of words. The clutterer may have to learn how to indicate differences in meaning, such as between "Where are you *going!*" spoken with falling inflection and "*Where* are you going?" spoken with rising inflection.

Finally, a general consideration. As Weiss (1964) stresses, clutterers tend to be heedless of what they do and how they sound when they speak. To offer help, one must get their attention, a potentially exasperating challenge. By recognizing the existence of a short attention span and by limiting the clutterer's therapeutic tasks to one or two at a time, the clinician can help the clutterer to achieve improvement by means of speech therapy. On the other hand, operant therapy is well suited to the clutterer because the responsibility for modifying behavior by controlling contingencies of reinforcement rests wholly with the clinician—and with this approach the clutterer's attention is desirable but not essential.

The answers—résumé

1. What assumptions underlie the therapy of disorders of speech?

A clinician must assume answers to at least six fundamental questions in each therapeutic encounter. First, is he responsible for the client's functioning as a whole, or for only part functions of speech? Second, should be view man behaviorally, as scientifically knowable, or phenomenologically, as unique, free, and hence unpredictable? Third, should he modify behavior for benefit of the client, the parents, or society? Fourth, whose value system should he follow in setting therapeutic goals, the client's or his own? Fifth, should he offer therapy for money, power, altruism, or as a solution for his own problems? Sixth, should he persist in traditional methods of therapy that prove unsuccessful or experiment with new methods? Each of these questions is thorny, some more obviously than others. None has a "right" answer. Yet every clinician in every therapeutic session assumes answers to every question by what he does, wittingly or blindly.

2. What modes of therapy are applicable to disorders of speech?

Four basic modes of therapy are available: (1) behavior therapy for explicit modification of speech (speech therapy and behavior modification); (2) behavior therapy for reduction of anxiety (reciprocal inhibition therapy and implosion therapy); (3) insight therapies to arouse irrational anxiety, which, when extinguished, improves personal adjustment (psychoanalytic therapies and nondirective therapies); (4) directive counseling to help the handicapped live gracefully with defects they cannot change and to instruct clients, parents, spouses, teachers, and friends in ways that they can facilitate rehabilitation.

Conceivably, speech pathologists may need to cope with four combinations of conditions to modify defective speech permanently:

1. Disorders that are "bad habits" (in which wrong patterns of speech were learned and persist because the correct pattern has not been learned) would require therapy for speech modification; counseling would be helpful.
2. Disorders that form a "vicious circle" (in which wrong patterns were learned and persist in part because of the speaker's struggles to avoid defective speech) would require therapy for speech modification; anxiety-reduction therapy and counseling would be helpful.
3. Disorders that are "bad habits with benefits" (in which wrong patterns were learned and persist in part because of reinforcing secondary benefits from them) would require therapy for speech modification and psychotherapeutic procedures to resolve resistance to modification; counseling and anxiety-reduction therapy would be helpful.
4. Disorders that are "symptomatic" (that are acquired and persist as psychoneurotic symptoms) require insight therapy; counseling, anxiety-reduction therapy, and speech therapy may be used as needed.

3. What therapeutic methods will modify disorders of speech?

Ideally, rehabilitative procedures would meet the following criteria: they would produce changes desired by the speech handicapped, they would modify observable behavior, they would be applications of learning principles, and they would be feasible for use by most clinicians. Although psychotherapy is necessary for some and probably desirable for treatment of most disorders of speech, the majority of speech pathologists are not trained to rely on it as the major method of effecting therapeutic change. On the other hand, speech therapy with its pragmatic procedures and behavior modification with its application of principles of learning are well suited to the purpose of improving defective speech. Both methods capitalize on the principle that obtainable behavior that can be explicitly specified can be consistently modified. Operant therapy, particularly, is rigorous in equally important matters of identifying desired terminal behavior, analyzing the progression of behavioral steps to be taught to reach the goal, and managing contingencies of reinforcement to be applied at each step. Methods of remediating speech are at hand; success depends largely on the ability to identify explicitly behavioral dimensions to be managed of language, articulation, phonation, and speech-flow, and on the ability to resolve resistance to permanent use of improved speech skills.

REFERENCES

Addison, R., and Homme, L., The reinforcing event (RE) menu. *NSPI Journal*, **4**, 8-9 (1966).

Agranowitz, A., and McKeown, M., *Aphasia Handbook for Adults and Children.* Springfield, Ill., Charles C Thomas, Publisher (1964).

Andrews, G., and Harris, M., *The Syndrome of Stuttering.* London: Heinemann (1964).

Andrews, G., and Ingham, R., An approach to the evaluation of stuttering therapy. *J. Speech Hearing Res.*, **15**, 296-302 (1972).

Aronson, A., Speech pathology and symptom therapy in the interdisciplinary treatment of psychogenic aphonia. *J. Speech Hearing Dis.*, **34**, 321-341 (1969).

Backus, O., Group structure in speech therapy. In Travis, L. (Ed.), *Handbook of Speech Pathology.* New York: Appleton-Century-Crofts (1957).

Backus, O., and Beasley, J., *Speech Therapy with Children.* New York: Houghton Mifflin Co. (1951).

Baer, D., Guess, D., and Sherman, J., Adventures in simplistic grammar. In Schiefelbusch, R. (Ed.), *Language of the Mentally Retarded.* Baltimore: University Park Press (1972).

Baltaxe, C., and Simmons, J., Language in childhood psychosis: a review. *J. Speech Hearing Dis.*, **40**, 439-458 (1975).

Baratz, J., Language in the economically disadvantaged child: a perspective. *Asha*, **10**, 143-145 (1968).

Barbara, D., *The Psychotherapy of Stuttering.* Springfield, Ill.: Charles C Thomas, Publisher (1962).

Bartak, L., and Rutter, M., Educational treatment of autistic children. In Rutter, M. (Ed.), *Infantile Autism: Concepts, Characteristics, and Treatment.* Edinburgh: Churchill, Livingstone, Ltd. (1971).

Bereiter, C., and Engelmann, S., *Teaching Disadvantaged Children in the Preschool.* Englewood Cliffs, N.J.: Prentice-Hall, Inc. (1966).

Berry, M., and Eisenson, J., *Speech Disorders.* New York: Appleton-Century-Crofts (1956).

Blakeley, R., *The Practice of Speech Pathology.* Springfield, Ill.: Charles C Thomas, Publisher (1972).

Bloodstein, O., *A Handbook on Stuttering.* Chicago: National Easter Seal Society for Crippled Children and Adults (1975a).

Bloodstein, O., Stuttering as tension and fragmentation. In Eisenson, J. (Ed.), *Stuttering: a Second Symposium.* New York: Harper & Row, Publishers (1975b).

Boone, D., *The Voice and Voice Therapy.* Englewood Cliffs, N.J.: Prentice-Hall, Inc. (1971).

Bradford, D., A framework of therapeusis for articulation therapy. In *Studies in Tachyphemia*, New York: Speech Rehabilitation Institute (undated).

Brady, J., Metronome-conditioned speech retraining for stuttering. *Behav. Ther.*, **2**, 129-150 (1971).

Bricker, W., A systematic approach to language training. In Schiefelbusch, R. (Ed.), *Language of the Mentally Retarded.* Baltimore: University Park Press (1972).

Briess, F., Voice therapy. (Part II) Essential treatment phases of specific laryngeal muscle dysfunction. *Arch. Otolaryng.*, **69**, 61-69 (1959).

Brodnitz, F., *Vocal rehabilitation.* Rochester, Minn.: American Academy of Ophthalmology and Otolaryngology (1965).

Brookshire, R., Speech pathology and the experimental analysis of behavior. *J. Speech Hearing Dis.*, **32**, 215-227 (1967).

Brookshire, R., Visual discrimination and response reversal learning by aphasic subjects. *J. Speech Hearing Res.*, **11**, 677-692 (1968).

Brookshire, R., and Eveslage, R., Verbal punishment of disfluency following augmentation of disfluency by random delivery of aversive stimuli. *J. Speech Hearing Res.*, **12**, 383-388 (1969).

Brutten, G., Stuttering: topography, assessment, and behavior change strategies. In Eisenson, J. (Ed.), *Stuttering: a Second Symposium.* New York: Harper & Row, Publishers (1975).

Brutten, E., and Shoemaker, D., *The Modification of Stuttering.* Englewood Cliffs, N.J.: Prentice-Hall, Inc. (1967).

Cherry, C., and Sayers, B., Experiments upon the total inhibition of stammering by external control, and some clinical results. *J. Psychosom. Res.*, **1**, 233-246 (1956).

Chomsky, N., *Language and Mind.* New York: Harcourt, Brace & World (1968).

Churchill, D., The relation of infantile autism and early childhood schizophrenia to developmental language disorders of childhood. *J. Autism Child. Schizo.*, **2**, 182-197 (1972).

Cooper, E., An inquiry into the use of interpersonal communication as a source for therapy with stutterers. In Barbara, D. (Ed.), *New Directions in Stuttering.* Springfield, Ill.: Charles C Thomas, Publisher (1965).

Cooper, M., *Modern Techniques of Vocal Rehabilitation.* Springfield, Ill.: Charles C Thomas, Publisher (1973).

Cooper, M., and Nahum, A., Vocal rehabilitation for contact ulcer of the larynx. *Arch. Otolaryng.*, **85**, 41-46 (1967).

Curlee, R., and Perkins, W., Conversational rate control therapy for stuttering. *J. Speech Hearing Dis.*, **34**, 245-250 (1969).

Dabul, B., and Hanson, W., The amount of language improvement in adult aphasics related to early and late treatment. Unpublished research, Los Angeles, 425 South Hill, Veterans Administration Outpatient Clinic (1975).

Diedrich, W., and Youngstrom, K., *Alaryngeal Speech.* Springfield, Ill.: Charles C Thomas, Publisher (1966).

Eisenson, J., *Aphasia in Children.* New York: Harper & Row, Publishers (1972).

Eisenson, J., *Adult Aphasia: Assessment and Treatment.* New York: Appleton-Century-Crofts (1973).

Eisenson, J., Language rehabilitation of aphasic adults: a review of some issues as to the state of the art. In Tower, D. (Editor-in-chief), *The Nervous System.* (Vol. 3) *Human Communication and Its Disorders.* New York: Raven Press (1975).

Eysenck, H. (Ed.), *Handbook of Abnormal Psychology.* New York: Basic Books, Inc. (1961).

Fairbanks, G., Systematic research in experimental phonetics. 1. A theory of the speech mechanism as a servosystem. *J. Speech Hearing Dis.*, **19**, 133-139 (1954).

Fairbanks, G., *Voice and Articulation Drillbook.* New York: Harper & Row, Publishers (1960).

Ford, F., and Urban, D., *Systems of Psychotherapy.* New York: John Wiley & Sons, Inc. (1963).

Froeschels, E., Chewing method as therapy. *Arch. Otolaryng.*, **56**, 427-434 (1952).

Gardner, W., Problems of laryngectomees. *Rehab. Rec.*, Jan.,-Feb., pp. 15-18 (1951).

Garrett, E., Speech pathology: some principles underlying therapeutic practices. *Asha*, **10**, 203-204 (1968).

Gearheart, B., *Learning Disabilities: Educational Strategies.* St. Louis: The C. V. Mosby Co. (1973).

Goda, S., *Articulation Therapy and Consonant Drill Book.* New York: Grune & Stratton, Inc. (1970).

Goldiamond, I., The maintenance of ongoing fluent verbal behavior and stuttering. *J. Mathetics*, **1**, 57-95 (1962a).

Goldiamond, I., Perception. In Bachrach, A. (Ed.), *Experimental Foundations of Clinical Psychology.* New York: Basic Books, Inc. (1962b).

Goldiamond, I., Stuttering and fluency as manipulable and operant response classes. In Krasner, L., and Ullmann, L. (Eds.), *Research in Behavior Modification.* New York: Holt, Rinehart & Winston, Inc. (1965).

Goldstein, A., Heller, K., and Sechrest, L., *Psychotherapy and the Psychology of Behavior Change.* New York: John Wiley & Sons, Inc. (1966).

Gray, B., and England, G., Stuttering: the measurement of anxiety during reciprocal inhibition. In Gray, B., and England, G. (Eds.), *Stuttering and the Conditioning Therapies.* Monterey, Calif.: Monterey Institute for Speech and Hearing (1969).

Gray, B., and England, G., Some effects of anxiety deconditioning upon stuttering frequency. *J. Speech Hearing Res.*, **15**, 114-122 (1972).

Gray, B., and Ryan, B., *Programmed Conditioning for Language: Program Book.* Palo Alto, Calif.: Monterey Learning Systems (1971).

Greene, M., *The Voice and Its Disorders.* London: Sir Isaac Pitman & Sons, Ltd. (1964).

Gregory, H., Applications of learning theory concepts in the management of stuttering. In Gregory, H. (Ed.), *Learning Theory and Stuttering Therapy.* Evanston, Ill.: Northwestern University Press (1968).

Gregory, H., An assessment of the results of stuttering therapy. *J. Commun. Dis.*, **5**, 320-334 (1972).

Gregory, H., *Stuttering: Differential Evaluation and Therapy.* New York: Bobbs-Merrill (1973).

Haney, R., Child therapy: relationship and process. In Travis, L. (Ed.), *Handbook of Speech Pathology and Audiology.* New York: Appleton-Century-Crofts (1971).

Harper, R., *Psychoanalysis and Psychotherapy: 36 Systems.* Englewood Cliffs, N.J.: Prentice-Hall, Inc. (1959).

Hejna, R., *Interviews With a Stutterer.* Danville, Ill.: The Interstate Printers & Publishers, Inc. (1963).

Hill, H., An experimental study of disorganization of speech and manual responses in normal subjects. *J. Speech Hearing Dis.*, **19**, 295-305 (1954).

Hirsch, R., and Silvertson, B., Preliminary report of language acquisition of twenty pupils in the Los Angeles County Autism Project. Unpublished research. Lawndale, Calif.: South Doty, Los Angeles County Autism Project (1975).

Hitt, W., Two models of man. *Am. Psychol.*, **24**, 651-658 (1969).

Hobbs, N., Sources of gain in psychotherapy. *Am. Psychol.*, **17**, 741-747 (1962).

Hodson, C., and Oswald, M., *Speech Recovery After Total Laryngectomy.* Baltimore: The Williams & Wilkins Co. (1958).

Holland, A., Some current trends in aphasia rehabilitation. *Asha*, **11**, 3-7 (1969).

Holland, A., Case studies in aphasia rehabilitation using programmed instruction. *J. Speech Hearing Dis.*, **35**, 377-390 (1970).

Holland, A., and Matthews, J., Application of teaching machine concepts to speech pathology and audiology. In Sloane, H., and MacAulay, B. (Eds.), *Operant Procedures in Remedial Speech and Language Training.* Boston: Houghton Mifflin Co. (1968).

Homme, L., Perspectives in psychology. XXIV. Control of coverants, the operants of the mind. *Psychol. Rec.*, **15**, 501-511 (1965).

Homme, L., Contiguity theory and contingency management. *Psychol. Rec.*, **16**, 233-241 (1966).

Ingham, R., Operant methodology in stuttering therapy. In Eisenson, J. (Ed.), *Stuttering: a Second Symposium.* New York: Harper & Row, Publishers (1975).

Ingham, R., and Andrews, G., The quality of fluency after treatment. *J. Commun. Dis.*, **4**, 279-288 (1971).

Ingham, R., and Andrews, G., Behavior therapy and stuttering: a review. *J. Speech Hearing Dis.*, **38**, 405-441 (1973).

Johnson, D., and Myklebust, H., *Learning Disabilities: Educational Principles and Practices.* New York: Grune & Stratton, Inc. (1967).

Johnson, W., and others, *Speech Handicapped School Children.* New York: Harper & Row, Publishers (1967).

Johnston, M., Echolalia and automatism in speech. In Sloane, H., and MacAulay, B. (Eds.), *Operant Procedures in Remedial Speech and Language Training.* Boston: Houghton Mifflin Co. (1968).

Johnston, M., and Harris, F., Observation and recording of verbal behavior in remedial speech work. In Sloane, H., and MacAulay, B. (Eds.), *Operant Procedures in Remedial Speech and Language Training.* Boston: Houghton Mifflin Co. (1968).

Kanfer, F., Issues and ethics in behavior manipulation. In Sloane, H., and MacAulay, B. (Eds.), *Operant Procedures in Remedial Speech and Language Training.* Boston: Houghton Mifflin Co. (1968).

Kirk, S., *Early Education of the Mentally Retarded.* Urbana: University of Illinois Press (1958).

Kirk, S., and Kirk, W., *Psycholinguistic and Learning Disabilities: Diagnosis and Remediation.* Urbana: University of Illinois Press (1971).

Lee, L., Recent studies in language acquisition. *Asha*, **11**, 272-274 (1969).

Lent, J., *Mimosa Cottage: Experiment in Hope. Psychology Today*, pp. 51-58 (June, 1968).

Liberman, A., and others, Perception of the speech code. *Psychol. Rev.*, **74**, 431-461 (1967).

Livingston, R., Reinforcement. In Quarton, G., Melnechuk, T., and Schmitt, F. (Eds.), *The Neurosciences.* New York: Rockefeller University Press (1967).

London, P., *The Modes and Morals of Psychotherapy.* New York: Holt, Rinehart & Winston, Inc. (1964).

Longerich, M., and Bordeaux, J., *Aphasia Therapeutics.* New York: The Macmillan Co. (1954).

Lovaas, O., A program for the establishment of speech in psychotic children. In Sloane, H., and MacAulay, B. (Eds.), *Operant Procedures in Remedial Speech and Language Training.* Boston: Houghton Mifflin Co. (1968).

Luper, H., An appraisal of learning theory concepts in understanding and treating stuttering in children. In Gregory, H. (Ed.), *Learning Theory and Stuttering Therapy.* Evanston, Ill.: Northwestern University Press (1968).

Luper, H., and Mulder, R., *Stuttering Therapy for Children.* Englewood Cliffs, N.J.: Prentice-Hall, Inc. (1964).

Luria, A., *The Role of Speech in the Regulation of Normal and Abnormal Behavior.* New York: Liveright Publishing Corp. (1961).

Luria, A., *Traumatic Aphasia: Its Syndromes, Psychology and Treatment.* The Hague: Mouton (1970).

Lyle, J., The effect of an institution environment upon the verbal development of imbecile children III. The Brooklands residential family unit. *J. Ment. Defic. Res.*, **4**, 14-23 (1960).

MacAulay, B., A program for teaching speech and beginning reading to nonverbal retardates. In Sloane, H., and MacAulay, B. (Eds.), *Operant Procedures in Remedial Speech and Language Training.* Boston: Houghton Mifflin Co. (1968).

Marks, M., Stuttering viewed as a sequence of responses. In Gray, B., and England, G., (Eds)., *Stuttering and the Conditioning Therapies.* Monterey, Calif.: Monterey Institute for Speech and Hearing (1969).

Marks, M., Taylor, M., and Rusk, H., Rehabilitation of the aphasic patient: a survey of three years' experience in a rehabilitation setting. *Arch. Phys. Med. Rehab.*, **38**, 219-226 (1957).

Martin, R., The experimental manipulation of stuttering behaviors. In Sloane, H., and MacAulay, B. (Eds.), *Operant Procedures in Remedial Speech and Language Training.* Boston: Houghton Mifflin Co. (1968).

Martin, R., and Siegel, G., The effects of response contingent shock on stuttering. *J. Speech Hearing Res.*, **9**, 340-352 (1966a).

Martin, R., and Siegel, G., The effects of simultaneously punishing stuttering and rewarding fluency. *J. Speech Hearing Res.*, **9**, 466-475 (1966b).

Martyn, M., and Sheehan, J., Onset of stuttering and recovery. *Behav. Res. Ther.*, **6**, 295-307 (1968).

McDearmon, J., Programmed learning instruction in phonics. In Sloane, H., and MacAulay, B. (Eds.), *Operant Procedures in Remedial Speech and Language Training.* Boston: Houghton Mifflin Co. (1968).

Meyer, V., and Comley, J., A preliminary report on the treatment of stammer by the use of rhythmic stimulation. In Gray, B., and England, G. (Eds.), *Stuttering and the Conditioning Therapies.* Monterey, Calif.: Monterey Institute for Speech and Hearing (1969).

Milisen, R., A rationale for articulation disorders. *J. Speech Hearing Dis.*, Monogr. Suppl. 4, pp. 5-17 (1954).

Milisen, R., Articulatory problems. In Reiber, R., and Brubaker, R. (Eds.), *Speech Pathology.* Amsterdam: North-Holland Publishing Co. (1966).

Moore, P., Voice disorders organically based. In Travis, L. (Ed.), *Handbook of Speech Pathology and Audiology.* New York: Appleton-Century-Crofts (1971).

Mowrer, D., Baker, R., and Schutz, R., Operant procedures in the control of speech articulation. In Sloane, H., and MacAulay, B. (Eds.), *Operant procedures in Remedial Speech and Language Training.* Boston: Houghton Mifflin Co. (1968).

Muma, J., The communication game: dump and play. *J. Speech Hearing Dis.*, **40**, 296-309 (1975).

Munroe, R., *Schools of Psychoanalytic Thought.* New York: The Dryden Press, Inc. (1955).

Murphy, A., *Functional Voice Disorders.* Englewood Cliffs, N.J.: Prentice-Hall, Inc. (1964).

Murphy, A., and FitzSimons, R., *Stuttering and Personality Dynamics.* New York: The Ronald Press Co. (1960).

Myklebust, H., Childhood aphasia: identification, diagnosis, remediation. In Travis, L. (Ed.), *Handbook of Speech Pathology and Audiology.* New York: Appleton-Century-Crofts (1971).

Myklebust, H., Learning disabilities and minimal brain dysfunctions in children. In Tower, D. (Editor-in-chief), *The Nervous System.* (Vol. 3) *Human Communication and Its Disorders.* New York: Raven Press (1975).

Palmer, M., Studies in clinical techniques. IV. Rapid repetitive manipulation of the mandible in dysphonia. *J. Speech Hearing Dis.*, **14**, 260-261 (1949).

Perkins, W., The challenge of functional disorders of voice. In Travis, L. (Ed.), *Handbook of Speech Pathology.* New York: Appleton-Century-Crofts (1957).

Perkins, W., Modification of stuttering by rate control. Final Report, Vocational Rehabilitation Administration Planning Grant RD-2180-S (1967).

Perkins, W., Vocal function: assessment and therapy. In Travis, L. (Ed.), *Handbook of Speech Pathology and Audiology.* New York: Appleton-Century-Crofts (1971).

Perkins, W., Replacement of stuttering with normal speech. I. Rationale, *J. Speech Hearing Dis.*, **38**, 283-294 (1973a).

Perkins, W., Replacement of stuttering with normal speech. II. Clinical procedures. *J. Speech Hearing Dis.*, **38**, 295-303 (1973b).

Perkins, W., Normal vocal tone generation: detection, diagnosis, and management of abnormal vocal tone generation. In Tower, D. (Editor-in-chief), *The Nervous System.* (Vol. 3) *Human Communication and Its Disorders.* New York: Raven Press (1975).

Perkins, W., and Curlee, R., Clinical impressions of portable masking unit effects in stuttering. *J. Speech Hearing Dis.*, **34**, 360-362 (1969).

Perkins, W., and others, Replacement of stuttering with normal speech. III. Clinical effectiveness. *J. Speech Hearing Dis.*, **39**, 416-428 (1974).

Peterson, R., Imitation: a basic behavioral mechanism. In Sloane, H., and MacAulay, B. (Eds.), *Operant Procedures in Remedial Speech and Language Training.* Boston: Houghton Mifflin Co. (1968).

Powers, M., Clinical and educational procedures in functional disorders of articulation. In Travis, L. (Ed.), *Handbook of Speech Pathology and Audiology.* New York: Appleton-Century-Crofts (1971).

Premack, D., Toward empirical behavioral laws. I. Positive reinforcement. *Psychol. Rev.*, **66**, 219-233 (1959).

Premack, D., Predicting instrumental performance from the independent rate of the contingent response. *J. exper. Psychol.*, **61**, 163-171 (1961).

Premack, D., Prediction of the comparative reinforcement values of running and drinking. *Science*, **139**, 1062-1063 (1963a).

Premack, D., Rate differential reinforcement in monkey manipulation. *J. exp. Anal. Behav.*, **6**, 81-89 (1963b).

Prins, D., Improvement and regression in stutterers following short-term intensive therapy. *J. Speech Hearing Dis.*, **35**, 123-135 (1970).

Richardson, S., Language training for mentally retarded children. In Schiefelbusch, R., Copeland, R., and Smith, J. (Eds.), *Language and Mental Retardation.* New York: Holt, Rinehart & Winston, Inc. (1967).

Risley, T., Hart, B., and Doke, L., Operant language development: the outline of a therapeutic technology. In Schiefelbusch, R. (Ed.), *Language of the Mentally Retarded.* Baltimore: University Park Press (1972).

Risley, T., and Wolf, M., Establishing functional speech in echolalic children. In Sloane, H., and MacAulay, B. (Eds.), *Operant Procedures in Remedial Speech and Language Training.* Boston: Houghton Mifflin Co. (1968).

Rogers, C., The necessary and sufficient conditions of therapeutic personality change. *J. consult. Psychol.*, **21**, 95-103 (1957).

Rubin, H., and Lehrhoff, I., Pathogenesis and treatment of vocal nodules. *J. Speech Hearing Dis.*, **27**, 150-161 (1962).

Rutter, M., and Bartak, L., Special educational treatment of autistic children: a comparative study. II. Follow-up findings and implications for services. *J. Child Psychol. Psychiatry & Allied Disciplines*, **14**, 241-270 (1973).

Ryan, B., Operant procedures applied to stuttering therapy for children. *J. Speech Hearing Dis.*, **36**, 264-280 (1971).

Sands, E., Sarno, M., and Shankweiler, D., Long-term assessment of language function in aphasia due to stroke. *Arch. phys. Med. Rehab.*, **50**, 202-206 (1969).

Sarno, M., Silverman, M., and Sands, E., Speech therapy and language recovery in severe aphasia. *J. Speech Hearing Res.*, **13**, 607-623 (1970).

Schiefelbusch, R., The development of communication skills. In Schiefelbusch, R., Copeland, R., and Smith, J. (Eds.), *Language and Mental Retardation*. New York: Holt, Rinehart & Winston, Inc. (1967).

Schiefelbusch, R., Language disabilities of cognitively involved children. In Irwin, J., and Marge, M. (Eds.), *Principles of Childhood Language Disabilities*. New York: Meredith Corp. (1972).

Schuell, H., Jenkins, J., and Jiminez-Pabon, E., *Aphasia in Adults*. New York: Harper & Row, Publisher (1964).

Schulz, M., *An Analysis of Clinical Behavior in Speech and Hearing*. Englewood Cliffs, N.J.: Prentice-Hall, Inc. (1972).

Shames, G., Operant conditioning and stuttering. In Eisenson, J. (Ed.), *Stuttering: a Second Symposium*. New York: Harper & Row, Publishers (1975).

Shames, G., and Egolf, D., *Operant Conditioning and the Management of Stuttering*. Englewood Cliffs, N.J.: Prentice-Hall, Inc. (1976).

Shames, G., Egolf, D., and Rhodes, R., Experimental programs in stuttering therapy. *J. Speech Hearing Dis.*, **34**, 30-47 (1969).

Shames, G., and Sherrick, C., A discussion of nonfluency and stuttering as operant behavior. *J. Speech Hearing Dis.*, **28**, 3-18 (1963).

Shearer, W., Cybernetics in the treatment of voice disorders. *J. Speech Hearing Dis.*, **24**, 280-282 (1959).

Sheehan, J., Stuttering as a self-role conflict. In Gregory, H. (Ed.), *Learning Theory and Stuttering Therapy*. Evanston, Ill.: Northwestern University Press (1968).

Sheehan, J., The role of role in stuttering. In Gray, B., and England, G. (Eds.), *Stuttering and the Conditioning Therapies*. Monterey, Calif.: Monterey Institute for Speech and Hearing (1969).

Sheehan, J., *Stuttering: Research and Therapy*. New York: Harper & Row, Publishers (1970).

Sheehan, J., Conflict theory and avoidance-reduction therapy. In Eisenson, J. (Ed.), *Stuttering: a Second Symposium*. New York: Harper & Row, Publishers (1975).

Shelton, R., Personal communication (1968).

Shriner, T., Economically deprived: aspects of language skills. In Travis, L. (Ed.), *Handbook of Speech Pathology and Audiology*. New York: Appleton-Century-Crofts (1971).

Shuy, R., Language problems of disadvantaged children. In Irwin, J., and Marge, M. (Eds.), *Principles of Childhood Language Disabilities*. New York: Meredith Corp. (1972).

Siegel, G., Book review of *The Modification of Stuttering*. *J. Commun. Dis.*, **2**, 174-180 (1969).

Siegel, G., and Martin, R., Experimental modification of disfluency in normal speakers. *J. Speech Hearing Res.*, **8**, 235-244 (1965).

Siegel, G., and Martin, R., Punishment of disfluencies in normal speakers. *J. Speech Hearing Res.*, **9**, 208-218 (1966).

Siegel, G., and Martin, R., Verbal punishment of disfluencies during spontaneous speech. *Language Speech*, **10**, 244-251 (1967).

Siegel, G., and Martin, R., The effects of verbal stimuli on disfluencies during spontaneous speech. *J. Speech Hearing Res.*, **11**, 358-364 (1968).

Sloane, H., Johnston, M., and Harris, F., Remedial procedures for teaching verbal behavior to speech deficient or defective young children. In Sloane, H., and MacAulay, B. (Eds)., *Operant Procedures in Remedial Speech and Language Training*. Boston: Houghton Mifflin Co. (1968).

Snidecor, J., *Speech Rehabilitation of the Laryngectomized*. Springfield, Ill.: Charles C Thomas, Publisher (1969).

Spradlin, J., Baer, D., and Butterfield, E., *Communications Research With Retarded Children*. HD 00870, to Bureau of Child Research. Lawrence: University of Kansas (1970).

Spreen, O., Psycholinguistic aspects of asphasia. *J. Speech Hearing Res.*, **11**, 467-480 (1968).

Stassi, E., Disfluency of normal speakers and reinforcement. *J. Speech Hearing Res.*, **4**, 358-361 (1961).

Stoll, B., Psychological factors determining the success or failure of the rehabilitation program of laryngectomized patients. *Ann. Otol. Rhinol. Laryng.*, **67**, 550-557 (1958).

Stromsta, C., A spectrographic study of dysfluencies labeled as stuttering by parents. De Therapia Vocis et Loquelae. (Vol. 1) Societatis Internationalis Logopaediae et Phoniatriae, XIII Congressus Vindobonae, Anno MCMLXV, *Acta*, August (1965).

Strupp, H., Patient-doctor relationships: psychotherapist in the therapeutic process. In Bachrach, A. (Ed.), *Experimental Foundations of Clinical Psychology*. New York: Basic Books, Inc. (1962).

Travis, L., The psychotherapeutical process. In Travis, L. (Ed.), *Handbook of Speech Pathology and Audiology*. New York: Appleton-Century-Crofts (1971a).

Travis, L., The unspeakable feelings of people with special reference to stuttering. In Travis, L. (Ed.), *Handbook of Speech Pathology and Audiology*. New York: Appleton-Century-Crofts (1971b).

Trotter, W., and Lesch, M., Personal experiences with a stutter-aid. *J. Speech Hearing Dis.*, **32**, 270-272 (1967).

Van Riper, C., The effect of penalty upon frequency of stuttering spasms. *J. genet. Psychol.*, **50**, 193-195 (1937).

Van Riper, C., *Speech Correction: Principles and Methods*. Englewood Cliffs, N.J.: Prentice-Hall, Inc. (1972).

Van Riper, C., *The Treatment of Stuttering*. Englewood Cliffs, N.J.: Prentice-Hall, Inc. (1973).

Van Riper, C., and Irwin, J., *Voice and Articulation*. Englewood Cliffs, N.J.: Prentice-Hall, Inc. (1958).

Van Thal, J., Vocal rehabilitation. *Br. J. Dis. Commun.*, **2**, 23-29 (1967).

Wann, T. (Ed.), *Behaviorism and Phenomenology: Contrasting Bases for Modern Psychology*. Chicago: The University of Chicago Press (1964).

Webster, E., Parent counseling by speech pathologists and audiologists. *J. Speech Hearing Dis.*, **31**, 331-340 (1966).

Webster, E., Procedures for group parent counseling in speech pathology and audiology. *J. Speech Hearing Dis.*, **33**, 127-131 (1968).

Webster, R., A behavioral analysis of stuttering: treatment and theory. In Calhoun, K., Adams, H., and Mitchell, K. (Eds.), *Innovative Treatment Methods in Psychopathology*. New York: John Wiley & Sons, Inc. (1974).

Weiss, D., *Cluttering*. Englewood Cliffs, N.J.: Prentice-Hall, Inc. (1964).

Weiss, D., and Beebe, H., *The Chewing Approach in Speech and Voice Therapy*. Basel: S. Karger AG (1951).

Wepman, J., *Recovery From Aphasia*. New York: The Ronald Press Co. (1951).

Wepman, J., A conceptual model for the processes involved in recovery from aphasia. *J. Speech Hearing Dis.*, **18**, 4-13 (1953).

Wepman, J., The relationship between self-correction and recovery from aphasia. *J. Speech Hearing Dis.*, **23**, 302-305 (1958).

Wepman, J., Approaches to the analysis of aphasia. In *Human Communication and Its Disorders*. 10. Bethesda, Md.: National Institutes of Health (1969).

West, R., and Ansberry, M., *The rehabilitation of Speech*. New York: Harper & Row, Publishers (1968).

Williams, D., A point of view about "stuttering." *J. Speech Hearing Dis.*, **22**, 390-397 (1957).

Williams, D., Stuttering therapy: an overview. In Gregory, H. (Ed.), *Learning Theory and Stuttering Therapy*. Evanston, Ill.: Northwestern University Press (1968).

Williams, D., Stuttering therapy for children. In Travis, L. (Ed.), *Handbook of Speech Pathology and Audiology*. New York: Appleton-Century-Crofts (1971).

Wing, J., Diagnosis, epidemiology, aetiology. In Wing, J. (Ed.), *Early Childhood Autism: Clinical, Educational and Social Aspects*. New York: Pergamon Press, Inc. (1966).

Winitz, H., *From Syllable to Conversation*. Baltimore: University Park Press (1975).

Wischner, G., Stuttering behavior, learning theory and behavior therapy: problems, issues and progress. In Gray, B., and England, G. (Eds.), *Stuttering and the Conditioning Therapies*. Monterey, Calif.: Monterey Institute of Speech and Hearing (1969).

Wolpe, J., The experimental foundations of some new psychotherapeutic methods. In Bachrach, A. (Ed.), *Experimental Foundations of Clinical Psychology*. New York: Basic Books, Inc. (1962).

Wolpe, J., Behavior therapy of stuttering: deconditioning the emotional factor. In Gray, B., and England, G. (Eds.), *Stuttering and the Conditioning Therapies*. Monterey, Calif.: Monterey Institute for Speech and Hearing (1969).

Wolpe, J., and Lazarus, A., *Behavior Therapy Techniques*. New York: Pergamon Press, Inc. (1966).

Wolpe, Z., Play therapy, psychodrama, and parent counseling. In Travis, L. (Ed.), *Handbook of Speech Pathology*. New York: Appleton-Century-Crofts (1957).

Wood, N., *Delayed Speech and Language Development*. Englewood Cliffs, N.J.: Prentice-Hall, Inc. (1964).

Yates, A., The relationship between theory and therapy in the clinical treatment of stuttering. In Gray, B., and England, G. (Eds.), *Stuttering and the Conditioning Therapies*. Monterey, Calif.: Monterey Institute for Speech and Hearing (1969).

Young, E., and Hawk, S., *Moto-kinesthetic Speech Training*. Palo Alto, Calif.: Stanford University Press (1955).

Appendixes

Requirements for the certificates of clinical competence

Effective March 1, 1975

The American Speech and Hearing Association issues Certificates of Clinical Competence to individuals who present satisfactory evidence of their ability to provide independent clinical services to persons who have disorders of communication (speech, language, and/or hearing). An individual who meets these requirements may be awarded a Certificate in Speech Pathology or in Audiology, depending upon the emphasis of his preparation; a person who meets the requirements for both professional areas may be awarded both Certificates.

I. STANDARDS

The individual who is awarded either, or both, of the Certificates of Clinical Competence must meet the following qualifications:

I,A. General background education

As stipulated below, applicants for a certificate should have completed specialized academic training and preparatory professional experience that provides an in-depth knowledge of normal communication processes, development and disorders thereof, evaluation procedures to assess the bases of such disorders, and clinical techniques that have been shown to improve or eradicate them. It is expected that the applicant will have obtained a broad general education to serve as a background prior to such study and experience. The specific content of this general background education is left to the discretion of the applicant and to the training program which he attends. However, it is highly desirable that it include study in the areas of human psychology, sociology, psychological and physical development, the physical sciences (especially those that pertain to acoustic and biological phenomena) and human anatomy and physiology, including neuroanatomy and neurophysiology.

I,B. Required education

A total of 60 semester hours[1] of academic credit must have been accumulated from accredited colleges or universities that demonstrate that the applicant has obtained a well-integrated program of course study dealing with the normal aspects of human communication, development thereof, disorders thereof, and clinical techniques for evaluation and management of such disorders.

Twelve (12) of these 60 semester hours must be obtained in courses that provide information that pertains to normal development and use of speech, language, and hearing.

Thirty (30) of these 60 semester hours must be in courses that provide (1) information relative to communication disorders, and (2) information about and training in evaluation and management of speech, language, and hearing disorders. At least 24 of these 30 semester hours must be in courses in the professional area (speech pathology or audiology) for which the certificate is requested, and no less than six (6) semester hours may be in audiology for the certificate in speech pathology or in speech pathology for the certificate in audiology. Moreover, no more than six (6) semester hours may be in courses that pro-

[1]In evaluation of credits, one quarter hour will be considered the equivalent of two-thirds of a semester hour. Transcripts that do not report credit in terms of semester or quarter hours should be submitted for special evaluation.

vide credit for clinical practice obtained during academic training.

Credit for study of information pertaining to related fields that augment the work of the clinical practitioner of speech pathology and/or audiology may also apply toward the total 60 semester hours.

Thirty (30) of the total 60 semester hours that are required for a certificate must be in courses that are acceptable toward a graduate degree by the college or university in which they are taken. Moreover, 21 of those 30 semester hours must be within the 24 semester hours required in the professional area (speech pathology or audiology) for which the certificate is requested or within the six (6) semester hours required in the other area.[2]

I,C. Academic clinical practicum

The applicant must have completed a minimum of 300 clock hours of supervised clinical experience with individuals who present a variety of communication disorders, and this experience must have been obtained within his training institution or in one of its cooperating programs.

I,D. The Clinical Fellowship Year

The applicant must have obtained the equivalent of nine (9) months of full-time professional experience (the Clinical Fellowship Year) in which bona fide clinical work has been accomplished in the major professional area (speech pathology or audiology) in which the certificate is being sought. The Clinical Fellowship Year must have begun after completion of the academic and clinical practicum experiences specified in Standards *I,A., I,B.,* and *I,C.* above.

I,E. The National Examinations in Speech Pathology and Audiology

The applicant must have passed one of the National Examinations in Speech Pathology and Audiology, either the National Exami-

nation in Speech Pathology or the National Examination in Audiology.

I,F. Membership in the American Speech and Hearing Association

In order to make initial application for and to obtain one of the Certificates of Clinical Competence, the individual must be a member of the American Speech and Hearing Association.

II. EXPLANATORY NOTES
II,A. General background education

While the broadest possible general educational background for the future clinical practitioner of speech pathology and/or audiology is encouraged, the nature of the clinician's professional endeavors suggests the necessity for some emphasis in his general education. For example, elementary courses in general psychology and sociology are desirable as are studies in mathematics, general physics, zoology, as well as human anatomy and physiology. These areas of introductory study that do not deal specifically with communication processes are not to be credited to the minimum 60 semester hours of education specified in Standard *I,B.*

II,B. Required education

II,B,1. Basic Communication Processes Area. The 12 semester hours in courses that provide information applicable to the normal development and use of speech, language, and hearing should be selected with emphasis upon the normal aspects of human communication in order that the applicant has a wide exposure to the diverse kinds of information suggested by the content areas given under the three broad categories that follow: (1) anatomic and physiologic bases for the normal development and use of speech, language, and hearing, such as anatomy, neurology, and physiology of speech, language, and hearing mechanisms; (2) physical bases and processes of the production and perception of speech and hearing, such as (a) acoustics or physics of sound, (b) phonology, (c) physiologic and acoustic phonetics, (d) perceptual processes, and (e) psychoacoustics; and (3) linguistic and psycholinguistic vari-

---

[2]This requirement may be met by courses completed as an undergraduate providing the college or university in which they are taken specifies that these courses would be acceptable toward a graduate degree if they were taken at the graduate level.

ables related to normal development and use of speech, language, and hearing, such as (a) linguistics (historical, descriptive, sociolinguistics, urban language), (b) psychology of language, (c) psycholinguistics, (d) language and speech acquisition, and (e) verbal learning or verbal behavior.

It is emphasized that the three broad categories of required education given above, and the examples of areas of study within these classifications, are not meant to be analogous with, nor imply, specific course titles. Neither are the examples of areas of study within these categories meant to be exhaustive.

At least two (2) semester hours of credit must be earned in each of the three categories.

Obviously, some of these 12 semester hours may be obtained in courses that are taught in departments other than those offering speech pathology and audiology programs. Courses designed to improve the speaking and writing ability of the student will not be credited.

II,B,2. Major professional area, Certificate in Speech Pathology. The 24 semester hours of professional education required for the Certificate of Clinical Competence in Speech Pathology should include mastery of information pertaining to speech and language disorders as follows: (1) understanding of speech and language disorders, such as (a) various types of disorders of communication, (b) their manifestations, and (c) their classifications and causes; (2) evaluation skills, such as procedures, techniques, and instrumentation used to assess (a) the speech and language status of children and adults, and (b) the bases of disorders of speech and language, and (3) management procedures, such as principles in remedial methods used in habilitation and rehabilitation for children and adults with various disorders of communication.

Within these categories at least six (6) semester hours must deal with speech disorders and at least six (6) hours must deal with language disorders.

II,B,3. Minor professional area, Certificate in Speech Pathology. For the individual

to obtain the Certificate in Speech Pathology, he must have not less than six (6) semester hours of academic credit in audiology. Where only this minimum requirement of six (6) semester hours is met, three (3) semester hours must be in habilitative/rehabilitative procedures with speech and language problems associated with hearing impairment, and three (3) semester hours must be in study of the pathologies of the auditory system and assessment of auditory disorders. However, when more than the minimum six (6) semester hours is met, study of habilitative/rehabilitative procedures may be counted in the *Major Professional Area for the Certificate in Speech Pathology (Section II,B,8).*

II,B,4. Major professional area, Certificate in Audiology. The 24 semester hours of professional education required for the Certificate of Clinical Competence in Audiology should be in the broad, but not necessarily exclusive, categories of study as follows: (1) auditory disorders, such as (a) pathologies of the auditory system, and (b) assessment of auditory disorders and their effect upon communication; (2) habilitative/rehabilitative procedures, such as (a) selection and use of appropriate amplification instrumentation for the hearing impaired, both wearable and group, (b) evaluation of speech and language problems of the hearing impaired, and (c) management procedures for speech and language habilitation and/or rehabilitation of the hearing impaired (that may include manual communication); (3) conservation of hearing, such as (a) environmental noise control, and (b) identification audiometry (school, military, industry); and (4) instrumentation, such as (a) electronics, (b) calibration techniques, and (c) characteristics of amplifying systems.

Not less than six (6) semester hours must be in the auditory pathology category, and not less than six (6) semester hours must be in the habilitation/rehabilitation category.

II,B,5. Minor professional area, Certificate in Audiology. For the individual to obtain the Certificate in Audiology, not less than six (6) semester hours must be obtained in the areas of speech and language pathology; of these three (3) hours must be in the area of speech pathology and three (3) hours in the area of language pathology. It is suggested that where only this minimum requirement of six (6) semester hours is met, such study be in the areas of evaluation procedures and management of speech and language problems that are not associated with hearing impairment.

II,B,6. Related areas. In addition to the 12 semester hours of course study in the Basic Communication Processes Area, the 24 semester hours in the Major Professional Area and the six (6) semester hours in the Minor Professional Area, the applicant may receive credit toward the minimum requirement of 60 semester hours of required education through advanced study in a variety of related areas. Such study should pertain to the understanding of human behavior, both normal and abnormal, as well as services available from related professions, and that, in general, should augment his background for a professional career. Examples of such areas of study are as follows: (a) theories of learning and behavior, (b) services available from related professions that also deal with persons who have disorders of communication, and (c) information from these professions about the sensory, physical, emotional, social and/or intellectual status of a child or an adult.

Academic credit that is obtained for practice teaching or practicum work in other professions will not be counted toward the minimum requirements.

In order that the future applicant for one of the certificates will be capable of critically reviewing scientific matters dealing with clinical issues relative to speech pathology and audiology, credit for study in the areas of statistics, beyond an introductory course, will be allowed to a maximum of three (3) semester hours. Academic study of the administrative organization of speech pathology and audiology programs also may be applied to a maximum of three (3) semester hours.

II,B,7. Education applicable to all areas. Certain types of course work may be acceptable among more than one of the areas of study specified above, depending upon the emphasis. For example, courses that provide an overview of research, e.g., introduction to graduate study or introduction to research, that consist primarily of a critical review of research in communication sciences, disorders, or management thereof, and/or a more general presentation of research procedures and techniques which will permit the clinician to read and evaluate literature critically will be acceptable to a maximum of three (3) semester hours. Such courses may be credited to the Basic Communication Processes Area, or one of the Professional Areas or the Related Areas, if substantive content of the course(s) covers material in those areas. Academic credit for a thesis or dissertation may be acceptable to a maximum of three (3) semester hours in the appropriate area. An abstract of the study must be submitted with the application if such credit is requested. In order to be acceptable, the thesis or dissertation must have been an experimental or descriptive investigation in the areas of speech and hearing science, speech pathology or audiology; that is, credit will not be allowed if the project was a survey of opinions, a study of professional issues, an annotated bibliography, biography, or a study of curricular design.

As implied by the above, the academic credit hours obtained for one course or one enrollment, may, and should be, in some instances divided among the Basic Communication Processes Area, one of the Professional Areas, and/or the Related Areas. In such cases, a description of the content of that course should accompany the application. This description should be extensive enough to provide the Clinical Certification Board with information necessary to evaluate the validity of the request to apply the content to more than one of the areas.

II,B,8. Major professional education applicable to both certificates. Study in the area of understanding, evaluation, and management of speech and language disorders associated with hearing impairment may apply to the 24 semester hours of Major Professional Area required for either certificate (speech pathology or audiology). However, no more than six (6) semester hours of that study will be allowed in that manner for the certificate in speech pathology.

II,C. Academic clinical practicum

It is highly desirable that students who anticipate applying for one of the Certificates of Clinical Competence have the opportunity, relatively early in their training program, to observe the various procedures involved in a clinical program in speech pathology and audiology, but this passive participation is not to be construed as direct clinical practicum during academic training. The student should participate in supervised, direct clinical experience during that training only after he has had sufficient course work to qualify him to work as a student clinician and only after he has sufficient background to undertake clinical practice under direct supervision. A minimum of 150 clock hours of the supervised clinical experience must be obtained during graduate study. Once this experience is undertaken, a substantial period of time may be spent in writing reports, in preparation for clinical sessions, in conferences with supervisors, and in class attendance to discuss clinical procedures and experiences; such time may not be credited toward the 300 minimum clock hours of supervised clinical experience required.

All student clinicians are expected to obtain direct clinical experience with both children and adults, and it is recommended that some of their direct clinical experience be conducted with groups. Although the student clinician should have experience with both speech and hearing disorders, at least 200 clock hours of this supervised experience must be obtained in the major professional area (speech pathology or audiology) in which he will seek certification, and not less than 35 clock hours must be obtained in the minor area.

For certification in speech pathology, the student clinician is expected to have experience in both the evaluation and management of a variety of speech and language problems. He must have no less than 50 clock hours of experience in evaluation of speech and language problems. He must also have no less than 75 clock hours of experience in management of language disorders of children and adults, and he must have no less than 25 clock hours each of experience in management of children and adults with whom disorders of (1) voice, (2) articulation, and (3) fluency are significant aspects of the communication handicap.[3]

Where only the minimum 35 clock hours of clinical practicum in audiology is met that is required for the persons seeking certification in speech pathology, that practicum must include 15 clock hours in assessment and/or management of speech and language problems associated with hearing impairment, and 15 clock hours must be in assessment of auditory disorders. However, where more than this minimum requirement is met, clinical practicum in assessment and/or management of speech and language problems associated with hearing impairment may be counted toward the minimum clock hours obtained with language and/or speech disorders.

For the student clinician who is preparing for certification in audiology, 50 clock hours of direct supervised experience must be obtained in identification and evaluation of hearing impairment, and 50 clock hours must be obtained in habilitation or rehabilitation of the communication handicaps of the hearing impaired. It is suggested that the 35 clock hours of clinical practicum in speech pathology required for certification in audiology be in evaluation and management of speech and language problems that are not related to a hearing impairment.

Supervisors of clinical practicum must be competent professional workers who hold a Certificate of Clinical Competence in the professional area (speech pathology or audiology) in which supervision is provided. This supervision must entail the personal and di-

---

[3]Work with multiple problems may be credited among these types of disorders. For example, a child with an articulation problem may also have a voice disorder. The clock hours of work with that child may be credited to experience with either articulation or voice disorders, whichever is most appropriate.

rect involvement of the supervisor in any and all ways that will permit him to attest to the adequacy of the student's performance in the clinical training experience. Knowledge of the student's clinical work may be obtained through a variety of ways such as conferences, audio and video tape recordings, written reports, staffings, discussions with other persons who have participated in the student's clinical training, and must include direct observation of the student in clinical sessions.

II,D. The Clinical Fellowship Year

Upon completion of his professional and clinical practicum education, the applicant must complete his Clinical Fellowship Year under the supervision of one who holds the Certificate of Clinical Competence in the professional area (speech pathology or audiology) in which that applicant is working (and seeking certification).

Professional experience is construed to mean direct clinical work with patients, consultations, record keeping, or any other duties relevant to a bona fide program of clinical work. It is expected, however, that a significant amount of clinical experience will be in direct clinical contact with persons who have communication handicaps. Time spent in supervision of students, academic teaching, and research, as well as administrative activity that does not deal directly with management programs of specific patients or clients will not be counted as professional experience in this context.

The Clinical Fellowship Year is defined as no less than nine months of full-time professional employment, with full-time employment defined as a minimum of 30 hours of work a week. This requirement also may be fulfilled by part-time employment as follows: (1) work of 15 to 19 hours per week over 18 months; (2) work of 20 to 24 hours per week over 15 months; or, (3) work of 25 to 29 hours per week over 12 months. In the event that part-time employment is used to fulfill a part of the Clinical Fellowship Year, 100 percent of the minimum hours of the part-time work per week requirement must be spent in di-

rect professional experience as defined above. The Clinical Fellowship Year must be completed within a maximum period of 36 consecutive months. Professional employment of less than 15 hours per week will not fulfill any part of this requirement.[4]

II,E. The National Examinations in Speech Pathology and Audiology

The National Examinations in Speech Pathology and Audiology are designed to assess, in a comprehensive fashion, the applicant's mastery of professional concepts as outlined above to which the applicant has been exposed throughout his professional education and clinical practicum.[5] The applicant must pass the National Examination, in either Speech Pathology or Audiology, that is appropriate to the certificate being sought. An applicant will be declared eligible for the National Examination on notification of the acceptable completion of the educational and clinical practicum requirements. The Examination must be passed within three years after the first administration for which an applicant is notified of his eligibility.

In the event the applicant fails the examination, he may retake it. If the examination is not successfully completed within the above mentioned three years, the person's application for certification will lapse. If the examination is passed at a later date, the person may reapply for clinical certification.[6]

---

[4]Further guidelines for the Clinical Fellowship Year are available, and, moreover, such guidelines are provided with application material for certification.

[5]An applicant for the Certificate of Clinical Competence ordinarily will be held to the requirements in effect two years prior to his completion of the required education and practicum requirements. Moreover, an applicant whose application has been rejected may reapply if changes in the requirements make his application acceptable as a result of such changes. However, if the Clinical Fellowship Year is not initiated within five years of the time academic and practicum requirements are completed, the applicant must meet academic and practicum requirements that are current when the Clinical Fellowship Year is begun.

[6]Upon such reapplication, the individual's application will be reviewed and current requirements will be applied. Appropriate fees will be charged for this review.

III. PROCEDURES FOR OBTAINING THE CERTIFICATES

III,A. Application for membership in the American Speech and Hearing Association and the initial application for certification may be made simultaneously and applicants are urged to follow this procedure.[7] However, applications for certification will not be evaluated until membership is approved and validated by the payment of dues.

III,B. The applicant must submit to the Clinical Certification Board, a description of his professional education and academic clinical practicum on forms provided for that purpose. The applicant should recognize that it is highly desirable to list upon this application form his entire professional education and academic clinical practicum training.

No credit may be allowed for courses listed on the application unless satisfactory completion is verified by an official transcript. *Satisfactory completion* is defined as the applicant's having received academic credit (i.e., semester hours, quarter hours, or other unit of credit) with a passing grade as defined by the training institution. If an applicant receives his training from a program accredited by the American Boards of Examiners in Speech Pathology and Audiology (ABESPA), approval of his educational requirements and academic clinical practicum will be automatic.

The applicant must request that the director of the training program where the majority of his graduate training was obtained sign the application. In the case where that training program is not accredited by ABESPA, that director, by his signature, (1) certifies that the application is correct, and (2) recommends that the applicant receive the certificate upon completion of all the requirements. In the case where the training program is accredited by ABESPA that director (1) certifies that the applicant has met the educational and clinical practicum requirements, and (2) recommends that the applicant receive the certificate upon completion of all the requirements.

In the event that the applicant cannot obtain the recommendation of the director of the training program, the applicant should send with his application a letter giving in detail the reasons he has been unable to do so. In such an instance he may wish to obtain letters of recommendations from other faculty members.

Application for approval of educational requirements and academic clinical practicum experiences should be made (1) as soon as possible after completion of those experiences, and (2) either before or shortly after the Clinical Fellowship Year is begun.

III,C. Upon completion of educational and academic clinical practicum training, the applicant should proceed to obtain professional employment and a supervisor for his Clinical Fellowship Year. The applicant and his supervisor must then submit to the Clinical Certification Board prior to the end of the first two months of employment a plan outlining how supervision of the Clinical Fellowship Year will be carried out. Assuming that this plan is approved, the applicant should then proceed to complete his Clinical Fellowship Year, after which an appropriate report should be submitted again to the Clinical Certification Board.

III,D. Upon notification by the Clinical Certification Board, of approval of the academic course work and clinical practicum requirements the applicant will be sent registration material for the National Examinations in Speech Pathology and Audiology. Upon approval of his Clinical Fellowship Year, achieving a passing score on the National Examination, and payment of all fees and current dues the applicant will become certified.

III,E. As mentioned in Footnote 7, a schedule of fees for certification may be obtained and payment of these fees is requisite for the various steps involved in obtaining a certificate. Checks should be made payable to the American Speech and Hearing Association.

---

[7]Application material for membership and certification, including a schedule of fees, may be obtained by writing to Manager, Professional Services Department, American Speech and Hearing Association, 9030 Old Georgetown Road, Washington, D.C. 20014.

IV. APPEALS

In the event that at any stage the Clinical Certification Board informs the applicant that his application has been rejected, the applicant has the right of formal appeal. In order to initiate such an appeal, the applicant must write to the Chairman of the Clinical Certification Board and specifically request a formal review of his application. If that review results, again, in rejection, the applicant has the right to request a review of his case by the American Boards of Examiners in Speech Pathology and Audiology (ABESPA) by writing to the Chairman of ABESPA at the National Office of the American Speech and Hearing Association.

Appendix B

Code of Ethics of the American Speech and Hearing Association

January 1, 1974

PREAMBLE

The preservation of the highest standards of integrity and ethical principles is vital to the successful discharge of the responsibilities of all Members. This Code of Ethics has been promulgated by the Association in an effort to highlight the fundamental rules considered essential to this basic purpose. The failure to specify any particular responsibility or practice in this Code of Ethics should not be construed as denial of the existence of other responsibilities or practices that are equally important. Any act that is in violation of the spirit and purpose of this Code of Ethics shall be unethical practice. It is the responsibility of each Member to advise the Ethical Practice Board of instances of violation of the principles incorporated in this Code.

Section A. The ethical responsibilities of the Member require that the welfare of the person he serves professionally be considered paramount.

1. The Member who engages in clinical work must possess appropriate qualifications. Measures of such qualifications are provided by the Association's program for certification of the clinical competence of Members.

(a) The Member must not provide services for which he has not been properly trained, i.e., had the necessary course work and supervised practicum.

(b) The Member who has not completed his professional preparation must not provide speech or hearing services except in a supervised clinical practicum situation as a part of his training. A person holding a full-time clinical position and taking part-time graduate work is not, for the purpose of this section, regarded as a student in training.

(c) The Member must not accept remuneration for providing services until he has completed the necessary course work and clinical practicum to meet certification requirements. The Member who is uncertified must not engage in private practice.

2. The Member must follow acceptable patterns of professional conduct in his relations with the persons he serves.

(a) He must not guarantee the results of any speech or hearing consultative or therapeutic procedure. A guarantee of any sort, expressed or implied, oral or written, is contrary to professional ethics. A reasonable statement of prognosis may be made, but successful results are dependent on many uncontrollable factors, hence, any warranty is deceptive and unethical.

(b) He must not diagnose or treat individual speech or hearing disorders by correspondence. This does not preclude follow-up by correspondence of individuals previously seen, nor does it preclude providing the persons served professionally with general information of an educational nature.

(c) He must not reveal to unauthorized persons any confidential information obtained from the individual he serves professionally without his permission.

(d) He must not exploit persons he serves professionally: (1) by accepting them for treatment where benefit cannot reasonably be expected to accrue; (2) by continuing treatment unnecessarily; (3) by charging exorbitant fees.

419

3. The Member must use every resource available, including referral to other specialists as needed, to effect as great improvement as possible in the persons he serves.

4. The Member must take every precaution to avoid injury to the persons he serves professionally.

Section B. The duties owed by the Member to other professional workers are many.

1. He should seek the freest professional discussion of all theoretical and practical issues but avoid personal invective directed toward professional colleagues or members of allied professions.

2. He should establish harmonious relations with members of other professions. He should endeavor to inform others concerning the services that can be rendered by members of the speech and hearing profession and in turn should seek information from members of related professions. He should strive to increase knowledge within the field of speech and hearing.

3. He must not accept fees, gifts, or other forms of gratuity for serving as a sponsor of applicants for clinical certification by the American Speech and Hearing Association.

Section C. The ASHA Member has other special responsibilities.

1. He must guard against conflicts of professional interest.

(a) He must not accept compensation in any form from a manufacturer or a dealer in prosthetic or other devices for recommending any particular product.

(b) The Member in private practice must not advertise: It is permissible only to employ a business card or similar announcement, and to list one's name, highest academic degree, type of services, and location in the classified section of the telephone directory in the manner customarily followed by physicians and attorneys. He may state that he holds the Certificate of Clinical Competence in the appropriate area (speech pathology and/or audiology) issued by the American Speech and Hearing Association.

(c) He must not engage in commercial activities that conflict with his responsibilities to the persons he serves professionally or to his colleagues. He must not permit his professional titles or accomplishments to be used in the sale or promotion of any product related to his professional field. He must not perform clinical services or promotional activity for any profit-making organization that is engaged in the retail sales of equipment, publications, or other materials. He may be employed by a manufacturer or publisher, provided that his duties are consultative, scientific, or educational in nature.

2. He should help in the education of the public regarding speech and hearing problems and other matters lying within his professional competence.

3. He should seek to provide and expand services to persons with speech and hearing handicaps, and to assist in establishing high professional standards for such programs.

4. He must not discriminate on the basis of race, religion, sex, or age in his professional relationships with his colleagues or clients.

Appendix C

A selected basic reference list for speech and hearing sciences, speech pathology, and audiology

Compiled by William Tiffany and students, Seattle, University of Washington Speech Science Laboratories, 1967; updated by author

JOURNALS

The very large number of journals in the areas related to studies in language and speech make it impractical to list all pertinent or significant ones in this reference guide. A few that are more or less directly "in" the areas of speech science and speech pathology and audiology are listed, as are some of the closely related journals. No attempt is made to be exhaustive.

For a more complete listing of pertinent journals, the lists normally reviewed by the more important abstracting services are readily available. See especially the following:

dsh Abstracts. Washington, D.C.: Deafness, Speech and Hearing Publications, Inc., American Speech and Hearing Association and Gallaudet College. Oct., 1966, issue contains a complete listing of journals currently abstracted.

LLBA: Language and Language Behavior Abstracts. New York: Appleton-Century-Crofts. *Each issue contains a complete listing of journals abstracted.*

Speech and hearing journals

American Annals of the Deaf. Washington, D.C.: Gallaudet College. Conference of Executives of American Schools for the Deaf, Convention of American Instructors of the Deaf.

Archives of Speech (no longer in publication). Iowa City: Department of Speech, State University of Iowa.

Asha: A Journal of the American Speech and Hearing Association. Washington, D.C.

Brain and Language. New York: Academic Press, Inc.

British Journal of Communication Disorders: the Journal of the College of Speech Therapists, London. London: E. & S. Livingstone. (Formerly *Speech Pathology and Therapy.*)

International Audiology. Leiden, Netherlands: The International Society of Audiology.

Journal of Auditory Research. Groton, Conn.: The C. W. Shilling Auditory Research Center, Inc.

Journal of Fluency Disorders. Tampa, Fla.: University of South Florida College of Social and Behavioral Sciences, Communicology Department.

Journal of Communication Disorders. New York: American Elsevier Publishing Co., Inc.

Journal of Speech and Hearing Disorders. Washington, D.C.: American Speech and Hearing Association.

Journal of Speech and Hearing Research. Washington, D.C.: American Speech and Hearing Association.

Language and Speech. Teddington, Middlesex, England: Robert Draper, Ltd.

Language Learning: a Journal of Applied Linguistics. Ann Arbor, Mich.: University of Michigan.

Language, Speech, and Hearing Services in Schools. Washington, D.C.: American Speech and Hearing Association.

Logos. New York: National Hospital for Speech Disorders.

Phonetica. Basel: S. Karger AG.

Quarterly Journal of Speech. Bloomington, Ill.: Speech Association of America.

Speech Monographs. Bloomington, Ill.: Speech Association of America.

Speech Pathology and Therapy. London: College of Speech Therapists.

Teacher of the Deaf. Newbury, Berks, England: National College for Teachers of the Deaf.

Volta Review. Washington, D.C.: Alexander Graham Bell Association for the Deaf, Volta Bureau.

Other selected journals

Acta Oto-Laryngologica. Stockholm: Almqvist & Wiksells.

American Journal of Mental Deficiency. Albany, N.Y.: American Association on Mental Deficiency.

American Journal of Physiology. Washington, D.C.: American Physiological Society.

American Speech. New York: Columbia University Press.

Annals of Otology, Rhinology and Laryngology. St. Louis: Annals Publishing Co.

Archives of Otolaryngology. Chicago: American Medical Association.

The Cleft Palate Journal: An International Journal of Craniofacial Anomalies. Baltimore: American Cleft Palate Association.

Folia Phoniatrica; International Journal of Phoniatrics. Basel: S. Karger AG.

Journal of Abnormal and Social Psychology. Washington, D.C.: American Psychological Association.

Journal of Experimental Psychology. Washington, D.C.: American Psychological Association.

Journal of Learning Disabilities. Chicago: Professional Press, Inc.

Journal of the Acoustical Society of America. New York: American Institute of Physics.

Journal of Verbal Learning and Verbal Behavior, New York: Academic Press, Inc.

Laryngoscope. St. Louis: American Otological Society.

Perception and Psychophysics. Austin, Texas: The Psychonomic Society.

Psychophysiology. Baltimore: Society for Psychophysiological Research.

Science. Washington, D.C.: American Association for the Advancement of Science.

ABSTRACTS AND YEARBOOKS

Abstracts of Japanese Medicine. Amsterdam, London, New York, Milan: Excerpta Medica Foundation.

Abstracts of Soviet Medicine. Amsterdam, London, New York, Milan: Excerpta Medica Foundation.

Abstracts of World Medicine. London: British Medical Association.

Biological Abstracts. Philadelphia: Biological Abstracts, Inc. Union of American Biological Societies.

Birth Defects: Abstracts of Selected Articles. New York: The National Foundation.

Child Development Abstracts and Bibliography. Lafayette, Ind.: Child Development Publications, Society for Research in Child Development, Inc., Purdue University.

Dental Abstracts. Crawfordsville, Ind.: American Dental Association. (Vol. 1) 1956-date. Monthly.

Dissertation Abstracts. Ann Arbor, Mich.: University Microfilm, Inc.

dsh Abstracts. Washington, D.C.: Deafness, Speech and Hearing Publications, Inc., American Speech and Hearing Association, and Gallaudet College.

Education Abstracts. Paris: Education Clearing House, United Nations Educational Scientific and Cultural Organization, 1950-1964. Title varies—before 1943—Albany, New York.

Educational Research Information Center—ERIC. Washington, D.C.: Document Reproduction Service, U.S. Department of Health, Education, and Welfare.

Excerpta Medica. Amsterdam, New York, London, Milan, Tokyo, Buenos Aires: Excerpta Medica Foundation.

International Abstracts of Biological Sciences. Oxford, London, New York, Paris: Pergamon Press for Biological and Medical Abstracts Limited. Vol. 1—to date, Jan., 1954.

International Abstracts of Surgery (supplementary to *Surgery, Gynecology, and Obstetrics*). Chicago: The Franklin H. Martin Memorial Foundation. (Vol. 16) 1913-date. Monthly.

Language Research in Progress. Washington, D.C.: Center for Applied Linguistics.

LLBA: Language and Language Behavior Abstracts. New York: Appleton-Century-Crofts.

Mental Measurements Yearbook. Buros, E. K., Jr. (Ed.). Highland Park, N.J.: Gryphon Press. Five editions from 1941 to 1959.

Mental Retardation Abstracts. Bethesda, Md.: National Clearinghouse for Mental Health Information, National Institute of Mental Health. (Vol. 2) 1965-date.

Modern Language Abstracts. Classified for shelves.

Psychological Abstracts. Washington, D.C.: American Psychological Association, Inc.

Rehabilitation Literature. Chicago: National Society for Crippled Children and Adults, Inc.

Year Book of Dentistry. Chicago: Year Book Medical Publishers, Inc.

Year Book of Education. London: Evans Brothers, Ltd.

Year Book of Medicine. Chicago: Year Book Medical Publishers, Inc.

Year Book of Neurology, Psychiatry, and Neurosurgery. Chicago: Year Book Medical Publishers, Inc.

Year Book of Pathology and Clinical Pathology. Chicago: Year Book Medical Publishers, Inc.

INDEXES AND CATALOGS

American Library Annual. New York: R. R. Bowker Co. 1911-date.

Applied Science and Technology Index. New York: The H. W. Wilson Co. 1958-date.

Auer, J. (Ed.), Doctoral dissertations in speech: work in progress. *Speech Monographs.* New York: The Speech Association of America. 1951-date. Annually.

Black, A. D., *Index of the Periodical Dental Literature Published in the English Language.* Buffalo: Dental Index Bureau. 1839-date.

Bibliographic Index: A Cumulative Bibliography of Bibliographies. New York: The H. W. Wilson Co. 1938-date.

Broadus, R. N., *The Research Literature of the Field of Speech.* ACRL Monographs No. 7. Chicago: Publication Committee of the Association of College and Reference Libraries, Jan. 1953, pp. 22-31.

Cumulative Book Index. New York: The H. W. Wilson Co. 1898-date.

Cumulative Indexes of the Journal of the American Speech and Hearing Association. Journal of Speech and Hearing Disorders, Vol. 1-26, 1936-1961. *Journal of Speech and Hearing Research,* Vol. 1-4, 1958-1961. *Asha,* Vol. 1-3, 1959-1961. Washington, D.C., 1962.

Cumulative Indexes of the Journals of the American Speech and Hearing Association. Journal of Speech and Hearing Disorders, Vol. 27-37, 1962-1972. *Monograph Supplements and Asha Monographs,* Nos. 10-17, 1962-1972. *Journal of Speech and Hearing Research,* Vol. 5-15, 1962-1972. *Language, Speech, and Hearing Services in Schools,* Vol. I-III, 1970-1972. *Asha Reports,* Nos. 1-7, 1965-1972. *Asha,* Vol. 4-14, 1962-1972. Washington, D.C. (1972).

Current List of Medical Literature. Washington, D.C.: National Library of Medicine, U.S. Department of Health, Education, and Welfare, January, 1942, to December, 1959.

Education Index. New York: The H. W. Wilson Co. 1929-date.

Gilchrist, D. B. (Ed.), *Doctoral dissertations accepted by American Universities.* New York: The H. W. Wilson Co. 1933-date.

Gregory, W. (Ed.), *Union List of Serials in Libraries of The United States and Canada.* (2nd ed.) New York: The H. W. Wilson Co. (1943).

Index Medicus, a quarterly classified record of the current medical literature of the world. Washington, D.C.: Carnegie Institute. 1927-date.

Index Psychoanalyticus. London: Hogarth Press and the Institute of Psycho-Analysis (1926).

Index to Dental Literature. Chicago: American Dental Association. 1939-date.

Index Translationum. Paris: UNESCO. 1955-date.

International Index: a guide to periodical literature in social science and humanities. 1907/1915 to date. New York: The H. W. Wilson Co. (1916).

Ireland, N. O. An index to indexes, a subject bibliography of published indexes. Boston: The F. W. Paxon Co. (1942).

Japanese Periodicals Index: Natural Sciences. Tokyo: National Diet Library. 1960-date.

Journal of the Acoustical Society of America. "Current Publications on Acoustics." New York: Acoustical Society of America. Vol 1-date.

Knower, F. H. (Ed.), *Graduate Thesis: an Index of Graduate Work in Speech*. Speech Monographs. New York: The Speech Association of America. 1935-date. Annually.

Library of Congress National Union Catalogue of Motion Pictures and Film Strips. New York: Rowman & Littlefield, Inc. Published periodically.

Poole's Index to Periodical Literature. (Rev. ed.) New York: Peter Smith (1938).

Rehabilitation Literature. Chicago: National Society for Crippled Children and Adults.

Research in Education. Washington, D.C.: ERIC—Educational Research Information Center, Superintendent of Documents, U.S. Department of Health, Education, and Welfare.

Science Citation Index, an International Index to the Literature of Science and Technology in Eight Parts. Philadelphia: Institute for Scientific Information, Inc. 1961-date.

The Index of Psychoanalytic Writings. New York: International Universities Press (1956). Revision and bringing to date of Index Psychoanalyticus. Author and subject index.

The Psychological Index. Princeton, N.J.: The American Psychological Association, Psychological Review Co. 1894-1935.

The Year Book of Education. London: Evans Brothers, Ltd. 1934-date.

U.S. Superintendent of Documents, monthly catalog of U.S. public documents. Washington, D.C.: Government Printing Office. 1895-date.

Walford, A. J. (Ed.), *Guide to Reference Material*. London: Library Association, 1959; Supplement, 1963.

Winchell, C. M., *Guide to Reference Books*. (7th ed.) Supplement, 1950-1952; 1953-1955; 1956-1958; 1959-June, 1962. Chicago: American Library Association (1951).

World List of Scientific Periodicals Published in Years 1900-1960. London: Butterworth (1965).

Year Book of Dentistry. Chicago: Year Book Medical Publishers. 1937-date.

Year Book of Neurology, Psychiatry, and Neurosurgery. Chicago: Year Book Medical Publishers. 1935-date.

Reader's Guide to Periodical Literature. New York: The H. W. Wilson Co. 1900-date.

BIBLIOGRAPHIES AND DICTIONARIES

Anderson, J., Bibliography on esophageal speech. *J. Speech Hearing Dis.*, **19**, 70-72 (1954).

Bibliographic Index: a Cumulated Bibliography of Bibliographies. New York: The H. W. Wilson Co. 1945-date.

Bibliography on Hearing. Harvard University Psycho-Acoustic Laboratory (1955).

Bibliography of Medical Reviews. Washington, D.C.: U.S. Department of Health, Education, and Welfare. Issued by the National Library of Congress (1961).

Bibliography of Medical Translations. U.S. Department of Commerce, Office of Technical Service (1963).

Broadus, R. N., Some sources of literature on speech disorders. *J. Speech Hearing Dis.*, **16**, 61-64 (1951).

Broadus, R. N., *The Research Literature in the Field of Speech*. Chicago: Publications Committee of the Association of College Reference Libraries (1953), p. 31.

DiCarlo, L. M., and Amster, W. M., The auditorily and speech handicapped. *Rev. Educat. Res.*, **23**, 453-475 (1953).

A Dictionary of Speech Pathology and Therapy. Cambridge, Mass.: Science-Art Publishers (1951).

Dorland, W. A. N., *Illustrated Medical Dictionary* (24th ed.) Philadelphia: W. B. Saunders Co. (1965). 1724 pages illustrated.

English, H. B., and English, A. C., *A Comprehensive Dictionary of Psychological and Psychoanalytical Terms*. New York: David McKay Co., Inc. (1964).

Frampton, M. E., and Gall, E. B. (Eds.), *Resources for Special Education*. Boston: P. Sargent (1956), 250 p.

Graham, E. C., and Mullen, M., *Rehabilitation Literature, 1950-1955*. New York: McGraw-Hill Book Co. (1956).

Harriman, P. L., *New Dictionary of Psychology*. New York: Philosophical Library, Inc. (1947).

Heber, R., and others, *Bibliography of World Literature in Mental Retardation, Jan., 1940–March, 1963*. Washington, D.C.: President's Panel of Mental Retardation, U.S. Department of Health, Education, and Welfare, Public Health Service (1963), 564 pages.

Knower, F. H., A selected bibliography of bibliographies for students of speech, *SSJ*, **17**, 141-153 (1951).

Landes, B. A., Selected bibliography on voice disorders. *J. Speech Hearing Dis.*, **24**, 285-299 (1957).

Leopold, W. F., *Bibliography of Child Language*. Evanston, Ill.: Northwestern University Studies, Humanities Series No. 28 (1952).

Leutnegger, R. R., A bibliography of aphasia. *J. Speech Hearing Dis.*, **16**, 280-292 (1951).

Loring, J. C. G., Selected bibliography on the effects of high-intensity on man. *JSHD Monograph Suppl.* No. 3 (Jan., 1954).

Martens, E. H., *An Annotated Bibliography on the Education and Psychology of Exceptional Children*. Washington, D.C.: U.S. Government Printing Office (1937), 42 pages.

McCroskey, R. L., and Bell, M. M., An annotated bibliography of publications on testing the hearing of infants. *Volta Rev.*, **67**, 548-593 (1965).

Mecham, M. J., Bibliography of publications of speech and hearing in cerebral palsy, 1933-1956. *JSHD*, **22**, 348-355 (1957).

Mulgrave, D., and others, *Bibliography of Speech and Allied Areas*. Philadelphia: Chilton Co. (1962).

National Society for Crippled Children and Adults, *A List of References on the Deaf and Hard of Hearing*. Chicago (1948).

National Society for Crippled Children and Adults, *A Selective Bibliography of Cerebral Palsy: an Author-Subject Index*. Chicago (1947).

National Society for Crippled Children and Adults, *A*

Special Education Bibliography: a Selection of Titles. Chicago (1948).

National Society for Crippled Children and Adults, *A Speech Correction Bibliography.* Chicago (1949).

Robbins, S. D., *A Dictionary of Speech Pathology and Therapy.* Cambridge, Mass.: Sci-Art Publishers (1951).

Rothstein, J., *Mental Retardation: Readings and Resources.* New York: Holt, Rinehart & Winston, Inc. (1962).

Thonssen, L., and Fatherson, E., *A Bibliography of Speech Education.* New York: The H. W. Wilson Co. (1939).

Thonssen, L., Fatherson, E., and Thonssen, D., *Bibliography of Speech Education, 1939-1948.* New York: The H. W. Wilson Co. (1950), pp. 259-304.

Weillon, E., *Medical Dictionary.* New York: Grune & Stratton, Inc. (1950).

Whitaker, B. L., Speech reading: a selected bibliography. *J. Speech Hearing Dis.*, **8**, 269-270 (1943).

ORGANIZATIONS

Alexander Graham Bell Association for the Deaf. 1537 35th St., N.W., Washington, D.C. 20007

American Academy for Cerebral Palsy. 1520 Louisiana Ave., New Orleans, La. 70115

American Academy of Physical Medicine and Rehabilitation. 30 North Michigan Ave., Chicago, Ill. 60602.

American Association for Cleft Palate Rehabilitation. Department of Otolaryngology, University Hospitals, Iowa City, Iowa 52240

American Association for Rehabilitation Therapy. 12012 Jean Dr., Pittsburgh, Pa. 15235

American Board of Otolaryngology. University Hospitals, Iowa City, Iowa 52240

American Board of Physical Medicine and Rehabilitation. 200 First St. S.W., Rochester, Minn.

American Child Guidance Foundation. 18 Tremont St., Boston, Mass. 02108

American Cleft Palate Association (ACPA). Department of Communicative Disorders, University of Florida, Gainesville, Fla. 32601

American Dental Association (ADA). 222 East Superior St., Chicago, Ill. 60611

American Group Psychotherapy Association. 1790 Broadway, New York, N.Y. 10003

American Hearing Society. 919 18th St., N.W., Washington, D.C. 20006

American Instructors of the Deaf (AID). Maryland School for the Deaf, Frederick, Md. 21701

American Laryngological Association (ALA). 12 Clovelly Rd., Wellesley Hills, Mass. 02181

American Laryngological, Rhinological & Otological Society (ALROS). 917 20th St. N.W., Washington, D.C. 20006

American Medical Association (AMA). 535 North Dearborn St., Chicago, Ill. 60610

American Neurological Association (ANA). 710 West 168th St., New York, N.Y. 10032

American Otological Society (AOS). 525 East 68th St., New York, N.Y. 10021

American Otorhinologic Society for Plastic Surgery (AOSPS). 75 Barberry Lane, Roslyn Heights, N.Y. 10115

American Psychiatric Association (APA). 1700 18th St., N.W., Washington, D.C. 20009

American Psychoanalytic Association (APA). 1 East 57th St., New York, N.Y. 10017

American Psychological Association (APA). 1200 Seventeenth St., N.W., Washington, D.C. 20036

American Public Health Association (APHA). 1790 Broadway, New York, N.Y. 10019

American Society of Oral Surgeons (ASOS). 919 North Michigan Ave., Chicago, Ill. 60611

American Speech and Hearing Association (ASHA). 9030 Old Georgetown Rd., Washington, D.C. 20014

Association for the Aid of Crippled Children (AACC). 345 East 46th St., New York, N.Y. 10017

Central States Speech Association. Columbia, Mo. 65201

Child Study Association of America. 9 East 89th St., New York, N.Y. 10028

Child Welfare League of America. 345 East 46th St., New York, N.Y. 10017

Conference of Church Workers Among the Deaf. P.O. Box 2751, West Durham, N.C.

Conference of Executives of American Schools for the Deaf (CEASD). % California School for the Deaf, 2601 Warring St., Berkeley, Calif. 94704

Council for Exceptional Children (CEC). 1201 16th St., N.W., Washington, D.C. 20006

Deafness Research Foundation. 310 Lexington Ave., New York, N.Y. 10016

Easter Seal Research Foundation of the National Society for Crippled Children and Adults. 2023 West Ogden Ave., Chicago, Ill. 60612

Hearing Aid Industry Conference (HAIC). 1 East 1st St., Duluth, Minn. 55802

Institute for the Crippled and Disabled. 400 1st Ave., New York, N.Y. 10010

Institute of Physical Medicine and Rehabilitation. 400 East 34th St., New York, N.Y. 10016

International Association of Laryngectomees. 521 West 57th St., New York, N.Y. 10019

National Association of Hearing and Speech Agencies (NAHSA). 919 18th St., N.W., Washington, D.C. 20006

National Association of the Deaf (NAD). 2495 Shattuck Ave., Berkeley, Calif. 94704

National Committee on Ethics of the Hearing Aid Industry. 10 Rockefeller Plaza, Room 509, New York, N.Y. 10020

National Health Council (NHC). 1790 Broadway, New York, N.Y. 10019

National Rehabilitation Association (NRA). 1029 Vermont Ave., N.W. Washington, D.C. 20005

National Society for Crippled Children and Adults. 2023 West Ogden Ave., Chicago, Ill. 60640

Society of Hearing Aid Audiologists (SHAA). 24202 Grand River Ave., Detroit, Mich. 48291

Southern Speech Association. % Dwight L. Freshley, University of Georgia, Athens, Ga.

Speech Association of American (SAA). Statler Hilton Hotel, New York, N.Y. 10001

United Cerebral Palsy Association (UCPA). 321 West 44th St., New York, N.Y. 10036

Western Speech Association. % Harold Livingston, Executive Secretary, Oregon State University, Corvallis, Ore. 97330

A glossary of terms for speech pathology as a behavioral science

Compiled by Jody Bell

abduct To draw away from the median line; opposite of adduct.

acoustic Relating to the physical properties of sound.

acuity Distinctness of sensation; sharpness, clearness.

adaptation effect The decrease of stuttering with successive readings of the same passage.

addition A type of articulatory defect in which extra phonemes are improperly added to words.

adduct To draw toward the median line; opposite of abduct.

aglossia Absence of the tongue.

agnosia Inability to recognize sensation in a sensory modality that can be recognized in other modalities.

agraphia Loss of the ability to write.

air-bone gap The difference between an individual's bone-conduction threshold and air-conduction threshold as revealed by pure-tone hearing testing.

alaryngeal speech Speech without a larynx.

allophone Subdivision of a phoneme.

ankyloglossia Tongue-tie.

anoxia Decreased amount of oxygen in organs and tissues, i.e., less than the physiologically normal amount.

aphasia Loss of the ability to speak or comprehend the spoken word due to central integrative disability; deficit in the ability to process symbolic materials irrespective of stimulus or response modality.

childhood aphasia General term applied to disturbance of language in children, presumably as a consequence of brain dysfunction in the auditory mechanism for processing speech. Acquired aphasia is impairment of speech after it is established. Congenital or developmental aphasia is impairment of normal acquisition of oral language in children whose disability does not seem to extend beyond the auditory system.

fluent aphasia According to the Boston Classification System, due to a posterior cerebral lesion in the dominant hemisphere, where auditory comprehension abilities are likely to be worse than expected. Articulation, prosody, and grammar are intact, but speech lacks content and meaning. Also called Wernicke's aphasia, sensory aphasia, receptive aphasia, pragmatic aphasia.

nonfluent aphasia According to the Boston Classification System, due to an anterior cerebral lesion in the dominant hemisphere, where auditory comprehension abilities are likely to be better than expected. Speech is labored, halting and telegraphic, with poor grammar and prominent misarticulations. Also called Broca's aphasia, motor aphasia, expressive aphasia, syntactic aphasia.

aphonia Loss of voice.

apraxia Disorder of voluntary movement not due to paralysis or muscular weakness.

articulation Vocal tract movements for speech sound production, synonymous with articulation-resonance; a jointing or connecting together loosely so as to allow motion between the parts.

articulation index An estimation of the severity of an articulatory disorder in which each sound is weighted to reflect its frequency in the language as a means of measuring therapeutic progress; in audiology, another term for speech discrimination score.

artificial larynx A device for generating substitute sound for lost vocal function that, when applied to the vocal tract, activates air in the resonators for speech modulation.

assessment Evaluation of behavioral disorder to determine nature, severity, prognosis, and appropriate treatment.

assimilation See *coarticulation*.

ataxia Inability to coordinate voluntary muscular movements.

athetosis Involuntary writhing movements that accompany purposeful or postural motion.

atrophy A wasting of tissues or organs.

audiologist A specialist in evaluation and rehabilitation of persons whose communication disorders center in whole or part in the hearing function.

audiology The study of the field of hearing, both normal and disordered.

audiometry Systematic testing of auditory acuity.

auditory Pertaining to perception of sound.

auditory discrimination Ability to distinguish among various speech sounds.

autism A form of childhood psychosis characterized by inability to form meaningful interpersonal relationships; self-absorption.

babbling Meaningless flow of sound making that characterizes vocal development in infants before the development of meaningful speech.

base rate Stable rate of response; also base line in operant conditioning.

behavior modification Application of principles of operant conditioning to clinical treatment.

behavior therapy Therapy that seeks to change observable behavior through systematic application of learning principles; reciprocal inhibition therapy.

behavioral model Theoretic framework within which phenomena are explained in terms of observable behavior without regard to underlying etiology.

benign Pertaining to the nonmalignant character of a neoplasm.

bilateral cleft A fissure in which the entire nasal cavity is open to the mouth because of the failure of the midline septum and vomer of the nose to fuse with the hard palate on both sides.

Boston Classification System Classification system for aphasia that seeks to correlate the area of the brain that has been injured and the resultant behavioral symptoms.

central hearing loss Impairment of hearing as a result of damage to auditory nerve pathways in the brain stem or in the centers of hearing in the cerebral cortex.

cerebral palsy Neurologic disability of children in which the primary symptoms of paralysis, weakness, and incoordination reflect motor damage.

character disorder A type of personality and emotional disturbance identified by asocial or antisocial behavior, not by specific symptoms.

chest register See *heavy voice.*

classical conditioning The connection between a response and its stimulus that is reinforced when stimulus and response occur together.

cleft palate A congenital fissure resulting from incomplete merging or fusion of embryonic processes that normally unite in the formation of the soft palate, the roof of the mouth, the premaxilla, or the upper lip.

clonic Pertaining to a form of movement marked by alternate successive contractions and relaxations of a muscle; in stuttering, repetitions.

cluttering Verbal manifestation of central language imbalance marked by symptoms such as lack of awareness of the disorder, short attention span, excessive rate, erratic rhythm, and garbled speech.

coarticulation Assimilative influence of one speech sound on another; overlap of motor commands for one sound while an articulator is still moving toward the position for a previous sound.

cognition Ability to think and reason; thinking.

conductive hearing loss Impairment of hearing due to abnormality in the mechanical system for transmitting acoustical waves to the inner ear.

confused language Neurologically based condition in which there is difficulty maintaining focus in verbal interaction.

congenital Existing at birth.

congenital aphasia See *aphasia, childhood.*

consistency effect The tendency for stuttering to occur on the same words during successive readings of a passage.

consonant A speech sound, produced with partial or complete occlusion of the vocal tract, that can release or arrest the vowellike syllable pulse.

constriction Binding or contraction of a part; a subjective sensation as if the body or any part were tightly bound or squeezed; in a behavioral model of voice, the behavior by which the feeling of openness of the throat is regulated along a scale from open to closed.

contingency of reinforcement In operant conditioning, the consequence attached to behavioral events.

control group In the experimental method, a group matched to the experimental group in which the independent variable is not present.

conversion reaction A major type of hysteria in which the distinguishing symptom is slight to total failure of a sensory or voluntary muscle mechanism when no organic disability exists.

correlation The way in which one variable relates to another; the statistic with which co-relations among variables are described.

damping Diminution of the amplitude of vibrations due to absorption of energy by the surrounding medium.

deaf Pertaining to a hearing loss that occurs prior to speech acquisition and is so severe that the child is unable to understand and learn speech normally by hearing.

deafened Pertaining to a severe loss of hearing after speech has been learned.

decode Translate; in speech, sorting out of speech signals from noise.

deep structure The infinitude of ideas that can be combined into spoken language.

deep test of articulation A test of sounds in all possible syllabic combinations.

delayed auditory feedback Delay of speaker's speech to his ears in excess of the time of arrival of air- or bone-conducted sound of his speech.

delayed language Failure to understand or speak the language code of the community at a normal age.

denasality Voice quality due to occlusion of nasal passages, preventing adequate nasal resonance.

dependent variable The variable in an experiment that the experimenter observes to determine whether it is affected by changes in the independent variable.

descriptive linguistics Set of linguistic rules with which to explain why certain speech sounds occur under certain conditions; structural linguistics.

descriptive method Method of study with which to describe observed relationships.

developmental aphasia See *aphasia, childhood.*

diadochokinesia Rapid repetition of movements.

diagnosis In medicine, the determination of the nature and etiology of a disease or a disorder.

diagnostic audiometry Evaluation of hearing in which pure-tone air and bone conduction, speech reception, and speech discrimination are tested.

diagnostic test of articulation An instrument used to make clinical decisions about the need for therapy, about which sounds should be treated therapeutically and in which order, and about the assessment of therapeutic progress.

diplophonia Double pitch, one usually normal and the other low, produced by two structures in the vocal tract vibrating at different rates.

disease model See *medical model.*

disfluency Disruption of smooth speech-flow.

disinhibition The inhibition of an inhibition; the removal of an inhibitory effect by a stimulus.

distinctive feature A linguistically distinguishable articulatory adjustment by which phonemes are produced and differentiated.

distortion In articulation, the correct phoneme is approximated, but the allophone is not close enough to be normally acceptable.

distraction effect Condition that draws attention away from anticipation of stuttering and thereby reduces stuttering.

duration Elapsed time of phonetic events.

dysarthria Incoordination in execution of the speech act due to paralysis or muscular weakness.

dyslexia Partial loss of ability to read with understanding.

ear training In speech therapy, the development of auditory discrimination of the error sound from the desired target sound.

echolalia Meaningless repetition of a word, phrase, or sentence just spoken by another person.

edema Swelling due to an accumulation of an excessive amount of fluid in cells or tissues.

ego The "I"; the central part of the personality that deals with reality and is influenced by social forces; the psychic structure that mediates among id, superego, and reality.

ego defense Unconscious adaptive and defensive adjustment by which the ego preserves control and protects itself from anxiety.

empirical Observable; founded on practical experience but not proved scientifically.

encode In psycholinguistics, selection of appropriate linguistic units of speech.

epigenesis Development involving gradual differentiation and diversification.

esophageal speech A type of speech achieved without a larynx, involving a method of inflating an air reservoir used to activate vibration of a neoglottis near the top of the esophagus.

etiology The cause of a disorder.

expansion Procedure used by parents to hasten progress of their child's language; involves repeating essentially what the child says but with a small improvement in grammar.

expectancy The ability of stutterers to anticipate their acts of stuttering.

experimental analysis of behavior System for a functional analysis of behavior in which the future of any behavior is determined by its consequences.

experimental group In the experimental method, a group in which the independent variable is present.

experimental method The equivalent in speech pathology of the classic scientific method, in which one formulates a hypothesis and tests it by observing the relationship between two variables when he manipulates one (the independent variable) to determine its effects on the other.

exteroception Pertaining to the surface of the body containing the end organs adapted to receive impressions of external environmental stimuli.

extinction Elimination of a response by failure to reinforce it.

extrinsic Originating outside of the part where found; from without.

falsetto See *light voice*.

flaccid paralysis Paralysis with loss of tone and absence of reflexes in the affected parts, producing a weak, flabby, and relaxed condition.

fluency Suprasegmental dimension of speech-flow having to do with how smoothly sounds, syllables, words, and phrases are joined together; the smoothness of speech sound initiation and articulatory transition from one phonetic position to another.

focus In vocal production, the sensation of the location of the focal placement of tone in the head or throat.

formant A band of frequencies at which acoustic energy is clustered in a tone.

functional Pertaining to the function of a structure or system; descriptive of a disorder caused by function, as with vocal nodules that are attributed to functional abuse.

functional aphonia Condition in which voice is absent and for which no organic cause is apparent; hysterical aphonia.

fundamental frequency Rate of glottal vibration; the main determinant of pitch perception.

generalization Clinically, the transfer of stimulus control over desired response to daily life; carryover.

generalized intellectual impairment Neurologically based condition in which memory for abstractions is disabled.

glottal fry See *pulsated voice*.

glottal vibration Opening and closing of the glottal space between the vocal cords.

habitual pitch The pitch around which the voice is typically produced.

haptic system Neural processes by which one perceives his body in relation to objects and space; includes sensations of touch and kinesthesis.

hard of hearing Auditory abnormality in which sufficient sensitivity remains to permit oral communication.

harmonics Components of complex sound whose frequencies are multiples of the fundamental frequency of that sound.

heavy voice The vocal mode used by most men, women, and children that is the most flexible and socially useful; chest register; modal register.

hertz Cycles per second.

hoarseness The sound of a voice that is breathy, rough, and relatively low in pitch.

homeostasis State of equilibrium in the body.

hyperactivity Excessive movement or muscular activity.

hyperfunction Excessive function; strained vocal production.

hypernasality Vowel quality characterized by excessive nasal resonance.

hypertrophy Overgrowth; general increase in bulk of a part or organ not due to tumor formation.

hypofunction Reduced, low, or inadequate function.

hypothesis Supposition or assumption advanced as a basis for reasoning or as a guide to experimental investigation; a small theory.

id In psychoanalysis, a part of the psychic or mental apparatus, the reservoir of psychic energy or libido.

identification audiometry A relatively quick gross test of auditory acuity for pure tones; screening audiometry.

idioglossia Idiosyncratic language of one's own, often spoken by twins.

incidence The amount or extent of an occurrence; the number of cases of a disorder. (Compare with *prevalence*.)

independent variable The variable in an experiment which the experimenter manipulates directly.

innervation Neural stimulation of a muscle.

instrumental conditioning The connection between a response and the stimulus conditions preceding that is strengthened by virtue of the reinforcing consequences that follow the response; operant conditioning.

intellect The capacity to reason and understand; the capacity to meet situations, especially new ones, successfully; the system of information processing.

interoral Within the mouth.

interval scale A scale of measurement in which distances between the units of measurement are equal.

intrinsic Inherent; belonging entirely to a part; denoting those muscles whose origins and insertions are within the same organ, e.g., intrinsic muscles of the larynx.

jitter Pitch perturbation; cycle-to-cycle variation in the periods of glottal cycles. It is basis for perceived roughness.

juncture A joining.

internal juncture The technique of putting joints between words in ways that control meaning, e.g., "ice cream" versus "I scream."

terminal juncture A technique of pauses and inflections, used by speakers to end phrases.

kernel sentence In transformational grammar, the basic sentence pattern.

kinesthesia Sense perception of movement.

language Symbolic formulation of ideas according to semantic and grammatical rules.

laryngeal paralysis Paralysis of vocal fold adduction-abduction functions.

laryngectomy Surgical removal of the larynx.

larynx The organ of voice production; the valve at the upper part of the respiratory tract between the pharynx and the trachea that protects the lungs and permits buildup of thoracic pressure.

lateral External; on the outer side as distinguished from medial.

learning disability Impairment of the ability of a seemingly normal child to learn because of conditions such as environmental deprivation, drugs, nutritional deficits, metabolic disorders, and brain damage.

light voice Falsetto; the vocal mode permitting highest pitches, produced when the vocalis muscles are stretched and thinned.

linguistic competence Knowledge of a language involving knowledge of the rules that relate sound and meaning.

linguistic performance Ability to phonetically organize spoken sounds into grammatical statements.

loudness Perception of the intensity of a sound.

malignant Cancerous; in the case of a neoplasm, having the property of uncontrollable growth.

malocclusion Condition in which the jaws or teeth do not fit together properly.

manic-depression Type of psychosis involving disturbances of mood and self-esteem in which the person may show either euphoria or melancholy of psychotic intensity.

masking The use of noise to occlude signal perception.

mean The central value of a set of measures computed by addition of all scores and division by their total number; average.

median A measure of central value computed by selecting the middle position in the rank order on an ordinal scale; average.

medical model Theoretic framework within which diagnosis or etiology of a disorder is essential to treatment of its cause.

mel In psychophysics, the unit of measure for the ratio scale of perceived pitch.

mental retardation Defective verbal and nonverbal intellectual functioning that originates during the developmental period and is associated with impairment in maturation, learning, and social adjustment.

metastasis The spreading of a malignant disease from one part of the body to another.

minimal brain dysfunction Presumed impairment of the brain of a young child inferred from disturbances of perception, thinking, language, and behavior.

modal register See *heavy voice*.

mode A measure of central value computed by selecting the category with the highest incidence on a nominal scale; average.

mode, vocal Vocal register; the basic laryngeal adjustment within which all other vocal behavior is controlled.

modulate The use and modification of transmitted energy; shaping of waves, pulses, and turbulence by vocal tract adjustments to produce vowels and consonants.

mongolism Syndrome of mental retardation associated with a chromosomal defect; Down's syndrome.

morpheme Smallest unit of language that has meaning; meaningful combinations of sounds from which words are built.

morphology In linguistics, the rules of word formation; in anatomy, structure of the parts.

motor phonetics The study of the production of speech sounds.

motor theory of speech perception A theory stating that the encoding process of speech production is used to decode speech for recognition and understanding.

myofunctional therapy Tongue thrust therapy.

nasality The quality of speech perceived as being hypernasal.

negative reinforcement Removal of an aversive condition (presumably unpleasant) contingent on a response, followed by an increase in frequency of that response.

neoglottis In alaryngeal speech, the new vibratory structure; pseudoglottis.

neonatal Relating to the period immediately succeeding birth and continuing through the first month of life.

neoplasm New growth; tumor; abnormal tissue that grows by cellular proliferation more rapidly than normal.

neurology The branch of medical science that has to do with the nervous system and its disorders.

neurophysiology Physiology of the nervous system.

neurosis Functional nervous disease characterized by overt or covert neurotic symptoms in which the ego function of reality testing is not impaired.

nominal scale Classification or naming of distinct and separate categories.

nondirective therapy A type of insight therapy in which the therapist selectively reflects implied feelings and responses to arouse and extinguish unrealistic anxieties.

nonstandard English The "native" language of a subculture, such as a black dialect.

normal distribution In statistics, a description of the distribution of scores that would be expected theoretically if an infinitely large, normally distributed population were measured; described by the bell-shaped curve.

null hypothesis In statistics, an alternate guess that something is nothing; a prediction that any difference is a result of chance. To test a research hypothesis, it is necessary to reject the probability that the null hypothesis is correct.

obturator Any structure that occludes an opening; a prosthesis used to close a congenital or acquired cleft in the palate.

occlusion The alignment of teeth in the upper and lower dental arches.

omission An articulation disorder in which phonemes included in normal pronunciation are absent.

operant conditioning See *experimental analysis of behavior*.

operational definition Observable operations that are defined as direct evidence of unobservable mental processes, such as palmar sweat as an operational measure of anxiety.

optimal pitch The pitch at which the voice functions most efficiently.

oral stereognosis Detection of forms of objects by feeling them in the mouth with tongue, lips, and jaw; oral form recognition.

ordinal scale A scale of measurement showing order or position in a series.

organic Relating to an organ; structural, as opposed to functional.

orofacial Relating to the mouth and face.

paramedian Near the middle line.

parameter A number that describes a characteristic of a population.

parametric statistics See *statistics, parametric*.

paranatal During and immediately following birth.

paranoia A type of psychosis marked by the presence of systematized delusions, often of a persecutory character, in an otherwise intact personality.

pathogenic Causing disease.

pathology The medical science that deals with all aspects of disease.

perception Awareness; consciousness; the process of becoming aware of or recognizing an object.

perceptual inconstancy Inability to maintain a balanced sensory input; a type of perceptual problem found in autism.

perseveration The constant repetition of a word, phrase, or act; the inability to appropriately change from one action to another.

personality The organized system of behavior and attitudes by which one establishes relationships with others.

perturbation, pitch See *jitter*.

phonation Generation of voice by means of the vocal cords.

phone Sound actually spoken that can be observed directly and measured physiologically and acoustically.

phoneme Abstract classification of groups of sounds that make differences in meaning.

phonemic regression Progressive distortion of perception of speech as damage in the auditory system is found higher in the neural auditory pathways.

phonetics The study of the production and perception of speech sounds.

phoniatrist Physician who studies voice and speech.

phonology The study of the sounds of a language.

pitch Perception of highness or lowness of a sound, determined by fundamental frequency.

positive reinforcement Presentation of an event (presumably pleasurable) contingent on a response, followed by an increase in frequency of that response.

postnatal Occurring after birth; during infancy.

prenatal Preceding birth; between conception and onset of labor.

presbycusis Loss of the ability to perceive or discriminate sounds as part of the aging process.

prevalence The percentage of a population affected by the disorder at a given time.

projective test Psychodynamic assessment of personality.

proprioception Stimuli and body information originating in muscles, tendons, joints, and other internal tissues.

prosody Stress, inflection, rhythm; the melody of speech.

prosthodontics Dental prosthetics; the science and art of providing suitable substitutes for teeth and associated parts in order that impaired function, appearance, comfort, and health of the patient may be restored.

psychoanalytic therapy A type of insight therapy

in which the freudian analyst interprets feelings in his search for the psychodynamic roots of a symptom.

psychodynamics The systematized study and theory of human behavior, emphasizing unconscious motivation and the functional significance of emotion.

psycholinguistics The joint study of psychology and linguistics which attempts to interrelate human behavior and culture with language.

psychophysics The relationship between psychologic response and the physical stimulus.

psychosexual development Various stages of ego development a child goes through which is thought to follow evolving sources of gratification for primitive id forces.

psychosis A severe emotional illness distinguished by grossly distorted perception of and response to reality.

psychosomatic Pertaining to the influence of the mind or higher functions of the brain (emotions, fears, desires, etc.) on the functions of the body, especially in relation to disease; psychophysiologic autonomic and visceral disorders.

pulsated voice Vocal fry; glottal fry; the vocal mode with the lowest fundamental frequency range produced by short, relaxed cords that close quickly and remain closed for a long portion of each glottal cycle.

pulse Type of sound generation in which there is abrupt release of closures in the vocal tract or larynx.

punishment Removal of a positive reinforcer (punishment I) or presentation of an aversive condition (punishment II) contingent on a response followed by a decrease in frequency of that response.

quality That aspect of perception of voice that is separate from pitch and loudness; perception of that aspect of sound determined acoustically by the frequency distribution of energy.

range In statistics, the difference between the highest and lowest score.

rate The speed of an utterance.

ratio scale A scale of measurement in which there is an absolute zero point above which the units are equal and proportional, and which allows addition, subtraction, multiplication, and division.

reciprocal inhibition A type of behavior therapy that uses systematic procedures for desensitizing anxiety by pairing deep relaxation with anxiety-producing situations.

recruitment In audiology, an abnormal increase of loudness with an increase of intensity.

register See *vocal mode.*

reliability Ability to obtain repeated stable measures.

resonance The natural or inherent frequency of any oscillating system; modification of the laryngeal tone by its passage through the cavities of the throat and head, so as to alter its quality.

retrocochlear hearing loss Hearing impairment due to a lesion beyond the cochlea in the auditory nerve carrying sensation to the first synaptic nucleus in the brain.

rhythm The pattern of timing of phonetic elements.

schedule of reinforcement In operant conditioning, a timetable for presentation of the sequence of reinforcement and the intervals between.

schizophrenia The most common type of psychosis, characterized by extensive withdrawal of the individual's interest from the outside world and distortion of perception and thinking.

scientific method See *experimental method.*

screening audiometry See *identification audiometry.*

screening test for articulation Gross, quick test to assess general adequacy of articulation and to separate persons who may need help from those who probably do not.

segmental phoneme Technical way of specifying speech sounds; the major unit used by all languages to change meaning.

semantic Relating to the study of meaning.

sensation A feeling; the translation into consciousness of the effects of a stimulus exciting any of the organs of sense.

sensorineural hearing loss Hearing impairment due to a lesion in the peripheral cochleoneural system.

sentence The basic unit of language necessary to express a complete idea.

sequence Temporal arrangement of phonetic elements.

shaping In operant conditioning, modification of an already existing response to the desired behavior.

shimmer The cycle-to-cycle variations in amplitude of glottal pulses that contribute to perception of roughness.

sign Announcement of an object that is close at hand.

sociopath Psychopathic individual whose behavior is asocial or antisocial.

somesthesia Bodily sensation; consciousness of the body.

sone Psychophysical unit for measurement of loudness.

spastic dysphonia Hyperfunctional disorder of voice, often called laryngeal stuttering, in which spasms of vocal constriction disrupt smooth production of tone.

speech Any aspect of oral communication, including covert thinking processes of language and overt phonetic processes of speaking.

speech discrimination The ability to distinguish one speech sound from another.

speech-flow Speech as it flows from phone to syllable, phrase, and sentence; behavioral dimensions of speech-flow include sequence, duration, rate, rhythm, and fluency.

speech pathology An applied interdisciplinary behavioral science.

speech reading The process of obtaining information about a speaker's message by observing him visually; lipreading.

speech reception threshold In audiology, the lowest level at which an individual is able to correctly repeat 50% of spondee words presented to him.

standard deviation In statistics, a description of how much the mean fails to be representative of all measures.

statistic A number derived from a sample that is an estimate of a characteristic of a population.

    descriptive statistic A single number that summarizes a characteristic of a collection of measurements of a group; characteristics described are central value, variability, and correlation.

    inferential statistic A number that predicts whether a factor is operating in enough people in a group to justify predicting its presence in a similar group.

    nonparametric statistics Statistics that make few, if any, assumptions about the form of distribution of scores in the population sampled; distribution-free statistics.

    parametric statistics Statistics based on the assumption that the sample chosen will give an accurate estimate of how people perform in the population sampled.

stimulus control In operant conditioning, extension of a response that occurs in some stimulus situations to other stimulus situations.

stoma An artificial opening, as in a tracheal stoma used in a laryngectomy.

stress In speech pathology, the increased pitch, loudness, or duration of some syllables as compared with others.

structural linguistics Descriptive linguistics; a description of language that takes into account the conception of structural relations among linguistic parts; it assumes that language is a system, and that the only observable evidence of how the system functions is seen in what happens to phones.

stuttering A disorder of speech-flow characterized by syllable disfluency; the abnormal timing of speech sound initiation.

subglottal Below the glottic opening between the vocal cords.

submucous cleft An orofacial disability in which the bones of the hard palate fail to unite to one extent or another, but the mucous membrane over the cleft is intact.

substitution An articulatory defect in which incorrect phonemes are substituted for those that would normally be heard.

successive approximation Selective reinforcement of closer approximations of the terminal goal in operant conditioning.

superego The part of the ego that aids in coping with the id; the conscience.

suprasegmental phoneme The use of stress, pitch, and juncture to change meaning.

surface structure Phonetic organization of sounds spoken and sounds heard in a language according to rules of a transformational grammar.

syllable The physiologic unit of speech; the minimum component consists of a vowel or vowel substitute that may be released or arrested with consonants.

symbol A sign for a conception that can exist independently of its referent.

syntax Arrangement of the words of a sentence in grammatical form; sentence structure.

terminal behavior In operant conditioning, the desired goal.

theory A reasoned explanation of the manner in which many factors are functionally related to each other; a larger explanation than a hypothesis that relates only two factors to each other.

tinnitus Noises (including ringing) in the ear.

tongue thrust A forward thrust of the tongue against the front teeth, coupled with tight lip closure in a kind of sucking movement.

tonic Pertaining to tension in muscles that exists independently of voluntary innervation; in stuttering, prolongations and hesitations.

transformational grammar The ability to convert deep structure to surface structure of a language.

trauma Physical or psychic wound.

tremor Trembling, shaking.

turbulence Speech friction sounds; release of the breath stream through constricted channels in the vocal tract.

unilateral cleft A fissure in the hard palate that opens one side of the nasal cavity directly to the oral cavity.

variable In experimentation, a dimension that can be measured directly or indirectly.

velopharyngeal competence The ability to separate the nasal from the oral cavity.

velopharyngeal insufficiency Inadequate velar or pharyngeal tissue or function to provide velopharyngeal competence.

ventricular dysphonia Hyperfunctional disorder of voice in which the primitive valving action of the false vocal folds intrudes on normal phonation.

virgules Slant lines that enclose phonemic symbols and indicate that broad differences are being transcribed.

vital capacity The greatest amount of air in the lungs that might be exhaled subsequent to maximal inhalation.

vocal fry See *pulsated voice*.

vocal hygiene Any form of vocalization that is not abusive to the larynx; freedom from vocal constriction.

vocal mode See *mode, vocal*.

vocal tract The buccal, oral, pharyngeal, and nasal cavities that are used to modulate the breath stream to produce sounds.

voiced sound A sound produced by vibration of the vocal cords.

voiceless sound A sound in which the larynx opens, as in breathing, but the vocal cords do not vibrate.

voicing A behavioral dimension basic to vocal production that ranges from voicelessness to a fully voiced tone; refers to behavioral management of the ac/dc balance of airflow.

vowel A voiced speech sound resonated by cavity adjustments of the vocal tract.

waves A series of pulses of air pressure generated by vocal cord vibrations and modulated by resonating characteristics of the vocal tract.

Author index

Subject index